Inflammation: The Cause of all Diseases 2.0

Inflammation: The Cause of all Diseases 2.0

Topic Editors

Vasso Apostolopoulos
Jack Feehan
Vivek P. Chavda

MDPI

Basel • Beijing • Wuhan • Barcelona • Belgrade • Novi Sad • Cluj • Manchester

Topic Editors
Vasso Apostolopoulos
Institute for Health and Sport
Victoria University
Melbourne
Australia

Jack Feehan
Institute for Health and Sport
Victoria University
Melbourne
Australia

Vivek P. Chavda
Department of Pharmaceutics
and Pharmaceutical
Technology
L M College of Pharmacy
Ahmedabad
India

Editorial Office
MDPI AG
Grosspeteranlage 5
4052 Basel, Switzerland

This is a reprint of the Topic, published open access by the journals *Cells* (ISSN 2073-4409), *Diseases* (ISSN 2079-9721), *Healthcare* (ISSN 2227-9032) and *International Journal of Molecular Sciences* (ISSN 1422-0067), freely accessible at: https://www.mdpi.com/topics/8P52MZ6248.

For citation purposes, cite each article independently as indicated on the article page online and as indicated below:

Lastname, A.A.; Lastname, B.B. Article Title. *Journal Name* **Year**, *Volume Number*, Page Range.

ISBN 978-3-7258-6183-5 (Hbk)
ISBN 978-3-7258-6184-2 (PDF)
https://doi.org/10.3390/books978-3-7258-6184-2

Contents

About the Editors

Vasso Apostolopoulos

Vasso Apostolopoulos AM is currently a Distinguished Professor at RMIT University, Melbourne Australia and the Director of Healthy Lifespan and Chronic Diseases. She is also the Immunology Program Director at the Australian Institute for Musculoskeletal Science Australia. Previously she has held several executive leadership roles including Pro Vice-Chancellor, Research Partnerships, Associate Provost, Deputy Vice-Chancellor Research, Vice-Chancellor's Distinguished Professorial Fellow, Director of Immunology and Translational Research Group at Victoria University, Immunology of Chronic Diseases Director at the Centre for Chronic Diseases, and Immunology and Vaccine Leader at the Burnet Institute and at the Austin Research Institute, Australia. She received her PhD majoring in immunology from the University of Melbourne, and the Advanced Certificate in Protein Crystallography from Birkbeck College, University of London. Professor Vasso Apostolopoulos is a world-renowned researcher who has been recognized with over 100 awards for the outstanding results of her research. She has more than 550 research publications and 22 patents to her credit, her interests are in vaccine and drug development for cancer, chronic, infectious and autoimmune diseases. She is also interested in understanding inflammation and how to manipulate the immune system to treat diseases.

Jack Feehan

Jack Feehan is a recipient of the Vice-Chancellor's Senior Research Fellowship at RMIT University, Melbourne Australia. Previously he was a senior research fellow at the Institute for Health and Sport, Victoria University. He has significant clinical and research expertise in the management of chronic diseases, particularly in older adults. Jack is a registered osteopath and received a Ph.D. from the University of Melbourne in geriatric immunology, and he now works on nutritional, exercise, and pharmacological interventions in chronic cardiometabolic, and musculoskeletal diseases. He also has a keen interest in inflammation and resulting diseases , such as type 2 diabetes and dementias. He has published over 70 papers, is an active supervisor of several PhD students and is an active presenter on topics of inflammation and chronic diseases.

Vivek P. Chavda

Vivek P. Chavda is an Assistant Professor (Selection Grade), Department of Pharmaceutics and Pharmaceutical Technology, L M College of Pharmacy, Ahmedabad, Gujarat, India. He is B Pharm and M Pharm Gold Medalist at Gujarat Technological University. Before joining academia, he served in the Biologics industry for almost 8 years in the Research and Development of Biologics. He has more than 250 peer-reviewed national and international publications, 38 book chapters, 10 book chapters under communication, 7 patents in the pipeline, and numerous newsletter articles to his credit. His research interests include development of biologics processes and formulations, medical device development, nano-diagnostics, non-carrier formulations, long-acting parenteral formulations, and nano-vaccines.

cells MDPI

Editorial

Inflammation: The Cause of All Diseases

Vivek P. Chavda [1], Jack Feehan [2] and Vasso Apostolopoulos [2,*]

1 Department of Pharmaceutics and Pharmaceutical Technology, L.M. College of Pharmacy, Ahmedabad 380009, Gujarat, India; vivek.chavda@lmcp.ac.in
2 School of Health and Biomedical Sciences, RMIT University, Melbourne, VIC 3083, Australia; jack.feehan@rmit.edu.au
* Correspondence: vasso.apostolopoulos@rmit.edu.au

1. Introduction

Inflammation is an essential biological process that serves as the body's first line of defence against harmful stimuli, including pathogens, damaged cells, and irritants. While acute inflammation is crucial for healing and recovery, chronic inflammation can lead to a variety of diseases, including cancer, cardiovascular disorders, and autoimmune conditions [1–3]. The recent Special Issue, 'Inflammation: The cause of all diseases 2.0' [4], along with the participating journals—*Cells*, *Diseases*, *Healthcare*, *International Journal of Molecular Sciences*, and *Vaccines*—sheds light on the complex interplay between inflammation and disease mechanisms, providing valuable insights into potential therapeutic strategies targeting inflammatory pathways [5–16]. Inflammation is characterized by a series of physiological responses involving immune cells, blood vessels, and molecular and cellular mediators. When cells are injured due to external or internal stimuli, an inflammatory response is initiated involving the secretion of pro-inflammatory cytokines, chemokines, and other signalling molecules [17]. This response aims to eliminate the initial cause of injury, remove damaged cells, and initiate the repair process. However, when inflammation becomes dysregulated or persists beyond its intended duration, it can contribute to chronic tissue damage, chronic inflammation, and the development of chronic diseases such as type-2 diabetes (T2D) [5,18], cancer [19,20], chronic obstructive pulmonary disease (COPD) [21], and cardiovascular diseases (CVD) [22]. The articles featured in this Special Issue explore various aspects of inflammation, including its molecular mechanisms and implications for different pathological conditions (Figure 1).

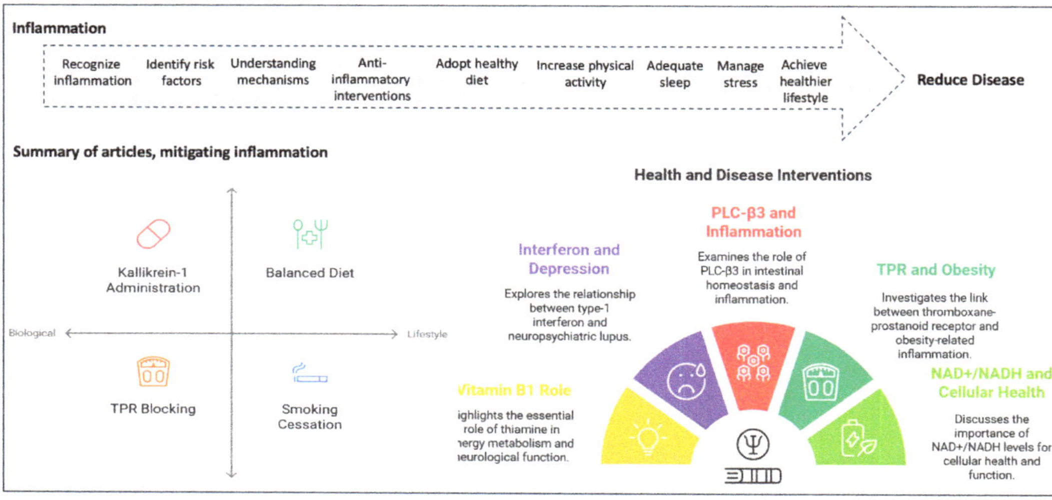

Figure 1. Process of managing chronic inflammation, and a summary of studies published in this Special Issue. Image was made using Biorender.com.

2. Chronic Inflammation Leading to Diseases

While chronic inflammation progresses quietly, it is a leading cause of many chronic diseases and poses a significant threat to individual health and longevity. Low-grade inflammation is increasingly recognized as a shared characteristic of metabolic, psychiatric, and neurodegenerative diseases [23,24]. Several factors promote low-level chronic inflammation, such as age, smoking, diet, sedentary lifestyle, obesity, hormones, stress, and irregular sleep patterns. Ageing correlates with an increase in inflammation due to the gradual decline in immune function with age (immune senescence), which leads to mitochondrial dysfunction, free radical accumulation, and increased visceral fat over time [25]. The chemicals in cigarette smoking stimulate the production of pro-inflammatory cytokines and reduce anti-inflammatory cytokines, contributing to chronic inflammation and leading to diseases such as cancer, chronic lung disorders, and vascular diseases [26]. Diet is well known to contribute to inflammation, especially highly processed foods and those rich in saturated fats, trans-fats, and refined sugar; the gut microbiota also play an important role in chronic inflammation [27]. In addition, sedentary patterns have been linked to low-grade inflammation and promote systemic chronic inflammation [28,29]. In a recent study, it was shown that regulatory T cells (Treg) suppress inflammation by enhancing exercise capacity and promoting muscle metabolic reprogramming by protecting mitochondria from interferon (IFN)-γ damage [30]. Physical activity has been shown to be beneficial in many disorders, including cancer, as well as in improving mental health and managing menopause symptoms [31,32]. Obesity leads to chronic low-grade inflammation, driven by pro-inflammatory immune cell activation and cytokine production, which contribute to insulin resistance and related diseases [33,34]. Both innate and adaptive immune responses, as well as adipokines, play significant roles in this process [35,36].

Twelve articles were published in this Special Issue, all of which discuss various molecular and cellular mechanisms through which inflammation drives chronic diseases. These are summarised as follows:

- Studies on chronic diseases: Excess type-1 interferon production is central to systemic lupus erythematosus, often resulting in neuropsychiatric lupus with depression. In this study, the administration of kallikrein-1 reduced type-1 interferon and improved depressive symptoms [7]. In another study, phospholipase C-β3 (PLC-β3), which plays a role in maintaining intestinal homeostasis, was shown to cause severe inflammation and lethality in PLC-β3 knockout mice [6]. This was observed after exposure to dextran sodium sulfate, which triggered inflammation in the small intestine due to disrupted Wnt/β-catenin signalling. Further, the reduced PLC-β3 levels in human ileal Crohn's biopsies also supports its role in chronic inflammation and disease progression [6].

- Studies on diet: A balanced diet is crucial for preventing inflammation, as poor nutrition and unhealthy eating habits contribute to chronic inflammation [37]. Consuming a variety of nutrient-rich foods helps maintain overall health and supports the body's ability to combat inflammatory processes, reducing the risk of chronic diseases associated with chronic inflammation. In the paper by Turrini et al., it was noted that vitamin B1 (thiamine) is essential for energy metabolism and neurological function, and thiamine deficiency can lead to Wernicke encephalopathy (WE). The authors reported a case of an 8-year-old girl with WE due to thiamine deficiency, presenting with ataxia, nystagmus, confusion, and other neurological symptoms, suggesting underlying chronic inflammation [16].
- Studies on obesity: In obesity-related diseases, there are elevated levels of several pro-inflammatory markers. As such, the link between thromboxane-prostanoid receptor (TPR) and obesity was evaluated, and it was noted that blocking TPR reduced lipopolysaccharide- and stearic acid-induced inflammation in human PBMCs; the activation of TPR enhanced these inflammatory effects [11]. In addition, in obesity, a high platelet–high-density lipoprotein ratio (PHR) is a potential marker of inflammation. Indeed, in 203 obese patients, higher PHR levels significantly correlated with the presence of T2D and glycaemic markers [5].
- Studies on smoking: Cigarette smoke from combustible cigarettes (CCs) contains harmful chemicals that impair immune cell function, exacerbating chronic inflammatory diseases. In contrast, heated tobacco products (HTPs) produce fewer harmful cytokines. The authors of this study found that both CCs and HTPs altered cytokine production in patients with ulcerative colitis, T2D, and COPD [9]. HTP, however, induced fewer pro-inflammatory cytokines but increased immunosuppressive IL-10, IL-35, and pro-fibrotic TGF-β [9]. In mice, exposure to cigarette smoke extracts, which induce inflammation in lung tissues, was mitigated by NADH supplementation [13]. NAD+/NADH levels are important for overall cellular health and function. This was shown by the improvements in lung antioxidant defences (superoxide dismutase, glutathione peroxidase, catalase, glutathione), reduced oxidative damage (malondialdehyde), and decreased pro-inflammatory markers (TNF-α, IL-17, IFN-γ, and myeloperoxidase activity) [13].
- Studies on immune/blood cells: In the paper by Tam et al. [15], genomic biomarkers were identified that are linked to high degranulation responses in primary human mast cells from 262 donors, suggesting that chronic inflammation, mediated by mast cell activation, can contribute to disease processes related to allergic responses. In addition, mild systemic inflammation increases erythrocyte fragility, potentially contributing to haemolysis. This was demonstrated in 9292 healthy participants where haemolysis was linked to high-sensitivity C-reactive proteins. A correlation with urinary neopterin/creatinine ratio and erythrocyte osmotic fragility was also noted in a mixed healthy population (n = 54) [14]. Both these findings link inflammation to impaired erythrocyte function. A review was published in this Special Issue describing the key players in rheumatoid arthritis pathogenesis. Immune cells, fibroblast-like synoviocytes, macrophages, monocytes, B cells, CD4+ T cells, Th1, Th17 cells, and pro-inflammatory mediators, CCR2, CX3CR1, RANKL, IL-1β, IL-6, and TNF-α, were described in the context of inflammatory responses associated with disease [12]. Another review described cellular senescence and mitochondrial dysfunction in CVD and provided advancements in therapies aimed at targeting mitochondrial dysfunction, such as energy starvation, oxidative stress, and mitophagy [8].
- Finally, a study by Popoca-Hernández et al. [10] evaluated non-surgical periodontal treatment in women with periodontitis and rheumatoid arthritis). The results showed

significant reductions in periodontal indices, inflammatory biomarkers, and disease activity after non-surgical periodontal treatment. The findings highlight the critical role of oral health in managing chronic diseases like rheumatoid arthritis [10].

All the published papers highlight the role of chronic inflammation in driving disease, necessitating a deeper understanding of how such products affect immune responses, resulting in chronic diseases (Figure 1).

3. Therapeutic Applications

Low-grade chronic inflammation is key in the development of many diseases [38]. Unlike acute inflammation, which is a protective response to injury or infection, chronic inflammation persists over time and damages healthy cells and tissues, contributing to disease progression. Therapeutic interventions targeting chronic inflammation aim to modulate the immune system, reduce inflammatory markers, and restore normal tissue function. Common strategies include the use of nonsteroidal anti-inflammatory drugs (NSAIDs) [39], corticosteroids [40], biologic agents, and lifestyle modifications, all of which have shown promise in alleviating symptoms and preventing further tissue damage in chronic inflammatory diseases. Novel approaches to alleviating inflammation have been developed in recent years, with the aim of reversing or minimising progression to disease formation. One approach targeted the NLRP3 inflammasome, a key protein involved in inflammatory response, with small-molecule inhibitors [41]. NLRP3 inhibitors were able to reduce neuroinflammation and improve cognitive function in a mouse model of Alzheimer's disease [42]. Metformin, an anti-diabetic drug, has been shown to have a dual purpose by downregulating the expression of pro-inflammatory markers (IL-1β, IL-6, TNF-α, COX-2, and TNF receptors) in cancer [43]. In addition, metformin reduces inflammation caused by air pollution in thrombosis [44], Parkinson's disease [45], and lung injury [46]. Monoclonal antibodies such as infliximab, etanercept, adalimumab, golimumab, and certolizumab, which target pro-inflammatory cytokines such as TNF-α in autoimmune/inflammatory diseases like lupus, rheumatoid arthritis, ulcerative colitis, ankylosing spondylitis, and uveitis, have increasingly become popular due to their ability to improve disease outcomes by reducing systemic inflammation [47]. Targeting the JAK-STAT pathway has been investigated to manage chronic inflammation [48]. Furthermore, bio-active compounds and dietary polyphenols have been shown to reduce inflammation, and could therefore be used as a complementary therapy for inflammation-related diseases [49]. The gut microbiota have been linked to inflammation and interventions are being developed to modulate the gut microbiome, such as probiotics or prebiotics, which could potentially reduce reliance on anti-inflammatory drugs, for example, in asthma treatment [50]. The therapeutic landscape for inflammation-driven diseases is advancing rapidly. New biologics targeting specific cytokines, inflammasomes, and inflammatory signalling pathways, such as JAK-STAT, bio-active compounds, and microbiome modulation, highlight the growing potential of precision medicine. These innovations are key to reducing the burden of chronic inflammatory conditions and improving patient outcomes.

4. Conclusions

While inflammation is crucial for the healing process, chronic inflammation can lead to significant health problems. Chronic inflammation is linked to numerous diseases ('all diseases'), ranging from CVD, T2D, metabolic diseases, cancer, autoimmunity, gastrointestinal disorders, respiratory diseases, neurodegenerative diseases, reproductive system disorders, allergies, skin disorders, and joint problems to headaches, food sensitivities, hormonal imbalances, and sleep disorders. The articles featured in this Special Issue provide valuable insights into the intricate relationship between inflammation and disease mechanisms, emphasizing how chronic inflammation underlies certain pathologies. Advancing the understanding of how inflammation drives various pathological conditions could pave the way for innovative therapeutic strategies, preventing the detrimental effects of chronic inflammation and ultimately improving health outcomes and quality of life. Addressing the core causes of inflammation may be crucial in preventing and treating many chronic diseases in the future.

Author Contributions: Conceptualization, V.A. and V.P.C.; methodology, V.A. and V.P.C.; Validation, V.A., J.F. and V.P.C.; formal analysis, V.A., J.F. and V.P.C.; data curation, V.A., J.F. and V.P.C.; writing—original draft preparation, V.A.; writing—review and editing, V.A., J.F. and V.P.C.; visualization, V.A. and V.P.C.; supervision, V.A.; project administration, V.A.; All authors have read and agreed to the published version of the manuscript.

Conflicts of Interest: The authors declare no conflicts of interest.

References

1. Alur, I. Low-Grade Inflammation: A Familiar Factor in Cardiovascular Diseases. *JACC Basic. Transl. Sci.* **2023**, *8*, 1475. [CrossRef] [PubMed]
2. Chaudhary, R.; Prasad, A.; Agarwal, V.; Rehman, M.; Kumar, A.; Kaushik, A.S.; Srivastava, S.; Srivastava, S.; Mishra, V. Chronic stress predisposes to the aggravation of inflammation in autoimmune diseases with focus on rheumatoid arthritis and psoriasis. *Int. Immunopharmacol.* **2023**, *125*, 111046. [CrossRef] [PubMed]
3. Holub, M.; Pottecher, J.; Herwald, H.; Pasupuleti, M.; Papareddy, P. Editorial: Systemic inflammation in severe infectious diseases. *Front. Immunol.* **2024**, *15*, 1483682. [CrossRef]
4. Inflammation: The Cause of all Diseases 2.0. 2024. Available online: https://www.mdpi.com/topics/8P52MZ6248 (accessed on 4 November 2024).
5. Alshuweishi, Y.; Abudawood, A.; Alfayez, D.; Almufarrih, A.A.; Alanazi, F.; Alshuweishi, F.A.; Almuqrin, A.M. Platelet/High-Density Lipoprotein Ratio (PHR) Predicts Type 2 Diabetes in Obese Patients: A Retrospective Study. *Healthcare* **2024**, *12*, 1540. [CrossRef]
6. Ando, T.; Takazawa, I.; Spencer, Z.T.; Ito, R.; Tomimori, Y.; Mikulski, Z.; Matsumoto, K.; Ishitani, T.; Denson, L.A.; Kawakami, Y.; et al. Ileal Crohn's Disease Exhibits Reduced Activity of Phospholipase C-beta3-Dependent Wnt/beta-Catenin Signaling Pathway. *Cells* **2024**, *13*, 986. [CrossRef]
7. Bhoj, P.S.; Nocito, C.; Togre, N.S.; Winfield, M.; Lubinsky, C.; Khan, S.; Mogadala, N.; Seliga, A.; Unterwald, E.M.; Persidsky, Y.; et al. Tissue Kallikrein-1 Suppresses Type I Interferon Responses and Reduces Depressive-Like Behavior in the MRL/lpr Lupus-Prone Mouse Model. *Int. J. Mol. Sci.* **2024**, *25*, 80. [CrossRef]
8. Camacho-Encina, M.; Booth, L.K.; Redgrave, R.E.; Folaranmi, O.; Spyridopoulos, I.; Richardson, G.D. Cellular Senescence, Mitochondrial Dysfunction, and Their Link to Cardiovascular Disease. *Cells* **2024**, *13*, 353. [CrossRef] [PubMed]
9. Kastratovic, N.; Zdravkovic, N.; Cekerevac, I.; Sekerus, V.; Harrell, C.R.; Mladenovic, V.; Djukic, A.; Volarevic, A.; Brankovic, M.; Gmizic, T.; et al. Effects of Combustible Cigarettes and Heated Tobacco Products on Systemic Inflammatory Response in Patients with Chronic Inflammatory Diseases. *Diseases* **2024**, *12*, 144. [CrossRef]
10. Popoca-Hernandez, E.A.; Martinez-Martinez, R.E.; Gonzalez-Amaro, R.F.; Nino-Moreno, P.D.C.; Ayala-Herrera, J.L.; Jerezano-Dominguez, A.V.; Espinosa-Cristobal, L.F.; Marquez-Corona, M.L.; Espinosa-de Santillana, I.A.; Medina-Solis, C.E. Impact of Non-Surgical Periodontal Treatment on the Concentration and Level of MRP-8/14 (Calprotectin) as an Inflammatory Biomarker in Women with Periodontitis and Rheumatoid Arthritis: A Quasi-Experimental Study. *Diseases* **2024**, *12*, 12. [CrossRef]
11. Rajamanickam, V.; Desouza, C.V.; Castillo, R.T.; Saraswathi, V. Blocking Thromboxane-Prostanoid Receptor Signaling Attenuates Lipopolysaccharide- and Stearic Acid-Induced Inflammatory Response in Human PBMCs. *Cells* **2024**, *13*, 1320. [CrossRef]
12. Salnikova, D.I.; Nikiforov, N.G.; Postnov, A.Y.; Orekhov, A.N. Target Role of Monocytes as Key Cells of Innate Immunity in Rheumatoid Arthritis. *Diseases* **2024**, *12*, 81. [CrossRef] [PubMed]
13. Slama, N.; Abdellatif, A.; Bahria, K.; Gasmi, S.; Khames, M.; Hadji, A.; Birkmayer, G.; Oumouna, M.; Amrani, Y.; Benachour, K. NADH Intraperitoneal Injection Prevents Lung Inflammation in a BALB/C Mice Model of Cigarette Smoke-Induced Chronic Obstructive Pulmonary Disease. *Cells* **2024**, *13*, 881. [CrossRef] [PubMed]
14. Stuart, C.M.; Jacob, C.; Varatharaj, A.; Howard, S.; Chouhan, J.K.; Teeling, J.L.; Galea, I. Mild Systemic Inflammation Increases Erythrocyte Fragility. *Int. J. Mol. Sci.* **2024**, *25*, 7027. [CrossRef] [PubMed]
15. Tam, I.Y.S.; Lee, T.H.; Lau, H.Y.A.; Tam, S.Y. Combinatorial Genomic Biomarkers Associated with High Response in IgE-Dependent Degranulation in Human Mast Cells. *Cells* **2024**, *13*, 1237. [CrossRef] [PubMed]
16. Turrini, I.; Guidetti, C.; Contaldo, I.; Pulitano, S.; Rigante, D.; Veredice, C. Wernicke Encephalopathy Caused by Avoidance-Restrictive Food Intake Disorder in a Child: A Case-Based Review. *Diseases* **2024**, *12*, 112. [CrossRef]
17. Pahwa, R.; Goyal, A.; Jialal, I. Chronic Inflammation. In *StatPearls*; StatPearls Publishing: Treasure Island, FL, USA, 2024.
18. Bosevski, M.; Stojanovska, L.; Apostolopoulos, V. Inflammatory biomarkers: Impact for diabetes and diabetic vascular disease. *Acta Biochim. Biophys. Sin.* **2015**, *47*, 1029–1031. [CrossRef]
19. Ephraim, R.; Feehan, J.; Fraser, S.; Nurgali, K.; Apostolopoulos, V. Cancer Immunotherapy: The Checkpoint between Chronic Colitis and Colorectal Cancer. *Cancers* **2022**, *14*, 6131. [CrossRef]
20. Ephraim, R.; Fraser, S.; Devereaux, J.; Stavely, R.; Feehan, J.; Eri, R.; Nurgali, K.; Apostolopoulos, V. Differential Gene Expression of Checkpoint Markers and Cancer Markers in Mouse Models of Spontaneous Chronic Colitis. *Cancers* **2023**, *15*, 4793. [CrossRef]

21. Xu, J.; Zeng, Q.; Li, S.; Su, Q.; Fan, H. Inflammation mechanism and research progress of COPD. *Front. Immunol.* **2024**, *15*, 1404615. [CrossRef]
22. Antoniades, C.; Chan, K. Calcification vs Inflammation: The Modern Toolkit for Cardiovascular Risk Assessment. *JACC Cardiovasc. Imaging* **2024**, *17*, 1225–1228. [CrossRef]
23. Lorenz, T.; Michels, N.; Slavich, G.M.; Giletta, M. Examining systemic inflammation as a pathway linking peer victimization to depressive symptoms in adolescence. *J. Child. Psychol. Psychiatry* **2024**. [CrossRef] [PubMed]
24. Perry, V.H. Contribution of systemic inflammation to chronic neurodegeneration. *Acta Neuropathol.* **2010**, *120*, 277–286. [CrossRef] [PubMed]
25. Feehan, J.; Tripodi, N.; Apostolopoulos, V. The twilight of the immune system: The impact of immunosenescence in aging. *Maturitas* **2021**, *147*, 7–13. [CrossRef] [PubMed]
26. Lee, J.; Taneja, V.; Vassallo, R. Cigarette smoking and inflammation: Cellular and molecular mechanisms. *J. Dent. Res.* **2012**, *91*, 142–149. [CrossRef]
27. Randeni, N.; Bordiga, M.; Xu, B. A Comprehensive Review of the Triangular Relationship among Diet-Gut Microbiota-Inflammation. *Int. J. Mol. Sci.* **2024**, *25*, 9366. [CrossRef]
28. Burini, R.C.; Anderson, E.; Durstine, J.L.; Carson, J.A. Inflammation, physical activity, and chronic disease: An evolutionary perspective. *Sports Med. Health Sci.* **2020**, *2*, 1–6. [CrossRef]
29. Falconer, C.L.; Cooper, A.R.; Walhin, J.P.; Thompson, D.; Page, A.S.; Peters, T.J.; Montgomery, A.A.; Sharp, D.J.; Dayan, C.M.; Andrews, R.C. Sedentary time and markers of inflammation in people with newly diagnosed type 2 diabetes. *Nutr. Metab. Cardiovasc. Dis.* **2014**, *24*, 956–962. [CrossRef]
30. Langston, P.K.; Sun, Y.; Ryback, B.A.; Mueller, A.L.; Spiegelman, B.M.; Benoist, C.; Mathis, D. Regulatory T cells shield muscle mitochondria from interferon-gamma-mediated damage to promote the beneficial effects of exercise. *Sci. Immunol.* **2023**, *8*, eadi5377. [CrossRef]
31. Apostolopoulos, V.; Borkoles, E.; Polman, R.; Stojanovska, L. Physical and immunological aspects of exercise in chronic diseases. *Immunotherapy* **2014**, *6*, 1145–1157. [CrossRef]
32. Stojanovska, L.; Apostolopoulos, V.; Polman, R.; Borkoles, E. To exercise, or, not to exercise, during menopause and beyond. *Maturitas* **2014**, *77*, 318–323. [CrossRef]
33. Sotak, M.; Clark, M.; Suur, B.E.; Borgeson, E. Inflammation and resolution in obesity. *Nat. Rev. Endocrinol.* **2024**, 1–17. [CrossRef] [PubMed]
34. Yende, A.S.; Sharma, D. Obesity, dysbiosis and inflammation: Interactions that modulate the efficacy of immunotherapy. *Front. Immunol.* **2024**, *15*, 1444589. [CrossRef]
35. Apostolopoulos, V.; de Courten, M.P.; Stojanovska, L.; Blatch, G.L.; Tangalakis, K.; de Courten, B. The complex immunological and inflammatory network of adipose tissue in obesity. *Mol. Nutr. Food Res.* **2016**, *60*, 43–57. [CrossRef] [PubMed]
36. Letukiene, A.; Hendrixson, V.; Gineviciene, V. Current knowledge and scientific trends in myokines and exercise research in the context of obesity. *Front. Med.* **2024**, *11*, 1421962. [CrossRef]
37. Margina, D.; Ungurianu, A.; Purdel, C.; Tsoukalas, D.; Sarandi, E.; Thanasoula, M.; Tekos, F.; Mesnage, R.; Kouretas, D.; Tsatsakis, A. Chronic Inflammation in the Context of Everyday Life: Dietary Changes as Mitigating Factors. *Int. J. Environ. Res. Public. Health* **2020**, *17*, 4135. [CrossRef]
38. Furman, D.; Campisi, J.; Verdin, E.; Carrera-Bastos, P.; Targ, S.; Franceschi, C.; Ferrucci, L.; Gilroy, D.W.; Fasano, A.; Miller, G.W.; et al. Chronic inflammation in the etiology of disease across the life span. *Nat. Med.* **2019**, *25*, 1822–1832. [CrossRef] [PubMed]
39. Wirth, T.; Lafforgue, P.; Pham, T. NSAID: Current limits to prescription. *Joint Bone Spine* **2024**, *91*, 105685. [CrossRef]
40. Mohlmann, J.E.; Ezzafzafi, S.; Lindemans, C.A.; Jansen, M.H.A.; Nierkens, S.; Huitema, A.D.R.; van Luin, M. Pharmacokinetics and Pharmacodynamics of Systemic Corticosteroids in Autoimmune and Inflammatory Diseases: A Review of Current Evidence. *Clin. Pharmacokinet.* **2024**, *63*, 1251–1270. [CrossRef] [PubMed]
41. Lackner, A.; Cabral, J.E.; Qiu, Y.; Zhou, H.; Leonidas, L.; Pham, M.A.; Macapagal, A.; Lin, S.; Armanus, E.; McNulty, R. Small molecule inhibitor binds to NOD-like receptor family pyrin domain containing 3 and prevents inflammasome activation. *iScience* **2024**, *27*, 110459. [CrossRef]
42. Lonnemann, N.; Hosseini, S.; Marchetti, C.; Skouras, D.B.; Stefanoni, D.; D'Alessandro, A.; Dinarello, C.A.; Korte, M. The NLRP3 inflammasome inhibitor OLT1177 rescues cognitive impairment in a mouse model of Alzheimer's disease. *Proc. Natl. Acad. Sci. USA* **2020**, *117*, 32145–32154. [CrossRef]
43. Bai, B.; Chen, H. Metformin: A Novel Weapon Against Inflammation. *Front. Pharmacol.* **2021**, *12*, 622262. [CrossRef] [PubMed]
44. Soberanes, S.; Misharin, A.V.; Jairaman, A.; Morales-Nebreda, L.; McQuattie-Pimentel, A.C.; Cho, T.; Hamanaka, R.B.; Meliton, A.Y.; Reyfman, P.A.; Walter, J.M.; et al. Metformin Targets Mitochondrial Electron Transport to Reduce Air-Pollution-Induced Thrombosis. *Cell Metab.* **2019**, *29*, 335–347.e335. [CrossRef] [PubMed]
45. Murata, H.; Barnhill, L.M.; Bronstein, J.M. Air Pollution and the Risk of Parkinson's Disease: A Review. *Mov. Disord.* **2022**, *37*, 894–904. [CrossRef] [PubMed]
46. Gao, J.; Yuan, J.; Wang, Q.; Lei, T.; Shen, X.; Cui, B.; Zhang, F.; Ding, W.; Lu, Z. Metformin protects against PM(2.5)-induced lung injury and cardiac dysfunction independent of AMP-activated protein kinase alpha2. *Redox Biol.* **2020**, *28*, 101345. [CrossRef] [PubMed]

47. Wajda, A.; Perricone, C.; Kashyap, A.; Iliyasu, M.Y. Editorial: Biological drugs and biosimilars in autoimmune diseases. *Front. Pharmacol.* **2023**, *14*, 1168972. [CrossRef]
48. Honap, S.; Agorogianni, A.; Colwill, M.J.; Mehta, S.K.; Donovan, F.; Pollok, R.; Poullis, A.; Patel, K. JAK inhibitors for inflammatory bowel disease: Recent advances. *Frontline Gastroenterol.* **2024**, *15*, 59–69. [CrossRef] [PubMed]
49. Zhang, J.; Cianciosi, D.; Islam, M.O.; Zhang, L. Editorial: Intervention effects of food-derived polyphenols and bioactive peptides on chronic inflammation. *Front. Nutr.* **2024**, *11*, 1493706. [CrossRef]
50. Aslam, R.; Herrles, L.; Aoun, R.; Pioskowik, A.; Pietrzyk, A. Link between gut microbiota dysbiosis and childhood asthma: Insights from a systematic review. *J. Allergy Clin. Immunol. Glob.* **2024**, *3*, 100289. [CrossRef]

cells

MDPI

Review

Proinflammatory Cytokines in Chronic Respiratory Diseases and Their Management

Vivek P. Chavda [1,*,†], Rajashri Bezbaruah [2,3,†], Nasima Ahmed [2], Shahnaz Alom [2,4], Bedanta Bhattacharjee [4], Lakshmi Vineela Nalla [5], Damanbhalang Rynjah [4], Laura Kate Gadanec [6] and Vasso Apostolopoulos [7]

1 Department of Pharmaceutics and Pharmaceutical Technology, L.M. College of Pharmacy, Ahmedabad 380009, Gujarat, India

2 Department of Pharmaceutical Sciences, Faculty of Science and Engineering, Dibrugarh University, Dibrugarh 786004, Assam, India; rajashribezbaruah@dibru.ac.in (R.B.); ahmed.nasima91@gmail.com (N.A.); shahnazalom1@gmail.com (S.A.)

3 Institute of Pharmacy, Assam Medical College and Hospital, Dibrugarh 786002, Assam, India

4 Girijananda Chowdhury Institute of Pharmaceutical Science-Tezpur, Sonitpur 784501, Assam, India; bedanta1994@gmail.com (B.B.); damanbhalangrynjah@gmail.com (D.R.)

5 Department of Pharmacology, GITAM School of Pharmacy, GITAM (Deemed to be University), Rushikonda, Visakhapatnam 530045, Andhra Pradesh, India; vineelavinni154@gmail.com

6 Institute for Health and Sport, Immunology and Translational Research Group, Victoria University, Werribee, VIC 3030, Australia; laura.gadanec@live.vu.edu.au

7 School of Health and Biomedical Sciences, RMIT University, Melbourne, VIC 3083, Australia; vasso.apostolopoulos@rmit.edu.au

* Correspondence: vivek7chavda@gmail.com

† These authors contributed equally to this work.

Abstract

Pulmonary homeostasis can be agitated either by external environmental insults or endogenous factors produced during respiratory/pulmonary diseases. The lungs counter these insults by initiating mechanisms of inflammation as a localized, non-specific first-line defense response. Cytokines are small signaling glycoprotein molecules that control the immune response. They are formed by numerous categories of cell types and induce the movement, growth, differentiation, and death of cells. During respiratory diseases, multiple proinflammatory cytokines play a crucial role in orchestrating chronic inflammation and structural changes in the respiratory tract by recruiting inflammatory cells and maintaining the release of growth factors to maintain inflammation. The issue aggravates when the inflammatory response is exaggerated and/or cytokine production becomes dysregulated. In such instances, unresolving and chronic inflammatory reactions and cytokine production accelerate airway remodeling and maladaptive outcomes. Pro-inflammatory cytokines generate these deleterious consequences through interactions with receptors, which in turn initiate a signal in the cell, triggering a response. The cytokine profile and inflammatory cascade seen in different pulmonary diseases vary and have become fundamental targets for advancement in new therapeutic strategies for lung diseases. There are considerable therapeutic approaches that target cytokine-mediated inflammation in pulmonary diseases; however, blocking specific cytokines may not contribute to clinical benefit. Alternatively, broad-spectrum anti-inflammatory approaches are more likely to be clinically effective. Herein, this comprehensive review of the literature identifies various cytokines (e.g., interleukins, chemokines, and growth factors) involved in pulmonary inflammation and the pathogenesis of respiratory diseases (e.g., asthma, chronic obstructive pulmonary, lung cancer, pneumonia, and pulmonary fibrosis) and investigates targeted therapeutic treatment approaches.

Cells **2025**, *14*, 400 https://doi.org/10.3390/cells14060400

Keywords: asthma; chemokines; chronic obstructive; COVID-19-associated lung disease; cystic fibrosis bronchiectasis; growth factors; interferons; interleukins; lung cancer; pneumonia; pulmonary fibrosis; proinflammatory cytokines; respiratory diseases

1. Introduction

Respiratory diseases remain one of the leading causes of death in underdeveloped nations [1,2]. Alarmingly, chronic respiratory diseases are the third leading cause of death worldwide, and are responsible for 4 million deaths annually [1,2]. Despite the 2021 Global Burden of Disease Study reporting a substantial decline in mortality caused by lower respiratory infections, a considerable number of deaths in infants and young children were associated with pneumonia and other lower respiratory tract diseases [3]. Recently, the World Health Organization (WHO) has shifted focus toward implementing strategies to facilitate the prevention of noncommunicable diseases (e.g., asthma, chronic obstructive pulmonary diseases (COPD), and chronic respiratory diseases) [4], as infectious respiratory disorders can be mitigated or controlled by vaccination and medication [3]. Asthma results in approximately 455,000 fatalities each year worldwide [5], and due to its chronicity and high morbidity burden causes great disruption to an individual's personal, social, and economic productivity, as well as quality of life [5]. Each year asthma accounts for more than 700,000 Emergency Department visits by children [6], and is believed to affect more than 350 million people globally [7]. Both developed and emerging nations have reported an increase in the prevalence of asthma [8], which may be attributed to air pollution, atmospheric chemical triggers, aeroallergens and traffic density in metropolitan areas [9,10], a lack of access to healthcare, and the availably and affordability of drugs in low-income and rural areas [11]. In addition to air pollution and workplace exposure to unhealthy air, tobacco smoke (active and passive smoke exposure) is a major contributor to the burden of respiratory diseases [12,13]. Indoor and outdoor air pollution expose almost 3 billion people to harmful consequences, resulting in 3 million avoidable deaths annually [14]. Furthermore, the frequency of lung cancer and COPD are also on the rise, with lung cancer representing the most common malignancy and the most common cause of deaths in people [15,16]. Millions of people lose their lives due to a lack of access to essential healthcare services, medications, vaccinations, and medical care [17,18]. Furthermore, as most respiratory infections are avoidable and prevention is often less expensive than the required treatment, global respiratory illness control and eradication depend on public health initiatives and surveillance, including raising awareness and increasing knowledge and education [1,19]. To find effective interventions, set targets, and effectively allocate finances and resources to minimize the burden of respiratory diseases, it is crucial to understand the socioeconomic load that these respiratory diseases place on healthcare resources [1,19]. Respiratory diseases, such as asthma, COPD, and acute respiratory distress syndrome (ARDS), are characterized by the excessive production of proinflammatory cytokines and chronic airway inflammation, which can lead to airway hyperresponsiveness, remodeling, and tissue damage [20].

Exposure to microorganisms, toxins, pollutants, irritants, and allergens causes airway inflammation [21]. Inflammatory receptors identify conserved molecular patterns displayed on pathogens, activating inflammatory cells such as macrophages, dendritic cells, natural killer (NK) cells, and T cells, which then release inflammatory mediators, including growth factors, chemokines, and proinflammatory cytokines [20–23]. Proinflammatory cytokines produced by immune cells in response to infection or injury, such as tumor necrosis factor (TNF) and interleukins (IL), play a significant role in the pathogenesis of respiratory diseases [20–23]. The release of cytokines triggers a cascade of events that lead to inflammation and damage to the airways and lung tissue, resulting in different respiratory illnesses and diseases [20–23]. Interestingly, while certain cytokines are proinflammatory and contribute to disease progression (e.g., IL-1, chemokines, and interferon (IFN)), others reduce inflammation and aid in the healing process (e.g., IL-4, IL-10, and IL-13), and have become of interest in cytokine biology and clinical research [24]. The mechanism of inflammation is dependent on genes (e.g., type II phospholipase A2 (PLA2), cyclooxygenase (COX)-2, and inducible nitric oxide synthase) that create small mediator molecules when inflammation occurs and that are upregulated during this process. These genes produce enzymes that boost the production of leukotrienes, prostanoids, nitric oxide (NO), and platelet-activating factor, which ultimately cause inflammation [25,26]. Endotoxins and other inflammatory products, such as histamines, reactive oxygen (ROS), and reactive nitrogen species (RNS), increase the expression of inflammatory genes and secrete IL-1 and TNF (and occasionally IFN-γ) [27] (Figure 1).

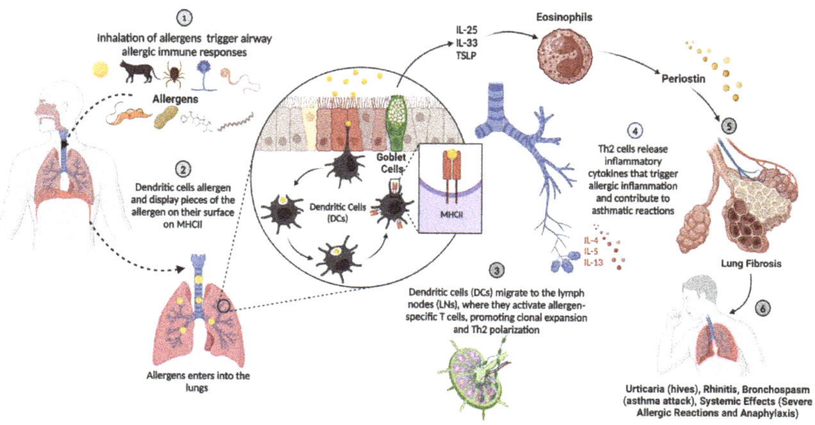

Figure 1. Schematic representation of the pathologic immune response in the airways. (1) Inhalation of allergens, such as pollen, dust mites, animal dander, and mold, triggers an immune reaction. (2) Dendritic cells (DCs) in the airway epithelium capture and process allergens, presenting them on MHC class II molecules [24]. (3) Activated DCs migrate to the lymph nodes, where they stimulate allergen-specific naïve T cells, leading to clonal expansion and differentiation into Th2 cells. (4) Th2 cells release inflammatory cytokines (IL-4, IL-5, IL-13), promoting eosinophilic inflammation, mucus hypersecretion, and bronchial hyper-responsiveness. (5) This cascade results in airway constriction, increased vascular permeability, and mucus production, leading to allergic asthma and, in severe cases, anaphylaxis [24]. Figure created using BioRender.com (Premium Version) (accessed on 28 February 2025).

The lungs are the fundamental organs of the respiratory system, and their most basic physiological role is to facilitate gas exchange and transport [28]; however, excessive inflammation, injury, and homeostatic imbalance can be fatal [29]. Pulmonary homeostasis depends on a careful balance between proinflammatory and anti-inflammatory responses [30]. It is believed that proinflammatory cytokines secreted by inflammatory cells play a crucial role in the pathogenesis of different lung diseases, such ARDS, asthma, cystic fibrosis bronchiectasis, and COPD [22,27]. The host's defense against pathological situations is strengthened by the proinflammatory cytokines released by macrophages [20,27]. Proinflammatory cytokines may be helpful in managing the pathology of inflammation, but when their levels increase and remain high, they can seriously harm tissue [27]. Coronavirus disease 2019 (COVID-19), caused by severe acute respiratory syndrome coronavirus-2 (SARS-CoV-2), poses a serious threat to global health [31]. Through immune system hyperactivation and uncontrolled cytokine release, COVID-19 has the ability to cause a cytokine storm in pulmonary tissues [32], similar to that observed in ARDS [33]. Therefore, managing cytokine release syndrome (CRS) and avoiding further infections may be a promising strategy for COVID-19 therapy [34]. Herein, we have attempted to establish the general role of cytokines in respiratory disorders, their signaling pathways, and their management strategies. Since most respiratory diseases, such as asthma, COPD, COVID-19-related ARDS, cystic fibrosis bronchiectasis, lung cancer, pneumonia, and pulmonary fibrosis, share similar proinflammatory cytokines, a comprehensive understanding of the inflammatory pathways related to their associated cytokines is essential to control and eradicate respiratory diseases [22].

2. Classification of Cytokines

Small signaling proteins generated by cells, referred to as cytokines, have a particular impact on the communication and interaction between cells [35]. These nonstructural proteins have a molecular weight that ranges from 8 to 40,000 Daltons and have an essential role in the immune system, inflammation, and healing after injury or disease [24]. Cytokines can exert their effect on the cells that release them (autocrine action), on cells that are close (paracrine action), or on cells that are far away (endocrine action) [36]. During physiological and pathological processes, immune cells, including macrophages, mast cells, T helper (Th) cells, endothelial cells, and Schwann cells, that are localized or migrate to the site of inflammation release cytokines in and via peripheral nerve tissue [37]. According to their structure, origin, and function, cytokines are classified into different types [38]. For example, (i) cytokines with chemotactic properties are called chemokines; (ii) cytokines produced by one leukocyte and acting on other leukocytes are known as ILs; (iii) cytokines with the ability to kill or inhibit tumor cells are referred to as TNF; (iv) cytokines that promote distinct stages of development and differentiation in pluripotent hematopoietic stem cells are called colony-stimulating factor (CSF); and (v) cytokines that can act by preventing lymphocyte proliferation are called transforming growth factor (TGF) [39].

2.1. Interleukins

Interleukins are a category of secreted proteins with a variety of forms and roles. They are predominantly produced by $CD4^+$ Th lymphocytes, monocytes, macrophages, and endothelial cells [25,26]. ILs, which are effective at thymocyte and T-cell activation, proliferation, and differentiation, can also improve the killing activity of cytotoxic T (Tc) and NK cells, causing fever, stimulating hematopoiesis, and encouraging immunological responses [25]. There are currently 40 known ILs, some of which are divided into subtypes (e.g., IL-1α and IL-1β) [40]. Moreover, based on commonalities in their receptor chains and sequences and other functional characteristics, ILs can be further categorized into families. The IL-1 family consists of 11 cytokines: 3 receptor antagonists (IL-1 receptor antagonist (Ra), IL-36Ra, and IL-38); 7 agonistic ligands (IL-1α, IL-1β, IL-18, IL-33, IL-36α, IL-36β, and IL-36γ); and 1 anti-inflammatory cytokine (IL-37) [41]. Autoimmune, viral, degenerative, and autoinflammatory disorders are all closely associated with IL-1. IL-2, IL-4, IL-7, IL-9, IL-15, and IL-21 create the IL-2 cytokine family, sometimes referred to as the common γ-chain family [42]. For progenitors and mature cells, these cytokines function as growth and proliferation factors. Although dendritic cells and NK cells can also express this cytokine, $CD4^+$ and $CD8^+$ T cells are the major producers of cytokines [24]. As a B-cell growth factor, IL-2 stimulates the production of antibodies, aids in the generation of regulatory T (Treg) cells, and encourages the growth and differentiation of NK and Th cells. In addition to sharing some of IL-2's properties, such as T-cell activation and NK cell proliferation stimulation, IL-15 also affects CD8$^+$ memory cells and NK cell homeostasis, and increased levels of IL-15 have also been observed in autoimmune diseases [41].

2.2. Tumor Necrosis Factor

The term "TNF" refers to a cytokine that was first identified as a tumor necrosis-inducing molecule in 1975 and possesses the ability to kill or inhibit tumor cells [41]. TNF acts on vascular endothelial cells, causing endothelial cell damage, vascular dysfunction and injury, thrombosis, and local blood flow blockade of the tumor tissue. The TNF superfamily, which also includes the TNF receptor superfamily, has more than 40 members [43], the most notable of which are TNF-α and TNF-β (also known as lymphotoxin) [43]. TNF-α induces inflammation and causes acute phase reactions and fever. Additionally, it induces neutrophil and endothelial cell activation and kills cells via apoptotic mechanisms. The type II transmembrane protein TNF-β plays a crucial role in the formation of Peyer's patches, in the lymph nodes, and in the maintenance of secondary lymphoid organs. Lymphocytes are primarily responsible for stimulating TNF-β expression [41].

2.3. Interferons

The pleiotropic characteristics of cytokines are further demonstrated by IFNs, which have the capacity to prevent viral replication [44–46]. Although it constitutes a broad-spectrum antiviral medication, IFN does not immediately kill or suppress an infiltrating virus. Rather, IFN induces cells to create antiviral proteins primarily through cell surface receptors, preventing hepatitis B virus from replicating [41,47]. Additionally, it can boost the health of T lymphocytes, macrophages, and NK cells, which have immunoregulatory effects, and improves the replication of antivirals [41,47]. Type I, II, and III IFNs are the three primary classes of IFNs. The two primary type I IFNs are IFN-α and IFN-β, and IFN-α is further divided into 13 distinct subtypes, including IFN-α1, IFN-α2, IFN-α4, IFN-α5, IFN-α6, IFN-α7, IFN-α8, IFN-α10, IFN-α13, IFN-α14, IFN-α16, IFN-α17, and IFN-α21 [48]. Type I IFNs have strong antiviral effects, especially against influenza, hepatitis B/C, and some RNA/DNA viruses, as well as having an important role in autoimmune diseases and cancer. IFN-α has been used therapeutically against hepatitis C, and more recently IFN-α was shown to protect against pulmonary tissue damage from the highly pathogenic avian influenza virus, H5N1 [49]. Lesser-known type I IFNs include IFN-δ, IFN-ε, IFN-ζ, IFN-κ, IFN-ω, and IFN-τ. IFN-δ is not a well-characterized IFN; however, it is expressed in response to viral infections. IFN-ε is involved in local immune responses against viruses in epithelial tissues and the mucosal surfaces of the lung and reproductive tract; IFN-ζ is expressed by dendritic cells in response to viral infections and cancer, and contributes to the stimulation of T cells; IFN-κ is expressed in keratinocytes and protects the skin against viral infections; IFN-ω is produced in response to viral infections; and IFN-τ plays an important role in pregnancy [50]. A type II IFN is IFN-γ, a proinflammatory cytokine involved in inflammation, defense against viruses, cancer, and immune regulation [50]; it also increases TNF activity and stimulates NO production [44]. Similar to type I IFNs, type III IFNs, such as IFN-λ1 (IL-29), IFN-λ2 (IL-28A), IFN-λ3 (IL-28B), and IFN-λ4, are vital in the host's defense against viral infections, with restricted expression on mucosal tissues (respiratory, gastrointestinal, and urogenital tracts). IFN-λ also plays important roles against hepatitis, cancer, and autoimmune diseases, and has been investigated for its role as a therapeutic against viral infections.

2.4. Colony-Stimulating Factor

CSF is a pro-inflammatory cytokine that initiates distinct stages of development and differentiation in pluripotent hematopoietic stem cells. CSF promotes hematopoiesis, which aids in the development of monocyte, neutrophil, eosinophil, and basophil progenitors, and in the activation of macrophages [41]. Alternatively, some CSFs have the ability to stimulate or augment the phagocytosis and killing activities of neutrophils and macrophages, in addition to their role in hematopoietic stem cell proliferation and differentiation during various developmental and differentiation phases [51]. Additionally, granulocyte–macrophage CSF (GM-CSF) and macrophage CSF (M-CSF) exhibit a connection between their expression and TNF, IL-1, IL-17, and IL-23 [52].

2.5. Chemokines

Chemokines, which are short peptides (8000 Daltons) that facilitate the movement of leukocytes from circulation into tissues, are another group of genes that promote inflammation [53]. There are approximately 50 known human chemokines, which are divided into four groups based on the location of their N-terminal cysteine residues [54]. The two main chemokine families are C-C motif (CC) and C-X-C motif (CXC). In general, CXC chemokines are more selective for neutrophils, while CC chemokines are chemotactic for monocytes and a small proportion of lymphocytes [54]. The most well-known chemokine is IL-8, also known as CXCL8, which is a member of the CXC chemokine family and is necessary for the recruitment of neutrophils and promoting and maintaining ongoing inflammatory responses [55]. However, CCL2 (also known as monocyte chemoattractant protein-1) and CCL11 (also referred to as eotaxin) are examples of CC chemokines that affect the recruitment of a range of leukocytes, particularly monocytes and eosinophils, respectively [56]. However, involvement in inflammatory responses is the most well-known function of chemokines. Chemokines actively promote macrophage, neutrophil, and T-cell recruitment to the site of inflammation and function as secondary proinflammatory mediators brought on by primary proinflammatory mediators, such as IL-1 or TNF [41].

2.6. Transforming Growth Factor

TGF-β is a polypeptide growth factor that is crucial for several functions, including cell growth and differentiation, extracellular matrix synthesis, angiogenesis, apoptosis, and immune system function [57]. Monocytes and macrophages are drawn to TGF-β by its chemo-attractive properties; however, it also has an anti-inflammatory impact by preventing lymphocyte proliferation [41].

2.7. Other Cytokines

In addition to the previously described cytokines, some other types of cytokines that play important roles in the pulmonary inflammatory process include leukemia inhibitory factor and oncostatin M, which cause the production of acute-phase proteins [58,59]. Moreover, osteopontin promotes the development of IL-2 and inhibits the production of IL-10 [41]. Table 1 summarizes the classifications of cytokines, along with their origins of secretion and roles during inflammation.

Table 1. Classification of cytokines, their origin of secretion, and roles during inflammation.

Cytokines	Key Secreting Cells	Roles During Inflammation	References
IL-1	Endothelial cells, epithelial cells, macrophages, monocytes, dendritic ells	Induces inflammation, fever, and acute phase response, and accelerates production of neutrophils	[25,41,60]
IL-2	$CD4^{+}$ and $CD8^{+}$ T cells	Activates NK cells and cytotoxic T cells and increases production of other cytokines	[25,41,60]
IL-3	$CD4^{+}$ T cells	Produces growth factor for hematopoietic stem cells	[41,60]

Table 1. *Cont.*

Cytokines	Key Secreting Cells	Roles During Inflammation	References
IL-4	CD4⁺ Th2 cells and mast cells	Promotes differentiation of Th2 cells and aids in growth and survival of mast cells, B cells, and T cells	[41,60]
IL-5	CD4⁺ Th2 cells	Stimulates growth and progression of eosinophil	[25,41]
IL-6	Endothelial cells, macrophages and T lymphocytes	Induces the liver to create acute-phase inflammatory response mediators	[41,60]
IL-7	Stromal cells of bone marrow	Plays a role in adaptive immunity by promoting the growth and division of thymocytes and pre-B cells	[41,60]
IL-8 (CXCL8)	Endothelial cells, macrophages, neutrophils	Plays a role in adaptive immunity, controls lymphocyte migration and neutrophil infiltration, and attracts neutrophils and T lymphocytes	[41,60]
IL-10	Macrophages, Th cells, regulatory T cells, dendritic cells	Reduces inflammation by preventing Th1 cells and the release of IL-12 from activated macrophages and dendritic cells	[41,60]
IL-12	Dendritic cells and macrophages	Increases the cytotoxicity of NK cells in innate immunity and triggers the development of Th1 cells in adaptive immunity	[41,60]
Type-I IFN (IFN-α, IFN-β)	Fibroblasts, macrophages, dendritic cells, endothelial cells, epithelial cells	NK cell activation, viral replication inhibition, and increases MHC-I molecule expression on virus-infected cells	[41,44,60–62]
IFN-γ	CD4⁺ and CD8⁺ T lymphocytes and NK cells	Promotes the production of MHC-I and II and the processing and presentation of antigens; activates macrophages in innate immune responses and adaptive cell-mediated immune responses	[41,44,61,62]
TNF-α	Macrophages and T cells	Brings about inflammation, causes acute phase reaction and fever, and induces neutrophil and endothelial cell activation and cellular apoptosis	[43,60]
TGF-β	T cells	Induces cytotoxicity and phagocytosis	[43,60]
Chemokines	Endothelial cells, macrophages and T cells	Leukocyte migration from the blood and tissues is controlled and stimulated by chemokines	[41,53,56]
G-CSF	Endothelial cells, fibroblast and macrophages	Encourages the production of growth factors and neutrophil maturation in inflammatory reactions	[41,52,60]
M-CSF	Macrophages and T cells	Encourages mononuclear phagocyte maturation and growth factors	[41,52,60]
GM-CSF	Endothelial cells, fibroblast, macrophages, and T cells	Activates mature granulocytes and encourages the maturation and expansion of neutrophil, eosinophil, and monocyte cells	[41,52,60]

Abbreviations: G-CSF, granulocyte colony-stimulating factor; GM-CSF, granulocyte monocyte colony-stimulating factor; IL, interleukin; IFN, interferon; M-CSF, monocyte colony-stimulating factor; MHC, major histocompatibility complex; NK, natural killer; Th, T-helper; TNF: tumor necrosis factor.

3. Pro-Inflammatory Cytokines in Respiratory Diseases

The lungs and airways are constantly exposed to external airborne insults comprising a mixture of harmless inhaled particles and detrimental pathogens, aeroallergens, and pollutants [20]. Cytokines play a pivotal role in the pulmonary equilibrium and have the ability to regulate host responses to damage or infections within the lungs, leading to the removal of injury, repair of lung tissue, and restoration of homeostasis [20]. However, as cytokine-mediated tissue damage can compromise gas exchange and transport, it is essential that pulmonary immunity is tightly controlled, enabling pathogenic clearance and the prompt restoration of homeostasis, while simultaneously avoiding unnecessary excessive and chronic inflammatory responses [20]. When the inflammatory response is unregulated or cytokine production becomes unbalanced, deleterious consequences occur, including airway remodeling, fibrosis, and undesired, maladaptive effects [63]. Proinflammatory cytokines secreted by inflammatory cells play a crucial role in the pathogenesis of different lung diseases, such as ARDS, asthma, cystic fibrosis bronchiectasis, and COPD (Table 2) [22]. Cytokines generated by Th2 cells appear crucial in directing inflammation, at least in mild-to-moderate illness [64]. Although there are many respiratory conditions that arise due to underlying inflammatory cytokine release, we have highlighted several major respiratory conditions, including COPD, asthma, pulmonary fibrosis, cystic fibrosis bronchiectasis, COVID-19, pneumonia, and lung cancer, that align with the major acting cytokines (Table 2).

Table 2. Major lung diseases and the corresponding cytokines that are involved in their pathogenesis and development.

Lung Disease	Cytokines Involved	References
Asthma	CCR2-5 agonist, CXCR2-3 agonist, EGF, eotaxin, GM-CSF, IL-1 β, IL-4, IL-5, IL-6, IL-8, IL-9, IL-13, IL-17, IL-25, IL-33, NGF, RANTES, SCF, TGF-β, TNF-α, TSLP, VEGF	[63,65–67]
COPD	CCR2 agonist, CCR3 agonist, CCR5 agonist, CXCR2 agonist, CXCR3 agonist, EGF, GM-CSF, IL-1β, IL-4, IL-6, IL-8, IL-12, IL-17, IL-18, IL-32, IFN-γ, TGF-β, TNF-α, TSLP	[63,65,68–71]
COVID-19-associated lung disease	IL-1β, IL-8, IL-6, IL-17, TNF-α	[72,73]
Cystic fibrosis bronchiectasis	IL-1β	[74–78]
Lung cancer	IFN-γ, IL-1β, IL-6, IL-8, IL-10, IL-17, IL-18, IL-22,TGF-β, TNF-α, VEGF	[79,80]
Pneumonia	IFN-γ, IL-lβ, IL-6, IL-8, IL-10, IL-33, MCP-1, TNF	[81–84]
Pulmonary fibrosis	CCL17, CCL18/PARC, CTGF, CXCL12/SDF-1, GM-CSF, IL-1, IL-4, IL-10, IL-13, IL-17, MCP-1, oncostatin M, PDGF, TGF- β	[63,65,72,85]
Pulmonary tuberculosis	TNF-α, IL-1β, IL-12, IL-18, IL- 23, IL-27, IL-10, IL-6, IL-17, IL-22, IFN-β, IFN- γ, TGF- β	[86]

Abbreviations: CTGF, connective tissue growth factor; EGF, epidermal growth factor; GM-CSF, granulocyte–macrophage colony-stimulating factor; IFN, interferon; IL, interleukin; MCP-1, monocyte chemotactic protein-1; PARC, pulmonary and activation-regulated chemokine; PDGF, platelet-derived growth factor; RANTES, regulated and normal T-cell expressed and secreted; SDF-1, stromal cell-derived factor-1; TGF, transforming growth factor; TNF, tumor necrosis factor; TSLP, thymic stromal lymphopoietin; VEGF: vascular endothelial growth factor.

In the context of chronic respiratory disease (asthma, COPD, etc.) extended exposition to inflammatory signals might eventually cause T-cell depletion and a decrease in responsiveness. High amounts of inhibitory receptors like PD-1, TIM-3, LAG-3, and TIGIT are frequently expressed by these cells' exhaustion. This also reduces the generation of cytokines such as IFN-γ, TNF-α, and IL-2, which are essential for efficient immune system responses. However, they may also cause low-to-no response to therapeutic treatments, for instance immunotherapy, which later depend on a vigorous immune response [64].

3.1. Chronic Obstructive Pulmonary Disease

Smoking and extended exposure to fumes, dust, or polluted air are the main causes of COPD, which manifests as chronic bronchial inflammation, lung tissue damage (emphysema), and some degree of lung fibrosis (Figure 2). The traditional proinflammatory cytokines (i.e., TNF-α, IFN-γ, IL-1, IL-6, IL-8, IL-18, and IL-32) drive the inflammatory process involving T cells, neutrophils, and macrophages; among these, IL-8 provides an integral function in the inflammatory reaction and stimulates neutrophils to the spot of inflammation in the lungs. Additionally, recent research has highlighted IL-17 in the pathophysiology of COPD [63]. Patients with COPD have elevated sputum IL-17 levels that are significantly more pronounced than those in patients with asthma [68]. Activated Th1 and Th2 cells were observed in COPD patients, suggesting that both may contribute to the disease processes, even though COPD is not often thought of as a Th2-mediated disease. Similarly, IL-13 may cause vascular remodeling, airway fibrosis, and mucus metaplasia in COPD [69]. Patients with COPD have an increased expression of the profibrotic cytokine TGF-β in their airways, and TGF-β is believed to help alter the structural composition of the lungs [63,65]. A new cytokine target in COPD that has gained notoriety is the D-dopachrome tautomerase (D-DT)/atypical chemokine-receptor-3 (ACKR3) ligand/receptor axis. Prior research has shown that D-DT and macrophage migration inhibitory factor (MIF) have conflicting roles in COPD. MIF also appears to have tissue-protective roles in myocardial ischemia, metabolic liver disease, and alveolar regeneration, although it is often believed to have proinflammatory, disease-exacerbating effects. Although D-DT has protective benefits against the inflammation of adipose tissue, heart failure, and myocardial ischemia, it also encourages endotoxemia, multiple sclerosis, and carcinogenesis. ACKR3, a new receptor for D-DT, was implicated by Melgert's group as having a protective role for D-DT in COPD. The findings have implications for utilizing pro-repair D-DT as a COPD treatment plan [70,71]. During clinical trials, IL-blocking antibodies have been reported to reduce the number of acute exacerbations and methods that inhibit upstream cytokines, such as thymic stromal lymphopoietin (TSLP), and have the potential to improve patient health in COPD [65].

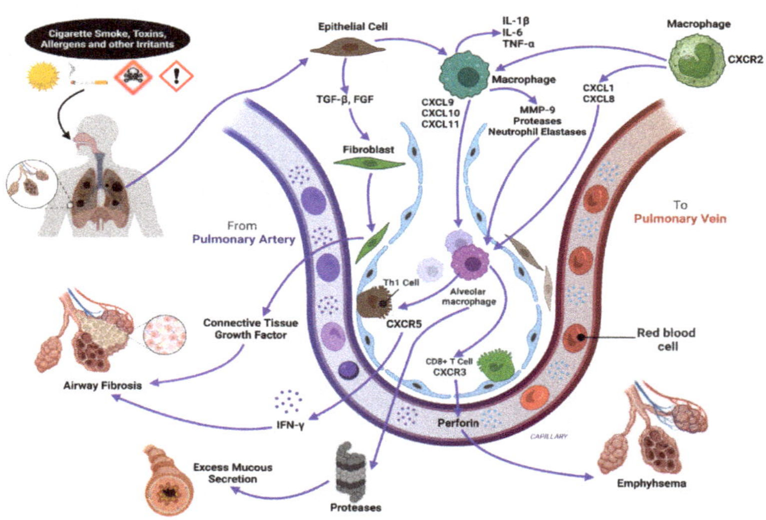

Figure 2. The role of cytokines in COPD. (1) Inhaled irritants, such as cigarette smoke, cause macrophages and epithelial cells to release several cytokines, including growth factors such as TGF-β and FGFs. These factors encourage fibroblast proliferation, which leads to fibrosis in the small airways. (2) These cells also release a number of chemokines that draw circulating cells into the lungs, as well as the proinflammatory cytokines TNF-α, IL-1β, and IL-6, all of which increase inflammation. (3) Monocytes are drawn to CCL2 via CCR2. (4) Neutrophils and monocytes are drawn to CXCL1 and CXCL8 via CXCR2. (5) Th1 cells and Tc1 cells are drawn to CXCL9, CXCL10, and CXCL11 via CXCR3;

both of these cell types release IFN-γ, which in turn promotes the production of further CXCR3-binding chemokines [87]. (6) Macrophages and neutrophils secrete neutrophil elastase MMP-9 to disrupt the pathogens and tissues of the host, which leads to emphysema and an excess secretion of mucus. Abbreviations: COPD, chronic obstructive pulmonary disease; CTGF, connective tissue growth factor; FGF, fibroblast growth factor; IFN, interferon; IL, interleukin; Tc, cytotoxic T cell; TGF; transforming growth factor; Th, T helper; TNF, tumor necrosis factor. Figure created using BioRender.com (Premium Version) (accessed on 21 February 2025).

3.2. *Asthma*

Asthma is a persistent inflammatory condition of the airways that is accompanied by structural alterations, such as an increase in smooth muscle and the remodeling of the airway wall [64]. Asthma is defined by significant fluctuations in airway function that are caused by significant interactions with the environment, such as exposure to allergens, pollutants, and viruses, in addition to underlying chronic mediator release (Figure 3) [64]. In mild-to-moderate allergic asthma, type 2 $CD4^+$ lymphocytes (Th2 cells) and their cytokines predominate, whereas severe steroid-resistant asthma has a more mixed Th2/Th1 phenotype with a Th17 component. Additionally, compared to eosinophilic and pauci-granulocytic asthma, neutrophilic asthma has been shown to have higher levels of IL-1β [66]. Other immune cells, such as neutrophils, macrophages, and dendritic cells, as well as structural cells, including the epithelium and smooth muscle cells in the airways, also release cytokines that lead to the initiation and progression of asthma. Asthma is distinct from other chronic inflammatory conditions, such as psoriasis, Crohn's disease, and rheumatoid arthritis, in that it displays a distinctive cytokine response characterized by Th2 cytokines, the bulk of which are encoded in a small cluster on chromosome 5q32-34. It has been proposed that the coordinated control of the immune response in favor of Th2 cytokines, such as IL-3, IL-4, IL-5, IL-6, IL-9, IL-13, and GM-CSF, is caused by a decrease in the inhibitory influence of Th1 cytokines, particularly IL-18, IL-12, and IFN. This imbalance between Th1- and Th2-type immunity appears early in childhood and may even start before birth in people who are predisposed to developing atopic dermatitis [67]. Clinical studies have shown elevated numbers of these immune cells and cytokines, and research employing asthma-prone mouse models has suggested their probable involvement in illness. In clinical trials using cytokine inhibitors, there have been reports of success in the treatment of inflammatory respiratory diseases. Combination medicines that inhibit several cytokines (such as corticosteroids) and a variety of redundant and disjointed pathways that each individually contribute to the pathophysiology of asthma may be the most efficient treatments for inflammatory diseases such as asthma, in contrast to acute diseases where inflammation is a transient reaction. Asthma entails persistent inflammation that, gradually, may result in immune cell exhaustion. This can lead to reduced therapeutic responses and prolonged appearances [64,65,88].

3.3. *Pulmonary Fibrosis*

The evolution of a number of lung disorders can ultimately lead to pulmonary fibrosis, defined as an excessive accumulation of scar tissue [89]. In contrast to acute respiratory situations, where inflammation is a transient reaction, pulmonary fibrosis is characterized by persistent inflammation that causes lung tissue to eventually scar (fibrosis). The inflammation in pulmonary fibrosis is characterized by the activation of fibroblasts through several pathways, like the TGF-β/Smad pathway, epithelial–mesenchymal transition, and oxidative stress, which causes tissue stiffening and scarring. The fibrotic process may be self-limiting in some instances; however, it can also become overt and irreversible, causing severe loss in lung function and gas exchange capacity [89]. While idiopathic pulmonary fibrosis patients have a median survival of just two to three years, pulmonary fibrosis is the primary cause of death in patients with the autoimmune disease scleroderma [90]. Collagen and extracellular matrix build up in the lungs in a variety of ways in pulmonary fibrosis [89]. Lung fibrosis is also influenced by the process known as epithelial–mesenchymal transition, which transforms lung epithelial cells into myofibroblasts [89]. All of these mechanisms are regulated by cytokines, either by directly attracting and activating cells that produce extracellular matrix or indirectly by regulating pulmonary inflammation, redox balance, and the activity of various enzymatic systems, such as matrix metalloproteinases (MMP) and their inhibiting and clotting enzymes [63].

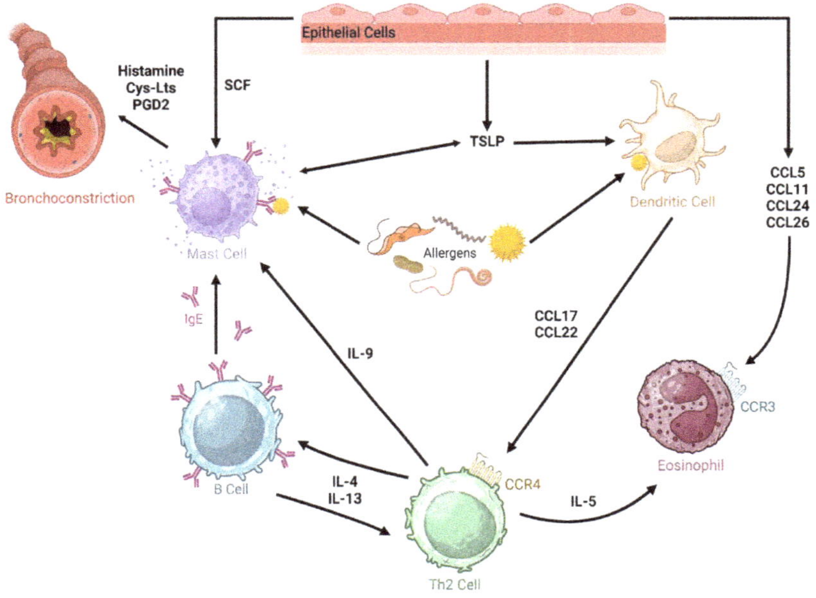

Figure 3. The role of cytokines in asthma. Due to the release of numerous cytokines, such as SCF (which keeps mast cells in the airways), TSLP (which acts on dendritic cells to release the Th2 chemoattractants CCL17 and CCL22 to act via CCR4), and several chemokines that attract eosinophils by activating CCR3, epithelial cells play a significant role in effectively managing inflammation in asthma. Th2 cells control the inflammatory response in asthma by releasing IL-4, IL-13, IL-5, and IL-9, which encourage eosinophilic inflammation and drive B cells to produce IgE, resulting in the stimulation of mast cell proliferation. By releasing histamine, Cys-LTs, and PGD2, mast cells are controlled by a number of interrelated cytokines and play a significant role in asthma [64]. Abbreviations: Cys-LTs, cysteinyl-leukotrienes; Ig, immunoglobulin; IL, interleukin; PGD_2, prostaglandin D 2; SCF, stem cell factor; Th, T helper; TSLP, thymic stromal lymphopoietin. Figure created using BioRender.com (Premium Version) (accessed on 17 November 2024).

Unquestionably, the most potent profibrotic cytokine is TGF-β. It is created in inactive form and typically kept in this state in tissues and the extracellular matrix; however, to exercise its functional impact, it must be activated [29]. The mechanism of fibrosis in the lungs is largely dependent on the activation of TGF-β by αV-containing integrins [63,85]. Together with TGF-β, connective tissue growth factor promotes fibrosis. Additionally, the Th2 cytokines IL-4 and IL-13 are powerful direct inhibitors of extracellular matrix deposition, whereas the Th1 cytokine IFN-γ is a direct promoter of fibrosis [63,72]. In contrast to scleroderma lung disease and idiopathic pulmonary fibrosis, patients suffer from a "profibrotic cytokine storm" with high levels of all cytokines. Th2 cytokines are the main drivers of fibrosis in asthma. In addition, TGF-β is a more potent profibrotic cytokine than IL-4 or IL-13, acting at considerably lower quantities. Utilizing both direct and indirect processes, the chemokine monocyte chemotactic protein (MCP)-1/CCL2, oncostatin M, and platelet-derived growth factor (PDGF) induce fibrosis. Pulmonary and activation-regulated chemokine (PARC)/CCL18 is a significant, primarily indirect, modulator of fibrosis and is elevated in association with various fibrotic lung diseases, including scleroderma, hypersensitivity pneumonitis, idiopathic pulmonary fibrosis, asthma, and sarcoidosis. Stromal cell-derived factor-1 and CXCL12 are other chemokines that cause fibrosis by attracting bone-marrow-derived fibroblast progenitors to the lung. The precise involvement of several other cytokines, including IL-1b, IL-17, IL-10, thymus and activation-regulated chemokine (CCL17), and GM-CSF, in the process of pulmonary fibrosis is still debatable or mechanistically unknown [63].

3.4. *Cystic Fibrosis Bronchiectasis*

Cystic fibrosis (CF) bronchiectasis is normally characterized by persistent and intense inflammation as a result of dysregulation in the inflammatory mediators, which begins early in life and develops throughout a patient's life [74,76]. The inflammation is also predominantly due to neutrophil stimulation and oxidative stress, which later exacerbate inflammation and tissue damage by activating the NF-κB pathway, leading to chronic inflammatory response. Additionally, the mitogen-activated protein kinase (MAPK) signaling pathways and the CFTR gene mutation contribute to the inflammatory response, oxidative stress, and inflammation on the affected site [76]. IL-1β is a proinflammatory mediator that is upregulated in respiratory conditions, such as cystic fibrosis bronchiectasis, COPD, and asthma [74]. In exposure to cigarette smoking, bronchial epithelial cells produce IL-1β, causing goblet cell hypertrophy, fibrosis, emphysema, and pulmonary inflammation in rodents [76]. IL-1β concentrations in bronchoalveolar lavage (BAL) fluid may be elevated in response to exposure to *Pseudomonas aeruginosa*, one of the primary therapeutically prominent microbes in cystic fibrosis bronchiectasis [76,91]. Furthermore, it has been shown that the intensity of the condition is correlated with mutations in IL-1β genes [78]. In contrast to these observations, Muselet-Charlier et al. reported a rapid IL-1β-induced stimulation of nuclear factor kappa-light-chain-enhancer of activated B cells (NF-κB) in a cystic fibrosis bronchial epithelial cell line [77]. Therefore, neutralizing or inhibiting IL-1β cytokines may be a successful treatment for different inflammatory respiratory diseases [77].

3.5. *COVID-19-Related Respiratory Disease*

SARS-CoV-2, which is responsible for causing the COVID-19 pandemic, has created devastating social and economic disruption and placed immense pressure on national and global healthcare systems [92]. Due to its ability to affect the respiratory tract, the SARS-CoV-2 virus typically causes pneumonia in the majority of patients and ARDS in 15% of cases [93]. One of the major causes of death in COVID-19 patients is ARDS, which has been attributed to a robust cytokine storm clinically defined as episodes of increased proinflammatory cytokine levels [34,94]. Acute lung injuries, cellular damage, microbial modification, severe lymphopenia, and a decrease in regulatory T cells are just a few of the serious effects of excessive cytokine production [95]. In patients with ARDS, the respiratory epithelium becomes compromised due to an increased release of pro-inflammatory cytokines in the lungs, such as IL-1β, IL-6, IL-17, and TNF-α, which play a critical role in lung injury [73].

Several proinflammatory cytokines, including IL-1β, IL-6, IL-8, IL-17, and TNF-α, contribute to the pathogenesis of CRS [96]. After infection with SARS-CoV-2, numerous cells, including epithelial cells, macrophages, T lymphocytes, neutrophils, and Th17 cells, release these proinflammatory cytokines in an unregulated manner, which worsens

SARS-CoV-2 infection [97]. The main receptor utilized by SARS-CoV-2 is angiotensin-converting enzyme-2, which initiates various signaling cascades that encourage the production of inflammatory cytokines [98,99]. Viral proteins have been shown to trigger the release of IL-6, which activates the transcription factor NF-κB [100]. Pro-inflammatory cytokines are released when the IL-6/soluble IL-6 receptor (sIL-6R) complex interacts with the gp130 protein, initiating a variety of intracellular signaling pathways, including Janus kinase (JAK)/signal transducer, transcription activation (STAT), and phosphatidylinositol 3-kinase (PI3K) [101]. This causes the release and transport of p65 and p50 proteins to the nucleus as a result of the phosphorylation of NF-κB inhibitor proteins, which then triggers NF-κB transcription and TNFα production [101]. Viral proteins, such as open reading frame 3a and protein E, activate the NLR-domain-containing protein 3 inflammasome, promoting the release of IL-1β [102]. $CD4^+$ T cells can differentiate into Th17 cells and produce IL-17 because of their association with IL-1β, IL-23, IL-6, and TGB-β. This differentiation may also be favored by hypoxia [103]. Activation of the C-Jun N-terminal kinase (JNK), p38, or extracellular signal-regulated kinase (ERK) initiates the translocation and activation of activator protein 1 (AP-1) on the IL-8 promoter, which results in the synthesis of IL-8. Neutrophils are drawn to the infectious site by the actions of the cytokines IL-8 and IL-17, which further causes inflammation and tissue damage [97]. Since there is no specific treatment for COVID-19 in critically ill patients, COVID-19 has yet to be completely eradicated; however, reducing the inflammatory response may be a viable option [73].

3.6. *Pneumonia*

In addition to other respiratory diseases, inflammatory cytokines are also responsible for the pathogenesis of pneumonia and lung cancer. Despite the availability of antibacterial medicines, diagnostic techniques, and sophisticated instruments, bacterial pneumonia remains a significant source of global morbidity and mortality [104]. The imbalance between proinflammatory and anti-inflammatory cytokines leads to the progression of pneumonia [83]. Macrophages are the first line of defense against pathogens, performing phagocytic activity, releasing a variety of pro- and anti-inflammatory cytokines, and shaping the tissue microenvironment [83]. Throughout the course of pneumonia, alveolar macrophages and infiltrating blood monocytes release increasing levels of cytokines, which not only activate antiviral or antibacterial immunity, but also raise the danger of a cytokine storm and tissue damage [83]. Pathogen-associated molecular patterns, such as lipopolysaccharide (LPS), bacterial or viral DNA, and some cytokines (i.e., IFN), induce polarization toward pro-inflammatory (M1-like) macrophages via STAT1, NF-κB, and IFN regulatory factor transcription factor signaling, resulting in augmented pro-inflammatory cytokine production (e.g., IL6, IL1β, IL8, IL33, TNF-α, and IFN-1) [105–107]. The attraction of other immune cell subsets, acute inflammation, antipathogen defense, and cytokine storms are all functions of M1-like monocytic cells. The cytokines IL4, IL13, and TGF induce the anti-inflammatory (M2-like) polarization of macrophages, which leads to inflammation resolution, tissue remodeling, and regeneration [107]. For optimal pathogen clearance and efficient structural and functional healing, the balance between M1/M2 states is necessary [108].

According to studies investigating community-acquired pneumonia, blood concentrations of TNF-α, IL-1β, IL-8, IFN-γ, and IL-6 were higher in infected individuals when compared to healthy volunteers, which indicates that they play a significant role in inflammatory responses [109,110]. While serum IL-6 levels were highest in patients with *pneumococcal pneumonia* and pneumonia caused by a *Legionella* species, serum TNF levels were higher in the majority of patients, regardless of the etiology [82]. None of the patients with *Chlamydia pneumoniae*, *Moraxella catarrhalis*, or *Haemophilus influenzae*-related pneumonia had serum IL-6 levels greater than 500 pg/mL [82]. The greatest levels of serum IFN-γ were observed in patients with pneumonia caused by Legionella species and Chlamydia pneumoniae. In contrast, serum IFN-γ concentrations were elevated in the majority of patients with viral or intracellular bacterial illness [82]. Moreover, Kragsbjerg et al. found that patients with bacteremic *Pneumococcal pneumonia* had significantly greater blood IL-8 levels on admission than patients with *Chlamydia pneumonia*, *Legionella pneumonia*, or influenza A virus infection [111]. Severe sepsis is another complication associated with community-acquired pneumonia. It has been found that the levels of IL-6 and TNF (proinflammatory cytokines) are higher in severe sepsis than those of IL-10 (anti-inflammatory cytokines) [81]. In non-acquired immunodeficiency syndrome immunocompromised patients with *Pneumocystis jirovecii* pneumonia (PcP), there was an imbalance between pro-inflammatory and anti-inflammatory cytokines in the BALF and blood [84]. In comparison to normal individuals, PcP patients exhibited significantly greater BALF levels of IL-1, TNF-α, IL-6, IL-8, and MCP-1, as well as significantly higher blood levels of IL-10, TGF-1 β, IL-8, IL-6, and MCP-1 [84].

3.7. Lung Cancer

Inflammation is a necessary reaction that is initiated in order to heal tissue injury and neutralize and eliminate pathogenic invaders; however, uncontrolled inflammation can become chronic, causing malignant cell changes in the surrounding tissue [112]. Inflammation increases the bioactive molecules in the tumor microenvironment, such as cytokines, chemokines, growth factors, and matrix-modifying enzymes (e.g., MMPs), which in turn raises the risk of cancer development [80]. Lung cancer remains one of the most prevalent types of cancer and has a high fatality rate [15,16]. Smoking and hereditary factors play a critical role in the development of lung cancer. Furthermore, the tumor microenvironment is also important in the growth and progression of lung cancer [113]. In lung cancer, cytokines are crucial in stimulating the body's immune system, and can either promote tumor growth (oncogenic cytokines) or inhibit tumor growth (antitumor cytokines) by influencing the signaling pathways involved in proliferation, growth, metastasis, and apoptosis [79]. There are several routes that drive lung cancer, including the NF-κB pathway, which produces pro-inflammatory cytokines that aid in the endurance and spread of tumor cells. Histone alterations and DNA methylation can control inflammatory pathways in lung cancer, whereas epigenetic modification and IL-6/STAT3 enhance tumor development, metastasis, and angiogenesis. These changes may cause inflammatory mediators to be overexpressed and promote the development of tumors. In lung cancer patients with carcinomatous pleurisy, the levels of IL-6 and IL-8 are higher, and the soluble form of sIL-6R is lower in effusion fluid compared to normal individuals [114]. TNF-α, IFN-γ, TGF-β, vascular endothelial growth factor, and ILs (e.g., IL-6, IL-17, IL-8, IL-10, IL-22, IL-1β, and IL-18) are the most relevant cytokines involved in lung cancer [80,115–117].

3.8. Tuberculosis

Tuberculosis (TB) is an airborne ailment triggered by the bacteria *Mycobacterium tuberculosis* (Mtb) and spread via tiny respiratory aerosols from an infected individual. The bacteria Mtb typically reaches the pulmonary alveolus via the aerosol delivery of particles ranging from 2 to 5 m. Mtb interacts with neutrophils, dendritic cells (DCs), alveolar macrophages, alveolar type II pneumocytes, and airway epithelial cells (AECs) in this microenvironment [118]. Both alveolar type II pneumocytes and AECs are expected to aid in the initial host immune defense after coming into interaction with Mtb by generating cytokines, chemokines, and other chemicals that may either promptly kill Mtb or improve the antimicrobial capabilities of infected macrophages. Furthermore, when infected DCs migrate to nearby lymph nodes, an innate immune response is triggered, which is crucial to halt the bacterium's development and convert it into a dormant form [119].

Multifunctional cytokines coordinate all of these responses, and some cytokines have been shown to have pro- or anti-inflammatory properties that lead to immune-mediated illness and infection. The cytokines that have been reported to produce Mtb infection are TNF-α, IL-1β, IL-18, IL-6, IL-17, and IL-22. The main producers of TNF-α in the case of Mtb infection are AECs, alveolar type II pneumocytes, NK T cells, macrophages, alveolar macrophages, DCs, neutrophils, $CD4^+$ (Th1), and $CD8^+$ T cells; similarly, IL-17 and IL-22 are produced by $CD4^+$ (Th17) T cells and NK T cells, which recruit and activate phagocytic cells and cause proinflammation in the lungs of infected individuals. Macrophages and DCs can produce IL-1β, IL-18, and IL-6, which stimulate the initiation of NK T cells. This results in IFN-γ secretion from Th1 cells and is followed by proinflammation at the infected site. However, several other cytokines are also produced, like TNF- β, IL-10, and IFN-γ, which are responsible for anti-inflammatory effects [86].

It is well recognized that immunosuppressive cytokines, such as IL-10, influence immune cells and encourage Mtb infection. Studies conducted on macrophages revealed that IL-10 levels decreased when Histone Deacetylase 6 (HDAC6) expression decreased and HDAC11 expression spiked, indicating that the former is a transcription activator while the latter type is an IL-10 suppressor [120].

During Mtb H37Rv infection, C-C chemokine receptor type 5 and extracellular signal-regulated kinase (CCR5/ERK)-regulated histone phosphorylation as well as acetylation reduce the development of MHC-II in macrophages. Without uncertainty, the absolute most recognized human immune factor that fights mycobacteria is TNF-α. As a result, Mtb might defeat a host's fight against TB by expressing certain mycobacterial proteins and lowering TNF-α production [121].

4. Characteristics of Cytokine Receptor Interactions

Numerous immunoregulatory effects of cytokines are vital to human biology and disease. However, the anticipated immunotherapeutic benefits of native cytokines are frequently diminished by toxicity or a lack of efficacy, either of which may occur from cytokine receptor pleiotropy and/or the unintentional activation of off-target cells [122]. Numerous crucial aspects of immunological function and many other facets of mammalian physiology are regulated by helical cytokines. The cytokine–receptor complex initiates the activation of intracellularly associated Janus kinases (JAKs) in the classical cytokine signaling pathway [123]. STAT factors are then phosphorylated and activated by JAKs to modify gene expression and ultimately influence cell fate. Some cytokines can activate the protein kinase B (Akt) and ERK pathways in addition to JAK/STAT signaling (Figure 4) [124,125]. Ligand-mediated dimerization is the standard method of cytokine receptor signaling. Regardless of cytokine receptors existing as dimers in their unliganded state, the signaling complex still requires two JAK-associated receptor subunits to bind to the cytokine at the same time to initiate signaling [122]. Tyrosine kinase (TK) receptors also exhibit a dimerization paradigm, and it appears that virtually all single-pass transmembrane receptors require ligand-mediated oligomerization or rearrangement to begin signaling [122]. The majority of cytokines form heterodimeric receptor complexes with a shared receptor subunit, such as the common gamma chain, gp130, and common beta chain (βc), together with a ligand-specific component (e.g., IL-2Rβ, IL-6Rα, or IL-3Rα) [126,127].

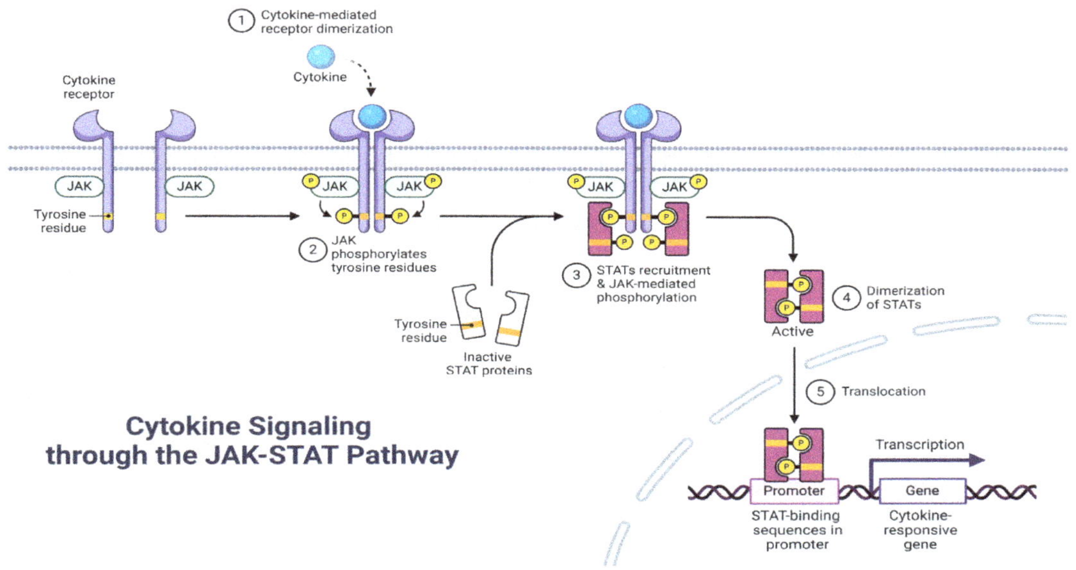

Figure 4. Schematic representation of cytokine signaling through the JAK/STAT cascade with a focus on cytokine receptor interactions. The process begins with cytokine-mediated receptor dimerization, where a cytokine binds to its receptor, leading to the dimerization of receptor subunits, a crucial step in intracellular signaling activation. Following this, JAK phosphorylates tyrosine residues on the intracellular domain of the receptor, creating docking sites for signaling proteins. Next, STAT proteins are recruited to the phosphorylated receptor and undergo JAK-mediated phosphorylation, enabling their activation. Once phosphorylated, STATs dimerize, a necessary step for their full activation. The active STAT dimers then translocate into the nucleus, where they bind to specific promoter sequences of cytokine-responsive genes, initiating transcription and driving various cellular responses. This pathway plays a fundamental role in immune regulation, inflammation, and cell growth. Figure created using BioRender.com (Premium Version) (accessed on 21 February 2025).

Cytokines interact with loops originating from conjoined fibronectin type III domains that make up the cytokine-binding homology regions (CHRs) of receptor chains by using the sides of their helical faces. The site 1/site 2 binding architecture, in which the cytokine binds to a first receptor subunit through site 1 and then recruits a second receptor subunit through site 2, was initially established in early structural studies on the human growth hormone system. This fundamental structural component can be seen in some form in every cytokine–receptor complex structure [128,129]. Erythropoietin and type I IFNs are two cytokines that, in contrast, activate each receptor chain in more energetically independent ways, as receptor–receptor stem interaction is minimal in these cytokine complexes [122]. There are numerous variants of the site 1/site 2 paradigm, as shown by the present database of crystal structures for cytokine–receptor complexes [130]. Site 3 is the third binding site identified in cytokines of the gp130/IL-6 class and is located at the tip of the α-helical bundle. It interacts with an immunoglobulin (Ig)-like domain on top of CHRs of the tall receptor class, for example, gp130, leukemic inhibitory factor (LIF) receptor, granulocyte colony-stimulating factor receptor (GCSF-R), IL-12Rβ2, and IL-23Rα. An interwoven c receptor dimer in the c family produces a site 2 interface that is a hybrid binding site created by the union of two head-to-head antiparallel βc chains. Gp130- and βc-class cytokines are able to build signaling complexes that are of a higher order than the typical

1:2 cytokine–receptor stoichiometry due to these structural differences. The fundamental cytokine–CHR recognition unit, for instance, is doubled by site 3 contact in the tetrameric GCSF/GCSF-R, viral IL-6/gp130, and hexameric IL-6/IL-6R/gp130 signaling complexes. Research targeting site 3, aimed at developing inhibitors of gp130 family cytokines such as IL-6, IL-23, and LIF, has been widespread. Instances where granulocyte–macrophage colony-stimulating factor (GM-CSF) is coupled to the GM-CSF receptor and βc appear to be driven by an extensive network of other interactions in the βc system. These interactions could be explicitly targeted when developing βc cytokines. A third Ig domain of their alpha receptors, which is positioned on top of the helical bundle and is present in a number of cytokines (e.g., IL-5 and IL-13), clearly represents an engineerable location [122,131,132]. IL-2 and IL-15 are the only ILs known to have a third receptor component (such as IL-2Rα and IL-15Rα, respectively) that is distinct from normal CHR-containing receptors in terms of both structure and cytokine interaction. These extra alpha subunits appear to be largely used to increase affinities and modify the target cell selectivity of their respective cytokines because they lack well-defined signaling activities. The helical bundle structures of type II IFN cytokines, such as IFN, IL-22, and IL-10, differ from those of type I four-helix cytokines in some situations, resulting in entangled dimers [122,133]. Nevertheless, the fundamental structural element of receptor CHR engaging with cytokine α-helical faces is seen in all of these various cytokine classes and continues to serve as the principal structural model for cytokine engineering investigations (Figure 5) [134].

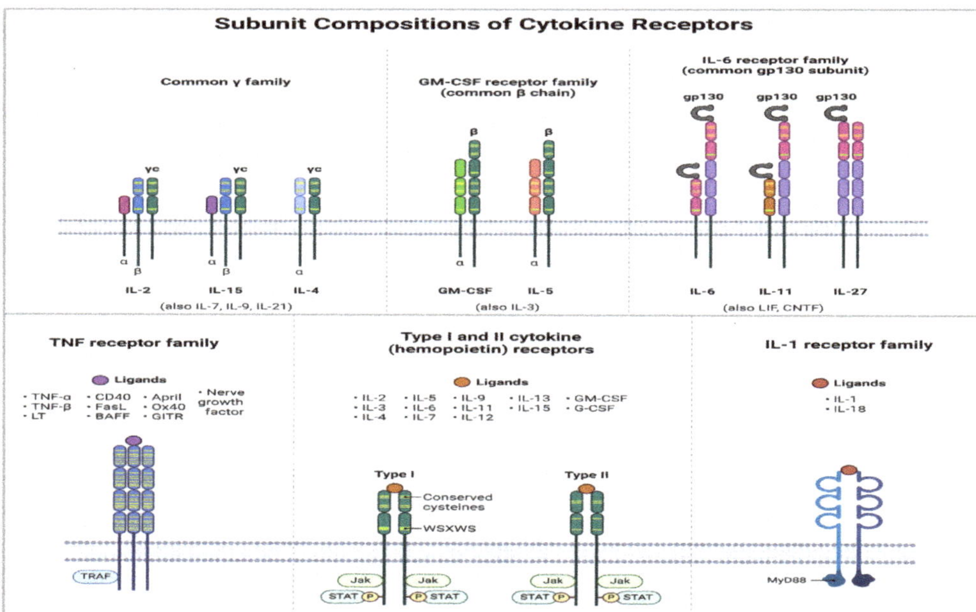

Figure 5. Fundamental structural elements of cytokine receptors. The figure provides a comprehensive overview of cytokine receptor subunit compositions, categorizing them into major receptor families based on their structural similarities and signaling mechanisms. The Common γ (gamma) Family includes receptors for IL-2, IL-15, and IL-4, which also interact with IL-7, IL-9, and IL-21. These receptors share a common γ-chain (γc) as a crucial signaling subunit, along with additional α and β subunits. The GM-CSF Receptor Family, also known as the Common β Chain family, consists of receptors for GM-CSF, IL-5, and IL-3, all of which rely on a shared β-chain for signal transduction.

The IL-6 Receptor Family, characterized by the common gp130 subunit, includes receptors for IL-6, IL-11, IL-27, as well as LIF and CNTF, which play significant roles in cytokine-mediated signaling. The TNF Receptor Family binds ligands such as TNF-α, TNF-β, FasL, BAFF, and nerve growth factor (NGF), and its signaling pathways often involve TRAF (TNF receptor-associated factor), which mediates inflammatory and apoptotic responses. Type I and II cytokine (Hemopoietin) receptors include type I receptors, which recognize cytokines such as IL-2, IL-3, IL-4, IL-5, IL-6, IL-7, IL-9, IL-11, IL-12, IL-13, IL-15, GM-CSF, and G-CSF, and type II receptors, which signal via the JAK-STAT pathway. Type I receptors are structurally defined by conserved cysteine residues and WSXWS motifs that are essential for function. Lastly, the IL-1 Receptor Family, which includes receptors for IL-1 and IL-18, signals through the MyD88 adaptor protein, contributing to innate immunity and inflammatory responses. Overall, these receptor families share common subunits that facilitate ligand binding and signaling, with JAK-STAT signaling being predominant in type I and II receptors, TNF receptors playing key roles in inflammation and apoptosis, and IL-1 receptors utilizing MyD88-dependent pathways for immune activation. Figure created using BioRender.com (Premium Version) (accessed on 21 February 2025).

5. Inflammatory Signaling Involved in Respiratory Diseases

Inflammatory molecules, such as matrix metalloproteinases, COX-2, cPLA2, intracellular adhesion molecule-1 (ICAM-1), and vascular cell adhesion molecule-1 (VCAM-1), are implicated in the pathophysiology of respiratory disorders, including asthma and COPD (Figures 1–3). The expression of these inflammatory molecules is also influenced by a range of inflammatory signaling cascades, including mitogen-activated protein kinases (MAPKs), protein kinase C (PKC), phosphatidylinositol-3-kinase (P13K)/Akt, Src family kinases (SFKs), ROS/Nicotinamide adenine dinucleotide phosphate oxidase (NADPH) oxidase (NOX), AP-1, epidermal growth factor receptor (EGFR), platelet-derived growth factor receptor (PDGFR), and NF-κB (Figure 6).

5.1. MAPKs

Growth factors, cytokines, neurotransmitters, and pharmacological and physical stimuli are significant mediators for the stimulation of MAPKs, which are pertinent aspects of the signaling network. These exogenous stimuli trigger transient reactions in the airway that alter smooth muscle activation, and they may also induce prolonged reactions that alter the integrity of the airway [135]. Transformations in the regulation of numerous genes that encode proteins that mediate cell–cell communication, cell-cycle regulation, intracellular signaling cascades, and extracellular matrix modification cause either transient or prolonged episodes in airway modification [136]. p38 MAPKs, c-Jun N-terminal kinases (JNKs), and ERKs are the three families of MAPKs that have been explored in mammals. Biochemical stressors, such as cytokines, LPS, UV radiation, and growth hormones, trigger JNK and p38 MAPK. ERK is triggered by a variety of stressors, such as cytokines and growth factors [137]. Therefore, it suppresses allergen-induced airway inflammatory responses by hindering MAPK activation via pharmaceutical or molecular strategies. Additionally, individuals with asthma revealed elevated immunostaining for phosphorylated (p)-JNK, p-ERK, and p-p38 MAPK, particularly in smooth muscle and airway epithelial cells [136]. The lateral region of the columnar epithelium is where p38 MAPK phosphorylation is most prominently exhibited. For this distinct cellular class, it is plausible that p38 MAPK regulates baseline metabolic functions. A preliminary investigation of p38 MAPK revealed that TNF-α and IL-1β cause monocytes to become activated [138]. Similarly, it has been established that restricting the p38 MAPK circuit has anti-inflammatory implications by reducing the production of TNF-α, IL-6, and IL-1β [139]. There is an intriguing possibility that IL-1β promotes prostaglandin E2 (PGE2) generation and COX-2 upregulation in airway smooth muscle cells via the p38 MAPK and ERK systems [140]. The JNK antagonist

SP600125 substantially reduced the levels of chemokine ligand 5, IL-13, IL-4, and TNF-α in lung supernatants from rats with allergen-induced prolonged lung inflammation [141]. Consequently, MAPKs are essential in modulating inflammation in the lungs and airways.

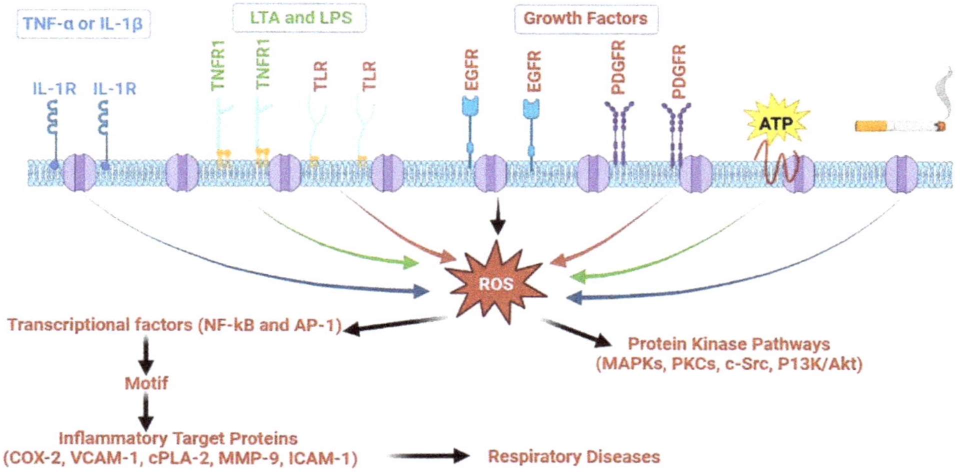

Figure 6. Graphical representation of the inflammatory signaling cascades in respiratory conditions. Numerous identified inflammatory targeting molecules (i.e., cPLA2, COX-2, VCAM-1, ICAM-1, and MMP-9), are linked to inflammation activation cascades triggered by diverse stimuli, including LPS, LTA, cigarette smoke, ATP, IL-1, and TNF-α. Additionally, by approaching transcription variables such as AP-1 and NF-κB in response to extracellular triggers, MAPKs, PI3K/Akt, NOX/ROS, GFTKR, PKCs, and SFKs constitute parts of signaling pathways that modulate the expression of inflammatory markers linked to respiratory conditions. Abbreviations: Akt, protein kinase B; AP-1, activator protein 1; ATP, adenosine triphosphate; COX, cyclooxygenase; EGFR, epidermal growth factor receptor; ICAM-1, intracellular adhesion molecule-1; IL, interleukin; LPS, lipopolysaccharide; LTA, lipoteichoic acid; MAPK, mitogen-activated protein kinases; MMP, matrix metalloproteinases; NOX, nicotinamide adenine dinucleotide phosphate oxidase; NF-κB, nuclear factor kappa-light-chain-enhancer of activated B cells; PDGFR, platelet-derived growth factor receptor; PKC, protein kinase C; PLA2, type II phospholipase A2; P13K, phosphatidylinositol-3-kinase; ROS, reactive oxygen species; SFK, Src family kinase; TLR, toll-like receptor; TNF, tumor necrosis factor; VCAM-1, vascular cell adhesion molecule-1. Figure created using BioRender.com (Premium Version) (accessed on 17 November 2024).

5.2. Protein Kinase C

PKCs have significant involvement in the contraction, apoptosis, flexibility, hypertrophy, migration, multiplication, and secretion of cells in the lungs [142]. PKC, an imperative group of enzymes implicated in transmission cascades, phosphorylates substrate preferentially at threonine/serine domains with a minimum of 11 distinct isoforms. The heterogeneous modulation of PKC isoforms by diacylglycerol, phospholipids, and calcium (Ca^{2+}) results in heterogeneity in their morphology, intracellular distribution, expression, precursor utilization, and stimulation mechanisms [142]. The three categories of PKC isoforms are atypical, novel, and conventional. The morphological and physiological alterations in the homologous motifs C1–C4 serve as the basis for this categorization [143]. PKCs are central regulatory gatekeepers in persistent respiratory disorders, including COPD and asthma. Inflammation of the bronchi, bronchoconstriction, and the formation of mucus have all been linked to PKCs [143]. Specifically. PKCδ modulates the generation of proinflammatory molecules via localized bronchi epithelium cells [144]. Improved PKCδ expression promotes the production of NF-κB-dependent proinflammatory mediators in human bronchial epithelial cells, whereas the presence of a dominant-negative PKC variant hinders this mechanism. In individual bronchial smooth muscle cells, PKCα, γ, μ, τ, βI, and ε are distributed in the cytoplasm, and PKC βII is expressed in the bilayer under baseline circumstances [145]. When administered to bronchial smooth muscle cells, the pro-inflammatory potent vasodilator peptide bradykinin (BK) triggers PKCα, ε, γ, and βI. Through a PKCε-dependent pathway, BK also triggers PGE2 deposition and COX-2 enzyme production in individual bronchial smooth muscle cells. COPD patients have elevated PKCα, which is suggested to contribute to the hypertrophy and multiplication of bronchial smooth muscle cells [143]. Propagating individual bronchial smooth muscle cells enhances PKCτ expression. However, PKC plays an integral role in modulating the actions of proinflammatory mediators by phosphorylating cytosolic PLA2 (cPLA2) and inducing the formation of arachidonic acid through phospholipids, which in response leads to the formation of functional eicosanoids in stimulated cells [146]. In individual bronchial interstitial fibroblasts, PKC is an important fibrosis modulator. Interstitial fibroblasts partially encode three PKCs, viz., PKCα, ε, and δ [143]. Proinflammatory mediators, including IL-6, IL-β, and TNF-α, are released in response to LPS activating specific PKCs [147]. Furthermore, thrombin stimulates intracellular Ca^{2+} and triggers selective PKCs [148]. TNF-α has been shown to augment MM-9 production in A549 cells via a PKCα-dependent mechanism [149]. This evidence suggests that PKCs are important in modulating inflammatory and respiratory disorders.

5.3. P13K/Akt

The PI3K protein series is associated with a comprehensive range of cellular processes, including expansion, migration, multiplication, and longevity. Therefore, PI3K deregulation has been attributed to the development or advancement of a number of clinical conditions, especially those involving the respiratory system [150]. PI3Ks are classified into three types based on their architecture and lipid target selectivity [151]. Category I PI3Ks have received the most experimental emphasis. Cellular membrane receptors (e.g., G-protein-coupled receptors (GPCRs)), insulin, and growth factors trigger category I PI3Ks. Category II PI3Ks include the isotypes α, β, and γ, which are distinguished by the inclusion of a C2 motif at the C-terminal. The single target for category III PI3Ks is phosphatidylinositol. Category IA and category IB PI3Ks are subcategories of category I PI3Ks. In the context of configuration, PI3K IA occurs as heterodimeric units that couple specific regulatory subunits with enzymatic p110 subunits [151]. Ras and receptor TKs are significant downstream regulatory pathways for PI3K IA. The p110 enzymatic subunit functionalized with the p101 regulatory subunit and the downstream signaling of Ras and GPCRs constitute the PI3K IB category [151]. Current information on the pharmacological activity of PI3K in pulmonary inflammation has been substantially advanced by the two clinically available PI3K blockers, LY294002 and Wortmannin [152]. Additionally, the intratracheal administration of LY294002 significantly attenuated ovalbumin (OVA)-induced increases in eosinophil numbers, cumulative cell numbers, and chemokine ligand 11, IL-13, and IL-15 concentrations in BAL fluid and markedly prevented OVA-induced bronchial mucous secretion and tissue eosinophilia [153]. Moreover, this experiment reported that LY294002 significantly restricted OVA-induced Akt serine phosphorylation, a downstream target of PI3K. Additionally, other investigations have shown that Wortmannin and LY294002 reduce bronchial hyperresponsiveness and eosinophilic bronchial inflammation in a mouse asthmatic paradigm [153]. Thus, it has been suggested that PI3K modulation may be advantageous in alleviating the inflammation of asthmatic bronchi. However, PI3K is also activated in response to ROS generation. LY294002 was reported to attenuate chemokine-induced ROS production in phagocytic cells, and investigations utilizing PI3K mutant rodents further validated this observation [152]. As a result, the PI3K group is extensively implicated in innumerable types of pulmonary and bronchial inflammation.

5.4. Src Family Kinases

Molecules known as signaling SFKs have traditionally been documented to modulate important cellular functions, such as metastasis, longevity, migration, and multiplication [154]. The Src tyrosine kinase (TK) family has nine components classified as nonreceptor TKs. Src, Yrk, Yes, and Fyn are abundantly distributed, while Lck, Fgr, Lyn, Hck, and Blk are distributed in relatively constrained sequences [155]. Components of the Src TK family are triggered by physiological stressors and the activation of a number of cellular membrane receptors, including GPCRs, integrin receptors, and TK receptors [155]. Additionally, we established that IL-1β or TNF-α promotes ICAM-1 and VCAM1 activity in human bronchial smooth muscle cells via a c-Src-dependent mechanism [154]. The modulation of IL-6/PGE2/COX-2-dependent bronchial aggravation by c-Src through ROS/NOX has also been reported [156]. The bilateral blockade of these kinases with both SU6656 and PP2 (selective small-molecule Src TK inhibitors) dramatically lowered LPS-induced serum and respiratory chemokine and cytokine concentrations and mitigated LPS-dependent microvascular permeability and respiratory damage [157]. Furthermore, an emerging avenue of exploration is the significance of Src family TKs in inflammatory reactions.

5.5. ROS/NOX

ROS, which are byproducts of regular biological metabolism, function as secondary mediators. To sustain cells safe from oxidative exposure throughout biological circumstances, ROS help maintain cellular "redox equilibrium". Additionally, the stimulation, longevity, multiplication, and organ activity of cells depend on the modulation of oxidative balance. Furthermore, exaggerated ROS generation, which is often induced by proinflammatory cytokine overstimulation, decreases either NOX or xanthine oxidase, and respiratory chain complexes lead to oxidative damage. Oxidative load is a destructive phenomenon that disrupts the lungs and bronchi, culminating in a variety of inflammatory respiratory injuries and disorders [154]. ROS are produced intracellularly by a variety of processes, such as those related to cytochrome P450, xanthine oxidase, the NOX complex, and mitochondrial biogenesis [158]. Being the predominant ROS-producing enzyme, NOX is a membrane-bound bifunctional enzymatic complex found in both nonphagocytic and phagocytic cells [159]. There are two primary functions for ROS generated by NOX. Initially, phagocytic cells demand superoxide radicals generated by NOX2 to undergo a respiratory surge that kills microorganisms. Considering the modulation of cellular signaling, NOX's second function is significant [159]. ROS produced by NOX can selectively and persistently modify half-life, protein function, and distribution [154]. In experiments conducted in vitro involving bronchial and airway epithelial cells and macrophages, it has been documented that ROS stimulate the genomic production of inflammatory markers, such as TNF-α and IL-1 [160,161]. Individuals experiencing asthma exhibit an augmented production of ROS, including hydroxyl radicals, hydrogen peroxide (H_2O_2), and superoxide anions. Multiple bronchial types of cells, especially antigen-presenting cells (i.e., eosinophils, neutrophils, and macrophages), have revealed an augmented generation of ROS in asthma [162]. The extent of bronchial hyperreactivity, as assessed by methacholine exposure, is linked with abnormal ROS generation. Therefore, oxidative load significantly modulates inflammatory pathways in respiratory and bronchial disorders by overexpressing dimeric signaling molecules, such as NF-κB and AP-1, and consequently the expression of proinflammatory markers, such as cPLA2, ICAM-1, MMP-9, COX-2, and VCAM-1 [162].

5.6. Activator Protein-1

AP-1 is a dimeric transcriptional regulator normally composed of Fos (Fra-1, Fra-2, Fos-B, c-Fos) and Jun (Jun B, c-Jun, Jun D) proteins that interact with specific promoter regions. Different cytokines (TNF-α and IL-1β) and PKC can trigger AP-1 through many forms of MAPKs and TKs, which in turn initiate a pathway of intracellular kinases [87]. Specific stimuli induce the Fos gene to be expressed more efficiently, which leads to more Fos protein synthesis. Additional stimuli induce c-Jun phosphorylation via triggered kinase enzymes, hence enhancing stimulation. Current findings show that c-Jun and sirtuin 1 (SIRT1) are effectively coupled, inhibiting the transcription function of AP-1 and lowering MMP-9 levels [163]. Most significantly, it was revealed that SIRT1 hindered the transcription function of AP-1, which led to the production of PGE2 and the upregulation of COX-2, reducing c-Jun/c-Fos acetylation mediated by p300 [164]. As a result, AP-1 could be essential in modulating the transcription of different inflammatory mediators. There is an indication that the epithelial cells in asthmatic bronchi exhibit c-Fos more invariably [165]. Thus, AP-1 is highlighted as a significant contributor to respiratory afflictions.

5.7. Growth Factor Tyrosine Kinase Receptor

Membrane-bound TK receptors are essential for effective cellular metabolism, tissue regeneration, and maturation. Asthma progression has also been attributed to abnormalities in receptor signaling and transcription mechanisms [154]. The PDGFR and epidermal growth factor receptor (EGFR) groups of TK receptors have gained interest as plausible therapy targets for respiratory afflictions, as these receptors have been shown to perform important functions in persistent tissue repair in respiratory fibrosis, bronchitis, and asthma [154]. Multiple morphological alterations, such as mesenchymal cell hypergenesis, maturation, and extracellular matrix formation, are triggered by the EGFR pathways of basal mesenchymal cells, including smooth muscle cells, myofibroblasts, and fibroblasts, as respiratory afflictions advance [154]. The PDGFR pathway transmits signaling for cell longevity, motility, and development, and is typically expressed in mesenchymal cells. Heparin-binding EGF-like growth factor, betacellulin, heregulin, amphiregulin, TGF-α, and EGF are examples of EGFR mediators that are identified in the individual bronchial epithelium [166]. Investigations have noted the overexpression of multiple EGFR mediators in conditions such as asthma and COPD. By stimulating EGFR, *Pseudomonas aeruginosa* bacterial homogenate triggers the synthesis of mucin in individual bronchial epithelial cells (NCI-H292) [166]. Additionally, it has been reported that ROS drives PDGFRα stimulation through c-Src group kinases [149]. Information is emerging that $p47^{phox}$ is phosphorylated by PKC in a manner necessary for the synthesis of ROS in response to PDGF, which is required for the regulation of MAPKs [154]. These investigations indicate that growth factor TK receptors may be significant for modulating the regulation of genes implicated in inflammation.

5.8. NF-κB

NF-κB is considered the key modulator of inflammatory conditions due to its crucial involvement in both the progression and clearance stages of inflammation [154]. Generally, the p65/RelA and p50 components of NF-κB form a heterodimeric structure. NF-κB is triggered by a variety of exogenous stressors, such as viruses, environmental particulates (PM10s), mitochondrial damage, and cytokines, including IL-1β and TNF-α [154]. In a mouse paradigm of ROS-induced transient airway damage, supplemental H_2O_2 also stimulated NF-κB. L-2-oxothiazolidine-4-carboxylate treatment markedly attenuated NF-κB trafficking into the nuclei and the production of cytokines, chemokines, and adhesion markers [167]. By restricting NF-κB stimulation in individual bronchial epithelial cells, a potential cyclin-dependent kinase antagonist has been indicated to attenuate the TNF-α-induced transcription of cellular adhesion markers [168]. Interestingly, researchers have also reported that heme oxygenase-1 upregulation suppresses NF-κB stimulation and oxidative load, which are sensitive to TNFR1 and prevent TNF-α-mediated bronchial aggravation [169]. These findings exemplify that NF-κB controls the synthesis of inflammatory proteins in bronchial and pulmonary inflammation and damage in a significant manner.

6. Current Cytokine-Targeted Therapeutic Implications

Targeted therapy is a novel therapeutic approach with considerable promise for treating severe chronic respiratory disorders, for which there are currently few effective therapeutic options [170]. Although the prognosis for many of these diseases is foreboding, targeted therapy shows promise for the subset of patients that respond to treatment and holds great potential for the future of medical care. The pathogenesis of several respiratory diseases, including asthma and COPD, has been linked to cytokine dysregulation [171]; however, less is known about the inflammatory mediators that are involved in COPD. Nevertheless, since the inflammatory process differs significantly from asthma, other cytokines and chemokines are likely involved, and therapeutic approaches need to be reformed. There is a current focus on finding novel drugs that inhibit the progression of airway limitation in COPD and establishing more specialized asthma treatments. These innovative therapeutic strategies are aimed at using cytokine and chemokine inhibitors and include glucocorticoids, tacrolimus, mycophenolate-helper lymphocyte (Th2)-selective inhibitors, humanized blocking antibodies against cytokines or their corresponding receptors, soluble receptors that bind secreted cytokines, low-molecular-weight receptor antagonists, and medications that obstruct the signal transduction pathways triggered by cytokines [172–174]. Alternatively, asthma and COPD may be treated with specific cytokines that decrease the allergic inflammatory process [175,176]. Due to the prevalence and severity of airway inflammation in chronic lung diseases, there is increased interest in identifying the factors that drive disease pathogenesis and development. Th2 cytokines are the primary targets for biological therapies for chronic airway diseases associated with eosinophilic inflammation. For example, as asthma is characterized by an eosinophilic inflammatory response orchestrated mainly by Th2-derived cytokines, this raises the possibility that limiting their release may be useful in producing therapeutic effects. Studies in experimental animals, such as mice with a deletion of Th2-specific cytokine genes, have supported this substantially. However, there are yet to be studies providing evidence that Th2 cytokine levels are elevated in the airways, and Th2 is unlikely to be relevant in COPD [177,178].

The eosinophilic inflammation associated with asthma is orchestrated by IL-5 [179,180]. The eosinophilic response to allergens and the resultant airway hyperresponsiveness (AHR) are significantly reduced in IL-5 gene knockout mice, confirming the efficacy of the method of suppressing IL-5. Anti-IL-5-blocking antibodies have been used to achieve this, and animal asthma models, including primates, are inhibited by these antibodies in terms of eosinophilic inflammation and AHR [181,182]. Clinical trials have been conducted since 2000 with the inhibitor mepolizumab, which was authorized for use in anti-IL-5 therapy for asthma by the Food and Drug Administration (FDA). Mepolizumab has been demonstrated to encourage a decrease in eosinophils, acute exacerbations, and the requirement for steroids [183,184]. Reslizumab and benralizumab are two additional anti-IL-5 antibodies that have recently received FDA approval for their safety and effectiveness in lowering asthma exacerbations [184,185]. The use of benralizumab and mepolizumab in phase 3 trials is being investigated as an IL-5 therapy for COPD indications. The initial findings revealed that mepolizumab treatment decreased COPD exacerbations, while benralizumab treatment had a modestly positive effect on lung function [186].

IgE production by B lymphocytes and eosinophil migration to the airways depend on IL-4 [187]. The distinct ability of IL-4 to induce Th2 differentiation places it at a pivotal and proximal point in the allergic response, making it an attractive target for inhibition. In mice, IL-4-blocking antibodies prevented allergen-induced AHR, goblet cell metaplasia, and pulmonary eosinophilia [188]. Therefore, blocking IL-4 may be useful in preventing allergy disorders, and soluble IL-4Rs are currently being tested in clinical settings. In individuals with moderately severe asthma, a single nebulized dosage of these receptors reverses the decline in lung function via inhaled corticosteroid cessation [189]. The IL-4 receptor inhibitor dupilumab has resulted in notable improvements in exacerbations and lung function in asthmatic patients who are already on dual therapy with inhaled corticosteroids and long-acting β adrenergic receptor agonists [190]. These findings are similar to the IL-5 treatment strategies for COPD. Dupilumab recently received FDA approval for its use in treating asthma; however, its effectiveness in treating COPD has not yet been evaluated.

There is mounting evidence that, irrespective of eosinophilic inflammation, IL-13 mimics many of the characteristics of asthma in mice, including AHR and mucus hypersecretion, and potently stimulates the release of eotaxin from airway epithelial cells [191,192]. IL-13 signals via the IL-4R chain, but can also activate several intracellular pathways by stimulating IL-13R1, making it a potential target for creating novel treatments. Lebrikizumab and tralokinumab, two anti-IL-13 therapies, were tested in phase 3 clinical asthma trials, but the inhibitors had little to no impact on lung function or reducing exacerbations [193].

Alternatively, proinflammatory cytokines, particularly IL-1β and TNF-α, may amplify the inflammatory response in asthma and COPD and corelate to disease severity. This suggests that blocking IL-1β or TNF-α may have beneficial effects, particularly in severe airway disease. Asthma-related airways express more IL-1, which activates several inflammatory genes [194]. There are no IL-1 inhibitors with low molecular weights, but IL-1RA, a naturally occurring cytokine, binds to IL-1R and inhibits IL-1 action [195]. In laboratory animals, IL-1RA lessens allergen-induced AHR; however, it does not appear that human recombinant IL-1RA is useful in managing asthma [196]. Studies on the function of IL1 in COPD have not yet been published. Through the activation of NF-κB, AP-1, and other transcription factors, TNF is produced in asthmatic airways and may be crucial in increasing asthmatic inflammation [197]. In asthma sufferers' provoked sputum, TNF levels are noticeably elevated [198]. Furthermore, there is scientific evidence that COPD patients who lose weight may exhibit increased TNF release from circulating cells, which may be due to TNF inducing skeletal muscle apoptosis, resulting in the distinctive cachexia seen in certain patients with severe COPD [199]. Even in patients who are comparatively insensitive to steroids, blocking humanized monoclonal antibodies directed against TNF (infliximab) and soluble TNF receptors (etanercept) has shown impressive clinical responses in rheumatoid arthritis and inflammatory bowel disease [200,201]. Clinical trials are currently being conducted on these antibodies and soluble TNF receptors as a logical approach to treating asthma, especially in patients with severe disease (Table 3). They may also help treat severe COPD, especially in patients with malaise and cachexia. Low-molecular-weight TNF inhibitors are being investigated due to the issues with antibody-based treatments. An MMP-related TNF-converting enzyme is essential for releasing TNF from the cell surface. Oral TNF inhibitors made of low-molecular-weight TNF-converting enzyme inhibitors are currently being developed [202].

Table 3. Description of available cytokine-targeted therapeutics for treating respiratory diseases that are in clinical trials (data were retrieved from ClinicalTrials.gov using search terms such as cytokine and respiratory disease) (accessed on 10 November 2024).

Targeted Cytokine	Intervention Molecule	Type of Antibody	Disease Condition	Clinical Efficacy	Status	Company/ Organization	Clinical Trials Associated
IL-5	Mepolizumab	Humanized, IgG1 monoclonal antibody	COPD, high levels of sputum eosinophils, and severe eosinophilic asthma	Reduces moderate and severe exacerbations	Phase III	GlaxoSmithKline	NCT02105961 NCT02555371 NCT01691859 NCT02135692
			Severe bilateral chronic rhinosinusitis	Improved nasal polyp size and nasal obstruction	Phase III	GlaxoSmithKline	NCT03085797
			Severe asthma and comorbid conditions	Controls asthma, improved lung function and health-related quality of life, as well as various comorbid pathologies	Phase II	GlaxoSmithKline	NCT01000506
					Phase III	GlaxoSmithKline	NCT01691521
					Phase III	GlaxoSmithKline	NCT01842607
					Phase III	GlaxoSmithKline	NCT02281318
			Hypereosinophilic syndrome	Decreased disease flares and blood eosinophil count	Phase III	GlaxoSmithKline	NCT03306043 NCT02836496
	Benralizumab	Humanized, afucosylated anti-IL-5 receptor α monoclonal antibody	Severe eosinophilic asthma, COPD	Reduced the exacerbations in severe COPD	Phase III	AstraZeneca	NCT01914757
					Phase III	AstraZeneca	NCT01928771
					Phase II	MedImmune LLC	NCT01227278
					Phase III	AstraZeneca	NCT02155660
					Phase III	AstraZeneca	NCT02138916
			Chronic rhinosinusitis	Reduced NP score, nasal blockage, and difficulty with sense of smell	Phase III	AstraZeneca	NCT03401229
			Severe eosinophilic asthma	Improved nasal polyposis and lung function	Phase III	AstraZeneca	NCT03170271
			Severe, uncontrolled asthma	Found to be safe and effective in long-term studies	Phase III	AstraZeneca	NCT02258542
			Severe asthma	Clinical remission is achievable and reduced exacerbation rates	Phase III	AstraZeneca	NCT02075255
	Reslizumab	Humanized monoclonal antibody	Eosinophilic granulomatosis with polyangiitis (EGPA)	Found to be safe and effective in EGPA	Phase II	National Jewish Health	NCT02947945
			Late-onset eosinophilic asthma	Reduction in asthma exacerbations and improved lung function	Phase III	Teva Branded Pharmaceutical Products R&D, Inc.	NCT01287039 NCT01285323
IL-4	Dupilumab	Human anti-interleukin-4 receptor α monoclonal antibody	Uncontrolled Asthma	Lower rates of severe asthma exacerbation, better lung function	Phase III	Sanofi	NCT02414854
			Glucocorticoid-dependent severe asthma	Decreased the rate of severe exacerbations and increased FEV1	Phase III	Sanofi	NCT02528214
			Chronic rhinosinusitis with nasal polyps	Improved upper and lower airway outcome measures	Phase III	Sanofi	NCT02912468 NCT02898454
			Persistent asthma	Improved lung function and decreased Th2-associated inflammatory markers	Phase II	Sanofi	NCT01312961

Table 3. *Cont.*

Targeted Cytokine	Intervention Molecule	Type of Antibody	Disease Condition	Clinical Efficacy	Status	Company/ Organization	Clinical Trials Associated
IL-13	Lebrikizumab	Anti-interleukin-13 monoclonal antibody	Uncontrolled asthma in adolescent patients	Reduced asthma exacerbation rates	Phase III	Hoffmann-La-Roche	NCT01875003
			Idiopathic pulmonary fibrosis	Benefits lung function	Phase II	Hoffmann-La-Roche	NCT01872689
			Adults with asthma	Improved lung function with high levels of serum periostin	Phase II	Genentech, Inc.	NCT00930163
	Tralokinumab	Anti-interleukin-13 monoclonal antibody	Moderate-to-severe asthma	Improved lung function with no improvement in ACQ-6	Phase IIa	MedImmune LLC	NCT00873860
TNF-α	Infliximab	Anti-TNF-α antibody	Asthma	Results are not posted	Phase II	Imperial College London	NCT00278083

Abbreviations: IL, interleukin; COPD, chronic obstructive pulmonary disease; EGPA, eosinophilic granulomatosis with polyangiitis; FEV1, forced expiratory volume; ACQ-6, asthma control questionnaire score 6.

6.1. Future Cytokine-Targeted Therapeutics for Respiratory Diseases

Respiratory conditions and diseases have been documented to have increased levels of a variety of proinflammatory mediators, which makes them ideal treatment candidates. The following sections further explore cytokine-targeted therapeutic implications in respiratory diseases.

6.1.1. Anti-IL-1β

IL-1β is a proinflammatory mediator that is upregulated in respiratory conditions (e.g., cystic fibrosis bronchiectasis, COPD, and asthma) [74]. Neutralizing IL-1β antibodies reduced the bacterial burden and pulmonary inflammation induced by *Pseudomonas aeruginosa* in cystic fibrosis rodents and enhanced IL-1β activation upon exposure to *Pseudomonas aeruginosa* [203]. In contrast to pauci-granulocytic and eosinophilic asthma, neutrophilic asthma has been reported to have elevated IL-1β levels [66]. He et al. explored the connection between the possibility of developing genomic variants and asthma in IL-1RA and IL-1-511C/T in a meta-analysis of 15 retrospective investigations [204]. The IL-1-511C/T variant was not identified; however, the IL-1RA variant was linked to an elevated incidence of asthma, which was irrespective of age or race [204]. The effectiveness of IL-β inhibitors for asthma and COPD has only been investigated in modest clinical experiments. Canakinumab is a human IgGκ monoclonal antibody with a high affinity that obliterates the biocompatibility of IL-1β. There has only been one randomized double-blind experiment in asthmatic individuals, and it used two single treatments on days 1 and 15 in moderately asthmatic individuals. Allergen exposures were undertaken on days 0 and 28, while individuals were permitted to continue consuming other anti-asthmatic therapeutics. The findings revealed that canakinumab reduced delayed asthmatic responsiveness by 28%. Canakinumab also markedly suppressed systemic IL-1 concentrations for the interval that was monitored after a single administration. Although this experiment was short and had a small sample size (16 individuals), the outcomes were favorable and optimistic [205]. The primary function of IL-1β is to trigger the inflammasome and promote resistance toward respiratory diseases; hence, precautions should be taken while employing IL-1 antagonistic therapies. Individuals with persistent inflammatory respiratory conditions may become more vulnerable to acute bronchial infection and relapses when IL-1 is blocked. As a result, it is important to extensively explore and implement specific treatments to decrease the inflammation process in definite individual categories.

6.1.2. Anti-IL-6

Primary human bronchial epithelial and inflammatory cells both have the ability to release IL-6 upon exposure to a spectrum of diverse stressors [206,207]. The impairment that advances with aging, pulmonary capacity decline, and a rise in the incidence of COPD are all hallmarks of "inflammaging" [208]. Proinflammatory mediators implicated in aging, particularly IL-6, have been related to poor medical conditions and fatality, and it is thought that they cause a sustained, moderate stimulation of long-term inflammation [209]. There are other hypotheses for age-related increases in systemic IL-6 concentrations, such as enhanced oxidative damage or chronic viral infestations (i.e., cytomegalovirus and herpes), which are reported in the weak and aged [210]. Nixon et al. revealed that in cystic fibrosis bronchiectasis, IL-6 mucus concentrations were inversely correlated with forced vital capacity and forced expiratory volumes for one second, with IL-6 declining following antibiotic therapy [211]. Serum concentrations of IL-6 and BAL fluid in asthmatic individuals were shown to be higher [212]. According to these investigations, IL-6 appears to have substantial involvement in the advancement of asthma and the subsequent gradual deterioration in pulmonary function. In various inflammatory conditions (mainly Crohn's disease and rheumatoid arthritis), inhibiting IL-6 receptors and their antibodies has been investigated. Tocilizumab, a neutralizing antibody for the IL-6 receptor, was reported in experimental studies to reduce IL-6 concentrations and ameliorate disease severity ratings and symptomatology in rheumatoid arthritis. The antibody was authorized in 2010; however, up to this point, it has not been investigated in persistent inflammatory bronchial disorders [213]. Accordingly, emphasizing IL-6 might be a noteworthy and effective therapeutic approach to reduce pulmonary capacity impairment, systemic inflammation linked to COPD, and persistent bronchial aggravation.

6.1.3. Anti-IL-8

Inflammatory airway epithelial cells are a key origin of IL-8, a cytokine that is pivotal for neutrophil trafficking [214]. Improvements in fibroblast growth factor-23 and TGF-β were shown to augment airway epithelial cell IL-8 expression [215]. The upregulation of IL-8 in cystic fibrosis bronchiectasis has also been found to be induced by NF-κB, with an augmentation during the initial stages of *Pseudomonas aeruginosa* invasion [216,217]. The airway epithelial cells of individuals with cystic fibrosis were also triggered by IL-1β to release IL-8 [218]. Additionally, IL-8 has been identified as a significant factor in the pathogenesis of COPD. COPD airway epithelial cells have greater initial concentrations of IL-8, which effectively causes mucous hypersensitivity by expressing the mucosal genes MUC5B and MUC5AC [219]. TNF-α and smoking cigarettes have both been detected to effectively augment macrophage IL-8 secretion [220]. This implies that smoking cigarettes is an effective promoter for abnormal IL-8 secretion in COPD passageways [221]. Moreover, it has been established that neutrophils and systemic IL-8 increases result in the acute exacerbation of COPD, with IL-8 having detrimental implications on pulmonary functioning [222]. The outcomes of inhibiting IL-8 have been investigated in COPD, but to date no appreciable therapeutic benefits in individuals have been reported [223]. Notably, CXC chemokine receptor 2 (CXCR2) is a neutrophil chemoattractant and has been proven to support IL-8 synthesis. It is a therapeutic candidate, since research has shown that its inhibitor suppresses IL-8 secretion. Individuals with asthma administered navarinxin (a CXCR2 receptor antagonist) showed a substantial decrease in serum and mucus neutrophils without any impairment in pulmonary functioning [224]. Navarinxin exhibited marginal pulmonary function changes in experimental COPD investigations [225]. Danirixin, an additional CXCR2 antagonist, is being explored for therapeutic application [65]. While these therapeutics appear intriguing, extensive investigation and validation are still required.

6.1.4. Anti-IL-4

Respiratory disease pathogenesis is regulated by IL-4, which promotes Th2 cell maturation and proliferation, the phenotypic switching of B cells to IgE production, eosinophil mobilization, mast cell growth, and mucosal fibroplasia [226]. Additionally, by augmenting the synthesis of fibronectin and collagen, IL-4 is directly implicated in the restructuring of the bronchi. Numerous studies examining the effectiveness of anti-IL-4 therapeutics in the management of asthma have produced contradictory findings [227]. The inhibition of IL-4 or its receptor in mouse paradigms of allergen-sensitized asthma has been demonstrated to reduce pulmonary swelling, blood IgE concentrations, and bronchial hyperactivity to cholinergic drugs (i.e., methacholine). It also suppresses IL-5 production from T cells and eosinophil infiltration into the bronchi [228,229]. Furthermore, although highly accepted, pascolizumab (humanized anti-IL-4 monoclonal antibody (mAb) IgG1) is ineffective in asthmatic individuals [230]. Individuals experiencing chronic, mild-to-extreme asthma and sputum or blood eosinophilia have recently been investigated with dupulimab (human mAbs that target the IL-4 receptor α subunit). In comparison to a sham group, dupilumab substantially reduced the rate of asthma complications throughout the discontinuation of inhaled β_2 sympathomimetics and corticosteroid treatment. This was followed by a significant improvement in pulmonary capacity and a decline in the concentrations of Th2 cell-linked biomarkers (e.g., eotaxin-3), exhaled NO, and eosinophils [190].

6.1.5. Anti-IL-5

IL-5 is essential for the development, differentiation, and stimulation of eosinophils [231]. As a result, pharmacological approaches that target anti-IL5 may be beneficial in therapy for eosinophilic asthma presentations [232]. Multiple preliminary investigations using asthmatic experimental animals have been performed in this direction. In addition, the administration of allergen-induced mice with the anti-IL-5 neutralizing antibody (TRFK-5) was effective in preventing eosinophil inflow through the bronchi [233]. Benralizumab, reslizumab, and mepolizumab are a few additional antibodies that have recently been discovered [234]. Mepolizumab (humanized recombinant IgG1-κ mAbs that target IL-5) has been demonstrated to be effective and efficacious in suppressing eosinophil counts in the serum and bronchi in a variety of clinical investigations conducted in diverse demographics of individuals with mild-to-severe recurrent obstructive asthma [235,236]. Furthermore, substantial refinements in asthma episodes, pulmonary capacity, and airway hyperactivity did not coincide with these outcomes.

Mepolizumab has recently been evaluated in a few subgroups of prolonged recurrent asthma, which is known for periodic relapses and bronchial eosinophilia that is resistant to systemic and/or inhaled corticosteroid treatments [237]. Collectively, the findings from these two short studies show that mepolizumab was highly sustained throughout the course of a 12-month therapy interval and significantly reduced asthmatic acute episodes and eosinophil concentrations in serum and produced mucus [238]. An intriguing humanized mAb (IgG4-κ), reslizumab, is a potential anti-IL-5 biosimilar agent in parallel to mepolizumab. Reslizumab has recently been demonstrated to dramatically enhance pulmonary capacity and reduce sputum eosinophils in individuals with eosinophilic asthma compared to sham treatment, producing a favorable shift toward superior asthmatic treatment. The greatest concentrations of blood and sputum eosinophils, which were linked to the existence of chronic rhinosinusitis, were prevalent in a subset of individuals, and these individuals were characterized by the strongest anti-asthmatic responses to reslizumab [239]. As a result, these studies highlight the significance of precise phenotypic screening in an effort to customize anti-asthmatic therapy to the unique biosimilar and symptomatic factors of various disease presentations.

6.1.6. Anti-IL-9

In respiratory diseases, IL-9 is upregulated and is responsible for promoting an increase in goblet cell numbers and mast cell proliferation [240]. Hyperactivity and inflammation of the bronchi were attenuated in mice following IL-9 suppression [241]. Additionally, MEDI-528 (humanized mAb that targets IL-9) demonstrated a satisfactory tolerability record in controlled phase 2a studies conducted in patients with moderate asthma and simultaneously elicited a signal favoring recovery in terms of asthma severity ratings and clinical recurrence patterns. The second of these experimental investigations demonstrated that 50 mg of MEDI-528, given subcutaneously biweekly, can exhibit a preventive response toward exercise-mediated bronchospasm [242].

6.1.7. Anti-IL-13

Since IL-13 is involved in numerous attributes of bronchial swelling and restructuring, such as the mobilization of basophils and eosinophils, the expansion of bronchial smooth muscle cells and pulmonary fibroblasts, IgE production, and extra mucus secretion, it has become a pivotal target for the advancement of novel anti-asthmatic targeted therapies. In preclinical experimental models of long-term allergic asthma, anti-IL-13 therapy significantly reduced bronchial morphological abnormalities, bronchial eosinophilia, and IgE production [243]. Anrukinzumab (humanized mAb anti-IL-13) effectively suppressed delayed asthmatic episodes triggered by allergens in clinical studies within 14 days, but not 35 days [244]. Lebrikizumab (humanized mAb inhibiting IL-13) has also been demonstrated to have a beneficial anti-asthmatic effect that is defined by the upregulation of IL-13-inducible genes, including periostin (matricellular protein) [245]. Lebrikizumab was effective in improving respiratory capacity in individuals with moderate-to-severe asthma who had elevated periostin serum concentrations. The percentage improvements in forced expiratory volume for one second recorded for 12 weeks were 5.5% overall in the lebrikizumab treatment group, 8.2% in the elevated-periostin group, and 1.6% in the low-periostin group, compared to reference data. This indicates potential readily observable biomarkers that may be regularly utilized in clinical practice to pinpoint unique asthmatic subtypes, marked by a prominent destructive involvement of IL-13 [246]. Tralokinumab (humanized mAb blocking IL-13), which is presently undergoing clinical investigation, has improved pharmacokinetic parameters and a satisfactory tolerability potential [247].

6.1.8. Anti-IL-17 and Anti-IL-23

In airway biopsies retrieved from individuals exhibiting chronic asthma, IL-17F and IL-17A (two proinflammatory mediators vitally implicated in neutrophilic activation and bronchial restructuring) are markedly elevated [248]. From this perspective, it has become interesting that anti-IL17 mAbs reduce the number of lymphocytes, eosinophils, and neutrophils found in BAL fluid in mouse models of allergen-induced asthma [249]. Currently, clinical phase II investigations are determining the effectiveness and stability of secukinumab (humanized mAb against IL-17A) and brodalumab (humanized mAb working specifically against the IL-17 receptor) in individuals with chronic asthma that is not satisfactorily managed by inhaled β_2-sympathomimetics and corticosteroids [250]. The application of antibodies against the mediator IL-23, which regulates the production of IL-17, may be an alternative and promising therapeutic treatment strategy. By suppressing this mediator, lymphocyte, eosinophil, and neutrophil migration into hypersensitive mouse bronchi was markedly reduced [251]. Risankizumab (humanized mAb blocking IL-23) is still undergoing clinical studies for the treatment of chronic asthma [65]. IL-17 is also implicated in immunological resistance toward pathogens and carcinogenesis. Therefore, inactivating this mediator may raise the incidence of secondary infestations, and the occurrence of cancer and experimental approaches must be carefully examined [252].

6.1.9. Anti-TSLP, Anti-IL-25, and Anti-IL-33

Respiratory conditions present elevated numbers of thymic stromal lymphopoietin (TSLP), IL-33, and IL-25, which are primarily expressed by the bronchial epithelium and are essential for triggering Th2-dependent inflammatory events [253]. Currently, it is hypothesized that these mediators may be promising candidates for innovative anti-asthmatic therapeutics. The attenuation of Th2-mediated sensitive airway swelling in mice by an anti-IL-25 monoclonal antibody has been documented [252]. Additionally, antibodies targeting the human IL-33 receptor have the potential to decrease the mouse allergen-induced inflammatory response and bronchial hyperactivity [254]. In adult airway epithelial cells, these antibodies may also significantly reduce the production of IL-17F [255]. A significant reduction in murine allergen-induced bronchial inflammation has also been documented as a result of antibody-mediated TSLP protein inactivation [256].

6.1.10. Anti-IL-27

IL-27 is a heterodimeric cytokine expressed by macrophages and monocytes that has been implicated in the etiopathogenesis of chronic corticosteroid-induced asthma. Similarly, IL-27 values in the bronchi of individuals with chronic neutrophilic asthma are augmented. Furthermore, glucocorticoid receptor nuclear trafficking, a crucial intracellular process for the pharmacological and biological effects of corticosteroids, was hindered by IL-27 in mouse pulmonary macrophages. IL-27 may be a promising candidate for novel treatment approaches designed to improve the management of chronic, corticosteroid-resistant asthma [256].

6.1.11. Anti-GM-CSF

Respiratory diseases upregulate the monomeric glycoprotein GM-CSF, which is essential for eosinophil viability and maturation [257]. An inhalant dose of a goat anti-mouse GM-CSF polyclonal antibody effectively reduced bronchial swelling, extra mucus secretion, and bronchoconstriction in a mouse paradigm of allergen-induced asthma [258]. Subsequently, namilumab (human IgG1 mAb blocking GS-CSF) was designed, and it has demonstrated its ability to rapidly reduce the survivability and stimulation of local adult eosinophils [259].

6.2. Safety of Anti-Cytokine Therapies

Randomized controlled trials have been used to evaluate adverse outcomes connected to drugs. Patients who received omalizumab and those who received a placebo saw similar rates of treatment-related adverse events. Even in a cohort of patients with chronic oral corticosteroid usage, mepolizumab was not linked to a higher incidence of adverse events when compared to a placebo [260]. Rare instances of hypersensitive reactions may occur. Anaphylactic responses following injections of reslizumab were uncommon and well tolerated [261]. Nasopharyngitis was the most frequent side effect seen with benralizumab, but its incidence was not appreciably different from that of the placebo group [185]. Injection-site reactions and upper respiratory tract infections were the most frequent side effects of dupilumab when compared to the placebo. There have been reports of persistent occurrences of symptomatic hypereosinophilia; this has been seen in 4–25% of individuals treated with dupilumab [262]. One explanation for this hypereosinophilia is that blocking the IL-4/IL-13 pathway inhibits the eotaxin-3, vascular cell adhesion protein 1, thymus, and activation-regulated chemokines without also blocking eosinophilopoiesis in the bone marrow. This decreases eosinophil migration and causes an increase in blood eosinophils. Therefore, it appears that the existence of hypereosinophilia (>1500 μL^{-1}) is advantageous when selecting the best biologic. Blood eosinophilia should be regularly checked in patients with severe asthma when dupilumab is started. Clinical and immunological responses to tocilizumab as an adjuvant treatment for severe pediatric persistent asthma were demonstrated in a recent case report with few side effects [263]. There was no discernible difference between the tezepelumab and placebo groups in terms of the types and rates of adverse events. The inclusion of patients with severe asthma in registries will provide clinicians with information on long-term safety, and the longer-term follow-up of patients treated with biologics is crucial to verify the lack of subsequent occurrences.

6.3. Ongoing and Completed Clinical Trials for the Management of Respiratory Diseases Based on Cytokine Therapy

The data for ongoing and completed clinical trials investigating the management of various respiratory diseases based on cytokine therapy are presented in Table 4 with the disease conditions and interventions.

Table 4. Clinical trials based on cytokine therapy for the management of respiratory diseases (data were retrieved from ClinicalTrials.gov using search terms such as cytokine and respiratory disease) (accessed on 10 November 2024).

NCT Number	Title	Conditions	Interventions	Phase	Status	Company/Organization
NCT00001908	T-Cell Cytokine Changes During IL-4 Receptor Treatment for Asthma	Asthma Hypersensitivity	--	--	Completed	National Institute of Allergy and Infectious Diseases
NCT00455767	Safety and Efficacy Study of Depelestat in ARDS Patients	Fibrosis Lung Disease Respiratory Disorders Acute Respiratory Distress Syndrome (ARDS) Pulmonary Fibrosis Inflammation	EPI-hNE4, Placebo	Phase II	Completed	Debiopharm International SA
NCT00753103	Anti-Cytokine Therapy for Vasculitis	Wegener's Granulomatosis Renal Limited Vasculitis Microscopic Polyangiitis	Infliximab, Cyclophosphamide, Prednisolone, Azathioprine, Mycophenolate Mofetil, Methylprednisolone	Phase II	Completed	University Hospital Birmingham NHS Foundation Trust
NCT01253941	Effects of Mud Bath Therapy in Chronic Obstructive Pulmonary Disease	COPD	Mud Bath Therapy	N/A	Completed	Fondazione Salvatore Maugeri
NCT02113072	Recurrent Wheezing in Infants: Risk Factors and Prevention With Probiotics	Respiratory Tract Diseases, Wheezing	Beclomethasone, Probiotics, Placebo	Phase III	Completed	Universidade Federal de Pernambuco
NCT02557958	Chronic Obstructive Pulmonary Disease Transcription Factor and Cytokine Study	COPD	Azithromycin, Placebo	Early Phase I	Completed	NYU Langone Health
NCT03595488	Dupilumab for Aspirin-exacerbated respiratory disease	Aspirin-Exacerbated Respiratory disease	Dupilumab	Phase II	Completed	Rochester General Hospital
NCT04102813	Deep Diaphragmatic Breathing: Neurobiological and Anti-inflammatory Effects	Unrecognized Condition	Functional Therapy	N/A	Completed	Azienda Ospedaliera Universitaria Policlinico Paolo Giaccone Palermo
NCT04374149	Therapeutic Plasma Exchange Alone or in Combination with Ruxolitinib in COVID-19-Associated CRS	Cytokine Release Syndrome COVID-19	Therapeutic Plasma Exchange Ruxolitinib	Phase II	Completed	Prisma Health Upstate

Table 4. *Cont.*

NCT Number	Title	Conditions	Interventions	Phase	Status	Company/Organization
NCT04445272	Clinical Trial to Evaluate the Effectiveness and Safety of Tocilizumab for Treating Patients With COVID-19 Pneumonia	COVID-19	Tocilizumab	Phase II	Completed	Fundacion SEIMC-GESIDA
NCT04457349	Therapeutic Plasma Exchange in Resistant Cytokine Storm of COVID-19	COVID-19	Therapeutic Plasma Exchange	N/A	Completed	Alexandria University
NCT04485169	Therapeutic Plasma Exchange for Coronavirus Disease-2019 Triggered Cytokine Release Storm	COVID-19 Cytokine Release Syndrome	Therapeutic Plasma Exchange	N/A	Completed	UNICEF
NCT05164692	Effects of Nasal-spraying LiveSpo Navax in Treatment of Acute Respiratory Infections in Children	Acute Respiratory Tract Infections	LiveSpo Navax, 0.9% NaCl Physiological Saline	N/A	Completed	National Children's Hospital, Vietnam
NCT05378022	Effects of Nasal-spraying LiveSpo Navax in Treatment of Influenza Virus in Children	Acute Respiratory Tract Infections	Combination Product: LiveSpo Navax, 0.9% NaCl Physiological Saline	N/A	Completed	National Children's Hospital, Vietnam
NCT05562843	Autologous Cellular Therapy With PRP-PC in Chronic Lung Diseases: An Observational Study LI-004	COPD ILD	Autologous Cellular Therapy with PRP-PC	N/A	Completed	H-CYTE

Abbreviations: ARDS, acute respiratory distress syndrome; COPD, chronic obstructive pulmonary disease; ILD, interstitial lung disease; COVID-19, coronavirus 2019; IL, interleukin; N/A, not applicable.

6.4. Future Therapeutic Options and Challenges

The notion of remission has been created recently, and several definitions have been applied. Remission is obviously defined as the absence of exacerbations, stopping systemic corticosteroid treatment, and controlling asthma symptoms [264]. The inclusion of the fourth criterion, improvement in lung function, is still open to controversy because certain patients with chronic illnesses and fixed airflow obstructions may not be able to normalize or improve their lung function while they are asymptomatic and free from exacerbations. Developing an agreement on the definition of remission also requires a consideration of the patient's perspective. Astegolimab, an anti-ST2 medication, has been the subject of current research [265]. In individuals with low blood eosinophil levels, this medication, which targets the IL-33 pathway, resulted in a marginally better reduction in exacerbation; this suggests that the IL-33 pathway may be more significant in type 2 low severe asthma. Itepekimab is an anti-IL-33 human IgG4P monoclonal antibody [266]. In one study, every 2 weeks for 12 weeks, 296 patients with moderate-to-severe asthma were randomly randomized to receive 300 mg subcutaneous itepekimab, itepekimab plus dupilumab (both at 300 mg), dupilumab (300 mg), or a placebo. Itepekimab and dupilumab together did not work better than either medication by itself. All four study groups had comparable rates of adverse events. In a phase 2a, multicenter, randomized, double-blind, placebo-controlled, 24-week trial, anti-IL-23 risankizumab was studied in moderate-to-severe asthma [267]. The findings of the study revealed that risankizumab exerted a biologic effect on airway immunity, which may have contributed to the poor clinical outcome. By stimulating the local release of neutrophil-mobilizing molecules, such as CXC chemokines, IL-17 plays a crucial part in the pulmonary host defense. There is debate about recent claims of IL-17's involvement in the onset of COPD. Similarly to the evidence on COPD, Th17 cells and the cytokines they produce (IL-17A and IL-17F) seem to have a role in the pathophysiology of severe and steroid-resistant asthma [268]. When it comes to chronic inflammatory airway illnesses, IL-17 regulation represents an appealing prospective therapeutic target. The efficacy of IL-17 and its receptor antagonist in treating COPD and asthma has been studied in small clinical trials. Regretfully, patients with either condition have not shown any improvements in lung function or disease symptoms. One of the major worries is whether mAbs are cost-effective for treating critically ill patients, especially in low-income nations. Another concern is whether health insurance companies will agree to pay for the treatment. According to a retrospective analysis, it normally takes seven to eight years to develop mAbs and an additional year to receive FDA approval; a priority review might shorten the approval process by around eight months [268].

7. Conclusions

The respiratory tract illustrates a distinctive interface with the external environment, and the induction of effective but rigidly regulated innate immune responses is pivotal to protect against pathologies and control and eliminate infections caused by invading pathogens, while simultaneously reducing the disturbance in the complex pulmonary anatomy. Proinflammatory cytokines produced by macrophages strengthen the host's defense against pathological conditions. Although pro-inflammatory cytokines might be favorable in controlling pathologies, their extreme rise in level can cause large-scale tissue damage. There has been viable realization regarding the contribution of similar cytokines in the expression of lung pathology among chronic pulmonary diseases.

Cytokines, including IL-4, IL-13, TGF-b, IL-17, and TSLP, assist in many chronic disease states. Increasing evidence has revealed the involvement of inflammatory proteins, including cPLA2, COX-2, VCAM-1, ICAM-1, and MMP-9, in the production and development of respiratory diseases. Additionally, these inflammatory proteins are regulated by various inflammatory signaling pathways, including PKCs, NOX/ROS, EGFR, PDGFR, c-Src, PI3K/Akt, MAPKs, AP-1, and NF-κB. However, multiple questions remain unanswered, although the general role of cytokines in respiratory diseases has been elucidated. There have been few studies investigating the role of transcription factors, such as the transcription factor NF-kB. In asthma, there is an increased expression of NF-κB in the airway epithelium, as well as alveolar macrophage expression and the generation of IL-8. Oxidative stress may also lead to the activation of NF-κB. Surprisingly, the expression of NF-κB is not increased in COPD, suggesting that NF-κB may not be needed for the transcription of cytokines. There may be important differences between asthma and COPD at the level of the transcriptional control of inflammatory cytokines [269]. Further studies are mandatory for the direct comparison of various pulmonary diseases and to concentrate on patients who show clinical features of any two respiratory disorders. Whether various respiratory disease conditions have common mechanisms or similar predisposing factors can be ascertained by the further investigation of cytokine expression. Additionally, this may reveal some common pathways in respiratory conditions. The functions of cytokines at the time of localized infection and systemic infection may have crucial differences. Several findings have stressed the emphasis of clinically relevant animal models to fully understand the role of cytokines in the pathogenesis of lung bacterial infection. The cytokine network can be locally modulated to serve as a significant addition to antibiotic therapy. The translation of exceedingly assuring experiments in animals into clinical trials fails to keep pace. It is important to note that the management of proinflammatory cytokines in respiratory diseases should be tailored to the specific disease and individual patient, taking into consideration factors such as the underlying cause of the disease, the severity of the symptoms, and the patient's overall health. One complication is that cytokines are functionally pleiotropic and redundant, and as a result, targeting an individual cytokine may have a less than expected effect or have undesired side effects. Another hardship is that animal models do not entirely mimic human disease. In addition, the exploration of the role of inflammatory proteins in widespread respiratory diseases is essential to identify possible therapeutic targets. Advancement in designing novel inhibitors with high specificity and no major adverse effects is essential. The option of targeted delivery of inflammatory protein inhibitors directly to the airway and lungs should also be explored, as it may have fewer side effects.

Thorough studies are needed to fully elucidate the role of inflammatory signaling molecules in pulmonary diseases to develop highly specific inhibitors. Until now, blocking specific cytokines or their receptors has been disappointing in clinical studies, which in turn suggests that a broader spectrum of anti-inflammatory effects is needed to treat individuals with severe respiratory diseases.

Author Contributions: Conceptualization, V.P.C.; writing—original draft preparation, V.P.C., R.B., N.A., S.A., B.B. and D.R.; writing—review and editing, V.P.C., R.B., B.B., L.V.N., L.K.G. and V.A. All authors have read and agreed to the published version of the manuscript.

Funding: This research received no funding.

Data Availability Statement: Not applicable.

Acknowledgments: L.K.G. would like to thank the Institute for Health and Sport, Victoria University, and V.A. would like to thank RMIT University for their support. L.K.G. is a recipient of the Victoria University postgraduate scholarship.

Conflicts of Interest: The authors declare no conflicts of interest.

References

1. Agusti, A.; Vogelmeier, C.F.; Halpin, D.M. Tackling the global burden of lung disease through prevention and early diagnosis. *Lancet Respir. Med.* **2022**, *10*, 1013–1015. [CrossRef] [PubMed]
2. Chen, X.; Zhou, C.-W.; Fu, Y.-Y.; Li, Y.-Z.; Chen, L.; Zhang, Q.-W.; Chen, Y.-F. Global, regional, and national burden of chronic respiratory diseases and associated risk factors, 1990–2019: Results from the Global Burden of Disease Study 2019. *Front. Med.* **2023**, *10*, 1066804. [CrossRef] [PubMed]
3. Yu, X.; Wang, H.; Ma, S.; Chen, W.; Sun, L.; Zou, Z. Estimating the global and regional burden of lower respiratory infections attributable to leading pathogens and the protective effectiveness of immunization programs. *Int. J. Infect. Dis.* **2024**, *149*, 107268. [CrossRef] [PubMed]
4. Das, M. WHO urges immediate action to tackle non-communicable diseases. *Lancet Oncol.* **2022**, *23*, 1361. [CrossRef]
5. Denton, E.; O'Hehir, R.E.; Hew, M. The changing global prevalence of asthma and atopic dermatitis. *Allergy* **2023**, *78*, 2079. [CrossRef]
6. Lee, M.O.; Sivasankar, S.; Pokrajac, N.; Smith, C.; Lumba-Brown, A. Emergency department treatment of asthma in children: A review. *J. Am. Coll. Emerg. Physicians Open* **2020**, *1*, 1552–1561. [CrossRef]
7. García-Marcos, L.; Chiang, C.-Y.; Asher, M.I.; Marks, G.B.; El Sony, A.; Masekela, R.; Bissell, K.; Ellwood, E.; Ellwood, P.; Pearce, N. Asthma management and control in children, adolescents, and adults in 25 countries: A Global Asthma Network Phase I cross-sectional study. *Lancet Glob. Health* **2023**, *11*, e218–e228. [CrossRef]
8. Yasaratne, D.; Idrose, N.S.; Dharmage, S.C. Asthma in developing countries in the Asia-Pacific Region (APR). *Respirology* **2023**, *28*, 992–1004. [CrossRef]
9. Cecchi, L.; Annesi-Maesano, I.; d'Amato, G. News on climate change, air pollution, and allergic triggers of asthma. *J. Investig. Allergol. Clin. Immunol.* **2018**, *28*, 91–97.
10. Kaya, A.B.; Çamur, K.C.; Çetin, H.M.; Kaya, S.B.; Erdoğanaras, F. The effects of urban areas, neighborhood and housing on urban health: A systematic review and meta-analysis on asthma. *Cities* **2023**, *143*, 104583. [CrossRef]
11. Mortimer, K.; Kurtulus, S.; Yorgancıoğlu, A.; Romero-Tapia, S.d.J.; Singh, N.; Ahmed, R.; Boladuadua, S.; Masekela, R. Living with Asthma in Low-and Middle-Income Countries in the Six WHO Regions. *NEJM Evid.* **2023**, *3*, EVIDpp2300292. [CrossRef] [PubMed]

12. Balan, I.; Mahmood, S.N.; Jaiswal, R.; Pleshkova, Y.; Manivannan, D.; Negit, S.; Shah, V.; Desai, P.; Akula, N.V.; Nawaz, M.U. Prevalence of active and passive smoking among asthma and asthma-associated emergency admissions: A nationwide prevalence survey study. *J. Investig. Med.* **2023**, *71*, 730–741. [CrossRef] [PubMed]
13. Tiotiu, A.; Ioan, I.; Wirth, N.; Romero-Fernandez, R.; González-Barcala, F.-J. The impact of tobacco smoking on adult asthma outcomes. *Int. J. Environ. Res. Public Health* **2021**, *18*, 992. [CrossRef] [PubMed]
14. Syed, M.; Folz, R.J.; Ali, U. Environmental factors and their impact on airway diseases: Exploring air pollution, indoor and outdoor allergens, and climate change. *Curr. Pulmonol. Rep.* **2023**, *12*, 162–170. [CrossRef]
15. Cai, Z.; Liu, Q. Understanding the Global Cancer Statistics 2018: Implications for cancer control. *Sci. China Life Sci.* **2021**, *64*, 1017–1020. [CrossRef]
16. Thandra, K.C.; Barsouk, A.; Saginala, K.; Aluru, J.S.; Barsouk, A. Epidemiology of lung cancer. *Contemp. Oncol. Współczesna Onkol.* **2021**, *25*, 45–52. [CrossRef]
17. Kruk, M.E.; Gage, A.D.; Arsenault, C.; Jordan, K.; Leslie, H.H.; Roder-DeWan, S.; Adeyi, O.; Barker, P.; Daelmans, B.; Doubova, S.V. High-quality health systems in the Sustainable Development Goals era: Time for a revolution. *Lancet Glob. Health* **2018**, *6*, e1196–e1252. [CrossRef]
18. Echeverria-Londono, S.; Li, X.; Toor, J.; de Villiers, M.J.; Nayagam, S.; Hallett, T.B.; Abbas, K.; Jit, M.; Klepac, P.; Jean, K. How can the public health impact of vaccination be estimated? *BMC Public Health* **2021**, *21*, 2049. [CrossRef]
19. Momtazmanesh, S.; Moghaddam, S.S.; Ghamari, S.-H.; Rad, E.M.; Rezaei, N.; Shobeiri, P.; Aali, A.; Abbasi-Kangevari, M.; Abbasi-Kangevari, Z.; Abdelmasseh, M. Global burden of chronic respiratory diseases and risk factors, 1990–2019: An update from the Global Burden of Disease Study 2019. *EClinicalMedicine* **2023**, *59*, 101936. [CrossRef]
20. Branchett, W.J.; Lloyd, C.M. Regulatory cytokine function in the respiratory tract. *Mucosal Immunol.* **2019**, *12*, 589–600. [CrossRef]
21. Moldoveanu, B.; Otmishi, P.; Jani, P.; Walker, J.; Sarmiento, X.; Guardiola, J.; Saad, M.; Yu, J. Inflammatory mechanisms in the lung. *J. Inflamm. Res.* **2008**, *2*, 1–11. [PubMed]
22. Aghasafari, P.; George, U.; Pidaparti, R. A review of inflammatory mechanism in airway diseases. *Inflamm. Res.* **2019**, *68*, 59–74. [CrossRef] [PubMed]
23. Robb, C.; Regan, K.; Dorward, D.; Rossi, A. Key Mechanisms Governing Resolution of Lung Inflammation. *Semin. Immunopathol.* **2016**, *38*, 425–448. [CrossRef] [PubMed]
24. Wang, T.; He, C. Pro-inflammatory cytokines: The link between obesity and osteoarthritis. *Cytokine Growth Factor Rev.* **2018**, *44*, 38–50. [CrossRef]
25. Antonelli, M.; Kushner, I. It's time to redefine inflammation. *FASEB J.* **2017**, *31*, 1787–1791. [CrossRef]
26. Chen, C.-M.; Lu, H.-C.; Tung, Y.-T.; Chen, W. Antiplatelet therapy for acute respiratory distress syndrome. *Biomedicines* **2020**, *8*, 230. [CrossRef]
27. Atamas, S.P.; Chapoval, S.P.; Keegan, A.D. Cytokines in chronic respiratory diseases. *F1000 Biol. Rep.* **2013**, *5*, 3. [CrossRef]
28. Bissonnette, E.Y.; Lauzon-Joset, J.-F.; Debley, J.S.; Ziegler, S.F. Cross-talk between alveolar macrophages and lung epithelial cells is essential to maintain lung homeostasis. *Front. Immunol.* **2020**, *11*, 583042. [CrossRef]
29. Fan, W.; Gui, B.; Zhou, X.; Li, L.; Chen, H. A narrative review on lung injury: Mechanisms, biomarkers, and monitoring. *Crit. Care* **2024**, *28*, 352. [CrossRef]
30. Holt, P.G.; Strickland, D.H.; Wikström, M.E.; Jahnsen, F.L. Regulation of immunological homeostasis in the respiratory tract. *Nat. Rev. Immunol.* **2008**, *8*, 142–152. [CrossRef]
31. Manirambona, E.; Okesanya, O.J.; Olaleke, N.O.; Oso, T.A.; Lucero-Prisno, D.E., III. Evolution and implications of SARS-CoV-2 variants in the post-pandemic era. *Discov. Public Health* **2024**, *21*, 16. [CrossRef]
32. Yang, L.; Xie, X.; Tu, Z.; Fu, J.; Xu, D.; Zhou, Y. The signal pathways and treatment of cytokine storm in COVID-19. *Signal Transduct. Target. Ther.* **2021**, *6*, 255. [CrossRef] [PubMed]
33. Swenson, K.E.; Swenson, E.R. Pathophysiology of acute respiratory distress syndrome and COVID-19 lung injury. *Crit. Care Clin.* **2021**, *37*, 749–776. [CrossRef] [PubMed]
34. Montazersaheb, S.; Hosseiniyan Khatibi, S.M.; Hejazi, M.S.; Tarhriz, V.; Farjami, A.; Ghasemian Sorbeni, F.; Farahzadi, R.; Ghasemnejad, T. COVID-19 infection: An overview on cytokine storm and related interventions. *Virol. J.* **2022**, *19*, 92. [CrossRef] [PubMed]
35. Vanderwall, A.G.; Milligan, E.D. Cytokines in pain: Harnessing endogenous anti-inflammatory signaling for improved pain management. *Front. Immunol.* **2019**, *10*, 3009. [CrossRef]
36. Altan-Bonnet, G.; Mukherjee, R. Cytokine-mediated communication: A quantitative appraisal of immune complexity. *Nat. Rev. Immunol.* **2019**, *19*, 205–217. [CrossRef]
37. Zhang, J.-M.; An, J. Cytokines, inflammation, and pain. *Int. Anesthesiol. Clin.* **2007**, *45*, 27–37. [CrossRef]
38. Mishra, A.K. Role of cytokines in the control of inflammation: A review. *Int. J. Ther. Innov.* **2023**, *1*, 5–8.
39. Turner, M.D.; Nedjai, B.; Hurst, T.; Pennington, D.J. Cytokines and chemokines: At the crossroads of cell signalling and inflammatory disease. *Biochim. Et Biophys. Acta (BBA) Mol. Cell Res.* **2014**, *1843*, 2563–2582. [CrossRef]

40. Harvanová, G.; Duranková, S.; Bernasovská, J. The role of cytokines and chemokines in the inflammatory response. *Alergol. Pol. Pol. J. Allergol.* **2023**, *10*, 210–219. [CrossRef]
41. Ferreira, V.L.; Borba, H.H.; Bonetti, A.d.F.; Leonart, L.; Pontarolo, R. Cytokines and interferons: Types and functions. *Autoantibodies Cytokines* **2018**, *13*, 1–25.
42. Akdis, M.; Burgler, S.; Crameri, R.; Eiwegger, T.; Fujita, H.; Gomez, E.; Klunker, S.; Meyer, N.; O'Mahony, L.; Palomares, O. Interleukins, from 1 to 37, and interferon-γ: Receptors, functions, and roles in diseases. *J. Allergy Clin. Immunol.* **2011**, *127*, 701–721. e770. [PubMed]
43. Ma, K.; Zhang, H.; Baloch, Z. Pathogenetic and therapeutic applications of tumor necrosis factor-α (TNF-α) in major depressive disorder: A systematic review. *Int. J. Mol. Sci.* **2016**, *17*, 733. [CrossRef] [PubMed]
44. Iwasaki, T.; Watanabe, R.; Ito, H.; Fujii, T.; Okuma, K.; Oku, T.; Hirayama, Y.; Ohmura, K.; Murata, K.; Murakami, K. Dynamics of type I and type II interferon signature determines responsiveness to anti-TNF therapy in rheumatoid arthritis. *Front. Immunol.* **2022**, *13*, 901437. [CrossRef]
45. Platanias, L.C. Mechanisms of type-I-and type-II-interferon-mediated signalling. *Nat. Rev. Immunol.* **2005**, *5*, 375–386. [CrossRef]
46. Utomo, B.S.R.; Hatta, M.; Sirait, R.H.; Pratiwi, S.; Massi, M.N. The role of cytokine interleukin-2, transcription factor of FoxP3 in the immunological regulation of allergic rhinitis. *Int. J. Otolaryngol. Head Neck Surg.* **2018**, *7*, 7–19. [CrossRef]
47. Dalskov, L.; Gad, H.H.; Hartmann, R. Viral recognition and the antiviral interferon response. *EMBO J.* **2023**, *42*, e112907. [CrossRef]
48. Moreau, T.R.; Bondet, V.; Rodero, M.P.; Duffy, D. Heterogeneity and functions of the 13 IFN-α subtypes–lucky for some? *Eur. J. Immunol.* **2023**, *53*, 2250307. [CrossRef]
49. Strayer, D.R.; Carter, W.A.; Stouch, B.C.; Stittelaar, K.J.; Thoolen, R.J.; Osterhaus, A.D.; Mitchell, W.M. Protection from pulmonary tissue damage associated with infection of cynomolgus macaques by highly pathogenic avian influenza virus (H5N1) by low dose natural human IFN-alpha administered to the buccal mucosa. *Antiviral Res.* **2014**, *110*, 175–180. [CrossRef]
50. Lee, A.J.; Ashkar, A.A. The Dual Nature of Type I and Type II Interferons. *Front. Immunol.* **2018**, *9*, 2061. [CrossRef]
51. Metcalf, D. The colony-stimulating factors and cancer. *Nat. Rev. Cancer* **2010**, *10*, 425–434. [CrossRef] [PubMed]
52. Hamilton, J.A.; Cook, A.D.; Tak, P.P. Anti-colony-stimulating factor therapies for inflammatory and autoimmune diseases. *Nat. Rev. Drug Discov.* **2017**, *16*, 53–70. [CrossRef] [PubMed]
53. Griffith, J.W.; Sokol, C.L.; Luster, A.D. Chemokines and chemokine receptors: Positioning cells for host defense and immunity. *Annu. Rev. Immunol.* **2014**, *32*, 659–702. [CrossRef] [PubMed]
54. Stone, M.J.; Hayward, J.A.; Huang, C.E.; Huma, Z.; Sanchez, J. Mechanisms of regulation of the chemokine-receptor network. *Int. J. Mol. Sci.* **2017**, *18*, 342. [CrossRef]
55. Alfaro, C.; Sanmamed, M.F.; Rodríguez-Ruiz, M.E.; Teijeira, Á.; Oñate, C.; González, Á.; Ponz, M.; Schalper, K.A.; Pérez-Gracia, J.L.; Melero, I. Interleukin-8 in cancer pathogenesis, treatment and follow-up. *Cancer Treat. Rev.* **2017**, *60*, 24–31. [CrossRef]
56. Hughes, C.E.; Nibbs, R.J. A guide to chemokines and their receptors. *FEBS J.* **2018**, *285*, 2944–2971. [CrossRef]
57. Deng, Z.; Fan, T.; Xiao, C.; Tian, H.; Zheng, Y.; Li, C.; He, J. TGF-β signaling in health, disease, and therapeutics. *Signal Transduct. Target. Ther.* **2024**, *9*, 61.
58. Yue, X.; Wu, L.; Hu, W. The regulation of leukemia inhibitory factor. *Cancer Cell Microenviron.* **2015**, *2*, e877.
59. Mozaffarian, A.; Brewer, A.W.; Trueblood, E.S.; Luzina, I.G.; Todd, N.W.; Atamas, S.P.; Arnett, H.A. Mechanisms of oncostatin M-induced pulmonary inflammation and fibrosis. *J. Immunol.* **2008**, *181*, 7243–7253. [CrossRef]
60. Akdis, M.; Aab, A.; Altunbulakli, C.; Azkur, K.; Costa, R.A.; Crameri, R.; Duan, S.; Eiwegger, T.; Eljaszewicz, A.; Ferstl, R. Interleukins (from IL-1 to IL-38), interferons, transforming growth factor β, and TNF-α: Receptors, functions, and roles in diseases. *J. Allergy Clin. Immunol.* **2016**, *138*, 984–1010. [CrossRef]
61. Li, L.; Xue, M.; Fu, F.; Yin, L.; Feng, L.; Liu, P. IFN-lambda 3 mediates antiviral protection against porcine epidemic diarrhea virus by inducing a distinct antiviral transcript profile in porcine intestinal epithelia. *Front. Immunol.* **2019**, *10*, 2394. [CrossRef] [PubMed]
62. Nam, S.; Lim, J.-S. Essential role of interferon regulatory factor 4 (IRF4) in immune cell development. *Arch. Pharmacal Res.* **2016**, *39*, 1548–1555. [CrossRef] [PubMed]
63. Cockx, M.; Gouwy, M.; Van Damme, J.; Struyf, S. Chemoattractants and cytokines in primary ciliary dyskinesia and cystic fibrosis: Key players in chronic respiratory diseases. *Cell. Mol. Immunol.* **2018**, *15*, 312–323. [CrossRef] [PubMed]
64. Ray, A.; Raundhal, M.; Oriss, T.B.; Ray, P.; Wenzel, S.E. Current concepts of severe asthma. *J. Clin. Investig.* **2016**, *126*, 2394–2403. [CrossRef]
65. Ying, S.; O'Connor, B.; Ratoff, J.; Meng, Q.; Fang, C.; Cousins, D.; Zhang, G.; Gu, S.; Gao, Z.; Shamji, B.; et al. Expression and Cellular Provenance of Thymic Stromal Lymphopoietin and Chemokines in Patients with Severe Asthma and Chronic Obstructive Pulmonary Disease. *J. Immunol.* **2008**, *181*, 2790–2798. [CrossRef]
66. Gao, P.; Gibson, P.G.; Baines, K.J.; Yang, I.A.; Upham, J.W.; Reynolds, P.N.; Hodge, S.; James, A.L.; Jenkins, C.; Peters, M.J. Anti-inflammatory deficiencies in neutrophilic asthma: Reduced galectin-3 and IL-1RA/IL-1β. *Respir. Res.* **2015**, *16*, 5. [CrossRef]

67. Robinson, D.; Humbert, M.; Buhl, R.; Cruz, A.A.; Inoue, H.; Korom, S.; Hanania, N.A.; Nair, P. Revisiting T ype 2-high and T ype 2-low airway inflammation in asthma: Current knowledge and therapeutic implications. *Clin. Exp. Allergy* **2017**, *47*, 161–175. [CrossRef]
68. Lai, T.; Tian, B.; Cao, C.; Hu, Y.; Zhou, J.; Wang, Y.; Wu, Y.; Li, Z.; Xu, X.; Zhang, M. HDAC2 suppresses IL17A-mediated airway remodeling in human and experimental modeling of COPD. *Chest* **2018**, *153*, 863–875. [CrossRef]
69. Kang, M.-J.; Choi, J.-M.; Kim, B.H.; Lee, C.-M.; Cho, W.-K.; Choe, G.; Kim, D.-H.; Lee, C.G.; Elias, J.A. IL-18 induces emphysema and airway and vascular remodeling via IFN-γ, IL-17A, and IL-13. *Am. J. Respir. Crit. Care Med.* **2012**, *185*, 1205–1217. [CrossRef]
70. Bernhagen, J. A new cytokine target for chronic obstructive pulmonary disease? *EBioMedicine* **2021**, *69*, 103479. [CrossRef]
71. Song, S.; Liu, B.; Habibie, H.; van den Bor, J.; Smit, M.J.; Gosens, R.; Wu, X.; Brandsma, C.-A.; Cool, R.H.; Haisma, H.J. D-dopachrome tautomerase contributes to lung epithelial repair via atypical chemokine receptor 3-dependent Akt signaling. *EBioMedicine* **2021**, *68*, 103479. [CrossRef] [PubMed]
72. Mao, Y.-M.; Zhao, C.-N.; Leng, J.; Leng, R.-X.; Ye, D.-Q.; Zheng, S.G.; Pan, H.-F. Interleukin-13: A promising therapeutic target for autoimmune disease. *Cytokine Growth Factor Rev.* **2019**, *45*, 9–23. [CrossRef] [PubMed]
73. Fara, A.; Mitrev, Z.; Rosalia, R.A.; Assas, B.M. Cytokine storm and COVID-19: A chronicle of pro-inflammatory cytokines. *Open Biol.* **2020**, *10*, 200160. [CrossRef] [PubMed]
74. Krick, S.; Grabner, A.; Baumlin, N.; Yanucil, C.; Helton, S.; Grosche, A.; Sailland, J.; Geraghty, P.; Viera, L.; Russell, D.W. Fibroblast growth factor 23 and Klotho contribute to airway inflammation. *Eur. Respir. J.* **2018**, *52*, 1800236. [CrossRef]
75. Wang, Y.; Xu, J.; Meng, Y.; Adcock, I.M.; Yao, X. Role of inflammatory cells in airway remodeling in COPD. *Int. J. Chronic Obstr. Pulm. Dis.* **2018**, *13*, 3341–3348. [CrossRef]
76. Harun, S.N.; Holford, N.H.; Grimwood, K.; Wainwright, C.E.; Hennig, S. Pseudomonas aeruginosa eradication therapy and risk of acquiring Aspergillus in young children with cystic fibrosis. *Thorax* **2019**, *74*, 740–748. [CrossRef]
77. Muselet-Charlier, C.; Roque, T.; Boncoeur, E.; Chadelat, K.; Clement, A.; Jacquot, J.; Tabary, O. Enhanced IL-1β-induced IL-8 production in cystic fibrosis lung epithelial cells is dependent of both mitogen-activated protein kinases and NF-κB signaling. *Biochem. Biophys. Res. Commun.* **2007**, *357*, 402–407. [CrossRef]
78. Sepahzad, A.; Morris-Rosendahl, D.J.; Davies, J.C. Cystic fibrosis lung disease modifiers and their relevance in the new era of precision medicine. *Genes* **2021**, *12*, 562. [CrossRef]
79. Abolfathi, H.; Sheikhpour, M.; Shahraeini, S.S.; Khatami, S.; Nojoumi, S.A. Studies in lung cancer cytokine proteomics: A review. *Expert Rev. Proteom.* **2021**, *18*, 49–64. [CrossRef]
80. Chanda, C. Role of inflammatory cytokines during lung cancer progression: A review. *Res. J. Pharm. Technol.* **2018**, *11*, 5163–5165. [CrossRef]
81. Kellum, J.A.; Kong, L.; Fink, M.P.; Weissfeld, L.A.; Yealy, D.M.; Pinsky, M.R.; Fine, J.; Krichevsky, A.; Delude, R.L.; Angus, D.C. Understanding the inflammatory cytokine response in pneumonia and sepsis: Results of the Genetic and Inflammatory Markers of Sepsis (GenIMS) Study. *Arch. Intern. Med.* **2007**, *167*, 1655–1663. [CrossRef] [PubMed]
82. Bacci, M.; Leme, R.; Zing, N.; Murad, N.; Adami, F.; Hinnig, P.; Feder, D.; Chagas, A.; Fonseca, F. IL-6 and TNF-α serum levels are associated with early death in community-acquired pneumonia patients. *Braz. J. Med. Biol. Res.* **2015**, *48*, 427–432. [CrossRef] [PubMed]
83. Dukhinova, M.; Kokinos, E.; Kuchur, P.; Komissarov, A.; Shtro, A. Macrophage-derived cytokines in pneumonia: Linking cellular immunology and genetics. *Cytokine Growth Factor Rev.* **2021**, *59*, 46–61. [CrossRef] [PubMed]
84. Chou, C.-W.; Lin, F.-C.; Tsai, H.-C.; Chang, S.-C. The importance of pro-inflammatory and anti-inflammatory cytokines in *Pneumocystis jirovecii* pneumonia. *Med. Mycol.* **2013**, *51*, 704–712. [CrossRef]
85. Bagnato, G.L.; Irrera, N.; Pizzino, G.; Santoro, D.; Roberts, W.N.; Bagnato, G.; Pallio, G.; Vaccaro, M.; Squadrito, F.; Saitta, A. Dual $\alpha v\beta 3$ and $\alpha v\beta 5$ blockade attenuates fibrotic and vascular alterations in a murine model of systemic sclerosis. *Clin. Sci.* **2018**, *132*, 231–242. [CrossRef]
86. Etna, M.P.; Giacomini, E.; Severa, M.; Coccia, E.M. Pro- and anti-inflammatory cytokines in tuberculosis: A two-edged sword in TB pathogenesis. *Semin. Immunol.* **2014**, *6*, 543–551. [CrossRef]
87. Defnet, A.E.; Shah, S.D.; Huang, W.; Shapiro, P.; Deshpande, D.A.; Kane, M.A. Dysregulated retinoic acid signaling in airway smooth muscle cells in asthma. *FASEB J. Off. Publ. Fed. Am. Soc. Exp. Biol.* **2021**, *35*, e22016. [CrossRef]
88. Gubernatorova, E.O.; Namakanova, O.A.; Gorshkova, E.A.; Medvedovskaya, A.D.; Nedospasov, S.A.; Drutskaya, M.S. Novel anti-cytokine strategies for prevention and treatment of respiratory allergic diseases. *Front. Immunol.* **2021**, *12*, 601842. [CrossRef]
89. Ortiz-Zapater, E.; Signes-Costa, J.; Montero, P.; Roger, I. Lung fibrosis and fibrosis in the lungs: Is it all about myofibroblasts? *Biomedicines* **2022**, *10*, 1423. [CrossRef]
90. Torrisi, S.E.; Ley, B.; Kreuter, M.; Wijsenbeek, M.; Vittinghoff, E.; Collard, H.R.; Vancheri, C. The added value of comorbidities in predicting survival in idiopathic pulmonary fibrosis: A multicentre observational study. *Eur. Respir. J.* **2019**, *53*, 1801587. [CrossRef]

91. Renema, P.; Hardy, K.S.; Housley, N.; Dunbar, G.; Annamdevula, N.; Britain, A.; Spadafora, D.; Leavesley, S.; Rich, T.; Audia, J.P. cAMP signaling primes lung endothelial cells to activate caspase-1 during Pseudomonas aeruginosa infection. *Am. J. Physiol. Lung Cell. Mol. Physiol.* **2020**, *318*, L1074–L1083. [CrossRef] [PubMed]
92. Ali, F.; Alom, S.; Shakya, A.; Ghosh, S.K.; Singh, U.P.; Bhat, H.R. Implication of in silico studies in the search for novel inhibitors against SARS-CoV-2. *Arch. Der Pharm.* **2022**, *355*, 2100360. [CrossRef] [PubMed]
93. Zhu, N.; Zhang, D.; Wang, W.; Li, X.; Yang, B.; Song, J.; Zhao, X.; Huang, B.; Shi, W.; Lu, R. A novel coronavirus from patients with pneumonia in China, 2019. *N. Engl. J. Med.* **2020**, *382*, 727–733. [CrossRef]
94. Karimi, A.; Hashemian, S.M.R. Cytokine storm in COVID-19 and the treatment simulacrum. *Biomed. Biotechnol. Res. J.* **2020**, *4*, S41–S48.
95. Zhang, C.; Wu, Z.; Li, J.-W.; Zhao, H.; Wang, G.-Q. Cytokine release syndrome in severe COVID-19: Interleukin-6 receptor antagonist tocilizumab may be the key to reduce mortality. *Int. J. Antimicrob. Agents* **2020**, *55*, 105954. [CrossRef]
96. Mehta, P.; McAuley, D.F.; Brown, M.; Sanchez, E.; Tattersall, R.S.; Manson, J.J. COVID-19: Consider cytokine storm syndromes and immunosuppression. *Lancet* **2020**, *395*, 1033–1034. [CrossRef]
97. Darif, D.; Hammi, I.; Kihel, A.; Saik, I.E.I.; Guessous, F.; Akarid, K. The pro-inflammatory cytokines in COVID-19 pathogenesis: What goes wrong? *Microb. Pathog.* **2021**, *153*, 104799. [CrossRef]
98. Lan, J.; Ge, J.; Yu, J.; Shan, S.; Zhou, H.; Fan, S.; Zhang, Q.; Shi, X.; Wang, Q.; Zhang, L. Structure of the SARS-CoV-2 spike receptor-binding domain bound to the ACE2 receptor. *Nature* **2020**, *581*, 215–220. [CrossRef]
99. Gadanec, L.K.; McSweeney, K.R.; Qaradakhi, T.; Ali, B.; Zulli, A.; Apostolopoulos, V. Can SARS-CoV-2 virus use multiple receptors to enter host cells? *Int. J. Mol. Sci.* **2021**, *22*, 992. [CrossRef]
100. Zhang, X.; Wu, K.; Wang, D.; Yue, X.; Song, D.; Zhu, Y.; Wu, J. Nucleocapsid protein of SARS-CoV activates interleukin-6 expression through cellular transcription factor NF-κB. *Virology* **2007**, *365*, 324–335. [CrossRef]
101. Ebihara, N.; Matsuda, A.; Nakamura, S.; Matsuda, H.; Murakami, A. Role of the IL-6 classic-and trans-signaling pathways in corneal sterile inflammation and wound healing. *Investig. Ophthalmol. Vis. Sci.* **2011**, *52*, 8549–8557. [CrossRef] [PubMed]
102. Kihel, A.; Hammi, I.; Darif, D.; Lemrani, M.; Riyad, M.; Guessous, F.; Akarid, K. The different faces of the NLRP3 inflammasome in cutaneous Leishmaniasis: A review. *Cytokine* **2021**, *147*, 155248. [CrossRef] [PubMed]
103. Orlov, M.; Wander, P.L.; Morrell, E.D.; Mikacenic, C.; Wurfel, M.M. A case for targeting Th17 cells and IL-17A in SARS-CoV-2 infections. *J. Immunol.* **2020**, *205*, 892–898. [CrossRef] [PubMed]
104. Anderson, R.; Feldman, C. The global burden of community-acquired pneumonia in adults, encompassing invasive pneumococcal disease and the prevalence of its associated cardiovascular events, with a focus on pneumolysin and macrolide antibiotics in pathogenesis and therapy. *Int. J. Mol. Sci.* **2023**, *24*, 11038. [CrossRef]
105. Gibbings, S.L.; Thomas, S.M.; Atif, S.M.; McCubbrey, A.L.; Desch, A.N.; Danhorn, T.; Leach, S.M.; Bratton, D.L.; Henson, P.M.; Janssen, W.J. Three unique interstitial macrophages in the murine lung at steady state. *Am. J. Respir. Cell Mol. Biol.* **2017**, *57*, 66–76. [CrossRef]
106. Schyns, J.; Bai, Q.; Ruscitti, C.; Radermecker, C.; De Schepper, S.; Chakarov, S.; Farnir, F.; Pirottin, D.; Ginhoux, F.; Boeckxstaens, G. Non-classical tissue monocytes and two functionally distinct populations of interstitial macrophages populate the mouse lung. *Nat. Commun.* **2019**, *10*, 3964. [CrossRef]
107. Robinson, K.M.; Ramanan, K.; Clay, M.E.; McHugh, K.J.; Rich, H.E.; Alcorn, J.F. Novel protective mechanism for interleukin-33 at the mucosal barrier during influenza-associated bacterial superinfection. *Mucosal Immunol.* **2018**, *11*, 199–208. [CrossRef]
108. Costantini, A.; Viola, N.; Berretta, A.; Galeazzi, R.; Matacchione, G.; Sabbatinelli, J.; Storci, G.; De Matteis, S.; Butini, L.; Rippo, M.R. Age-related M1/M2 phenotype changes in circulating monocytes from healthy/unhealthy individuals. *Aging* **2018**, *10*, 1268. [CrossRef]
109. Fernandez-Botran, R.; Uriarte, S.M.; Arnold, F.W.; Rodriguez-Hernandez, L.; Rane, M.J.; Peyrani, P.; Wiemken, T.; Kelley, R.; Uppatla, S.; Cavallazzi, R.; et al. Contrasting Inflammatory Responses in Severe and Non-severe Community-acquired Pneumonia. *Inflammation* **2014**, *37*, 1158–1166. [CrossRef]
110. Paats, M.S.; Bergen, I.M.; Hanselaar, W.E.; van Zoelen, E.C.G.; Hoogsteden, H.C.; Hendriks, R.W.; Van der Eerden, M.M. Local and systemic cytokine profiles in nonsevere and severe community-acquired pneumonia. *Eur. Respir. J.* **2013**, *41*, 1378–1385. [CrossRef]
111. Kragsbjerg, P.; Jones, I.; Vikerfors, T.; Holmberg, H. Diagnostic value of blood cytokine concentrations in acute pneumonia. *Thorax* **1995**, *50*, 1253–1257. [CrossRef] [PubMed]
112. Lee, H.-M.; Lee, H.-J.; Chang, J.-E. Inflammatory cytokine: An attractive target for cancer treatment. *Biomedicines* **2022**, *10*, 2116. [CrossRef] [PubMed]
113. Landskron, G.; De la Fuente, M.; Thuwajit, P.; Thuwajit, C.; Hermoso, M.A. Chronic inflammation and cytokines in the tumor microenvironment. *J. Immunol. Res.* **2014**, *2014*, 149185. [CrossRef]
114. Brenner, D.R.; Fanidi, A.; Grankvist, K.; Muller, D.C.; Brennan, P.; Manjer, J.; Byrnes, G.; Hodge, A.; Severi, G.; Giles, G.G. Inflammatory cytokines and lung cancer risk in 3 prospective studies. *Am. J. Epidemiol.* **2017**, *185*, 86–95. [CrossRef] [PubMed]

115. Shang, G.-S.; Liu, L.; Qin, Y.-W. IL-6 and TNF-α promote metastasis of lung cancer by inducing epithelial-mesenchymal transition. *Oncol. Lett.* **2017**, *13*, 4657–4660. [CrossRef]
116. Lin, Q.; Xue, L.; Tian, T.; Zhang, B.; Guo, L.; Lin, G.; Chen, Z.; Fan, K.; Gu, X. Prognostic value of serum IL-17 and VEGF levels in small cell lung cancer. *Int. J. Biol. Markers* **2015**, *30*, 359–363. [CrossRef]
117. Timperi, E.; Focaccetti, C.; Gallerano, D.; Panetta, M.; Spada, S.; Gallo, E.; Visca, P.; Venuta, F.; Diso, D.; Prelaj, A. IL-18 receptor marks functional CD8+ T cells in non-small cell lung cancer. *Oncoimmunology* **2017**, *6*, e1328337. [CrossRef]
118. Lee, H.-M.; Yuk, J.-M.; Shin, D.-M.; Jo, E.-K. Dectin-1 is Inducible and Plays an Essential Role for Mycobacteria-Induced Innate Immune Responses in Airway Epithelial Cells. *J. Clin. Immunol.* **2009**, *6*, 795–805. [CrossRef]
119. Roy, S.; Sharma, S.; Sharma, M.; Aggarwal, R.; Bose, M. Induction of nitric oxide release from the human alveolar epithelial cell line A549: An in vitro correlate of innate immune response to *Mycobacterium tuberculosis*. *Immunology* **2004**, *3*, 471–480. [CrossRef]
120. Wang, X.; Wu, Y.; Jiao, J.; Huang, Q. Mycobacterium tuberculosis infection induces IL-10 gene expression by disturbing histone deacetylase 6 and histonedeacetylase 11 equilibrium in macrophages. *Tuberculosis* **2018**, *108*, 118–123. [CrossRef]
121. Olsen, A.; Chen, Y.; Ji, Q.; Zhu, G.; De Silva, A.D.; Vilchèze, C.; Weisbrod, T.; Li, W.; Xu, J.; Larsen, M.; et al. Targeting Mycobacterium tuberculosis Tumor Necrosis Factor Alpha-Downregulating Genes for the Development of Antituberculous Vaccines. *mBio* **2016**, *7*, 10–1128. [CrossRef] [PubMed]
122. Spangler, J.B.; Moraga, I.; Mendoza, J.L.; Garcia, K.C. Insights into cytokine–receptor interactions from cytokine engineering. *Annu. Rev. Immunol.* **2015**, *33*, 139–167. [CrossRef] [PubMed]
123. Mohan, K.; Ueda, G.; Kim, A.R.; Jude, K.M.; Fallas, J.A.; Guo, Y.; Hafer, M.; Miao, Y.; Saxton, R.A.; Piehler, J. Topological control of cytokine receptor signaling induces differential effects in hematopoiesis. *Science* **2019**, *364*, eaav7532. [CrossRef] [PubMed]
124. Murray, P.J. The JAK-STAT signaling pathway: Input and output integration. *J. Immunol.* **2007**, *178*, 2623–2629. [CrossRef]
125. Schindler, C.; Levy, D.E.; Decker, T. JAK-STAT signaling: From interferons to cytokines. *J. Biol. Chem.* **2007**, *282*, 20059–20063. [CrossRef]
126. Murakami, M.; Kamimura, D.; Hirano, T. Pleiotropy and specificity: Insights from the interleukin 6 family of cytokines. *Immunity* **2019**, *50*, 812–831. [CrossRef]
127. Hercus, T.R.; Dhagat, U.; Kan, W.L.; Broughton, S.E.; Nero, T.L.; Perugini, M.; Sandow, J.J.; D'Andrea, R.J.; Ekert, P.G.; Hughes, T. Signalling by the βc family of cytokines. *Cytokine Growth Factor Rev.* **2013**, *24*, 189–201. [CrossRef]
128. Pestka, S.; Krause, C.D.; Walter, M.R. Interferons, interferon-like cytokines, and their receptors. *Immunol. Rev.* **2004**, *202*, 8–32. [CrossRef]
129. Kossiakoff, A.A.; de Vos, A.M. Structural basis for cytokine hormone-receptor recognition and receptor activation. *Adv. Protein Chem.* **1998**, *52*, 67–108.
130. Fields, J.K.; Günther, S.; Sundberg, E.J. Structural basis of IL-1 family cytokine signaling. *Front. Immunol.* **2019**, *10*, 1412. [CrossRef]
131. Scheide-Noeth, J.-P.; Rosen, M.; Baumstark, D.; Dietz, H.; Mueller, T.D. Structural basis of interleukin-5 inhibition by the small cyclic peptide AF17121. *J. Mol. Biol.* **2019**, *431*, 714–731. [CrossRef] [PubMed]
132. Jiang, X.; Gao, J.; Xue, Y.; Qin, Y.; Li, X.; Sun, Z.; Xie, H.; Chang, M.; Nie, P.; Zou, J. Identification and expression analysis of IL-4/13 receptors in grass carp Ctenopharyngodon idella. *Fish Shellfish. Immunol.* **2019**, *87*, 254–264. [CrossRef] [PubMed]
133. Walter, M.R. The role of structure in the biology of interferon signaling. *Front. Immunol.* **2020**, *11*, 606489. [CrossRef] [PubMed]
134. Kim, J.W.; Cochran, J.R. Targeting ligand–receptor interactions for development of cancer therapeutics. *Curr. Opin. Chem. Biol.* **2017**, *38*, 62–69. [CrossRef]
135. Deshpande, D.A.; Guedes, A.G.; Graeff, R.; Dogan, S.; Subramanian, S.; Walseth, T.F.; Kannan, M.S. CD38/cADPR signaling pathway in airway disease: Regulatory mechanisms. *Mediat. Inflamm.* **2018**, *2018*, 8942042. [CrossRef]
136. Santana, F.P.; da Silva, R.C.; Ponci, V.; Pinheiro, A.J.; Olivo, C.R.; Caperuto, L.C.; Arantes-Costa, F.M.; Claudio, S.R.; Ribeiro, D.A.; Tibério, I.F. Dehydrodieugenol improved lung inflammation in an asthma model by inhibiting the STAT3/SOCS3 and MAPK pathways. *Biochem. Pharmacol.* **2020**, *180*, 114175. [CrossRef]
137. Pelaia, C.; Vatrella, A.; Gallelli, L.; Lombardo, N.; Sciacqua, A.; Savino, R.; Pelaia, G. Role of p38 mitogen-activated protein kinase in asthma and COPD: Pathogenic aspects and potential targeted therapies. *Drug Des. Dev. Ther.* **2021**, 1275–1284. [CrossRef]
138. Soni, S.; Anand, P.; Padwad, Y.S. MAPKAPK2: The master regulator of RNA-binding proteins modulates transcript stability and tumor progression. *J. Exp. Clin. Cancer Res.* **2019**, *38*, 121. [CrossRef]
139. Verma, A.K.; Singh, M.F.; Awasthi, A. Role of p38 MAP Kinase Inhibitor (SB239063) and Vitamin B 12 against Neuroinflammation. *Int. J. Pharm. Investig.* **2021**, *11*, 94–98. [CrossRef]
140. Che, L.; Yu, C.; Chen, G.; Lin, J.; Xie, Z.; Xia, T.; Luo, W.; Cai, X.; Liu, S. The inflammatory response induced by RELMβ upregulates IL-8 and IL-1β expression in bronchial epithelial cells in COPD. *Int. J. Chronic Obstr. Pulm. Dis.* **2021**, 2503–2513. [CrossRef]
141. Popmihajlov, Z.; Sutherland, D.J.; Horan, G.S.; Ghosh, A.; Lynch, D.A.; Noble, P.W.; Richeldi, L.; Reiss, T.F.; Greenberg, S. CC-90001, a c-Jun N-terminal kinase (JNK) inhibitor, in patients with pulmonary fibrosis: Design of a phase 2, randomised, placebo-controlled trial. *BMJ Open Respir. Res.* **2022**, *9*, e001060. [CrossRef] [PubMed]

142. Brunner, J.; Borchard, G.; Peptide Structure Optimisation. UnrTablavelling the Modulation of Tight Junctions: Molecular Mechanisms and Permeation Enhancement. 2022. Available online: https://m2.mtmt.hu/api/citation/32564792?&format=xml (accessed on 21 February 2025).
143. Mehta, M.; Dhanjal, D.S.; Satija, S.; Wadhwa, R.; Paudel, K.R.; Chellappan, D.K.; Mohammad, S.; Haghi, M.; Hansbro, P.M.; Dua, K. Advancing of cellular signaling pathways in respiratory diseases using nanocarrier based drug delivery systems. *Curr. Pharm. Des.* **2020**, *26*, 5380–5392. [CrossRef] [PubMed]
144. Page, K.; Li, J.; Zhou, L.; Iasvoyskaia, S.; Corbit, K.C.; Soh, J.-W.; Weinstein, I.B.; Brasier, A.R.; Lin, A.; Hershenson, M.B. Regulation of airway epithelial cell NF-κB-dependent gene expression by protein kinase Cδ. *J. Immunol.* **2003**, *170*, 5681–5689. [CrossRef] [PubMed]
145. Nakano, R.; Kitanaka, T.; Namba, S.; Kitanaka, N.; Sugiya, H. Protein kinase Cε regulates nuclear translocation of extracellular signal-regulated kinase, which contributes to bradykinin-induced cyclooxygenase-2 expression. *Sci. Rep.* **2018**, *8*, 8535. [CrossRef]
146. Wu, T.; Han, C.; Shelhamer, J.H. Involvement of p38 and p42/44 MAP kinases and protein kinase C in the interferon-γ and interleukin-1α-induced phosphorylation of 85-kDa cytosolic phospholipase A2 in primary human bronchial epithelial cells. *Cytokine* **2004**, *25*, 11–20. [CrossRef]
147. Lien, C.-F.; Chen, S.-J.; Tsai, M.-C.; Lin, C.-S. Potential role of protein kinase C in the pathophysiology of diabetes-associated atherosclerosis. *Front. Pharmacol.* **2021**, *12*, 716332. [CrossRef]
148. Lin, C.-H.; Cheng, H.-W.; Ma, H.-P.; Wu, C.-H.; Hong, C.-Y.; Chen, B.-C. Thrombin induces NF-κB activation and IL-8/CXCL8 expression in lung epithelial cells by a Rac1-dependent PI3K/Akt pathway. *J. Biol. Chem.* **2011**, *286*, 10483–10494. [CrossRef]
149. Lee, I.T.; Lin, C.C.; Wu, Y.C.; Yang, C.M. TNF-α induces matrix metalloproteinase-9 expression in A549 cells: Role of TNFR1/TRAF2/PKCα-dependent signaling pathways. *J. Cell. Physiol.* **2010**, *224*, 454–464. [CrossRef]
150. Basu, B.; Ghosh, S.; Das, S.; Das, A. Implications of Phosphoinositide 3-Kinase (PI3K) Signalling in Cellular and Molecular Mechanisms of Respiratory Diseases. In *Targeting Cellular Signalling Pathways in Lung Diseases*; Springer: Berlin/Heidelberg, Germany, 2021; pp. 601–623.
151. Wang, J.; Hu, K.; Cai, X.; Yang, B.; He, Q.; Wang, J.; Weng, Q. Targeting PI3K/AKT signaling for treatment of idiopathic pulmonary fibrosis. *Acta Pharm. Sin. B* **2022**, *12*, 18–32. [CrossRef]
152. Khezri, M.R.; Varzandeh, R.; Ghasemnejad-Berenji, M. The probable role and therapeutic potential of the PI3K/AKT signaling pathway in SARS-CoV-2 induced coagulopathy. *Cell. Mol. Biol. Lett.* **2022**, *27*, 6. [CrossRef]
153. Shimizu, T.; Saito, T.; Aoki-Saito, H.; Okada, S.; Ikeda, H.; Nakakura, T.; Fukuda, H.; Arai, S.; Fujiwara, K.; Nakajima, Y. Resolvin E3 ameliorates high-fat diet-induced insulin resistance via the phosphatidylinositol-3-kinase/Akt signaling pathway in adipocytes. *FASEB J.* **2022**, *36*, e22188. [CrossRef] [PubMed]
154. Traina, G.; Bolzacchini, E.; Bonini, M.; Contini, D.; Mantecca, P.; Caimmi, S.M.E.; Licari, A. Role of air pollutants mediated oxidative stress in respiratory diseases. *Pediatr. Allergy Immunol.* **2022**, *33*, 38–40. [CrossRef] [PubMed]
155. Li, H.; Zhao, C.; Tian, Y.; Lu, J.; Zhang, G.; Liang, S.; Chen, D.; Liu, X.; Kuang, W.; Zhu, M. Src family kinases and pulmonary fibrosis: A review. *Biomed. Pharmacother.* **2020**, *127*, 110183. [CrossRef] [PubMed]
156. Agraval, H.; Sharma, J.R.; Prakash, N.; Yadav, U.C. Fisetin suppresses cigarette smoke extract-induced epithelial to mesenchymal transition of airway epithelial cells through regulating COX-2/MMPs/β-catenin pathway. *Chem. Biol. Interact.* **2022**, *351*, 109771. [CrossRef]
157. Severgnini, M.; Takahashi, S.; Tu, P.; Perides, G.; Homer, R.J.; Jhung, J.W.; Bhavsar, D.; Cochran, B.H.; Simon, A.R. Inhibition of the Src and Jak kinases protects against lipopolysaccharide-induced acute lung injury. *Am. J. Respir. Crit. Care Med.* **2005**, *171*, 858–867. [CrossRef]
158. van der Vliet, A. Nox enzymes in allergic airway inflammation. *Biochim. Biophys. Acta (BBA) General. Subj.* **2011**, *1810*, 1035–1044. [CrossRef]
159. Albano, G.D.; Gagliardo, R.P.; Montalbano, A.M.; Profita, M. Overview of the mechanisms of oxidative stress: Impact in inflammation of the airway diseases. *Antioxidants* **2022**, *11*, 2237. [CrossRef]
160. Mumby, S.; Adcock, I.M. Recent evidence from omic analysis for redox signalling and mitochondrial oxidative stress in COPD. *J. Inflamm.* **2022**, *19*, 10. [CrossRef]
161. Kyo, M.; Zhu, Z.; Nanishi, M.; Shibata, R.; Ooka, T.; Freishtat, R.J.; Mansbach, J.M.; Camargo Jr, C.A.; Hasegawa, K. Association of nasopharyngeal and serum glutathione metabolism with bronchiolitis severity and asthma risk: A prospective multicenter cohort study. *Metabolites* **2022**, *12*, 674. [CrossRef]
162. Van der Vliet, A.; Janssen-Heininger, Y.M.; Anathy, V. Oxidative stress in chronic lung disease: From mitochondrial dysfunction to dysregulated redox signaling. *Mol. Asp. Med.* **2018**, *63*, 59–69. [CrossRef]
163. Gao, Z.; Ye, J. Inhibition of transcriptional activity of c-JUN by SIRT1. *Biochem. Biophys. Res. Commun.* **2008**, *376*, 793–796. [CrossRef] [PubMed]
164. Zhang, R.; Chen, H.-Z.; Liu, J.-J.; Jia, Y.-Y.; Zhang, Z.-Q.; Yang, R.-F.; Zhang, Y.; Xu, J.; Wei, Y.-S.; Liu, D.-P. SIRT1 suppresses activator protein-1 transcriptional activity and cyclooxygenase-2 expression in macrophages. *J. Biol. Chem.* **2010**, *285*, 7097–7110. [CrossRef] [PubMed]

165. Michaeloudes, C.; Abubakar-Waziri, H.; Lakhdar, R.; Raby, K.; Dixey, P.; Adcock, I.M.; Mumby, S.; Bhavsar, P.K.; Chung, K.F. Molecular mechanisms of oxidative stress in asthma. *Mol. Asp. Med.* **2022**, *85*, 101026. [CrossRef] [PubMed]
166. Kohri, K.; Ueki, I.; Shim, J.; Burgel, P.; Oh, Y.; Tam, D.; Dao-Pick, T.; Nadel, J. Pseudomonas aeruginosa induces MUC5AC production via epidermal growth factor receptor. *Eur. Respir. J.* **2002**, *20*, 1263–1270. [CrossRef]
167. Lee, Y.C.; Lee, K.S.; Park, S.J.; Park, H.S.; Lim, J.S.; Park, K.H.; Im, M.J.; Choi, I.W.; Lee, H.K.; Kim, U.H. Blockade of airway hyperresponsiveness and inflammation in a murine model of asthma by a prodrug of cysteine, L-2-oxothiazolidine-4-carboxylic acid. *FASEB J.* **2004**, *18*, 1917–1919. [CrossRef]
168. Oh, J.H.; Park, E.J.; Park, J.-W.; Lee, J.; Lee, S.H.; Kwon, T.K. A novel cyclin-dependent kinase inhibitor down-regulates tumor necrosis factor-α (TNF-α)-induced expression of cell adhesion molecules by inhibition of NF-κB activation in human pulmonary epithelial cells. *Int. Immunopharmacol.* **2010**, *10*, 572–579. [CrossRef]
169. Lee, I.-T.; Luo, S.-F.; Lee, C.-W.; Wang, S.-W.; Lin, C.-C.; Chang, C.-C.; Chen, Y.-L.; Chau, L.-Y.; Yang, C.-M. Overexpression of HO-1 protects against TNF-α-mediated airway inflammation by down-regulation of TNFR1-dependent oxidative stress. *Am. J. Pathol.* **2009**, *175*, 519–532. [CrossRef]
170. Lin, H.-C.; Tu, Y.-F.; Hwang, G.-J.; Huang, H. From precision education to precision medicine. *Educ. Technol. Soc.* **2021**, *24*, 123–137.
171. Coverstone, A.M.; Seibold, M.A.; Peters, M.C. Diagnosis and management of T2-high asthma. *J. Allergy Clin. Immunol. Pract.* **2020**, *8*, 442–450. [CrossRef]
172. Tashkin, D.P.; Lipworth, B.; Brattsand, R. Benefit: Risk profile of budesonide in obstructive airways disease. *Drugs* **2019**, *79*, 1757–1775. [CrossRef]
173. Proboszcz, M.; Goryca, K.; Nejman-Gryz, P.; Przybyłowski, T.; Górska, K.; Krenke, R.; Paplińska-Goryca, M. Phenotypic variations of mild-to-moderate obstructive pulmonary diseases according to airway inflammation and clinical features. *J. Inflamm. Res.* **2021**, 2793–2806. [CrossRef] [PubMed]
174. Breiteneder, H.; Peng, Y.Q.; Agache, I.; Diamant, Z.; Eiwegger, T.; Fokkens, W.J.; Traidl-Hoffmann, C.; Nadeau, K.; O'Hehir, R.E.; O'Mahony, L. Biomarkers for diagnosis and prediction of therapy responses in allergic diseases and asthma. *Allergy* **2020**, *75*, 3039–3068. [CrossRef] [PubMed]
175. Parnes, J.R.; Molfino, N.A.; Colice, G.; Martin, U.; Corren, J.; Menzies-Gow, A. Targeting TSLP in asthma. *J. Asthma Allergy* **2022**, 749–765. [CrossRef] [PubMed]
176. Allam, V.S.R.R.; Pavlidis, S.; Liu, G.; Kermani, N.Z.; Simpson, J.; To, J.; Donnelly, S.; Guo, Y.-K.; Hansbro, P.M.; Phipps, S. Macrophage migration inhibitory factor promotes glucocorticoid resistance of neutrophilic inflammation in a murine model of severe asthma. *Thorax* **2023**, *78*, 661–673. [CrossRef]
177. Lunding, L.P.; Skouras, D.B.; Vock, C.; Dinarello, C.A.; Wegmann, M. The NLRP3 Inflammasome Inhibitor OLT1177® Ameliorates Experimental Allergic Asthma in Mice. *J. Immunol.* **2022**, *208*, 109.102. [CrossRef]
178. Uysal, P. Novel Applications of Biomarkers in Chronic Obstructive Pulmonary Disease. In *Biomarkers in Medicine*; Bentham Science Publishers: Sharjah, United Arab Emirates, 2022; p. 425.
179. Gevaert, P.; Han, J.K.; Smith, S.G.; Sousa, A.R.; Howarth, P.H.; Yancey, S.W.; Chan, R.; Bachert, C. The Roles of Eosinophils and Interleukin-5 in the Pathophysiology of Chronic Rhinosinusitis with Nasal Polyps. In *International Forum of Allergy & Rhinology*; Willey: Hoboken, NJ, USA, 2022; pp. 1413–1423.
180. Hameed, R.M.; Abood, H.A.A.N.; Ahmed, M.M. *Interleukin-5 and Interleukin-5 Receptor Polymorphism in Asthma*; IntechOpen: London, UK, 2022.
181. Pelaia, C.; Paoletti, G.; Puggioni, F.; Racca, F.; Pelaia, G.; Canonica, G.W.; Heffler, E. Interleukin-5 in the pathophysiology of severe asthma. *Front. Physiol.* **2019**, *10*, 1514. [CrossRef]
182. Kay, A.B.; Hamid, Q.; Robinson, D.S.; Bentley, A.M.; Tsicopoulos, A.; Ying, S.; Moqbel, R.; Corrigan, C.J.; Durham, S.R. Asthma, Eosinophils, and Interleukin-5. In *Eosinophils in Allergy and Inflammation*; CRC Press: Boca Raton, FL, USA, 2019; pp. 395–406.
183. Hearn, A.P.; Kent, B.D.; Jackson, D.J. Biologic treatment options for severe asthma. *Curr. Opin. Immunol.* **2020**, *66*, 151–160. [CrossRef]
184. Shrimanker, R.; Keene, O.; Hynes, G.; Wenzel, S.; Yancey, S.; Pavord, I.D. Prognostic and predictive value of blood eosinophil count, fractional exhaled nitric oxide, and their combination in severe asthma: A post hoc analysis. *Am. J. Respir. Crit. Care Med.* **2019**, *200*, 1308–1312. [CrossRef]
185. FitzGerald, J.M.; Bleecker, E.R.; Nair, P.; Korn, S.; Ohta, K.; Lommatzsch, M.; Ferguson, G.T.; Busse, W.W.; Barker, P.; Sproule, S.; et al. Benralizumab, an anti-interleukin-5 receptor α monoclonal antibody, as add-on treatment for patients with severe, uncontrolled, eosinophilic asthma (CALIMA): A randomised, double-blind, placebo-controlled phase 3 trial. *Lancet* **2016**, *388*, 2128–2141. [CrossRef]
186. Brightling, C.E.; Bleecker, E.R.; Panettieri, R.A.; Bafadhel, M.; She, D.; Ward, C.K.; Xu, X.; Birrell, C.; van der Merwe, R. Benralizumab for chronic obstructive pulmonary disease and sputum eosinophilia: A randomised, double-blind, placebo-controlled, phase 2a study. *Lancet Respir. Med.* **2014**, *2*, 891–901. [CrossRef]

187. Wu, A.Y.; Sur, S.; Grant, J.A.; Tripple, J.W. Interleukin-4/interleukin-13 versus interleukin-5: A comparison of molecular targets in biologic therapy for the treatment of severe asthma. *Curr. Opin. Allergy Clin. Immunol.* **2019**, *19*, 30–37. [CrossRef] [PubMed]
188. Bai, J.-y.; Li, Y.; Xue, G.-h.; Li, K.-r.; Zheng, Y.-F.; Zhang, Z.-q.; Jiang, Q.; Liu, Y.-y.; Zhou, X.-z.; Cao, C. Requirement of Gαi1 and Gαi3 in interleukin-4-induced signaling, macrophage M2 polarization and allergic asthma response. *Theranostics* **2021**, *11*, 4894. [CrossRef] [PubMed]
189. Husna, S.M.N.; Shukri, N.M.; Ashari, N.S.M.; Wong, K.K. IL-4/IL-13 axis as therapeutic targets in allergic rhinitis and asthma. *PeerJ* **2022**, *10*, e13444. [CrossRef] [PubMed]
190. Wenzel, S.; Ford, L.; Pearlman, D.; Spector, S.; Sher, L.; Skobieranda, F.; Wang, L.; Kirkesseli, S.; Rocklin, R.; Bock, B. Dupilumab in persistent asthma with elevated eosinophil levels. *N. Engl. J. Med.* **2013**, *368*, 2455–2466. [CrossRef]
191. Shastri, M.D.; Allam, V.S.R.R.; Shukla, S.D.; Jha, N.K.; Paudel, K.R.; Peterson, G.M.; Patel, R.P.; Hansbro, P.M.; Chellappan, D.K.; Dua, K. Interleukin-13: A pivotal target against influenza-induced exacerbation of chronic lung diseases. *Life Sci.* **2021**, *283*, 119871. [CrossRef]
192. Scott, G.; Asrat, S.; Allinne, J.; Lim, W.K.; Nagashima, K.; Birchard, D.; Srivatsan, S.; Ajithdoss, D.K.; Oyejide, A.; Ben, L.-H. IL-4 and IL-13, not eosinophils, drive type 2 airway inflammation, remodeling and lung function decline. *Cytokine* **2023**, *162*, 156091. [CrossRef]
193. Wechsler, M.E. Current and emerging biologic therapies for asthma and COPD. *Respir. Care* **2018**, *63*, 699–707. [CrossRef]
194. Osei, E.T.; Brandsma, C.-A.; Timens, W.; Heijink, I.H.; Hackett, T.-L. Current perspectives on the role of interleukin-1 signalling in the pathogenesis of asthma and COPD. *Eur. Respir. J.* **2020**, *55*, 1900563. [CrossRef]
195. Behzadi, P.; Sameer, A.S.; Nissar, S.; Banday, M.Z.; Gajdács, M.; García-Perdomo, H.A.; Akhtar, K.; Pinheiro, M.; Magnusson, P.; Sarshar, M. The Interleukin-1 (IL-1) superfamily cytokines and their single nucleotide polymorphisms (SNPs). *J. Immunol. Res.* **2022**, *2022*, 2054431. [CrossRef]
196. Ma, Y.; Thornton, S.; Boivin, G.P.; Hirsh, D.; Hirsch, R.; Hirsch, E. Altered susceptibility to collagen-induced arthritis in transgenic mice with aberrant expression of interleukin-1 receptor antagonist. *Arthritis Rheum.* **1998**, *41*, 1798–1805. [CrossRef]
197. Zhang, Y.-L.; Zhang, R.-G.; Chen, F.-Y.; Qiu, Z.-E.; Chen, L.; Huang, Z.-X.; Huang, J.; Zhu, Y.-X.; Zhao, L.; Zhou, W.-L. Cellular mechanism underlying the facilitation of contractile response induced by tumor necrosis factor-α in mouse tracheal smooth muscle. *Am. J. Pathol.* **2022**, *192*, 104–111. [CrossRef] [PubMed]
198. Liu, H.; Li, Y.; Zhang, X.; Shi, M.; Meng, X.; Li, D. Clinical Efficacy of Qizhi Yifei Granules on Patients with High Peripheral Blood Eosinophil-Type Acute Exacerbation of Chronic Obstructive Pulmonary Disease. *Curr. Top. Nutraceutical Res.* **2022**, *20*, 298. [CrossRef]
199. Ghosh, A.J.; Hobbs, B.D.; Yun, J.H.; Saferali, A.; Moll, M.; Xu, Z.; Chase, R.P.; Morrow, J.; Ziniti, J.; Sciurba, F. Lung tissue shows divergent gene expression between chronic obstructive pulmonary disease and idiopathic pulmonary fibrosis. *Respir. Res.* **2022**, *23*, 97. [CrossRef] [PubMed]
200. Karampitsakos, T.; Papaioannou, O.; Sampsonas, F.; Tzouvelekis, A. Infliximab-induced interstitial lung disease. *BMJ Case Rep. CP* **2021**, *14*, e245726. [CrossRef] [PubMed]
201. Velthuis, K.; Jessurun, N.T.; Nguyen, T.D.; Scholl, J.; Jansen, J.R.; van Lint, J.A.; Kosse, L.J.; Ten Klooster, P.M.; Vonkeman, H.E. First-time adverse drug reactions, survival analysis, and the share of adverse drug reactions in treatment discontinuation in real-world rheumatoid arthritis patients: A comparison of first-time treatment with adalimumab and etanercept. *Expert Opin. Drug Saf.* **2023**, *22*, 485–492. [CrossRef]
202. Osipov, V.N.; Khachatryan, D.S.; Balaev, A.N. Biologically active quinazoline-based hydroxamic acids. *Med. Chem. Res.* **2020**, *29*, 831–845. [CrossRef]
203. Henderson, A.G.; Davis, J.M.; Keith, J.D.; Green, M.E.; Oden, A.M.; Rowe, S.M.; Birket, S.E. Static mucus impairs bacterial clearance and allows chronic infection with Pseudomonas aeruginosa in the cystic fibrosis rat. *Eur. Respir. J.* **2022**, *60*, 2101032. [CrossRef]
204. He, Y.; Peng, S.; Xiong, W.; Xu, Y.; Liu, J. Association between Polymorphism of Interleukin-1beta and Interleukin-1 Receptor Antagonist Gene and Asthma Risk: A Meta-Analysis. *Sci. World J.* **2015**, *2015*, 685684. [CrossRef]
205. Rogliani, P.; Calzetta, L.; Ora, J.; Matera, M.G. Canakinumab for the treatment of chronic obstructive pulmonary disease. *Pulm. Pharmacol. Ther.* **2015**, *31*, 15–27. [CrossRef]
206. Croasdell Lucchini, A.; Gachanja, N.N.; Rossi, A.G.; Dorward, D.A.; Lucas, C.D. Epithelial cells and inflammation in pulmonary wound repair. *Cells* **2021**, *10*, 339. [CrossRef]
207. Nieri, D.; Daniele, M.; Lombardi, S.; Bazzan, E.; Santerini, S.; De Cusatis, G.; Vagaggini, B.; Cosio, M.G.; Saetta, M.; Paggiaro, P. Circulating extracellular vesicles are associated with disease severity and interleukin-6 levels in COPD: A Pilot study. *J. Clin. Med.* **2021**, *10*, 5014. [CrossRef] [PubMed]
208. Santoro, A.; Bientinesi, E.; Monti, D. Immunosenescence and inflammaging in the aging process: Age-related diseases or longevity? *Ageing Res. Rev.* **2021**, *71*, 101422. [CrossRef] [PubMed]
209. Agrawal, A.; Tay, J.; Ton, S.; Agrawal, S.; Gupta, S. Increased reactivity of dendritic cells from aged subjects to self-antigen, the human DNA. *J. Immunol.* **2009**, *182*, 1138–1145. [CrossRef] [PubMed]

210. Mehrotra, N.; Freire, A.X.; Bauer, D.C.; Harris, T.B.; Newman, A.B.; Kritchevsky, S.B.; Meibohm, B.; Study, H.A. Predictors of mortality in elderly subjects with obstructive airway disease: The PILE score. *Ann. Epidemiol.* **2010**, *20*, 223–232. [CrossRef]
211. Nixon, L.S.; Yung, B.; Bell, S.C.; Stuart Elborn, J.; Shale, D.J. Circulating immunoreactive interleukin-6 in cystic fibrosis. *Am. J. Respir. Crit. Care Med.* **1998**, *157*, 1764–1769. [CrossRef]
212. Corren, J. New targeted therapies for uncontrolled asthma. *J. Allergy Clin. Immunol. Pract.* **2019**, *7*, 1394–1403. [CrossRef]
213. Kishimoto, T. IL-6: From its discovery to clinical applications. *Int. Immunol.* **2010**, *22*, 347–352. [CrossRef]
214. Voynow, J.A.; Shinbashi, M. Neutrophil elastase and chronic lung disease. *Biomolecules* **2021**, *11*, 1065. [CrossRef]
215. Krick, S.; Baumlin, N.; Aller, S.P.; Aguiar, C.; Grabner, A.; Sailland, J.; Mendes, E.; Schmid, A.; Qi, L.; David, N.V. Klotho inhibits interleukin-8 secretion from cystic fibrosis airway epithelia. *Sci. Rep.* **2017**, *7*, 14388. [CrossRef]
216. Lampronti, I.; Manzione, M.G.; Sacchetti, G.; Ferrari, D.; Spisani, S.; Bezzerri, V.; Finotti, A.; Borgatti, M.; Dechecchi, M.C.; Miolo, G. Differential Effects of Angelicin Analogues on NF-κB Activity and IL-8 Gene Expression in Cystic Fibrosis IB3-1 Cells. *Mediat. Inflamm.* **2017**, *2017*, 2389487. [CrossRef]
217. Jaudszus, A.; Arnold, C.; Hentschel, J.; Hünniger, K.; Baier, M.; Mainz, J.G. Increased cytokines in cystic fibrosis patients' upper airways during a new P. aeruginosa colonization. *Pediatr. Pulmonol.* **2018**, *53*, 881–887. [CrossRef] [PubMed]
218. Weber, A.; Wasiliew, P.; Kracht, M. Interleukin-1 (IL-1) pathway. *Sci. Signal.* **2010**, *3*, cm1. [CrossRef] [PubMed]
219. Schneider, D.; Ganesan, S.; Comstock, A.T.; Meldrum, C.A.; Mahidhara, R.; Goldsmith, A.M.; Curtis, J.L.; Martinez, F.J.; Hershenson, M.B.; Sajjan, U. Increased cytokine response of rhinovirus-infected airway epithelial cells in chronic obstructive pulmonary disease. *Am. J. Respir. Crit. Care Med.* **2010**, *182*, 332–340. [CrossRef] [PubMed]
220. Sarir, H.; Mortaz, E.; Janse, W.T.; Givi, M.E.; Nijkamp, F.P.; Folkerts, G. IL-8 production by macrophages is synergistically enhanced when cigarette smoke is combined with TNF-α. *Biochem. Pharmacol.* **2010**, *79*, 698–705. [CrossRef]
221. Zhang, X.; Zheng, H.; Zhang, H.; Ma, W.; Wang, F.; Liu, C.; He, S. Increased interleukin (IL)-8 and decreased IL-17 production in chronic obstructive pulmonary disease (COPD) provoked by cigarette smoke. *Cytokine* **2011**, *56*, 717–725. [CrossRef]
222. Huang, A.-X.; Lu, L.-W.; Liu, W.-J.; Huang, M. Plasma inflammatory cytokine IL-4, IL-8, IL-10, and TNF-α levels correlate with pulmonary function in patients with asthma-chronic obstructive pulmonary disease (COPD) overlap syndrome. *Med. Sci. Monit. Int. Med. J. Exp. Clin. Res.* **2016**, *22*, 2800. [CrossRef]
223. Mahler, D.A.; Huang, S.; Tabrizi, M.; Bell, G.M. Efficacy and safety of a monoclonal antibody recognizing interleukin-8 in COPD: A pilot study. *Chest* **2004**, *126*, 926–934. [CrossRef]
224. Lazaar, A.L.; Miller, B.E.; Tabberer, M.; Yonchuk, J.; Leidy, N.; Ambery, C.; Bloomer, J.; Watz, H.; Tal-Singer, R. Effect of the CXCR2 antagonist danirixin on symptoms and health status in COPD. *Eur. Respir. J.* **2018**, *52*, 1801020. [CrossRef]
225. Rennard, S.I.; Dale, D.C.; Donohue, J.F.; Kanniess, F.; Magnussen, H.; Sutherland, E.R.; Watz, H.; Lu, S.; Stryszak, P.; Rosenberg, E. CXCR2 antagonist MK-7123. A phase 2 proof-of-concept trial for chronic obstructive pulmonary disease. *Am. J. Respir. Crit. Care Med.* **2015**, *191*, 1001–1011. [CrossRef]
226. Almikhlafi, M.A.; Haghayeghi, K.; Gardner, A. Endothelin A (ETA) and Endothelin B (ETB) Receptor Subtypes Potentiate Epidermal Growth Factor (EGF)-Mediated Proliferation in Human Asthmatic Bronchial Airway Smooth Muscle. *Cureus* **2022**, *14*, e28333. [CrossRef]
227. Dyneva, M.E.; Aminova, G.E.; Kurbacheva, O.; Ilina, N.I. Dupilumab: New opportunities for the treatment of asthma and chronic rhinosinusitis with nasal polyps. *Russ. J. Allergy* **2021**, *18*, 18–31. [CrossRef]
228. Ijaz, B.; Shabbir, A.; Shahzad, M.; Mobashar, A.; Sharif, M.; Basheer, M.I.; Tareen, R.B. Amelioration of airway inflammation and pulmonary edema by Teucrium stocksianum via attenuation of pro-inflammatory cytokines and up-regulation of AQP1 and AQP5. *Respir. Physiol. Neurobiol.* **2021**, *284*, 103569. [CrossRef] [PubMed]
229. Naz, S.; Ashraf, S.; Parvez, M.K.; Al-Dosari, M.S.; Ul-Haq, Z. Structure and ligand-based drug discovery of IL-4 inhibitors via interaction-energy-based learning approaches. *J. Biomol. Struct. Dyn.* **2022**, *40*, 6503–6521. [CrossRef] [PubMed]
230. Pelaia, G.; Canonica, G.W.; Matucci, A.; Paolini, R.; Triggiani, M.; Paggiaro, P. Targeted therapy in severe asthma today: Focus on immunoglobulin E. *Drug Des. Dev. Ther.* **2017**, *11*, 1979–1987. [CrossRef]
231. Doran, E.; Cai, F.; Holweg, C.T.; Wong, K.; Brumm, J.; Arron, J.R. Interleukin-13 in asthma and other eosinophilic disorders. *Front. Med.* **2017**, *4*, 139. [CrossRef]
232. Nwaru, B.I.; Ekerljung, L.; Rådinger, M.; Bjerg, A.; Mincheva, R.; Malmhäll, C.; Axelsson, M.; Wennergren, G.; Lotvall, J.; Lundbäck, B. Cohort profile: The West Sweden Asthma Study (WSAS): A multidisciplinary population-based longitudinal study of asthma, allergy and respiratory conditions in adults. *BMJ Open* **2019**, *9*, e027808. [CrossRef]
233. Maskey, A.; Srivastava, K.; Soffer, G.; Dunkin, D.; Yuan, Q.; Li, X.-M. Induction of severe eosinophilic esophagitis and multi-organ inflammation by airborne allergens is associated with IL-4/IL-13 and CCL11 but not IgE in genetic susceptible mice. *J. Inflamm. Res.* **2022**, *15*, 5527–5540. [CrossRef]
234. Yanagibashi, T.; Satoh, M.; Nagai, Y.; Koike, M.; Takatsu, K. Allergic diseases: From bench to clinic-Contribution of the discovery of interleukin-5. *Cytokine* **2017**, *98*, 59–70. [CrossRef]

235. Farah, C.S.; Badal, T.; Reed, N.; Rogers, P.G.; King, G.G.; Thamrin, C.; Peters, M.J.; Seccombe, L.M. Mepolizumab improves small airway function in severe eosinophilic asthma. *Respir. Med.* **2019**, *148*, 49–53. [CrossRef]
236. Van Toor, J.J.; van der Mark, S.C.; Kappen, J.H.; In't Veen, J.; Braunstahl, G.J. Mepolizumab add-on therapy in a real world cohort of patients with severe eosinophilic asthma: Response rate, effectiveness, and safety. *J. Asthma* **2021**, *58*, 651–658. [CrossRef]
237. Simpson, J.; Bafadhel, M. Alternatives to induced sputum for identifying inflammatory subtypes of asthma. *Respirology* **2017**, *22*. [CrossRef] [PubMed]
238. Mukherjee, M.; Aleman Paramo, F.; Kjarsgaard, M.; Salter, B.; Nair, G.; LaVigne, N.; Radford, K.; Sehmi, R.; Nair, P. Weight-adjusted intravenous reslizumab in severe asthma with inadequate response to fixed-dose subcutaneous mepolizumab. *Am. J. Respir. Crit. Care Med.* **2018**, *197*, 38–46. [CrossRef] [PubMed]
239. Vatrella, A.; Maglio, A.; Pelaia, C.; Ciampo, L.; Pelaia, G.; Vitale, C. Eosinophilic inflammation: An appealing target for pharmacologic treatments in severe asthma. *Biomedicines* **2022**, *10*, 2181. [CrossRef] [PubMed]
240. Rayees, S.; Din, I.; Rayees, S.; Din, I. Cytokine-Based Therapies. In *Asthma: Pathophysiology, Herbal and Modern Therapeutic Interventions*; Springer: Berlin/Heidelberg, Germany, 2021; pp. 27–32.
241. Gong, F.; Pan, Y.H.; Huang, X.; Zhu, H.Y.; Jiang, D.L. From bench to bedside: Therapeutic potential of interleukin-9 in the treatment of asthma. *Exp. Ther. Med.* **2017**, *13*, 389–394. [CrossRef]
242. Oh, C.K.; Leigh, R.; McLaurin, K.K.; Kim, K.; Hultquist, M.; Molfino, N.A. A randomized, controlled trial to evaluate the effect of an anti-interleukin-9 monoclonal antibody in adults with uncontrolled asthma. *Respir. Res.* **2013**, *14*, 93. [CrossRef]
243. Pera, T.; Penn, R.B. G Protein-Coupled Receptors in Airway Smooth Muscle Function and Obstructive Lung Disease. In *Signal Transduction and Smooth Muscle*; CRC Press: Boca Raton, FL, USA, 2018; pp. 205–243.
244. Iftikhar, I.H.; Schimmel, M.; Bender, W.; Swenson, C.; Amrol, D. Comparative efficacy of anti IL-4, IL-5 and IL-13 drugs for treatment of eosinophilic asthma: A network meta-analysis. *Lung* **2018**, *196*, 517–530. [CrossRef]
245. Jain, M.; Doughty, D.; Clawson, C.; Li, X.; White, N.; Agoram, B.; van der Merwe, R. Tralokinumab pharmacokinetics and tolerability when administered by different subcutaneous injection methods and rates. *Int. J. Clin. Pharmacol. Ther.* **2017**, *55*, 606. [CrossRef]
246. Shaikh, S.B.; Prabhu, A.; Bhandary, Y.P. Interleukin-17A: A potential therapeutic target in chronic lung diseases. *Endocr. Metab. Immune Disord. Drug Targets* **2019**, *19*, 921–928. [CrossRef]
247. Van Lommel, A.T.; Bollé, T.; Hellings, P.W. Pulmonary neuroepithelial bodies as hypothetical immunomodulators: Some new findings and a review of the literature. In *Airway Chemoreceptors in Vertebrates*; Taylor & Francis Group: Abingdon, UK, 2019; pp. 311–330.
248. Pelaia, C.; Crimi, C.; Vatrella, A.; Busceti, M.T.; Gaudio, A.; Garofalo, E.; Bruni, A.; Terracciano, R.; Pelaia, G. New treatments for asthma: From the pathogenic role of prostaglandin D2 to the therapeutic effects of fevipiprant. *Pharmacol. Res.* **2020**, *155*, 104490. [CrossRef]
249. Moermans, C.; Damas, K.; Guiot, J.; Njock, M.-S.; Corhay, J.-L.; Henket, M.; Schleich, F.; Louis, R. Sputum IL-25, IL-33 and TSLP, IL-23 and IL-36 in airway obstructive diseases. Reduced levels of IL-36 in eosinophilic phenotype. *Cytokine* **2021**, *140*, 155421. [CrossRef]
250. Hatta, M.; Surachmanto, E.E.; Islam, A.A.; Wahid, S. Expression of mRNA IL-17F and sIL-17F in atopic asthma patients. *BMC Res. Notes* **2017**, *10*, 202. [CrossRef] [PubMed]
251. Fowler, P.C.; Naluai, Å.T.; Oscarsson, M.; Torkzadeh, S.; Bohman, A.; Bende, M.; Harandi, A.M. Differential expression of angiotensin-converting enzyme 2 in nasal tissue of patients with chronic rhinosinusitis with nasal polyps. *medRxiv* **2021**. [CrossRef]
252. Naji AL-Hasnawi, A.T.; Jabbar AL-Hasnawi, S.M. Role of interleukin 25 and interleukin 33 as immunological markers in pediatric asthma. *Eur. Asian J. Biosci.* **2020**, *14*, 4625–4630.
253. Bonser, L.R.; Erle, D.J. The airway epithelium in asthma. *Adv. Immunol.* **2019**, *142*, 1–34.
254. Kearley, J.; Buckland, K.F.; Mathie, S.A.; Lloyd, C.M. Resolution of allergic inflammation and airway hyperreactivity is dependent upon disruption of the T1/ST2–IL-33 pathway. *Am. J. Respir. Crit. Care Med.* **2009**, *179*, 772–781. [CrossRef]
255. Ádám, D.; Arany, J.; Tóth, K.F.; Tóth, B.I.; Szöllősi, A.G.; Oláh, A. Opioidergic signaling—A neglected, yet potentially important player in atopic dermatitis. *Int. J. Mol. Sci.* **2022**, *23*, 4140. [CrossRef]
256. Nguyen, T.H.; Maltby, S.; Tay, H.L.; Eyers, F.; Foster, P.S.; Yang, M. Identification of IFN-γ and IL-27 as critical regulators of respiratory syncytial virus–induced exacerbation of allergic airways disease in a mouse model. *J. Immunol.* **2018**, *200*, 237–247. [CrossRef]
257. Plichta, J.; Kuna, P.; Panek, M. Biologic drugs in the treatment of chronic inflammatory pulmonary diseases: Recent developments and future perspectives. *Front. Immunol.* **2023**, *14*, 1207641. [CrossRef]
258. Yamashita, N.; Tashimo, H.; Ishida, H.; Kaneko, F.; Nakano, J.; Kato, H.; Hirai, K.; Horiuchi, T.; Ohta, K. Attenuation of airway hyperresponsiveness in a murine asthma model by neutralization of granulocyte–macrophage colony-stimulating factor (GM-CSF). *Cell. Immunol.* **2002**, *219*, 92–97. [CrossRef]

259. Dhagat, U.; Hercus, T.R.; Broughton, S.E.; Nero, T.L.; Cheung Tung Shing, K.S.; Barry, E.F.; Thomson, C.A.; Bryson, S.; Pai, E.F.; McClure, B.J. The mechanism of GM-CSF inhibition by human GM-CSF auto-antibodies suggests novel therapeutic opportunities. *MAbs* **2018**, *10*, 1018–1029. [CrossRef]
260. Ortega, H.G.; Liu, M.C.; Pavord, I.D.; Brusselle, G.G.; FitzGerald, J.M.; Chetta, A.; Humbert, M.; Katz, L.E.; Keene, O.N.; Yancey, S.W.; et al. Mepolizumab treatment in patients with severe eosinophilic asthma. *N. Engl. J. Med.* **2014**, *371*, 1198–1207. [CrossRef] [PubMed]
261. Castro, M.; Zangrilli, J.; Wechsler, M.E.; Bateman, E.D.; Brusselle, G.G.; Bardin, P.; Murphy, K.; Maspero, J.F.; O'Brien, C.; Korn, S. Reslizumab for inadequately controlled asthma with elevated blood eosinophil counts: Results from two multicentre, parallel, double-blind, randomised, placebo-controlled, phase 3 trials. *Lancet Respir. Med.* **2015**, *3*, 355–366. [CrossRef] [PubMed]
262. Wenzel, S.; Castro, M.; Corren, J.; Maspero, J.; Wang, L.; Zhang, B.; Pirozzi, G.; Sutherland, E.R.; Evans, R.R.; Joish, V.N.; et al. Dupilumab efficacy and safety in adults with uncontrolled persistent asthma despite use of medium-to-high-dose inhaled corticosteroids plus a long-acting β2 agonist: A randomised double-blind placebo-controlled pivotal phase 2b dose-ranging trial. *Lancet* **2016**, *388*, 31–44. [CrossRef] [PubMed]
263. Esty, B.; Harb, H.; Bartnikas, L.M.; Charbonnier, L.M.; Massoud, A.H.; LeonAstudillo, C.; Visner, G.; Subramaniam, M.; Phipatanakul, W.; Chatila, T.A. Treatment of Severe Persistent Asthma With IL-6 Receptor Blockade. *J. Allergy Clin. Immunol. Pract.* **2019**, *7*, 1639–1642.e4. [CrossRef] [PubMed]
264. Menzies-Gow, A.; Bafadhel, M.; Busse, W.W. An expert consensus framework for asthma remission as a treatment goal. *J. Allergy Clin. Immunol.* **2020**, *145*, 757–765. [CrossRef]
265. Kelsen, S.G.; Agache, I.O.; Soong, W. Astegolimab (anti-ST2) efficacy and safety in adults with severe asthma: A randomized clinical trial. *J. Allergy Clin. Immunol.* **2021**, *148*, 790–798. [CrossRef]
266. Wechsler, M.E.; Ruddy, M.K.; Pavord, I.D. Efficacy and safety of itepekimab in patients with moderate-to-severe asthma. *N. Engl. J. Med.* **2021**, *385*, 1656–1668. [CrossRef]
267. Brightling, C.E.; Nair, P.; Cousins, D.J. Risankizumab in severe asthma–A phase 2a, placebo-controlled trial. *N. Engl. J. Med.* **2021**, *385*, 1669–1679. [CrossRef]
268. Alcorn, J.F.; Crowe, C.R.; Kolls, J.K. TH17 cells in asthma and COPD. *Annu. Rev. Physiol.* **2010**, *72*, 495–516. [CrossRef]
269. Barnes, P.J. The cytokine network in asthma and chronic obstructive pulmonary disease. *J. Clin. Investig.* **2008**, *11*, 3546–3556. [CrossRef]

cells

MDPI

Review

Role of Protein Tyrosine Phosphatases in Inflammatory Bowel Disease, Celiac Disease and Diabetes: Focus on the Intestinal Mucosa

Claudia Bellomo [1,†], Francesca Furone [1,†], Roberta Rotondo [2,‡], Ilaria Ciscognetti [1,‡], Martina Carpinelli [1], Martina Nicoletti [1], Genoveffa D'Aniello [3], Leandra Sepe [4], Maria Vittoria Barone [1,3,*] and Merlin Nanayakkara [5]

1 Department of Translational Medical Science, Section of Pediatrics, University Federico II, Via S. Pansini 5, 80131 Naples, Italy; claudia.bellomo@unina.it (C.B.); francesca.furone@gmail.com (F.F.); ilariaciscognetti@gmail.com (I.C.); martinacarpinelli@gmail.com (M.C.); martina.nicoletti0@gmail.com (M.N.)
2 Department of Medicine and Surgery, University of Parma, 43121 Parma, Italy; robertarot.97@gmail.com
3 ELFID (European Laboratory for the Investigation of Food-Induced Diseases), University Federico II, Via S. Pansini 5, 80131 Naples, Italy; jedaniello1998@gmail.com
4 Department of Molecular Medicine and Medical Biotechnology, University of Naples Federico II, 80131 Naples, Italy; leandra.sepe@unina.it
5 Federico II University Hospital, 80131 Naples, Italy; merlin.nanayakka@unina.it
* Correspondence: mv.barone@unina.it
† These authors contributed equally to the manuscript.
‡ These authors contributed equally to the manuscript.

Abstract: Protein tyrosine phosphatases (PTPs) are a family of enzymes essential for numerous cellular processes, such as cell growth, inflammation, differentiation, immune-mediated responses and oncogenic transformation. The aim of this review is to review the literature concerning the role of several PTPs—PTPN22, PTPN2, PTPN6, PTPN11, PTPσ, DUSP2, DUSP6 and PTPRK—at the level of the intestinal mucosa in inflammatory bowel disease (IBD), celiac disease (CeD) and type 1 diabetes (T1D) in both in vitro and in vivo models. The results revealed shared features, at the level of the intestinal mucosa, between these diseases characterized by alterations of different biological processes, such as proliferation, autoimmunity, cell death, autophagy and inflammation. PTPs are now actively studied to develop new drugs. Also considering the availability of organoids as models to test new drugs in personalized ways, it is very likely that soon these proteins will be the targets of useful drugs.

Keywords: protein tyrosine phosphatases; celiac disease; diabetes; inflammatory bowel diseases; intestinal mucosa

1. Introduction

Protein tyrosine phosphatases (PTPs) are enzymes that remove phosphate groups from tyrosine residues on other proteins. Tyrosine kinases are, on the other hand, enzymes that add phosphates to tyrosine residues. Owing to the activity carried out by protein kinases and phosphatases, the regulation of phospho-tyrosine signalling is possible, so the cells are ready to respond to external signals, inducing changes in the intracellular environment. When receptors on the cell surface bind to ligands, this results in the transduction of external signals within the cell. Therefore, RTKs (receptor tyrosine kinases) can dimerise upon ligand binding, leading to trans autophosphorylation of the receptor. This event leads to the recruitment of proteins that bind phospho-tyrosine residues to the receptor, which propagates and amplifies a variety of signal cascades [1]. The kinases and phosphatases have complementary functions in regulating cell signalling with the kinases controlling the amplitude of a signalling response and the phosphatases controlling the rate and duration of the response. PTPs are a super family with 100 circa different genes while the kinases are circa 90 genes, indicating the same level of complexity for the two families [2]. Moreover, they reach a higher level of complexity considering post-transcriptional modifications, alternative promoters or alternative splicing. Such diversity, on the one hand, makes a neat classification hard; on the other hand, it points to a wide range of biological functions that are not completely clarified. Understanding the "phosphatome", is currently a real challenge to understand the specificity and roles of all phosphatases. In fact, it is not possible to generalize the function of each phosphatase: some of them are very selective, whereas others are more promiscuous [3]. Therefore, PTPs are signalling molecules that regulate a variety of cellular processes, such as cell growth, differentiation, the cell cycle, oncogenic transformation, embryonic development, immune response, inflammation, proliferation, differentiation, cell adhesion and autophagy [4–7].

PTP1B was the first phosphatase identified. This protein has a sequence analogous to a segment of the receptor protein CD45 (Cluster of Differentiation 45) [8]. Owing to this structural analogy, it is possible to identify the existence of a conserved catalytic domain, with a cysteine amino acid residue, that has become the main feature of the PTP gene family [9].

Members of the PTP family are classified according to their structural and biochemical properties.

Human PTPs are classified into four categories depending on the substrate specificity and amino acid sequence. Class 1 consists of the classical PTPs, including the receptor-type protein tyrosine phosphatases (RPTPs) and non-receptor-type protein tyrosine phosphatases (nRPTPs). Class 2 comprises the dual-specificity phosphatases (DSPs) that target phosphorylated tyrosine, serine and threonine residues. The low-molecular-weight phosphatases (LMW-PTPs) belong to class 3 and the CDC25 class phosphatases form class 4 [10] (Figure 1). At the cellular level, the PTP proteins are mainly cytosolic, nucleo-cytosolic and receptor proteins. Although, at the tissue level, they are expressed mainly in the developing embryo, the immune system and the nervous system, they are also expressed at the level of the intestine [11].

The importance of tyrosine phosphorylation in normal cell physiology is highlighted by the fact that many human diseases are the result of aberrant protein tyrosine kinase (PTK) or protein tyrosine phosphatase (PTP) function [12]. PTP mutations that cause hereditary disease phenotypes have been described to date for T-cell Leukemia, Rheumatoid arthritis, Hashimoto thyroiditis, Addison Disease, Noonan and Leopard syndrome and others [13]. Interestingly, both loss-of-function and gain-of-function mutations in these genes may underlie the reported disease. Most studies in the literature have described both the molecular mechanisms and the therapeutic target of PTPs in cancer [14,15].

Moreover, the role of PTPs in inflammatory diseases such as inflammatory bowel disease (IBD), celiac disease (CeD) and type 1 diabetes (T1D) has been established [9,16–18].

IBD, CeD and T1D share genetic alterations of genes involved mainly in the pathways of intestinal barrier dysfunction, immune/inflammatory pathways and autophagy [19,20]. A notable aspect of these three diseases is the presence of increased intestinal permeability that precedes the onset of inflammation [21]. Moreover, both T1D and IBD patients have an increased risk of CeD [19].

IBD and CeD share a specific target organ, the intestine. Both are complex diseases in which genetics and the environment contribute to the dysregulation of innate and adaptive immune responses, leading to chronic inflammation and disease. T1D has as an organ target not only pancreatic β-cells but also the intestinal mucosa. In fact, clinical and experimental research has revealed that diabetes mellitus is characterized by intestinal hypomotility, gut microbial dysbiosis, increased gut permeability and dysfunction of intestinal stem cells, which may be linked to inflammation of the intestinal mucosa [22–24].

All previously described conditions are characterized by the presence of genetic and environmental factors and inflammation. Among the environmental factors that trigger inflammation, nutrients play a significant role in inducing low-grade inflammation, which is considered a "common background" for various diseases, including diabetes,

IBD and CeD [25]. A new concept emerging in the recent literature suggests that genetic predisposition can increase the susceptibility of cells to inflammatory triggers, leading to cellular vulnerability and autoimmunity [25,26]. How this cellular vulnerability is characterized is not yet clear, but signalling molecules, including PTPs, are emerging as possible culprits.

The aim of this review is to review the recent literature on the role of PTPs at the level of the intestine in inflammatory diseases, such as CeD, IBD and T1D.

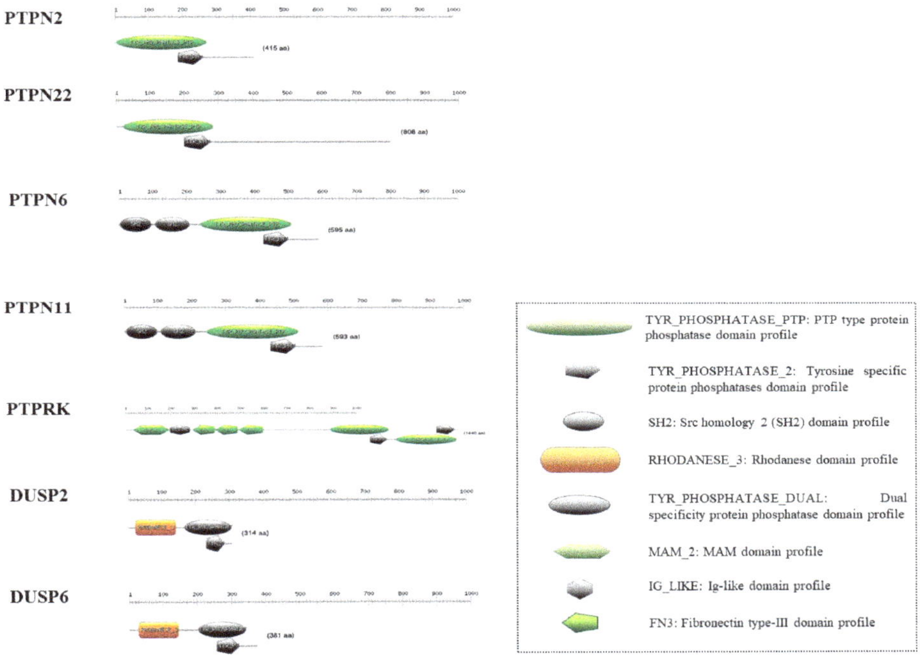

Figure 1. Graphical representation of the PTP domain profile.

2. Materials and Methods

We selected the most recent literature on IBD, T1D and CeD, which are correlated with/associated with PTP proteins. Citing 72/103 manuscripts from the last 20 years, 51/103 are from the last 10 years, 36/103 are from the last 5 years and only 3 are from between 1993 and 1998 as they are the original references for the PTP described.

The software used to create the figures were Clustal, Microsoft Power Point and BioRender. In particular, Clustal was used to create Figure 1; BioRender was used for Figure 2; and Microsoft Power Point was used for the graphical abstract, Figure 3.

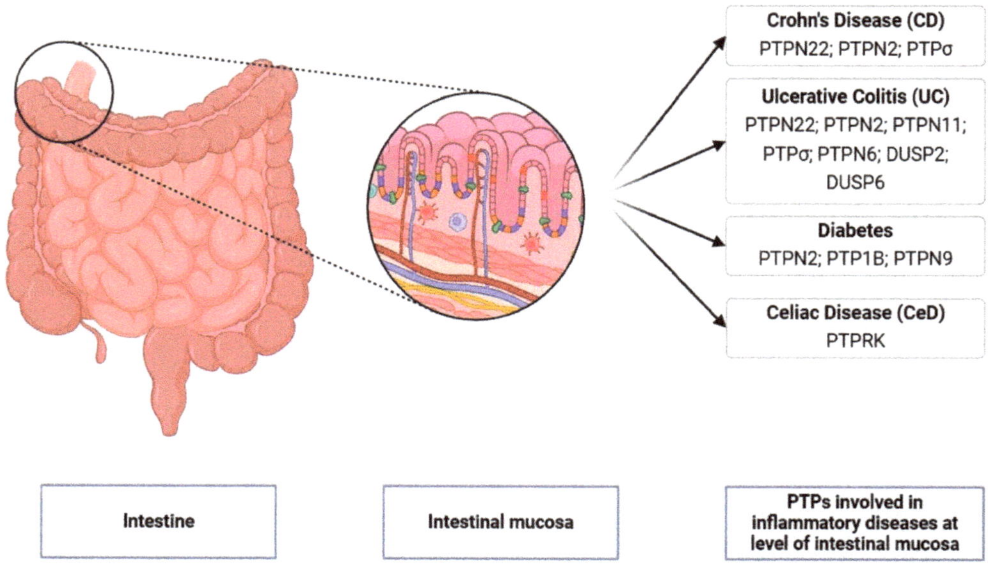

Figure 2. Schematic representation of PTPs (PTPN22; PTPN2; PTPσ; PTPN11; PTPN6; DUSP2; DUSP6; PTPRK) involved in Crohn's disease, ulcerative colitis, diabetes and celiac disease at level of intestinal mucosa.

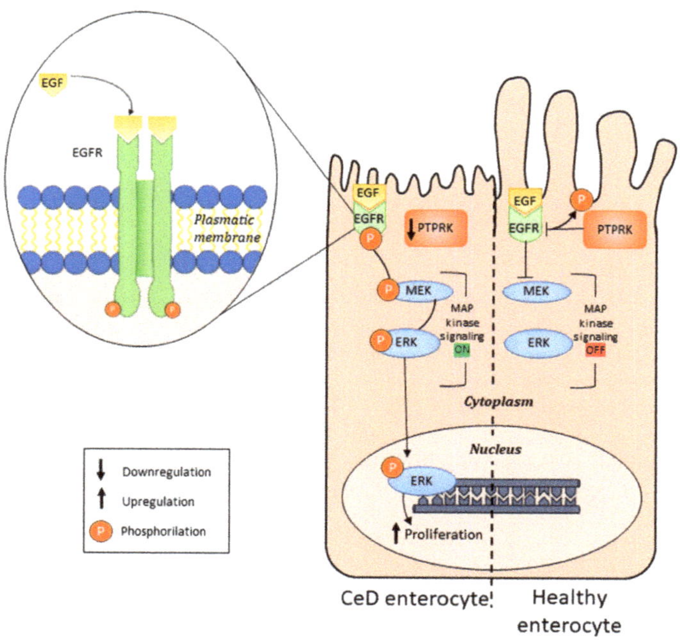

Figure 3. Schematic representation of CeD (**left**) and healthy (**right**) enterocytes with a description of the role of PTPRK in the regulation of the EGF pathway. In CeD enterocytes, with respect to healthy enterocytes, the downregulation of PTPRK leads to the upregulation of EGFR, and MAP-kinase signalling is always switched ON, increasing proliferation.

3. PTPs and Inflammatory Bowel Disease

In this section, we describe the role of the PTPs involved in the development of IBDs (Crohn's disease (CD) and ulcerative colitis (UC)) at the level of the intestine, namely PTPN22, PTPN2, PTPN6, PTPN11, PTPσ DUSP2, and DUSP6 (Figure 2) (Table 1).

PTPN22 (Protein tyrosine phosphatase non-receptor 22) is expressed mainly in haematopoietic cells and is associated with multiple inflammatory disorders [1,9,27]. A gene association study demonstrated that SNPs generating the loss-of-function variant in PTPN22 were associated, respectively, with CD and UC [28–30]. In mouse models of experimental arthritis and DSS (dextran sulphate sodium)-induced colitis, PTPN22 deficiency resulted in increased intestinal susceptibility to inflammatory agents and pronounced disease progression, indicating that PTPN22 is required to protect individuals from systemic and gastrointestinal inflammation. Katakura et al. [31] and Yarilina et al. [32] reported that, in mice, PTPN22 promotes intestinal inflammation suppression in models of colitis and can ameliorate intestinal mucosa injury [33]. In mouse models, PTPN22 represses acute inflammatory immune responses in the gut in the presence of IL-10 (interleukin-10) but promotes acute gut inflammation in the absence of IL-10. During chronic intestinal inflammation, however, PTPN22 promotes gut inflammation irrespective of the presence of IL-10 [34]. In addition, PTPN22 at the level of the intestine is involved in autophagy and inflammatory regulation through the dephosphorylation of NOD-like receptor protein 3 (NLRP3) to allow for efficient inflammasome activation. The loss of functional autophagy counteracts the reduction in NLRP3 activation observed in PTPN22-deficient cells, leading to increased IL-1β secretion [35,36]. Defects in autophagy result in impaired goblet cell function, and variants in genes involved in autophagy are associated with an increased risk of developing IBD [37] (Figure 2 and Table 1).

The PTPN2 protein has the highest expression levels in lymphoid tissue. Previous studies in mice have provided insight into the crucial role of PTPN2 in intestinal homeostasis, including the regulation of pro-inflammatory cytokine secretion, autophagy, intestinal epithelial barrier function and gut microbiota homeostasis [38,39]. The anti-inflammatory role of PTPN2 is highlighted by the fact that PTPN2-deficient mice die a few weeks after birth because of systemic inflammation and severe colitis [40]. PTPN2 crucially contributes to normal macrophage-IEC (intestinal epithelial cell) interactions that govern macrophage differentiation and epithelial barrier function and represents a target for therapeutic intervention in IBD. PTPN2 has also been shown to play an important role in Paneth cell regulation. PTPN2 knockout (KO) mice presented a reduced number of Paneth cells, increased Paneth cell endoplasmic reticulum stress and dysbiosis [38,41].

Clinically relevant loss-of-function mutations in the PTPN2 gene contribute to the etiopathogenesis of chronic inflammatory intestinal disease, at least in part through the dysregulation of epithelial barrier properties. As well as PTPN22, PTPN2 was also shown to regulate inflammasome activation, IL-1B secretion and autophagy regulation [40]. Consistent with these findings, PTPN2 levels were increased in the intestinal epithelium in active CD patients. [21,42,43]. In fact, PTPN2 protects the intestinal barrier by restricting the capacity of INF gamma to increase epithelial permeability and TNFα-induced signalling and cytokine secretion in human intestinal epithelial cells [21,42–44] (Figure 2 and Table 1).

PTPN11 was upregulated in both UC patients and a colitis model in mice [45–47]. It is a cytoplasmic protein tyrosine phosphatase that functions as a positive regulator of the Ras–mitogen-activated protein kinase (MAPK) signalling pathway downstream of various growth factors and cytokines, contributing to the regulation of cell proliferation and differentiation. Yamashita et al. demonstrated that mice lacking PTPN11 specifically in IECs developed severe colitis and alterations in the intestinal mucosa, with the numbers of absorptive enterocytes and goblet cells markedly reduced in the small intestine and colon with respect to controls [48]. Abnormal development of the intestinal epithelium and disrupted host–microbiota equilibrium was also described in PTPN11-deficient mice [49,50]. Moreover, Xiao et al. demonstrated that PTPN11 expressed in the monocyte/macrophage lineage serves as a pro-inflammatory factor in the intestine [51]. However, the precise role of PTPN11 in the regulation of gastrointestinal stem cell and progenitor functions, especially in vivo, has remained unclear (Figure 2 and Table 1).

PTPσ (protein tyrosine phosphatase receptor S) consists of a cell adhesion molecule-like domain, a transmembrane domain and a cytosolic region. PTPσ expression is developmentally regulated and found primarily in the nervous system and specific epithelia. PTPσ $-/-$ mice presented high neonatal mortality. Analysis of the intestinal tissue of surviving mice revealed the presence of mucosal inflammation, intestinal crypt branching and villus blunting associated with human IBD. Additionally, PTPσ targets apical junction complex proteins in the intestine and regulates epithelial permeability [52,53] (Figure 2 and Table 1).

PTPN6 is predominantly expressed in hematopoietic and epithelial cells. It was associated with increased proliferation and altered goblet and Paneth cell differentiation. Previous studies demonstrate that the levels of PTPN6 were reduced in active UC and CD with respect to controls [54]. In another study, two PTPN6 SNPs were genotyped in a population of 107 IBD patients from Southern Tunisia and a weak association with UC was identified [55]. For this reason, a link between PTPN6 and IBD still needs to be defined (Figure 2 and Table 1).

DUSP2 was first identified as a mitogen-inducible gene in human T cells. DUSP2 is a nuclear protein phosphatase regulated by extracellular signal-regulated kinase 1/2 (ERK1/2) and p38 MAPKs. DUSP2 is a positive mediator of inflammation [56]. DUSP2 $-/-$ mice exhibit increased mucosal hyperaemia, increased colonic ulceration and high levels of pro-inflammatory cytokines, including IL-6, IL-17, Tumour necrosis factor α (TNFα) and IL-1β. In a study of UC patients, the level of blood DUSP2 mRNA expression was reduced [57] (Figure 2 and Table 1).

DUSP6 is a cytoplasmic phosphatase specific to the ERK protein kinase [58]. The signal transduction pathway regulated by ERK is responsible for the regulation of multiple cellular responses. DUSP6 KO mice have shown CD4+ T cell polarization; altered differentiation of T-helper 1 (TH1), TH2 and TH17 cells; and an increased rate of cell proliferation and of cell death. This depletion also causes severe inflammation in mouse models of IBD with intestinal epithelial hyperplasia, the depletion of caliciform cells and infiltration of mononuclear cells. Furthermore, colon explants secrete increased levels of TNF-α and Interferon-γ (IFN-γ). In these mice, ERK inhibition significantly reduces colitis. Additionally, Beaudry K. et al., using ex vivo DUSP6 KO organoid cultures, demonstrated that the loss of DUSP6 caused an increase in crypt depth and epithelial cell proliferation [59] (Figure 2 and Table 1).

In conclusion, PTPs have a nodal role in IBD pathogenesis. It is notable that they play an important role in the intestinal epithelium, mostly regulating its homeostasis. This indicates that the intestinal epithelium compartment could be the key both to the understanding the of the molecular pathways responsible for the mucosal alterations and to find new targets for therapeutic intervention. In this context, it is important to highlight the role of intestinal organoids derived from staminal cells that represent the intestinal epithelium not only of a specific disease, but also of a specific patient, opening the door for precision medicine in these diseases.

Table 1. PTP proteins involved in inflammatory intestinal diseases and their function at the level of the intestine investigated in several study models.

PTP Protein	Disease	Alteration in the Disease	Models of Study	Function at the Level of the Intestine	Reference
PTPN22	CD-UC	Loss of function	Mice [31–34]; Cell culture [35–37]	(1) PTPN22 has a dual context-dependent role: -in acute gut inflammation, PTPN22 together with IL-10 is a repressor of inflammtory response; PTPN22 minus IL-10 is a promoter -during chronic inflammation, PTPN22 promotes gut inflammation irrespective of the presence of IL-10 (2) protections from systemic and gastrointestinal inflammation (3) autophagy regulation (4) inflammasoma regulation	[1,9,27–37]
PTPN2	CD-UC	Loss of function	Mice [38–41] Intestinal epithelial cell (IEC) lines (T84;HT29cl.19a) [42,44]	INTESTINAL HOMEOSTASIS -regulation of pro-inflammatory cytokine secretion -autophagy -intestinal epithelial barrier function -Paneth cell regulation -autophagy regulation -inflammasoma activation -gut microbiota homeostasis	[21,38–44]
PTPN2	Diabetes	Minor allele frequency	Patients	Involved in many leaky gut-associated diseases	[60–62]
PTPN11	UC	Up-regulated and Down-regulated	Mice [45–50] Cell culture [51]	Homeostasis of IECs of absorptive enterocytes and goblet cells; microbiota equilibrium; positive regulator of MAPK signalling pathway; regulation of cell proliferation and differentiation	[45–51]
PTPσ	UC	Down-regulated	Mice [52,53]	PTPσ is a regulator of mucosal inflammation, intestinal epithelial development and permeability	[52,53]
PTPN6	UC	Down-regulated	Patients	PTPN6 is associated with increased proliferation and altered goblet and Paneth cell differentiation	[54,55]
DUSP2	UC	Low levels (mRNA)	Mice [46]	DUSP2 is a regulator of mucosal inflammation and colonic ulceration	[56,57]
DUSP6	UC	Down-regulated	Mice [47] HT29 and HCT116 colorectal carcinoma cells [47]	DUSP6 is a modulator of CD4+ T cell activation and epithelial cell proliferation	[58,59]
PTPRK	CeD	Down-regulated	Intestinal organoids [9]	PTPRK is a regulator of epithelial inflammation and enterocyte proliferation	[18,63–77]

4. PTPs and Diabetes

T1D is an autoimmune disease characterized by the destruction of insulin-producing β-cells in the pancreas. The onset of T1D is thought to be due to a complex interplay of genetic and environmental factors. The primary genetic risk factors include specific human leukocyte antigen (HLA) alleles, particularly HLA-DQ and HLA-DR, which are essential for immune regulation. Environmental triggers, such as viral infections and certain dietary components, can act as catalysts in genetically predisposed individuals. Autoreactive T cells, activated by these environmental factors, infiltrate the pancreatic islets, triggering an immune response against β-cells. This response leads to the release of pro-inflammatory cytokines and chemokines, resulting in the destruction of β-cells [78–80]. Several studies have focused on the autoimmune processes involved in pathogenesis, which are described in depth in the literature [16,17]. On the other hand, recent studies indicate that, in addition to this mechanism, altered intestinal permeability, impaired barrier function and the intestinal microbiota can significantly influence the development of diabetes [22,23]. Changes in the intestinal mucosa, such as reduced cytokine production (IL-17A, IL-22 and IL-23A) and shifts in microbiota composition (e.g., a decrease in SFB), have been observed in various mouse models of T1D. These changes do not seem to depend solely on hyperglycemia but are associated with intestinal inflammation and compromised epithelial cell integrity [22,23].

Studies suggest that treating intestinal inflammation could restore the microbiota balance and improve the condition of intestinal epithelial cells, potentially positively influencing T1D. In particular, the use of anti-TNFα therapies, which are common in inflammatory bowel diseases such as Crohn's disease, has been shown to reduce intestinal inflammation and improve diabetic pathology [23].

Gastrointestinal (GI) symptoms are generally more common in people with diabetes than in the general population, with prevalence rates varying widely. GI complications are commonly nausea, vomiting, abdominal pain, heartburn, dysphagia, constipation, diarrhea and fecal incontinence [81]. Diabetes disrupts intestinal homeostasis through insulin-like growth factor binding protein 3 (IGFBP3). Chronic hyperglycemia and inflammation alter liver function, reducing insulin-like growth factor 1 (IGF-I) and increasing IGFBP3 levels. Elevated IGFBP3 targets intestinal crypts, leading to the apoptosis of intestinal stem cells (ISCs). The remaining ISCs struggle to differentiate into essential cell types, impairing crypt turnover and causing mucosal atrophy, which results in malabsorption. This, in turn, worsens hyperglycemia and inflammation, creating a feedback loop that further disrupts intestinal homeostasis [22,23]. Meanwhile, the role of the enteric nervous system and its neurotransmitters is gaining attention. Damage to this system can lead to specific GI motility disorders, such as diabetic gastroparesis, constipation and diarrhea. These complications increase diabetes-related morbidity and reduce patients' quality of life [82].

In summary, GI dysfunction significantly increases morbidity in diabetes and creates a vicious cycle of malabsorption, inflammation and impaired GI motility, all of which severely impact patients' quality of life.

PTPs are crucial regulators of cellular signalling pathways and have also been implicated in the pathogenesis of T1D. PTPs serve as pivotal negative regulators of multiple signalling pathways, influencing both immune responses and glucose metabolism [17,60,83–88]. Understanding the specific roles and mechanisms of different PTPs offers valuable insights into their potential as targets for therapeutic strategies aimed at modulating autoimmune responses and managing T1D.

The loss of PTPN2 function seems to be associated with increased intestinal permeability and increased expression of pro-inflammatory mediators, indicating that PTPN2 plays a protective role in maintaining intestinal barrier integrity and regulating the inflammatory response. A polymorphism in the PTPN2 rs2542151 GT or GG genotype is associated with an earlier onset of type 1 diabetes [61]. In addition, PTPN2 rs2542151 has been linked to a higher prevalence of type 2 diabetes (T2DM) and greater severity of non-alcoholic fatty liver disease (NAFLD) [60]. PTPN2 is known for its role as a negative regulator of IFN-γ-mediated pro-inflammatory signalling. IFN-γ increases intestinal permeability and promotes inflammation. This is a process that PTPN2 appears to counteract by limiting the expression of proteins such as claudin-2, which is involved in the formation of pores in the epithelial barrier. These changes may facilitate the access of intestinal antigens to the immune system, contributing to chronic inflammation and insulin resistance [60]. A recent study revealed that reduced expression of the T1D candidate gene PTPN2 exacerbates damage caused by IFN-α and TNF-α. PTPN2 seems to provide protection against both factors, revealing a shared downstream signalling pathway between them. The inhibition of PTPN2 also impairs PDX1 (pancreatic and duodenal homeobox 1) expression and insulin production after TNF-α exposure [62].

PTPN2 is a crucial regulator of the harmful effects of TNF-α in human β-cells, suggesting that patients with PTPN2 risk polymorphisms may benefit from therapies targeting

TNF-α. PTPN2 may also influence T1D development through its role in regulating intestinal permeability.

Further research is needed to explore the specific molecular mechanisms underlying T1D progression and, also, what the role of PTPs is in both the development and the progression of the disease. Targeting PTPs could provide new perspectives for therapeutic intervention and disease management [62] (Figure 2 and Table 1).

Interestingly, tissue transglutaminase (TTg), one of the major players in CeD autoimmunity, can modify PTEN, a phosphatase of the PTP family, also increasing the activity binding of the auto-antibodies (IA-2; anti-islet antibodies) participating in the autoimmune response in type 1 diabetes [89]. Moreover, TTg participates in the inflammatory response by activating NFk-β [90]. Considering, also, that in CeD as well as in type 1 diabetes deposits of TTg/anti-TTg are present at the level of the intestinal mucosa [91,92], these two diseases share more common elements than previously thought.

In addition to PTPN2, two other PTPs have only been associated with T2D: PTP-1B and PTPN9 (PTP-MEG2). They are protein tyrosine phosphatases implicated in regulating insulin and leptin signalling pathways, both of which play critical roles in metabolic processes [93,94].

PTP-1B acts as a negative regulator of insulin and leptin receptor pathways. It deactivates insulin and leptin signalling by dephosphorylating key pathway components, impacting downstream effects on glucose metabolism and fatty acid oxidation. As such, PTP-1B inhibition has been identified as a promising strategy for managing type 2 diabetes and related complications, including obesity. Interestingly, metformin can inhibit PTP1B tyrosine phosphatase activity to stimulate the insulin receptor tyrosine kinase [95]. Still, the development of specific PTP-1B inhibitors remains in preliminary stages, with challenges in achieving selectivity and bioavailability due to the conserved structure of PTP active sites [93].

PTPN9 also plays a role in metabolic regulation, with recent studies highlighting its involvement in the pathology of polycythemia vera and its modulation of insulin and ErbB2 receptor signalling. PTPN9 depletion in diabetic mouse liver tissues has been shown to increase insulin sensitivity and normalize blood glucose, indicating that its inhibition could be an effective approach for diabetes treatment. Through an innovative library-based approach, researchers have developed highly selective PTPN9 inhibitors that enhance insulin action and improve glucose homeostasis in cell cultures and diabetic mouse models. This strategy involves targeting peripheral binding pockets near the active site to achieve the necessary specificity and efficacy [94,96].

Together, these findings suggest that selective inhibition of PTP-1B and PTPN9 could offer new therapeutic targets for type 2 diabetes. However, overcoming challenges such as the PTP active site's high conservation and achieving cell permeability are essential for developing effective small-molecule PTP inhibitors. The research thus lays important groundwork for future PTP-targeted therapies aimed at improving metabolic health and managing diabetes.

5. PTP and Celiac Disease

CeD is a multifactorial disease in which environmental triggers combined with genetic predispositions determine its onset. Repeated GWASs (genome-wide association studies) were able to identify 39 non-HLA (human leukocyte antigen) susceptibility loci associated with CeD, and, together, these loci can explain approximately 10–14% of CeD heritability [63]. Combined with the HLA locus, only 50% of CeD heritability is explained. Among these 39 non-HLA loci (Rho involved in CeD), 4 were not directly involved in immunological processes. C1ORF106 (C1 Orfan 106), ARHGAP31 (GTPase activating protein 31), LPP (lipoma-preferred partner) and PTPRK (protein tyrosine phosphatase receptor-type K) play roles in actin rearrangement in the cytoskeleton, in the cell-cell adhesion process and in the maintenance of intestinal epithelial barrier function [63]. PTPRK also regulates EGFR (epidermal growth factor receptor) signalling through dephosphorylation of catalytic sites and inactivation of the receptor.

The PTPRK gene is located on the long arm of chromosome 6 [64]. PTPRK mRNA is widely expressed, except in the immune cells, skeletal muscles and testes, and it is up-regulated by the transforming growth factor β (TGF-β) signal transduction pathway.

PTPRK is a receptor-type PTP that consists of an extracellular region, a single transmembrane region and two tandem catalytic domains [65]. Many functions are performed by the PTPRK gene [66–70], including the regulation of EGFR activation [66,67,71]. Altered regulation of EGFR has been shown to promote uncontrolled cell proliferation, angiogenesis and metastasis development. Proliferation is also a marker of CeD pathogenesis, mainly through the signalling of EGFR [72]. In biopsies and fibroblasts from patients with CeD, there is a delay in EGFR trafficking in early endocytic vesicles such that the receptor remains activated longer than that in controls [73]. Gliadin further delays the endocytic pathway and can prolong the activation of the EGFR/ERK (extracellular signal-regulated kinase) signalling pathway and cell proliferation in biopsies from controls and patients with CeD [74,75]. Elevated activation of the EGFR/MAPK pathway is also found in the enterocytes of patients with CeD, resulting in alterations in the cytoskeleton. Furthermore, altered expression of genes involved in autophagy and the regulation of the EGFR pathway are also observed in patients with CeD [73].

The effects of PTPRK in regulating the proliferation of enterocytes and keratinocytes have also been studied via biopsies and organoids [18,76,77]. PTPRK phosphatase expression levels are reduced in biopsies from patients with a gluten-containing diet (GCD) and from potential patients with CeD (Pot-CeD), whereas EGFR phosphorylation, ERK and cell proliferation levels are increased compared with those in biopsies from controls (CTRs). These findings suggest that the reduction in PTPRK protein expression levels is independent of intestinal villous atrophy [18].

Another study found a region on chromosome 6 through a GWAS that includes two genes, the THEMIS gene, which codes for a molecule involved in the selection of thymocytes, and the PTPRK gene. Both genes perform immuno-related functions and are involved in the pathogenesis of CeD. Gene expression analysis of duodenal biopsies from patients with CeD revealed higher mRNA levels in the THEMIS gene than those in samples taken from the same patients after gluten-free diet (GFD) treatment or from CTRs. These findings point to the correlation between low PTPRK expression levels in the CeD and increased permeability of the intestinal barrier, and PTPRK inhibition may promote enterocyte hyper-proliferation in intestinal crypts. Moreover, compared with CTR patients, patients with CeD have similar mRNA levels, indicating that adhesion to a GFD is sufficient to restore the transcriptional activity of the THEMIS and PTPRK genes to normal levels [77].

Altered function of the intestinal epithelium plays an important role in the pathogenesis of inflammatory diseases [97]. Intestinal organoids, derived from intestinal stem cells, recreate the crypt/villus axis in vitro, allowing the role of the intestinal epithelium in various pathologies to be studied [98–102]. CeD intestinal organoids reproduce the low-grade inflammation of CeD intestinal biopsies [103]. In CeD organoids, low PTPRK levels are associated with increased EGFR/ERK phosphorylation and proliferation. Nanayakkara et al. conducted functional experiments on intestinal organoids from patients with CeD and controls to study the role of PTPRK in intestinal epithelial cell proliferation. In control organoids, the silencing of PTPRK induces the increase in the phosphorylation of EGFR and ERK and proliferation. On the other hand, overexpressing PTPRK in CeD organoids was able to reduce the phosphorylation of EGFR and ERK and proliferation to normal levels. PTPRK expression in intestinal organoids from patients with CeD and controls can modulate the phosphorylation of EGFR and ERK and proliferation [18] (Figures 2 and 3 and Table 1).

The discovery of the role of PTPRK in CeD organoids is exemplary of how organoids can be used to understand specific features of intestinal diseases. In fact, they can allow for the study of an important feature of CeD, such as proliferation, which is a hallmark of CeD, and also the role of PTPs in the pathogenesis of CeD. This shifts the attention from T-cell response to the intestinal epithelium in this disease.

6. Conclusions

In conclusion, the involvement of PTP phosphatases in diseases such as IBD, T1D and CeD implicates the nodal role of the signalling mediated by phospho-tyrosines in these diseases. PTPs are signalling molecules that operate in almost all cells of the body and are able to regulate a variety of cellular processes, such as cell growth, differentiation, the cell cycle and oncogenic transformation. The generation of different diseases is likely due to the fragility of specific cell tissues induced by a combination of exogenous and endogenous factors. Moreover, these data point to an emerging role of the intestinal epithelium not only in inflammatory chronic intestinal diseases, including IBD and CeD, but also in T1D, where PTP alterations have been found both at the level of pancreatic β-cells and at the level of intestinal epithelial cells. Taken together, these data link IBD, T1D and CeD, which were previously regarded as unrelated and mediated by independent pathogenetic events. Moreover, although previously considered "undraggable", PTPs are now actively studied to develop new drugs. Considering also the availability of organoids as models to test new drugs in personalized way, it is very likely that, soon, these proteins will be the targets of useful drugs.

Author Contributions: C.B. and F.F. equally contributed to the investigation, data curation and writing; F.F. also contributed to graphic representation; R.R. and I.C. equally contributed to data curation, the initial draft and editing; M.C. contributed to the investigation of PTPN2 and PTPN22 and the table representation; G.D. contributed to the investigation of PTPRK and PTPN1 and revision of the manuscript; M.N. (Martina Nicoletti) contributed to the investigation of PTPN6, Dusp2 and 6 and she took part in the original draft preparation and conceptualization. L.S. contributed to alignment of the PTP domain profile and contributed to general description of PTP as requested by reviewers. M.N. (Merlin Nanayakkara) and M.V.B. contributed to the methodology, investigation, data curation, resources and writing of the manuscript. All authors have read and agreed to the published version of the manuscript.

Funding: This research received no external funding.

Data Availability Statement: Not applicable.

Acknowledgments: The authors wish to thank Francesco Silvestro, Violeta Catalina Greu, Francesca Natasha Hewa Munasinghege and Majed Mordaa for their technical support.

Conflicts of Interest: The authors declare no conflicts of interest.

References

1. Hunter, T. Tyrosine phosphorylation: Thirty years and counting. *Curr. Opin. Cell Biol.* **2009**, *21*, 140–146. [CrossRef] [PubMed]
2. Tautz, L.; Critton, D.A.; Grotegut, S. Protein tyrosine phosphatases: Structure, function, and implication in human disease. *Methods Mol. Biol.* **2013**, *1053*, 179–221. [CrossRef] [PubMed]
3. Chen, M.J.; Dixon, J.E.; Manning, G. Genomics and evolution of protein phosphatases. *Sci. Signal* **2017**, *10*, eaag1796. [CrossRef] [PubMed]
4. Hendriks, W.J.; Elson, A.; Harroch, S.; Pulido, R.; Stoker, A.; den Hertog, J. Protein tyrosine phosphatases in health and disease. *FEBS J.* **2013**, *280*, 708–730. [CrossRef]
5. Welsh, C.L.; Pandey, P.; Ahuja, L.G. Protein Tyrosine Phosphatases: A new paradigm in an old signaling system? *Adv. Cancer Res.* **2021**, *152*, 263–303. [CrossRef]
6. Yang, B.; Gan, M.S.; Lin, Z.Y.; Wang, Z.F. Identification of autophagy-related genes as potential biomarkers for type 1 diabetes mellitus. *Ann. Transl. Med.* **2022**, *10*, 637. [CrossRef] [PubMed]
7. Spalinger, M.R.; McCole, D.F.; Rogler, G.; Scharl, M. Role of protein tyrosine phosphatases in regulating the immune system: Implications for chronic intestinal inflammation. *Inflamm. Bowel Dis.* **2015**, *21*, 645–655. [CrossRef]
8. Liu, R.; Mathieu, C.; Berthelet, J.; Zhang, W.; Dupret, J.M.; Rodrigues Lima, F. Human Protein Tyrosine Phosphatase 1B (PTP1B): From Structure to Clinical Inhibitor Perspectives. *Int. J. Mol. Sci.* **2022**, *23*, 7027. [CrossRef]
9. Pike, K.A.; Tremblay, M.L. Protein Tyrosine Phosphatases: Regulators of CD4 T Cells in Inflammatory Bowel Disease. *Front. Immunol.* **2018**, *9*, 2504. [CrossRef]

10. Li, H.; Zhang, P.; Liu, C.; Wang, Y.; Deng, Y.; Dong, W.; Yu, Y. The Structure, Function and Regulation of Protein Tyrosine Phosphatase Receptor Type J and Its Role in Diseases. *Cells* **2022**, *12*, 8. [CrossRef]
11. Forrest, A.R.; Taylor, D.F.; Fink, J.L.; Gongora, M.M.; Flegg, C.; Teasdale, R.D.; Suzuki, H.; Kanamori, M.; Kai, C.; Hayashizaki, Y.; et al. PhosphoregDB: The tissue and sub-cellular distribution of mammalian protein kinases and phosphatases. *BMC Bioinform.* **2006**, *7*, 82. [CrossRef] [PubMed]
12. Kramer, I.M. Chapter 18—Protein Phosphatases. In *Signal Transduction*, 3rd ed.; Kramer, I.M., Ed.; Academic Press: Boston, MA, USA, 2016; pp. 935–995. [CrossRef]
13. Hendriks, W.J.A.J.; Pulido, R. Protein tyrosine phosphatase variants in human hereditary disorders and disease susceptibilities. *Biochim. Biophys. Acta (BBA) Mol. Basis Dis.* **2013**, *1832*, 1673–1696. [CrossRef] [PubMed]
14. Sivaganesh, V.; Sivaganesh, V.; Scanlon, C.; Iskander, A.; Maher, S.; Lê, T.; Peethambaran, B. Protein Tyrosine Phosphatases: Mechanisms in Cancer. *Int. J. Mol. Sci.* **2021**, *22*, 12865. [CrossRef] [PubMed]
15. Zhao, M.; Shuai, W.; Su, Z.; Xu, P.; Wang, A.; Sun, Q.; Wang, G. Protein tyrosine phosphatases: Emerging role in cancer therapy resistance. *Cancer Commun.* **2024**, *44*, 637–653. [CrossRef] [PubMed]
16. Tizaoui, K.; Shin, J.I.; Jeong, G.H.; Yang, J.W.; Park, S.; Kim, J.H.; Hwang, S.Y.; Park, S.J.; Koyanagi, A.; Smith, L. Genetic Polymorphism of PTPN22 in Autoimmune Diseases: A Comprehensive Review. *Medicina* **2022**, *58*, 1034. [CrossRef]
17. Anderson, W.; Barahmand-Pour-Whitman, F.; Linsley, P.S.; Cerosaletti, K.; Buckner, J.H.; Rawlings, D.J. PTPN22 R620W gene editing in T cells enhances low-avidity TCR responses. *eLife* **2023**, *12*, e81577. [CrossRef]
18. Nanayakkara, M.; Bellomo, C.; Furone, F.; Maglio, M.; Marano, A.; Lania, G.; Porpora, M.; Nicoletti, M.; Auricchio, S.; Barone, M.V. PTPRK, an EGFR Phosphatase, Is Decreased in CeD Biopsies and Intestinal Organoids. *Cells* **2022**, *12*, 115. [CrossRef]
19. Pinto-Sanchez, M.I.; Seiler, C.L.; Santesso, N.; Alaedini, A.; Semrad, C.; Lee, A.R.; Bercik, P.; Lebwohl, B.; Leffler, D.A.; Kelly, C.P.; et al. Association Between Inflammatory Bowel Diseases and Celiac Disease: A Systematic Review and Meta-Analysis. *Gastroenterology* **2020**, *159*, 884–903.e31. [CrossRef] [PubMed]
20. Strakova, V.; Elblova, L.; Johnson, M.B.; Dusatkova, P.; Obermannova, B.; Petruzelkova, L.; Kolouskova, S.; Snajderova, M.; Fronkova, E.; Svaton, M.; et al. Screening of monogenic autoimmune diabetes among children with type 1 diabetes and multiple autoimmune diseases: Is it worth doing? *J. Pediatr. Endocrinol. Metab.* **2019**, *32*, 1147–1153. [CrossRef]
21. McCole, D.F. Phosphatase regulation of intercellular junctions. *Tissue Barriers* **2013**, *1*, e26713. [CrossRef]
22. D'Addio, F.; Fiorina, P. Type 1 Diabetes and Dysfunctional Intestinal Homeostasis. *Trends Endocrinol. Metab.* **2016**, *27*, 493–503. [CrossRef] [PubMed]
23. Rouland, M.; Beaudoin, L.; Rouxel, O.; Bertrand, L.; Cagninacci, L.; Saffarian, A.; Pedron, T.; Gueddouri, D.; Guilmeau, S.; Burnol, A.F.; et al. Gut mucosa alterations and loss of segmented filamentous bacteria in type 1 diabetes are associated with inflammation rather than hyperglycaemia. *Gut* **2022**, *71*, 296–308. [CrossRef] [PubMed]
24. Auricchio, R.; Paparo, F.; Maglio, M.; Franzese, A.; Lombardi, F.; Valerio, G.; Nardone, G.; Percopo, S.; Greco, L.; Troncone, R. In vitro-deranged intestinal immune response to gliadin in type 1 diabetes. *Diabetes* **2004**, *53*, 1680–1683. [CrossRef] [PubMed]
25. Barone, M.V.; Auricchio, R.; Nanayakkara, M.; Greco, L.; Troncone, R.; Auricchio, S. Pivotal Role of Inflammation in Celiac Disease. *Int. J. Mol. Sci.* **2022**, *23*, 7177. [CrossRef]
26. Liston, A.; Todd, J.A.; Lagou, V. Beta-Cell Fragility As a Common Underlying Risk Factor in Type 1 and Type 2 Diabetes. *Trends Mol. Med.* **2017**, *23*, 181–194. [CrossRef]
27. Cloutier, J.F.; Veillette, A. Association of inhibitory tyrosine protein kinase p50csk with protein tyrosine phosphatase PEP in T cells and other hemopoietic cells. *EMBO J.* **1996**, *15*, 4909–4918. [CrossRef] [PubMed]
28. Diaz-Gallo, L.M.; Medrano, L.M.; Gómez-García, M.; Cardeña, C.; Rodrigo, L.; Mendoza, J.L.; Taxonera, C.; Nieto, A.; Alcain, G.; Cueto, I.; et al. Analysis of the influence of two CD24 genetic variants in Crohn's disease and ulcerative colitis. *Hum. Immunol.* **2011**, *72*, 969–972. [CrossRef]
29. Sadr, M.; Moazzami, B.; Soleimanifar, N.; Elhamian, N.; Rezaei, A.; Ebrahimi Daryani, N.; Rezaei, N. Single Nucleotide Polymorphisms of PTPN22 Gene in Iranian Patients with Ulcerative Colitis. *Fetal Pediatr. Pathol.* **2019**, *38*, 8–13. [CrossRef]
30. Waterman, M.; Xu, W.; Stempak, J.M.; Milgrom, R.; Bernstein, C.N.; Griffiths, A.M.; Greenberg, G.R.; Steinhart, A.H.; Silverberg, M.S. Distinct and overlapping genetic loci in Crohn's disease and ulcerative colitis: Correlations with pathogenesis. *Inflamm. Bowel Dis.* **2011**, *17*, 1936–1942. [CrossRef] [PubMed]
31. Katakura, K.; Lee, J.; Rachmilewitz, D.; Li, G.; Eckmann, L.; Raz, E. Toll-like receptor 9-induced type I IFN protects mice from experimental colitis. *J. Clin. Investig.* **2005**, *115*, 695–702. [CrossRef] [PubMed]
32. Yarilina, A.; DiCarlo, E.; Ivashkiv, L.B. Suppression of the effector phase of inflammatory arthritis by double-stranded RNA is mediated by type I IFNs. *J. Immunol.* **2007**, *178*, 2204–2211. [CrossRef] [PubMed]
33. Wang, Y.; Shaked, I.; Stanford, S.M.; Zhou, W.; Curtsinger, J.M.; Mikulski, Z.; Shaheen, Z.R.; Cheng, G.; Sawatzke, K.; Campbell, A.M.; et al. The autoimmunity-associated gene PTPN22 potentiates toll-like receptor-driven, type 1 interferon-dependent immunity. *Immunity* **2013**, *39*, 111–122. [CrossRef]
34. Jofra, T.; Galvani, G.; Cosorich, I.; De Giorgi, L.; Annoni, A.; Vecchione, A.; Sorini, C.; Falcone, M.; Fousteri, G. Experimental colitis in IL-10-deficient mice ameliorates in the absence of PTPN22. *Clin. Exp. Immunol.* **2019**, *197*, 263–275. [CrossRef] [PubMed]
35. Spalinger, M.R.; Lang, S.; Gottier, C.; Dai, X.; Rawlings, D.J.; Chan, A.C.; Rogler, G.; Scharl, M. PTPN22 regulates NLRP3-mediated IL1B secretion in an autophagy-dependent manner. *Autophagy* **2017**, *13*, 1590–1601. [CrossRef] [PubMed]

36. Larabi, A.; Barnich, N.; Nguyen, H.T.T. New insights into the interplay between autophagy, gut microbiota and inflammatory responses in IBD. *Autophagy* **2020**, *16*, 38–51. [CrossRef]
37. Spalinger, M.R.; Schmidt, T.S.; Schwarzfischer, M.; Hering, L.; Atrott, K.; Lang, S.; Gottier, C.; Geirnaert, A.; Lacroix, C.; Dai, X.; et al. Protein tyrosine phosphatase non-receptor type 22 modulates colitis in a microbiota-dependent manner. *J. Clin. Investig.* **2019**, *129*, 2527–2541. [CrossRef]
38. Theiss, A.L. Ptpn2: A Critical Regulator of Paneth Cell Homeostasis. *Cell Mol. Gastroenterol. Hepatol.* **2023**, *16*, 163–164. [CrossRef] [PubMed]
39. Glas, J.; Wagner, J.; Seiderer, J.; Olszak, T.; Wetzke, M.; Beigel, F.; Tillack, C.; Stallhofer, J.; Friedrich, M.; Steib, C.; et al. PTPN2 gene variants are associated with susceptibility to both Crohn's disease and ulcerative colitis supporting a common genetic disease background. *PLoS ONE* **2012**, *7*, e33682. [CrossRef]
40. Spalinger, M.R.; Sayoc-Becerra, A.; Santos, A.N.; Shawki, A.; Canale, V.; Krishnan, M.; Niechcial, A.; Obialo, N.; Scharl, M.; Li, J.; et al. PTPN2 Regulates Interactions Between Macrophages and Intestinal Epithelial Cells to Promote Intestinal Barrier Function. *Gastroenterology* **2020**, *159*, 1763–1777.e14. [CrossRef]
41. Canale, V.; Spalinger, M.R.; Alvarez, R.; Sayoc-Becerra, A.; Sanati, G.; Manz, S.; Chatterjee, P.; Santos, A.N.; Lei, H.; Jahng, S.; et al. PTPN2 Is a Critical Regulator of Ileal Paneth Cell Viability and Function in Mice. *Cell Mol. Gastroenterol. Hepatol.* **2023**, *16*, 39–62. [CrossRef]
42. Scharl, M.; McCole, D.F.; Weber, A.; Vavricka, S.R.; Frei, P.; Kellermeier, S.; Pesch, T.; Fried, M.; Rogler, G. Protein tyrosine phosphatase N2 regulates TNFα-induced signalling and cytokine secretion in human intestinal epithelial cells. *Gut* **2011**, *60*, 189–197. [CrossRef] [PubMed]
43. Scharl, M.; Paul, G.; Weber, A.; Jung, B.C.; Docherty, M.J.; Hausmann, M.; Rogler, G.; Barrett, K.E.; McCole, D.F. Protection of Epithelial Barrier Function by the Crohn's Disease Associated Gene Protein Tyrosine Phosphatase N2. *Gastroenterology* **2009**, *137*, 2030–2040.e35. [CrossRef] [PubMed]
44. McCole, D.F. Regulation of epithelial barrier function by the inflammatory bowel disease candidate gene, PTPN2. *Ann. N. Y Acad. Sci.* **2012**, *1257*, 108–114. [CrossRef]
45. Spalinger, M.R.; Manzini, R.; Hering, L.; Riggs, J.B.; Gottier, C.; Lang, S.; Atrott, K.; Fettelschoss, A.; Olomski, F.; Kündig, T.M.; et al. PTPN2 Regulates Inflammasome Activation and Controls Onset of Intestinal Inflammation and Colon Cancer. *Cell Rep.* **2018**, *22*, 1835–1848. [CrossRef]
46. Wang, M.; Li, J.; Yin, Y.; Liu, L.; Wang, Y.; Qu, Y.; Hong, Y.; Ji, S.; Zhang, T.; Wang, N.; et al. Network pharmacology and in vivo experiment-based strategy to investigate mechanisms of JingFangFuZiLiZhong formula for ulcerative colitis. *Ann. Med.* **2022**, *54*, 3219–3233. [CrossRef]
47. Jiang, X.; Guo, H.; Wu, J.; He, Q.; Li, Y.; Wang, M.; Pan, H.; Li, W.; Wang, J.; Wang, Q.; et al. Critical role of SHP2 (PTPN11) signaling in germinal center-derived lymphoma. *Haematologica* **2014**, *99*, 1834–1845. [CrossRef]
48. Yamashita, H.; Kotani, T.; Park, J.H.; Murata, Y.; Okazawa, H.; Ohnishi, H.; Ku, Y.; Matozaki, T. Role of the protein tyrosine phosphatase Shp2 in homeostasis of the intestinal epithelium. *PLoS ONE* **2014**, *9*, e92904. [CrossRef]
49. Heuberger, J.; Kosel, F.; Qi, J.; Grossmann, K.S.; Rajewsky, K.; Birchmeier, W. Shp2/MAPK signaling controls goblet/paneth cell fate decisions in the intestine. *Proc. Natl. Acad. Sci. USA* **2014**, *111*, 3472–3477. [CrossRef] [PubMed]
50. Coulombe, G.; Leblanc, C.; Cagnol, S.; Maloum, F.; Lemieux, E.; Perreault, N.; Feng, G.S.; Boudreau, F.; Rivard, N. Epithelial tyrosine phosphatase SHP-2 protects against intestinal inflammation in mice. *Mol. Cell Biol.* **2013**, *33*, 2275–2284. [CrossRef] [PubMed]
51. Xiao, P.; Zhang, H.; Zhang, Y.; Zheng, M.; Liu, R.; Zhao, Y.; Zhang, X.; Cheng, H.; Cao, Q.; Ke, Y. Phosphatase Shp2 exacerbates intestinal inflammation by disrupting macrophage responsiveness to interleukin-10. *J. Exp. Med.* **2019**, *216*, 337–349. [CrossRef] [PubMed]
52. Murchie, R.; Guo, C.-H.; Persaud, A.; Muise, A.; Rotin, D. Protein tyrosine phosphatase σ targets apical junction complex proteins in the intestine and regulates epithelial permeability. *Proc. Natl. Acad. Sci. USA* **2014**, *111*, 693–698. [CrossRef] [PubMed]
53. Muise, A.M.; Walters, T.; Wine, E.; Griffiths, A.M.; Turner, D.; Duerr, R.H.; Regueiro, M.D.; Ngan, B.Y.; Xu, W.; Sherman, P.M.; et al. Protein-tyrosine phosphatase sigma is associated with ulcerative colitis. *Curr. Biol.* **2007**, *17*, 1212–1218. [CrossRef] [PubMed]
54. Leblanc, C.; Langlois, M.; Perreault, N.; Rivard, N. A28 shp-1 regulates intestinal epithelium homeostasis by controlling activation of both pi3k/akt and wnt/β-catenin pathways. *J. Can. Assoc. Gastroenterol.* **2018**, *1* (Suppl. S2), 46. [CrossRef]
55. Bouzid, D.; Fourati, H.; Amouri, A.; Marques, I.; Abida, O.; Haddouk, S.; Ben Ayed, M.; Tahri, N.; Penha-Gonçalves, C.; Masmoudi, H. Association of ZAP70 and PTPN6, but Not BANK1 or CLEC2D, with Inflammatory Bowel Disease in the Tunisian Population. *Genet. Test. Mol. Biomark.* **2013**, *17*, 321–326. [CrossRef] [PubMed]
56. Jeffrey, K.L.; Brummer, T.; Rolph, M.S.; Liu, S.M.; Callejas, N.A.; Grumont, R.J.; Gillieron, C.; Mackay, F.; Grey, S.; Camps, M.; et al. Positive regulation of immune cell function and inflammatory responses by phosphatase PAC-1. *Nat. Immunol.* **2006**, *7*, 274–283. [CrossRef]
57. Lu, D.; Liu, L.; Ji, X.; Gao, Y.; Chen, X.; Liu, Y.; Liu, Y.; Zhao, X.; Li, Y.; Li, Y.; et al. The phosphatase DUSP2 controls the activity of the transcription activator STAT3 and regulates TH17 differentiation. *Nat. Immunol.* **2015**, *16*, 1263–1273. [CrossRef]
58. Maillet, M.; Purcell, N.H.; Sargent, M.A.; York, A.J.; Bueno, O.F.; Molkentin, J.D. DUSP6 (MKP3) null mice show enhanced ERK1/2 phosphorylation at baseline and increased myocyte proliferation in the heart affecting disease susceptibility. *J. Biol. Chem.* **2008**, *283*, 31246–31255. [CrossRef]

59. Beaudry, K.; Langlois, M.J.; Montagne, A.; Cagnol, S.; Carrier, J.C.; Rivard, N. Dual-specificity phosphatase 6 deletion protects the colonic epithelium against inflammation and promotes both proliferation and tumorigenesis. *J. Cell Physiol.* **2019**, *234*, 6731–6745. [CrossRef]
60. Miele, L.; Giorgio, V.; Liguori, A.; Petta, S.; Pastorino, R.; Arzani, D.; Alberelli, M.A.; Cefalo, C.; Marrone, G.; Biolato, M.; et al. Genetic susceptibility of increased intestinal permeability is associated with progressive liver disease and diabetes in patients with non-alcoholic fatty liver disease. *Nutr. Metab. Cardiovasc. Dis.* **2020**, *30*, 2103–2110. [CrossRef]
61. Espino-Paisan, L.; de la Calle, H.; Fernández-Arquero, M.; Figueredo, M.Á.; de la Concha, E.G.; Urcelay, E.; Santiago, J.L. A polymorphism in PTPN2 gene is associated with an earlier onset of type 1 diabetes. *Immunogenetics* **2011**, *63*, 255–258. [CrossRef]
62. Roca-Rivada, A.; Marín-Cañas, S.; Colli, M.L.; Vinci, C.; Sawatani, T.; Marselli, L.; Cnop, M.; Marchetti, P.; Eizirik, D.L. Inhibition of the type 1 diabetes candidate gene PTPN2 aggravates TNF-α-induced human beta cell dysfunction and death. *Diabetologia* **2023**, *66*, 1544–1556. [CrossRef] [PubMed]
63. Kumar, V.; Gutierrez-Achury, J.; Kanduri, K.; Almeida, R.; Hrdlickova, B.; Zhernakova, D.V.; Westra, H.J.; Karjalainen, J.; Ricaño-Ponce, I.; Li, Y.; et al. Systematic annotation of celiac disease loci refines pathological pathways and suggests a genetic explanation for increased interferon-gamma levels. *Hum. Mol. Genet.* **2015**, *24*, 397–409. [CrossRef] [PubMed]
64. Zhang, Y.; Siebert, R.; Matthiesen, P.; Yang, Y.; Ha, H.; Schlegelberger, B. Cytogenetical assignment and physical mapping of the human R-PTP-kappa gene (PTPRK) to the putative tumor suppressor gene region 6q22.2-q22.3. *Genomics* **1998**, *51*, 309–311. [CrossRef] [PubMed]
65. Jiang, Y.P.; Wang, H.; D'Eustachio, P.; Musacchio, J.M.; Schlessinger, J.; Sap, J. Cloning and characterization of R-PTP-kappa, a new member of the receptor protein tyrosine phosphatase family with a proteolytically cleaved cellular adhesion molecule-like extracellular region. *Mol. Cell Biol.* **1993**, *13*, 2942–2951. [CrossRef]
66. Kose, H.; Sakai, T.; Tsukumo, S.; Wei, K.; Yamada, T.; Yasutomo, K.; Matsumoto, K. Maturational arrest of thymocyte development is caused by a deletion in the receptor-like protein tyrosine phosphatase kappa gene in LEC rats. *Genomics* **2007**, *89*, 673–677. [CrossRef]
67. Erdenebayar, N.; Maekawa, Y.; Nishida, J.; Kitamura, A.; Yasutomo, K. Protein-tyrosine phosphatase-kappa regulates CD4+ T cell development through ERK1/2-mediated signaling. *Biochem. Biophys. Res. Commun.* **2009**, *390*, 489–493. [CrossRef]
68. Anders, L.; Mertins, P.; Lammich, S.; Murgia, M.; Hartmann, D.; Saftig, P.; Haass, C.; Ullrich, A. Furin-, ADAM 10-, and gamma-secretase-mediated cleavage of a receptor tyrosine phosphatase and regulation of beta-catenin's transcriptional activity. *Mol. Cell Biol.* **2006**, *26*, 3917–3934. [CrossRef] [PubMed]
69. Novellino, L.; De Filippo, A.; Deho, P.; Perrone, F.; Pilotti, S.; Parmiani, G.; Castelli, C. PTPRK negatively regulates transcriptional activity of wild type and mutated oncogenic beta-catenin and affects membrane distribution of beta-catenin/E-cadherin complexes in cancer cells. *Cell Signal.* **2008**, *20*, 872–883. [CrossRef]
70. Schnekenburger, J.; Mayerle, J.; Krüger, B.; Buchwalow, I.; Weiss, F.U.; Albrecht, E.; Samoilova, V.E.; Domschke, W.; Lerch, M.M. Protein tyrosine phosphatase kappa and SHP-1 are involved in the regulation of cell-cell contacts at adherens junctions in the exocrine pancreas. *Gut* **2005**, *54*, 1445–1455. [CrossRef]
71. Asano, A.; Tsubomatsu, K.; Jung, C.G.; Sasaki, N.; Agui, T. A deletion mutation of the protein tyrosine phosphatase kappa (Ptprk) gene is responsible for T-helper immunodeficiency (thid) in the LEC rat. *Mamm. Genome* **2007**, *18*, 779–786. [CrossRef]
72. Barone, M.V.; Troncone, R.; Auricchio, S. Gliadin peptides as triggers of the proliferative and stress/innate immune response of the celiac small intestinal mucosa. *Int. J. Mol. Sci.* **2014**, *15*, 20518–20537. [CrossRef] [PubMed]
73. Lania, G.; Nanayakkara, M.; Maglio, M.; Auricchio, R.; Porpora, M.; Conte, M.; De Matteis, M.A.; Rizzo, R.; Luini, A.; Discepolo, V.; et al. Constitutive alterations in vesicular trafficking increase the sensitivity of cells from celiac disease patients to gliadin. *Commun. Biol.* **2019**, *2*, 190. [CrossRef] [PubMed]
74. Nanayakkara, M.; Lania, G.; Maglio, M.; Kosova, R.; Sarno, M.; Gaito, A.; Discepolo, V.; Troncone, R.; Auricchio, S.; Auricchio, R.; et al. Enterocyte proliferation and signaling are constitutively altered in celiac disease. *PLoS ONE* **2013**, *8*, e76006. [CrossRef] [PubMed]
75. Barone, M.V.; Nanayakkara, M.; Paolella, G.; Maglio, M.; Vitale, V.; Troiano, R.; Ribecco, M.T.; Lania, G.; Zanzi, D.; Santagata, S.; et al. Gliadin peptide P31-43 localises to endocytic vesicles and interferes with their maturation. *PLoS ONE* **2010**, *5*, e12246. [CrossRef]
76. Xu, Y.; Xue, S.; Zhou, J.; Voorhees, J.J.; Fisher, G.J. Notch and TGF-β pathways cooperatively regulate receptor protein tyrosine phosphatase-κ (PTPRK) gene expression in human primary keratinocytes. *Mol. Biol. Cell* **2015**, *26*, 1199–1206. [CrossRef] [PubMed]
77. Bondar, C.; Plaza-Izurieta, L.; Fernandez-Jimenez, N.; Irastorza, I.; Withoff, S.; Wijmenga, C.; Chirdo, F.; Bilbao, J.R. THEMIS and PTPRK in celiac intestinal mucosa: Coexpression in disease and after in vitro gliadin challenge. *Eur. J. Hum. Genet.* **2014**, *22*, 358–362. [CrossRef]
78. Törn, C.; Hadley, D.; Lee, H.S.; Hagopian, W.; Lernmark, Å.; Simell, O.; Rewers, M.; Ziegler, A.; Schatz, D.; Akolkar, B.; et al. Role of Type 1 Diabetes-Associated SNPs on Risk of Autoantibody Positivity in the TEDDY Study. *Diabetes* **2015**, *64*, 1818–1829. [CrossRef]

79. Knip, M.; Simell, O. Environmental triggers of type 1 diabetes. *Cold Spring Harb. Perspect. Med.* **2012**, *2*, a007690. [CrossRef]
80. Atkinson, M.A.; Bluestone, J.A.; Eisenbarth, G.S.; Hebrok, M.; Herold, K.C.; Accili, D.; Pietropaolo, M.; Arvan, P.R.; Von Herrath, M.; Markel, D.S.; et al. How does type 1 diabetes develop?: The notion of homicide or β-cell suicide revisited. *Diabetes* **2011**, *60*, 1370–1379. [CrossRef]
81. Du, Y.T.; Rayner, C.K.; Jones, K.L.; Talley, N.J.; Horowitz, M. Gastrointestinal Symptoms in Diabetes: Prevalence, Assessment, Pathogenesis, and Management. *Diabetes Care* **2018**, *41*, 627–637. [CrossRef]
82. Rodrigues, M.L.; Motta, M.E. Mechanisms and factors associated with gastrointestinal symptoms in patients with diabetes mellitus. *J. Pediatr.* **2012**, *88*, 17–24. [CrossRef] [PubMed]
83. Menard, L.; Saadoun, D.; Isnardi, I.; Ng, Y.S.; Meyers, G.; Massad, C.; Price, C.; Abraham, C.; Motaghedi, R.; Buckner, J.H.; et al. The PTPN22 allele encoding an R620W variant interferes with the removal of developing autoreactive B cells in humans. *J. Clin. Investig.* **2011**, *121*, 3635–3644. [CrossRef] [PubMed]
84. Kim, Y.K.; Kim, Y.R.; Wells, K.L.; Sarbaugh, D.; Guney, M.; Tsai, C.F.; Zee, T.; Karsenty, G.; Nakayasu, E.S.; Sussel, L. PTPN2 Regulates Metabolic Flux to Affect β-Cell Susceptibility to Inflammatory Stress. *Diabetes* **2024**, *73*, 434–447. [CrossRef] [PubMed]
85. Gurzov, E.N.; Tran, M.; Fernandez-Rojo, M.A.; Merry, T.L.; Zhang, X.; Xu, Y.; Fukushima, A.; Waters, M.J.; Watt, M.J.; Andrikopoulos, S.; et al. Hepatic oxidative stress promotes insulin-STAT-5 signaling and obesity by inactivating protein tyrosine phosphatase N2. *Cell Metab.* **2014**, *20*, 85–102. [CrossRef]
86. Ashton, M.P.; Eugster, A.; Dietz, S.; Loebel, D.; Lindner, A.; Kuehn, D.; Taranko, A.E.; Heschel, B.; Gavrisan, A.; Ziegler, A.G.; et al. Association of Dendritic Cell Signatures With Autoimmune Inflammation Revealed by Single-Cell Profiling. *Arthritis Rheumatol.* **2019**, *71*, 817–828. [CrossRef] [PubMed]
87. Yeung, W.C.; Rawlinson, W.D.; Craig, M.E. Enterovirus infection and type 1 diabetes mellitus: Systematic review and meta-analysis of observational molecular studies. *BMJ* **2011**, *342*, d35. [CrossRef] [PubMed]
88. Sandholm, N.; Rubio García, A.; Pekalski, M.L.; Inshaw, J.R.J.; Cutler, A.J.; Todd, J.A. Thymocyte regulatory variant alters transcription factor binding and protects from type 1 diabetes in infants. *Sci. Rep.* **2022**, *12*, 14137. [CrossRef] [PubMed]
89. Donnelly, C.; Williams, A. Investigating the potential impact of post translational modification of auto-antigens by tissue transglutaminase on humoral islet autoimmunity in type 1 diabetes. *Metabol. Open* **2020**, *8*, 100062. [CrossRef] [PubMed]
90. Wang, Y.; Ande, S.R.; Mishra, S. Phosphorylation of transglutaminase 2 (TG2) at serine-216 has a role in TG2 mediated activation of nuclear factor-kappa B and in the downregulation of PTEN. *BMC Cancer* **2012**, *12*, 277. [CrossRef]
91. Borrelli, M.; Maglio, M.; Korponay-Szabó, I.R.; Vass, V.; Mearin, M.L.; Meijer, C.; Niv-Drori, H.; Ribes-Koninckx, C.; Roca, M.; Shamir, R.; et al. Intestinal anti-transglutaminase 2 immunoglobulin A deposits in children at risk for coeliac disease (CD): Data from the PreventCD study. *Clin. Exp. Immunol.* **2018**, *191*, 311–317. [CrossRef]
92. Maglio, M.; Troncone, R. Intestinal Anti-tissue Transglutaminase2 Autoantibodies: Pathogenic and Clinical Implications for Celiac Disease. *Front. Nutr.* **2020**, *7*, 73. [CrossRef] [PubMed]
93. Behl, T.; Gupta, A.; Sehgal, A.; Albarrati, A.; Albratty, M.; Meraya, A.M.; Najmi, A.; Bhatia, S.; Bungau, S. Exploring protein tyrosine phosphatases (PTP) and PTP-1B inhibitors in management of diabetes mellitus. *Biomed. Pharmacother.* **2022**, *153*, 113405. [CrossRef] [PubMed]
94. Zhang, S.; Liu, S.; Tao, R.; Wei, D.; Chen, L.; Shen, W.; Yu, Z.H.; Wang, L.; Jones, D.R.; Dong, X.C.; et al. A highly selective and potent PTP-MEG2 inhibitor with therapeutic potential for type 2 diabetes. *J. Am. Chem. Soc.* **2012**, *134*, 18116–18124. [CrossRef] [PubMed]
95. Beysel, S.; Unsal, I.O.; Kizilgul, M.; Caliskan, M.; Ucan, B.; Cakal, E. The effects of metformin in type 1 diabetes mellitus. *BMC Endocr. Disord.* **2018**, *18*, 1. [CrossRef] [PubMed]
96. Wu, J.; Sun, Y.; Zhou, H.; Ma, Y.; Wang, R. Design, synthesis, biological evaluation and molecular dynamics simulation studies of (R)-5-methylthiazolidin-4-One derivatives as megakaryocyte protein tyrosine phosphatase 2 (PTP-MEG2) inhibitors for the treatment of type 2 diabetes. *J. Biomol. Struct. Dyn.* **2020**, *38*, 3156–3165. [CrossRef]
97. Pietz, G.; De, R.; Hedberg, M.; Sjöberg, V.; Sandström, O.; Hernell, O.; Hammarström, S.; Hammarström, M.L. Immunopathology of childhood celiac disease-Key role of intestinal epithelial cells. *PLoS ONE* **2017**, *12*, e0185025. [CrossRef]
98. Watson, C.L.; Mahe, M.M.; Múnera, J.; Howell, J.C.; Sundaram, N.; Poling, H.M.; Schweitzer, J.I.; Vallance, J.E.; Mayhew, C.N.; Sun, Y.; et al. An in vivo model of human small intestine using pluripotent stem cells. *Nat. Med.* **2014**, *20*, 1310–1314. [CrossRef]
99. Okita, K.; Ichisaka, T.; Yamanaka, S. Generation of germline-competent induced pluripotent stem cells. *Nature* **2007**, *448*, 313–317. [CrossRef]
100. Wallach, T.E.; Bayrer, J.R. Intestinal Organoids: New Frontiers in the Study of Intestinal Disease and Physiology. *J. Pediatr. Gastroenterol. Nutr.* **2017**, *64*, 180–185. [CrossRef]
101. Finkbeiner, S.R.; Freeman, J.J.; Wieck, M.M.; El-Nachef, W.; Altheim, C.H.; Tsai, Y.H.; Huang, S.; Dyal, R.; White, E.S.; Grikscheit, T.C.; et al. Generation of tissue-engineered small intestine using embryonic stem cell-derived human intestinal organoids. *Biol. Open* **2015**, *4*, 1462–1472. [CrossRef]

102. Banerjee, P.; Senapati, S. Translational Utility of Organoid Models for Biomedical Research on Gastrointestinal Diseases. *Stem Cell Rev. Rep.* **2024**, *20*, 1441–1458. [CrossRef] [PubMed]
103. Porpora, M.; Conte, M.; Lania, G.; Bellomo, C.; Rapacciuolo, L.; Chirdo, F.G.; Auricchio, R.; Troncone, R.; Auricchio, S.; Barone, M.V.; et al. Inflammation Is Present, Persistent and More Sensitive to Proinflammatory Triggers in Celiac Disease Enterocytes. *Int. J. Mol. Sci.* **2022**, *23*, 1973. [CrossRef] [PubMed]

International Journal of
Molecular Sciences

MDPI

Article

Tissue Kallikrein-1 Suppresses Type I Interferon Responses and Reduces Depressive-Like Behavior in the MRL/lpr Lupus-Prone Mouse Model

Priyanka S. Bhoj [1], Cassandra Nocito [1], Namdev S. Togre [1], Malika Winfield [1], Cody Lubinsky [1], Sabeeya Khan [1], Nikhita Mogadala [1], Alecia Seliga [1], Ellen M. Unterwald [2], Yuri Persidsky [1] and Uma Sriram [1,*]

1 Department of Pathology and Laboratory Medicine, Lewis Katz School of Medicine, Temple University, Philadelphia, PA 19140, USA; priyanka.bhoj@temple.edu (P.S.B.); cassandra.nocito@gmail.com (C.N.); namdev.togre@temple.edu (N.S.T.); malika.winfield@temple.edu (M.W.); codylubinsky@gmail.com (C.L.); sabeeyakj@gmail.com (S.K.); nikhita.mogadala@gmail.com (N.M.); aleciaseliga.as@gmail.com (A.S.); yuri.persidsky@temple.edu (Y.P.)

2 Center for Substance Abuse Research, Lewis Katz School of Medicine, Temple University, Philadelphia, PA 19140, USA; ellen.unterwald@temple.edu

* Correspondence: uma.sriram@temple.edu

Abstract: Excessive production and response to Type I interferons (IFNs) is a hallmark of systemic lupus erythematosus (SLE). Neuropsychiatric lupus (NPSLE) is a common manifestation of human SLE, with major depression as the most common presentation. Clinical studies have demonstrated that IFNα can cause depressive symptoms. We have shown that the kallikrein–kinin system (KKS) [comprised of kallikreins (Klks) and bradykinins] and angiotensin-converting enzyme inhibitors suppressed Type I IFN responses in dendritic cells from lupus-prone mice and human peripheral blood mononuclear cells. Tissue Klk genes are decreased in patients with lupus, and giving exogenous Klk1 ameliorated kidney pathology in mice. We retro-orbitally administered mouse *klk1* gene-carrying adenovirus in the Murphy Roths Large lymphoproliferative (MRL/lpr) lupus-prone mice at early disease onset and analyzed immune responses and depressive-like behavior. Klk1 improved depressive-like behavior, suppressed interferon-responsive genes and neuroinflammation, and reduced plasma IFNα levels and proinflammatory cytokines. Klk1 also reduced IFNAR1 and JAK1 protein expression, important upstream molecules in Type I IFN signaling. Klk1 reduced bradykinin B1 receptor expression, which is known to induce proinflammatory response. Together, these findings suggest that Klk1 may be a potential therapeutic candidate to control IFNα production/responses and other inflammatory responses in SLE and NPSLE.

Keywords: neuropsychiatric lupus; type I interferons; kallikrein–kinin system; tissue kallikreins; depression

1. Introduction

Neuropsychiatric lupus (NPSLE) [1,2] is one of the common manifestations of human systemic lupus erythematosus (SLE). NPSLE symptoms include anxiety, depression, and cognitive impairment. NPSLE pathogenesis includes ischemic and neuroinflammatory mechanisms [3]. The symptoms present within the first year of lupus diagnosis [4] suggest that early factors contributing to peripheral autoimmunity may promote NPSLE.

Extensive studies in the past two decades have highlighted IFNα as a central player in lupus pathogenesis [5,6]. Elevated IFNα levels in the cerebrospinal fluid (CSF) are associated with lupus psychosis [7]. Moreover, IFNα administration in chronic viral infections and some cancers [8,9] causes depression in a high percentage of patients. Recent studies show that systemic immune responses—including Type I IFNs—affect neuroinflammation and neuropsychiatric responses [10]. Our recent publication [11] shows an increased IFN signature in the brain and increased depressive-like behavior in the Murphy Roths Large lymphoproliferative (MRL/lpr) lupus-prone mouse model at a young age compared to the age-matched wild-type strain. We hypothesize that excess IFNα (produced in the brain or coming from the periphery) causes NPSLE symptoms, and reducing this response is important to ameliorate the disease.

We discovered that the kallikrein–kinin system (KKS) can suppress the Type I IFN response [12]. The KKS [comprised of kallikreins (Klks), bradykinins (BKs)] and angiotensin-converting enzyme inhibitors (ACEi), which bridge the KKS–renin–angiotensin (RAS) pathway, suppressed the Type I IFN responses in murine dendritic cells (DCs) from normal and lupus-prone mice and in human peripheral blood mononuclear cells [12]. Tissue Klks [13], an important component of the KKS, are a family of 15 secreted serine proteases that are emerging as important regulators of neurological diseases [14–16], including Alzheimer's disease [17], Parkinson's disease [18], and multiple sclerosis [19]. Tissue Klk converts low molecular weight kininogen to kinin peptide [20], in turn activating bradykinin B1 and B2 receptors and triggering a host of biological effects [15,21,22]: blood pressure regulation, smooth muscle contraction/relaxation, vascular cell growth, vascular permeability, inflammatory cascade inactivation, and neuroprotective effects. It has been shown that ACE from the RAS pathway affects BK production and downstream signaling in cardiovascular models [15,23]; we demonstrated similar effects in our NPSLE model [11]. We hypothesize that Klks also act via signaling BK to bring about the effects in this model. They may also act via protease-activated receptors (PARs) to bring about the effects [24–29].

Kallikrein 1 (Klk1), a widely expressed tissue Klk [13,30], is decreased in lupus patients and lupus mouse models [31]; administration of exogenous Klk1 ameliorated lupus nephritis in mice [31,32]. Earlier studies have shown that Klk1 only affects the kidneys [31,32]. Organ-specific responses vary in lupus, and for the first time, we demonstrate the effects of Klk1 in regulating IFN responses in vivo in the periphery and in the central nervous system (CNS) (neuroinflammation and behavior) in lupus. Using the MRL/lpr mice, a popularly used lupus-prone model, we show in a short-term study that exogenous *Klk1* administration reduced depressive-like behavior, key interferon responsive genes (IRGs), and proinflammatory responses. *Klk1* administration transformed the microglia to a less inflammatory state. It also normalized the expression of key genes associated with depression.

2. Results

2.1. Adenoviral Vector Delivery of Mouse Klk1 Increases Tissue Protein Expression

Chandra Mohan's group has shown [32] that mouse *klk1* gene delivery using an adenoviral vector via the tail vein was able to infect and express Klk1 protein in the peripheral organs. We used a retro-orbital injection route to administer the vector and analyzed Klk1 expression by western blot and immunohistochemical analyses (Figure 1A,B). Klk1 protein expression was higher in the kidneys of the Ad-Klk1 group than in those of the Ad-GFP group.

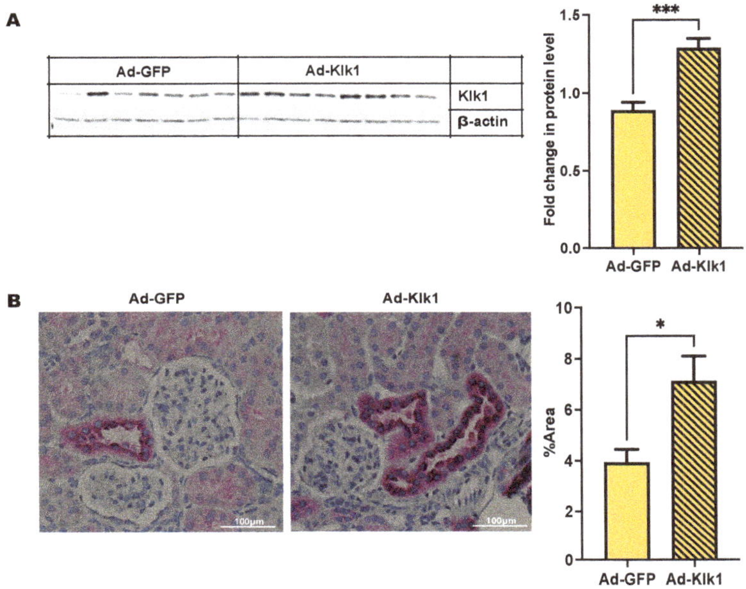

Figure 1. Administration of *Ad-klk1* increases Klk1 protein expression (**A**) Western blot of Klk1 protein (MW: 28 kDa) and (**B**) immunohistochemical results (indicated by pink staining) of Klk1 protein expression in the kidney of the spontaneous cohort. Images were taken at 40× magnification and analyzed using ImageJ (1.54f software). The results are expressed as mean ±SEM. An unpaired *t*-test was used; * $p \leq 0.05$ and *** $p \leq 0.001$ compared to the Ad-GFP group; n = 7–8 mice/group.

2.2. Tissue Klk1 Decreases IRG and hmgb1 Gene Expression in the Brain and Periphery

In the spontaneous MRL/lpr cohort, *Ad-klk1* delivery significantly decreased interferon-stimulated gene 15 (*isg15*) and high-mobility group box 1 (*hmgb1*) expression in the brain and spleen compared to those in the respective tissues of Ad-GFP group. Although not significantly different, the expression of C-X-C motif chemokine ligand 10 (*cxcl10*; $p = 0.2$), myxovirus resistance gene (*mx1*; $p = 0.06$), and interferon regulatory factor 7 (*irf7*; $p = 0.07$) was also lower in the brain of the Ad-Klk1 group than in the Ad-GFP group (Figure 2A). *Ad-klk1* administration also suppressed IRGs in the IFNα-induced MRL/lpr cohort. Gene expression of *isg15* and *mx1* were significantly lower in the brain and spleen of the Ad-Klk1 group than those in the respective tissues of the Ad-GFP group. Moreover, *cxcl10* and *irf7* expression were significantly reduced in the brain of the Ad-Klk1 group, with a similar, though not significant, trend observed in the spleen (Figure 2B), suggesting profound effects of Klk1 on Type I IFN responses in the periphery and brain. Expression of *hmgb1*, a proinflammatory danger signal that is shown to be increased during the course of the disease, was also reduced significantly in the spontaneous cohort (Figure 2A) but remained unchanged in the IFNα-induced cohort (Figure 2B). Overall, Ad-Klk1 reduced the expression of IRGs and proinflammatory genes in the brain and spleen of both spontaneous and IFNα-induced MRL/lpr mice.

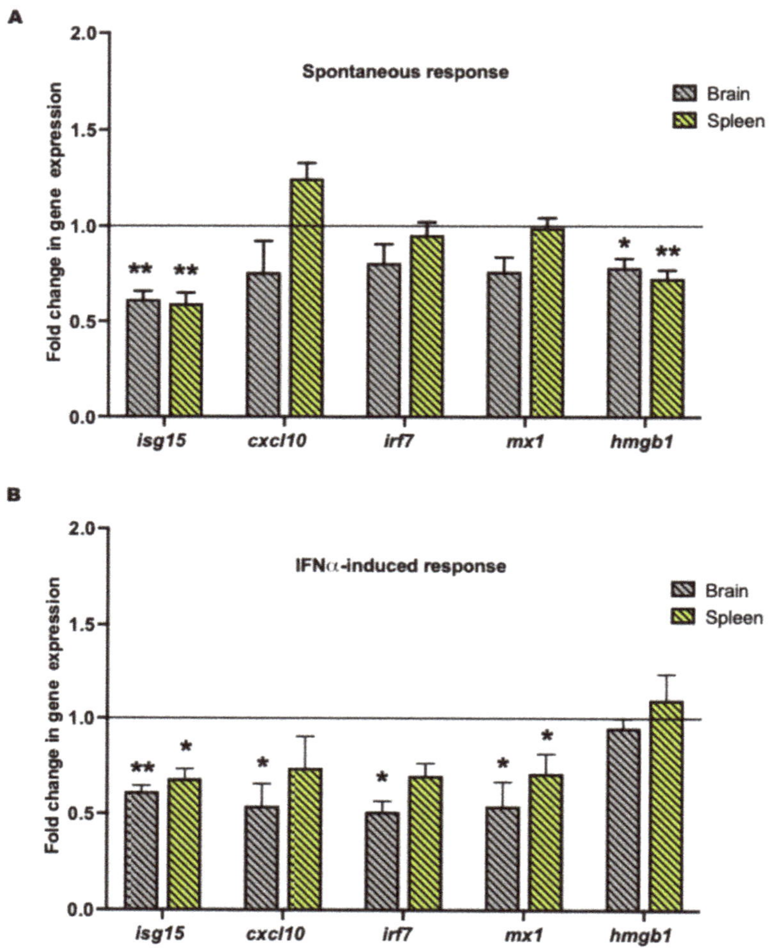

Figure 2. Tissue Klk1 decreases IRGs and *hmgb1* gene expression in the brain and periphery: (**A**) Spontaneous MRL/lpr mice and (**B**) IFNα-induced MRL/lpr mice. The data, obtained by qPCR, were analyzed using an unpaired *t*-test and are expressed as the mean ±SEM of the fold change in gene expression in the Ad-Klk1 group compared to the Ad-GFP group (marked as a solid black line at 1.0 on the Y axis). * $p \leq 0.05$ and ** $p \leq 0.01$ compared to the Ad-GFP group; n = 7–8 mice/group in the spontaneous cohort, and n = 5 mice/group in the IFNα-induced cohort.

2.3. Tissue Klk1 Reduces Inflammatory Cytokine Levels in Plasma

We next investigated whether Klk1 suppresses the inflammatory response in the plasma of spontaneous and IFNα-induced MRL/lpr mice. Klk1 administration significantly reduced the levels of tumor necrosis factor-α (TNFα), IL (interleukin)-10, monocyte chemoattractant protein-1 (MCP-1), IL-33, IL-5, and IL-2 in the spontaneous cohort (Figure 3A), and IL-33 and IL-5 in the IFNα-induced cohort (Figure 3B). Other proinflammatory cytokines and chemokines were unaffected or showed decreasing levels (not statistically significant) in the Ad-Klk1 group compared to Ad-GFP controls (Table S1).

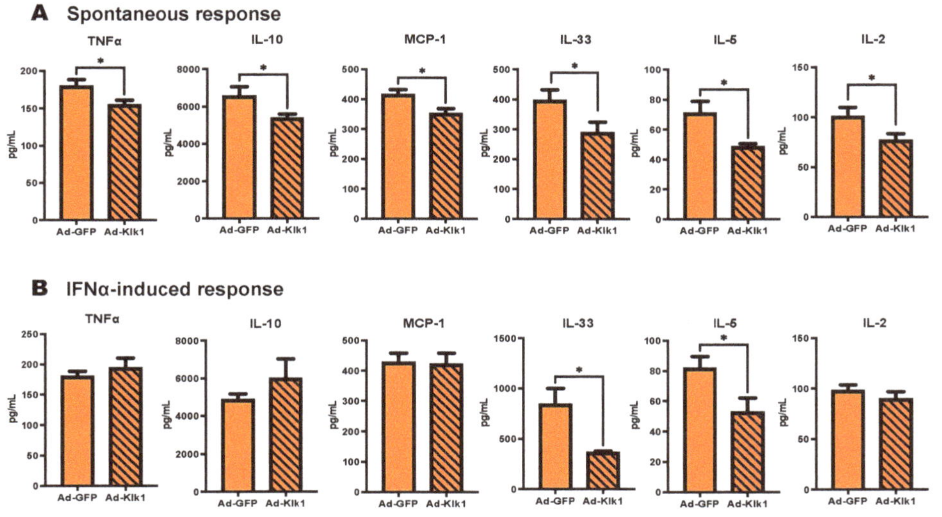

Figure 3. Tissue Klk1 reduces inflammatory cytokine levels in the plasma: (**A**) Spontaneous MRL/lpr mice and (**B**) IFNα-induced MRL/lpr mice. Multiplex cytokine analysis was performed using the MSD ELISA kit. The data were analyzed using an unpaired t-test and are expressed as the mean ±SEM. * $p \leq 0.05$ compared to the Ad-GFP group; n = 7–8 mice/group in the spontaneous cohort, and n = 5 mice/group in the IFNα-induced cohort.

2.4. Klk1 Decreases Plasma IFNα Levels and Proteins in Type I IFN Signaling

Increased IFNα levels in patients with SLE are a hallmark of the disease [33,34]. We tested whether Klk1 could reduce IFNα levels in the MRL/lpr mice. Circulating IFNα levels were lower in the Ad-Klk1 group than in the Ad-GFP group in both spontaneous ($p = 0.03$) and IFNα-induced ($p = 0.06$) MRL/lpr mice (Figure 4A). Type I IFN signaling follows an autocrine feedback loop via their receptor IFNAR1 that refuels and amplifies the signal [35]. We tested whether *klk1* administration can reduce IFNAR1 expression. The protein expression of IFNAR1 and JAK1, an IFNAR1-associated kinase, were significantly decreased in the kidneys (Figure 4B) and spleen (Figure 4C) following *Ad-Klk1* administration.

2.5. Tissue Klk1 Reduces Depressive-Like Behavior in Lupus-Prone Mice

Depression is a common psychiatric manifestation in patients with NPSLE [36]. We have previously confirmed [11] that it is an early disease manifestation in lupus-prone MRL/lpr mice [37]. Tail suspension test (TST) [38] was used to assess depressive-like behavior in our cohorts. Immobility time during the TST, a measure of depressive-like behavior, was significantly lower in the Ad-Klk1 group than in the Ad-GFP group in both spontaneous (Figure 5A) and IFNα-induced (Figure S1A) MRL/lpr mice. Notably, there was no difference in locomotor function between the groups (as measured by a rotarod test [39] for assessment of motor skills, coordination, and balance; Figure S1B), indicating that the reduced immobility time in TST is not due to a defect in locomotion but rather an indication of decreased depressive-like behavior. Although not significantly different, plasma serotonin levels, known as the body's "feel good" neurotransmitter [40], were higher in the Ad-Klk1 group than in the Ad-GFP group (Figure 5B). The gene expression of the serotonin transporter (*5htt*), 5-hydroxytryptamine 2A receptor (*htr2a*), and tryptophan hydroxylase 2 (*tph-2*), which are the homeostatic regulators of serotonin levels in the brain, was higher in the Ad-Klk1 group than in the Ad-GFP group. However, the expression of brain-derived neurotrophic factor (*bdnf*), which also regulates depressive-like behavior, was unaltered between the groups (Figure 5C).

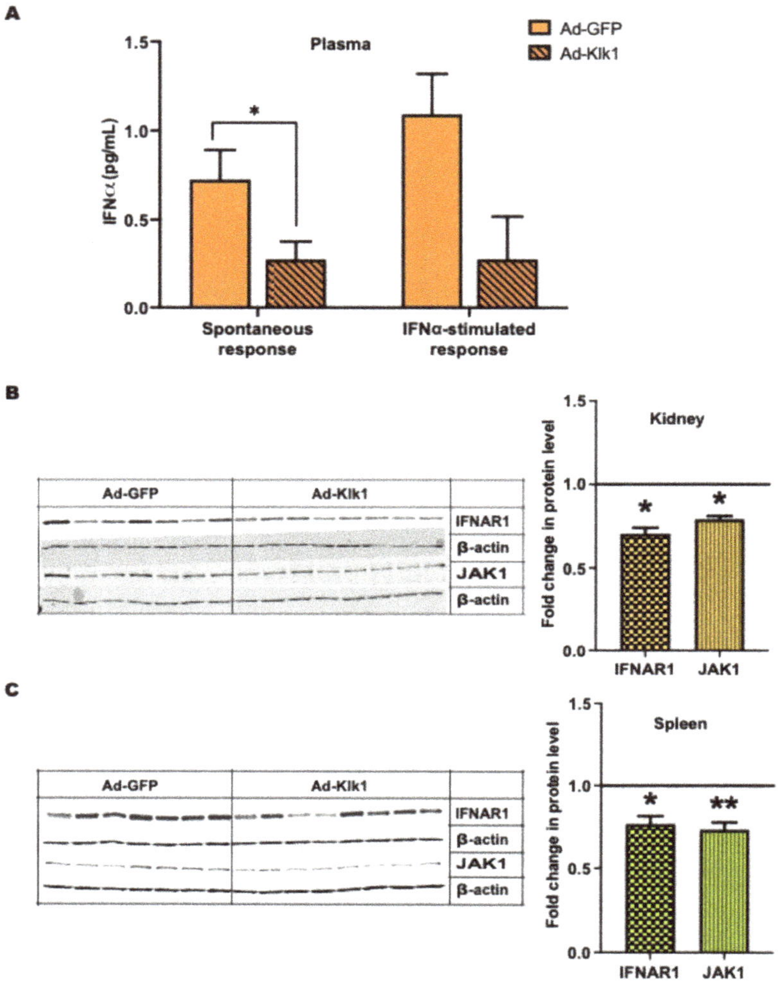

Figure 4. Tissue Klk1 decreases plasma IFNα levels and proteins in Type I IFN signaling: (**A**) Plasma IFNα levels in the spontaneous MRL/lpr mice were measured using the high sensitivity Verikine ELISA kit and are expressed as the mean ±SEM of IFNα levels (pg/mL). Western blot analysis of IFNAR1 (MW: 64 kDa) and JAK1 (MW: 80 kDa) protein levels in the (**B**) kidney and (**C**) spleen of spontaneous MRL/lpr mice. Data were analyzed using an unpaired *t*-test and are expressed as the mean ±SEM of the fold change in protein levels in the Ad-Klk1 group compared to the Ad-GFP group (marked as a solid black line at 1.0 on the Y axis). * $p \leq 0.05$ and ** $p \leq 0.01$ compared to the Ad-GFP group; n = 7–8 mice/group.

We further analyzed the correlation between TST immobility time and IFN-α levels, IRGs, and serotonin-related markers. Specifically, we selected markers that exhibited a significant difference between the Ad-Klk1 and Ad-GFP groups of the spontaneous cohort. Markers presented in Figure 5D showed significant correlations. TST immobility time was found to correlate positively with plasma IFN-α levels and brain *isg15* gene expression. As expected, TST immobility time was negatively correlated with the expression of the *5htt* and *tph-2* genes, both of which are key regulators of serotonin synthesis and transport.

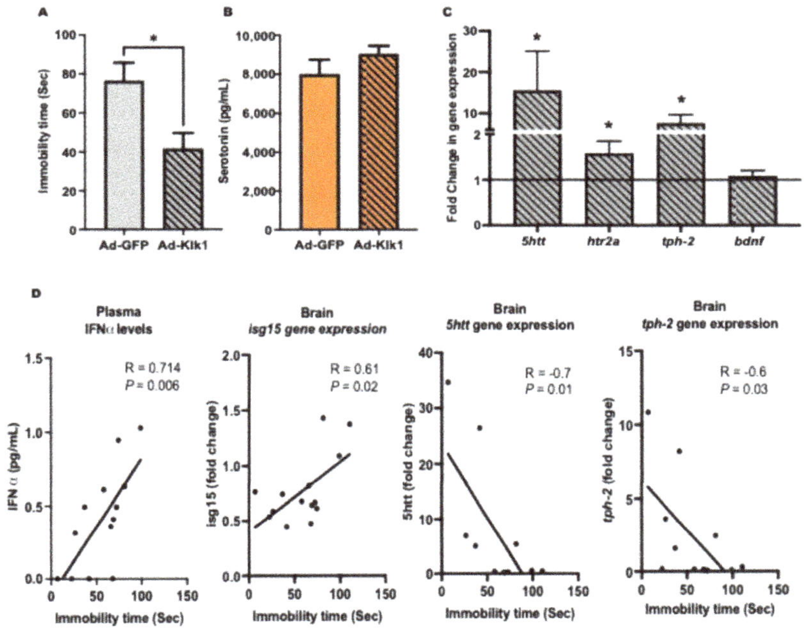

Figure 5. Tissue Klk1 decreases depressive-like behavior and depression-related gene expression in the spontaneous MRL/lpr mice: (**A**) Tail suspension test (TST). (**B**) Plasma serotonin levels were estimated by using the ELISA kit. (**C**) Gene expression analysis of serotonin regulators in the brain; the results are expressed as the mean ±SEM of the fold change in gene expression in the Ad-Klk1 group compared to the Ad-GFP group (marked as a solid black line at 1.0 on the Y axis). (**D**) Correlation of the immobility time in the TST with plasma IFNα levels and serotonin-related markers (brain *isg15*, *5htt*, and *tph-2*). The data were analyzed using an unpaired *t*-test and * $p \leq 0.05$ compared to the Ad-GFP group; n = 7–8 mice/group.

2.6. Klk1 Administration Reduces Microglial Inflammatory State in the Brain

To study the effects of Klk1 on microglia in lupus-prone mice, we analyzed the expression of IBA-1, a well-established marker of microglia. We found that Klk1 transformed the microglia to a less inflammatory state (with a reduction in IBA-1 staining in Figure 6), as described elegantly by Paolicelli et al. [41].

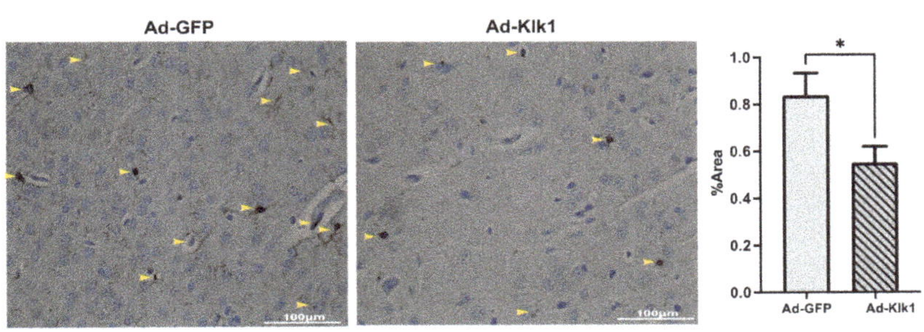

Figure 6. Tissue Klk1 reduced microglial inflammatory state and number. Immunohistochemical staining of IBA-1 in microglia. Data were analyzed using an unpaired *t*-test and are expressed as the mean ±SEM of the percentage area of IBA-1 staining in the cortex region of the brain at 40× magnification (brown staining, indicated by yellow arrows) using ImageJ (1.54f software). * $p \leq 0.05$ compared to Ad-GFP group; n = 7–8 mice/group.

2.7. *Klk1* Administration Reduces C3 and IgG Expression in the Kidney

Complement and immune complex deposition in the kidney glomeruli is an early pathological hallmark of lupus nephritis [42]. Compared to *Ad-gfp* administration, *Ad-klk1* administration significantly reduced C3 and IgG protein levels in the kidneys in the spontaneous MRL/lpr cohort (Figure 7).

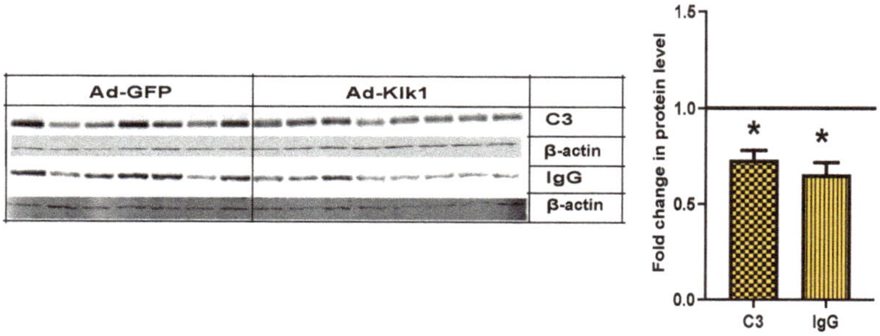

Figure 7. Tissue Klk1 decreases C3 and IgG protein levels in the kidney: Western blot analysis of C3 (MW: 50 kDa) and IgG (MW: 50 kDa) protein levels in the kidney of spontaneous MRL/lpr mice. Data were analyzed using an unpaired *t*-test and are expressed as the mean ±SEM of the fold change in protein levels in the Ad-Klk1 group compared to the Ad-GFP group (marked as a solid black line at 1.0 on the Y axis). * $p \leq 0.05$ compared to the Ad-GFP group; n = 7–8 mice/group.

We also analyzed autoantibodies against dsDNA and chromatin in the plasma in both MRL/lpr cohorts (Figure S2A,B). *Ad-klk1* administration resulted in reduced autoantibody levels, with a significant decrease in anti-dsDNA levels in the spontaneous cohort. Proteinuria and blood urea nitrogen (BUN) scores were unaltered between the groups, suggesting that a longer treatment duration may be required to observe significant changes in pathological scores.

2.8. *Klk1* Alters BK and PAR2 Receptor Expression

Klk catalyzes the conversion of kininogen into BK, which activates BK receptors B1R and B2R [20]. B1R blockade has been shown to mitigate systemic autoimmunity and renal inflammation in MRL/lpr mice [43]. Therefore, we studied the effect of *Ad-klk1* administration on BK receptors' expression. Strikingly, *b1r* gene expression was significantly lower in the brain (Figure 8A) and spleen (Figure 8C) of the Ad-Klk1 group than in the Ad-GFP group of the spontaneous MRL/lpr mice. However, no change in renal *b1r* expression was observed between the Ad-Klk1 and Ad-GFP groups (Figure 8B). Moreover, *b2r* expression was non-significantly altered in all three tissues of both groups (Figure 8); a trend in the increase in B2R gene expression was found in the brain.

Klk also signals via protease-activated receptors (PARs) [24]. Klk activation via PAR2 has been shown in various inflammatory diseases [27]. We found a significant increase in *par2* gene expression in the spleen but not in the brain and kidneys of spontaneous MRL/lpr mice after *Ad-Klk1* administration (Figure S3).

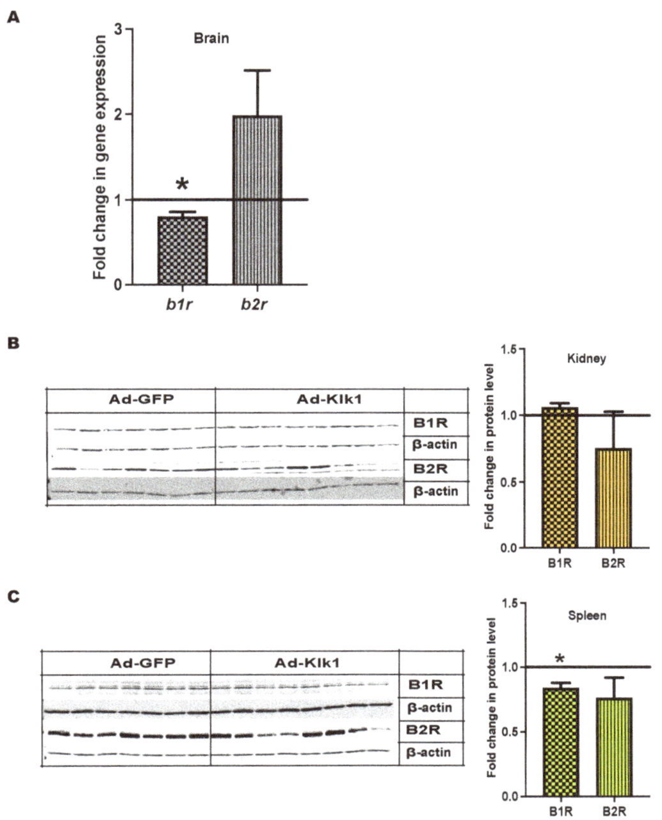

Figure 8. Tissue Klk1 alters BK receptor expression in the spontaneous MRL/lpr mice: (**A**) Fold change in *b1r* and *b2r* gene expression in the brain of the Ad-Klk1 group compared to those of the Ad-GFP group (marked as a solid black line at 1.0 on the Y axis), as measured by qPCR. Fold change in B1R (MW: 40 kDa) and B2R (MW: 50 kDa) protein levels in the (**B**) kidneys and (**C**) spleen of the Ad-Klk1 group compared to those of the Ad-GFP group (marked as a solid black line at 1.0 on the Y axis), as measured by western blot. The results are expressed as mean ±SEM. An unpaired *t*-test was used; * $p \leq 0.05$ and $p \leq 0.001$ compared to the Ad-GFP group; n = 7–8 mice/group.

3. Discussion

Administration of tissue kallikrein (*klk1*) has been shown to ameliorate experimental nephritis [31,32,44]. We, for the first time, showed in this short-term study that *klk1* administration reduced Type I IFN response in the periphery and brain and normalized depressive-like behavior in the MRL/lpr mice, a popularly used NPSLE model. Klk1 also reduced autoantibody levels in the spontaneous model. The FDA recently approved anti-IFNAR treatment (anifrolumab) [45] only for severe systemic lupus treatment. Based on the rigor of previous studies in the kidney [31,32] and our data in the brain, it is evident that this molecule of the KKS could potentially be developed as a therapeutic for systemic lupus and NPSLE.

Attenuating the production and response to Type I IFNs—called the "IFN signature"—has been the goal for therapeutic development in lupus for several decades [46]. Tissue *klk1* administration could significantly suppress some of the key IRGs (IRF7 and CXCL10) both in the periphery and in the brain in this short-term analysis. In particular, *isg15* was significantly suppressed in the spontaneous and IFNα-induced cohorts. Administration of IFNα is known to induce depression in many patients with chronic viral hepatitis infection and has been an established model of inflammation-induced depression [8]. *Isg15* is one of the few genes shown to be elevated in the blood of patients with chronic viral hepatitis treated with IFNα [47]. HMGB1, released from apoptotic or necrotic cells, acts as a damage-associated molecular pattern and exerts proinflammatory effects on many cells of the innate immune system. HMGB1 has been found to play an important role in mediating inflammation and has been implicated in multiple disease phenotypes in SLE, including lupus nephritis and NPSLE [48]. In our study, Klk1 significantly reduced hmgb1 gene expression in the brain and spleen. In a recent study, a long-acting tissue Klk has been shown to reduce HMGB1 release by neurons and microglial cells after ischemic stroke [49].

SLE is a complex and heterogeneous disease, and NPSLE manifestations in lupus have been investigated seriously only in the last couple of decades [3]. After several clinical trials, blocking the IFNAR1 using an antagonist (anifrolumab) has only been approved recently by the FDA and only for systemic lupus [50]. Clinical trials are being revisited to understand the effects of IFNAR1 blocking, and individual case reports about the efficacy of NPSLE have been published recently [51,52]. We show in this report that *klk1* administration significantly reduced IFNAR1 as well as JAK1 signaling molecules that are upstream of Type I IFN signaling [35]. JAK inhibitors have also been independently tested in clinical trials for rheumatic diseases [53], and some are approved for rheumatoid arthritis. Our study interestingly revealed that tissue Klk1 can effectively inhibit the key signaling molecules in the Type I IFN pathway, suggesting that this is a potential candidate to develop as a biologic not only for lupus but for other IFN-mediated diseases.

Depression and anxiety are the major psychological manifestations of NPSLE and cause severe loss of quality of life for lupus patients [3]. An estimated 40% of lupus patients suffer from the symptoms of NPSLE. Evidence from several lupus-prone mouse models has indicated IFNα as a contributor to lupus pathogenesis [10]. We have reported a constitutive increase in the IRGs of the brains of young MRL/lpr mice and an increase in depressive-like behaviors of these mice at a young age [11]. Putterman's group has also shown [37] depression as an early and major behavioral characteristic in the MRL/lpr mice even before autoantibodies begin to develop. We have earlier reported that depressive-like behavior was the most prominent characteristic in the MRL/lpr model at an early age and sought to analyze this psychological function only in this study. Many recent studies have indicated that chronic inflammation is related to depression and mood disorders in patients [40,54]. IFNα is a well-known inducer of depression and has been studied in various models [55,56]. IFN triggers the induction of indolamine 2,3-dioxygenase (IDO) and results in higher tryptophan metabolism along the kynurenine pathway and less being available for conversion to 5-hydroxytryptophan that induces the serotonin pathway; decreased serotonin levels lead to depression. Reduced serum serotonin levels in SLE patients were related to severe disease phenotype [57,58], including nephritis, suggesting an involvement of important immunopathological processes. A Type I IFN-mediated skewing of the tryptophan metabolism and up-regulation of IDO and platelet activation were identified as possible underlying mechanisms of decreased serotonin in SLE patients [57]. While there was not a significant decrease in the circulating serotonin levels in our analysis, we observed that tissue Klk1 was able to normalize the expression of molecules in the serotonin pathway, increasing the expression of *5htt*, *htr2a*, and *tph-2*. Moreover, there was a negative correlation between immobility time and the expression of brain *5htt* and *tph-2* genes. As expected, we also found a positive correlation between circulating IFNα levels and *isg15* gene expression, which were significantly down-regulated by Klk1 administration with time of immobility in TST. BDNF, a member of the neurotrophin family, has been receiving increasing attention in SLE [59], with varied observations in patients in different studies. Studies by Zheng et al. [60] showed that decreased serum BDNF levels aggravated depression, while increased BDNF improved depression in SLE. Another report indicated that plasma BDNF levels were consistently lower in patients with NPSLE with irreversible organic brain damage than in healthy controls, and the levels increased with disease improvement. We found that in this short-term study, Klk1 increased the *bdnf* gene expression. We expect that a longer duration of treatment may lead to significant effects.

Increased IFNα levels have been detected in the blood of SLE patients and correlate with disease activity, especially in juvenile SLE [61]. Increased IFNα has also been shown in the CSF of NPSLE patients and mouse models to be a leading effector of NPSLE. IFNα production within the CNS and increased IFNα levels in the CSF were found in patients with NPSLE. Klk1 significantly reduced circulating IFNα levels and IRGs in the brain in our short-term study. Klk1 administration also significantly reduced other key cytokines/chemokines implicated in SLE and NPSLE, such as TNFα, IL-10, and MCP-1. We have previously shown [11] a constitutive increase in proinflammatory cytokines levels, including TNFα and IL-10, in the MRL/lpr than in the MRL/wt. Effects were more pronounced in the spontaneous cohort than in the IFNα-induced cohort in this short-term study; a longer treatment period may be needed to suppress inflammation with an ongoing IFN response. Literature shows increased TNFα in patients with SLE that correlated with disease activity and has been proposed to contribute to SLE immunopathogenesis [62]. The IL-10 cytokine is specifically known for its suppressive function; however, in lupus, IL-10 is pathogenic, promoting direct differentiation of activated B cells into plasma cells [63,64]. MCP-1 has been discovered as an important biomarker for lupus nephritis activity that was high in both serums and urines of patients with lupus [65–67]. TNFα, IL-10, and MCP-1 (CCL2), biomarkers of inflammation, are also increased in people with depression. Interestingly, cytokines IL-33 and IL-5 were both significantly suppressed in both cohorts. We found that IL-33 was more highly induced in the IFNα-administered cohort than in the spontaneous cohort. Nonetheless, Klk1 significantly reduced the levels in both groups. IL-33, a nuclear alarmin released during cell death, elicits potent inflammatory responses. It is also implicated in lupus autoimmunity [68], and elevated serum concentrations of IL-33 and the soluble form of the IL-33 receptor, ST2L, have been reported in patients with SLE [69]. MRL/lpr lupus-prone mice treated with anti-IL-33 antibodies had reduced renal inflammation and serum autoantibodies. A recent study shows that extracellular IL-33 complexed with NETs may represent an important source of IL-33 alarmin, contributing to excessive Type I IFN [70]. Patients with lupus nephritis, an organ-specific autoimmune disease, have increased levels of IL-5 in their urine, suggesting that IL-5 may be involved in eosinophil recruitment in these patients [71]. A study reported that keratinocytes in skin lesions from patients with SLE often overexpressed IL-5 and found that higher cytokine levels correspond to more severe lesions [72]. We observed that IL-2 levels were decreased by Klk1 in the spontaneous model, while no effect was observed in the IFNα-induced cohort. IL-2 cytokine level is typically low in SLE [73]. Our observations may be an independent Klk1 response affecting T cells, probably via PARs, which needs to be investigated further.

We have demonstrated that microglia are important players in NPSLE [74]. Microglia regulate dendrite pruning and are important for memory functions. A disease-associated microglia (DAM) population has been identified in NPSLE mouse models [75]. We have previously shown that captopril (ACEi) was able to reduce microglial activation in the MRL/lpr mice [11]. We observed that Klk1 significantly reduced the inflammatory state of microglia. We used IBA-1 as one of the markers to analyze this response, as we also showed the effects of ACE inhibitors in an earlier study [11]. As more recent studies elucidate more definitive roles of microglia [41], a further in-depth investigation is required to understand the exact role of these microglia in NPSLE. Also, whether the effects are brought about by BK that is common to both pathways remains to be investigated.

Tissue Klk generates BK via kininogen breakdown that probably signals via the BK receptors (B1R and B2R). Des-Arg-9-BK, a breakdown product of the BK peptide (from both plasma and tissue Klk pathways) that signals via B1R, is high in rheumatic autoimmune diseases [43,76]. B1R is shown to be proinflammatory in lupus nephritis [43], and the effects can be due to stimulation with the Des-Arg-9-BK peptide. Opposing roles of kinin B1 (inflammatory) [77] and B2 receptors (protective) [78] are shown in different models. In this study, we show that Klk1 reduced B1R expression and increased B2R expression (in the brain). This can be one of the mechanisms by which Klk1 ameliorates the inflammatory effects of lupus. We showed earlier [12] in dendritic cells that blocking the BK receptors did not completely revert IFN suppression, indicating that Klk1 may act via other pathways. PARs are G protein-coupled serine protease receptors that have been shown to induce pro- and anti-inflammatory effects [24]. One of the PAR receptors, PAR2, has been reported in lupus. Recent studies [79,80] using lupus-prone mice show opposite effects via PAR2 to induce kidney disease; A PAR2 agonist has been shown to suppress IRF5 [28] (an important IFN regulatory factor implicated in lupus) in macrophages. PAR2 activation blocked apoptosis in intestinal epithelial cells [81]. We tested PAR2 expression in our cohorts and observed that *klk1* administration increased it. The elimination of inflammatory and IFN responses may be mediated via PAR2; the mechanisms need to be studied in detail.

4. Materials and Methods

4.1. Mice

MRL/lpr female mice were purchased from the Jackson Laboratory (Bar Harbor, ME, USA) and used in experiments starting at 8 weeks (baseline). It has been shown that MRL/lpr mice start to develop autoantibodies beginning at 9 weeks of age; therefore, we started treatment in our cohort at this age. All animals were maintained in the animal facility of Temple University, an American Association for the Accreditation of Laboratory Animal Care-accredited facility, following the guidelines of the Institutional Animal Care and Use Committee of Temple University under a fully approved protocol (IACUC protocol number 5052).

4.2. In Vivo Gene Delivery of Ad-klk1 and Administration of IFNα

The effects of tissue Klk1 were analyzed by using the adenovirus vector carrying the mouse *klk1* gene (*Ad-klk1*) with a GFP reporter in the spontaneous as well as IFNα-induced MRL/lpr model (Figure 9). The *Ad-klk1* was obtained from Vector Biolabs (Malvern, PA, USA) and synthesized as described previously [32]. The control vector only carried the *gfp* gene (*Ad-gfp*).

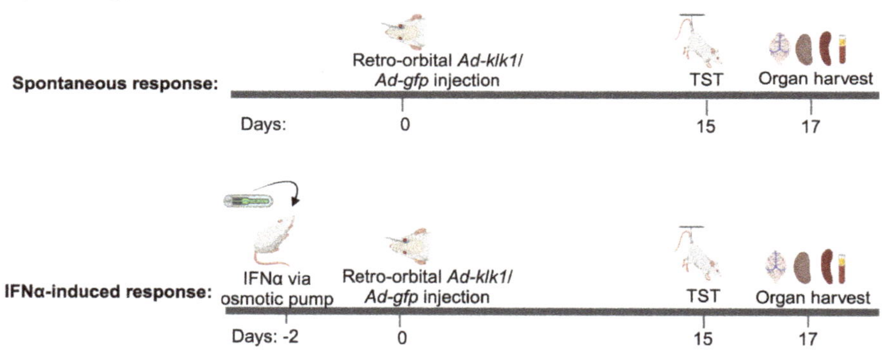

Figure 9. Scheme of the experiment: One cohort of nine-week-old MRL/lpr mice was administered with IFNα- or saline-carrying osmotic pump (IFNα-induced response) on day −2, followed by the retro-orbital administration of *Ad-klk1* or *Ad-gfp* vector on day 0. The spontaneous cohort received *Ad-klk1* or control (*Ad-gfp*) vector only. Behavioral studies were performed on day 15, and the mice were sacrificed on day 17 to collect the brain, spleen, kidneys, and blood.

For the spontaneous model, the mice were administered retro-orbitally (r.o.) with 1×10^7 PFU (in 100 μL PBS/mouse) *Ad-klk1* or *Ad-gfp* on day 0. On days 15 and 16, a tail suspension test was performed. All mice were euthanized on day 17. For the IFNα-induced model, recombinant IFNα (5×10^5 U/mouse) was administered to the mice via osmotic pumps (ALZET® Osmotic Pumps, Cupertino, CA, USA) that were inserted subcutaneously following sterile procedures. Osmotic pumps were first weighed and primed with recombinant human IFNα (PBL Assay Science, Piscataway NJ, USA) or PBS for 48 h before being surgically inserted into the mice. All the pumps had a reservoir of 200 μL, which pumped 0.25 μL/h over the course of 14 days. In these experiments, *Ad-klk1* or *Ad-gfp* was administered r.o. 2 days after IFNα pump implantation. The TST was performed on day 15, and the mice were euthanized on day 17. At the terminal time point in each experiment, mice were perfused with saline, and the brain, spleen, and kidneys were harvested and stored at −80 °C for gene and protein analysis in their respective storage reagents. On day 0 and 17, blood was collected in EDTA-treated tubes for the baseline and for terminal plasma measurements, respectively. Cells were removed from the plasma by centrifugation for 10 min at 1000–2000× *g* at 4 °C.

4.3. Proteinuria Measurement

Proteinuria was measured using the dipstick method (Multistix 10 SG; Siemens Healthcare, Malvern, PA, USA). Briefly, mice were sacrificed using excess isoflurane. The urine was collected using a pipette and applied to dipsticks. Color was scored as per the kit instructions (a score of 1 is 30 mg/dL, 2 is 100 mg/dL, 3 is 300 mg/dL, and 4 is 2000 mg/dL) [11].

4.4. Blood Urea Nitrogen Analysis

After sacrificing the mice, blood was collected by sub-mandibular bleeding. BUN levels were analyzed by dipsticks (Azostix reagent strips, Siemens Healthcare, Malvern, PA, USA) and scored per manufacturer's instructions as 1: 5–15 mg/dL, 2: 15–25 mg/dL, 3: 30–40 mg/dL, and 4: 50–80 mg/dL). Strips were scored by two personnel in a blinded fashion [11].

4.5. RNA Extraction and qPCR

Gene expression in the kidney, spleen, and whole-brain samples was analyzed using TaqMan probes and real-time quantitative PCR (qPCR). RNA was extracted using TriZol (Thermo Fisher Scientific, Waltham, MA, USA) following the manufacturer's protocol. DNA removal was performed using the DNA-free™ Kit (Thermo Fisher Scientific, Waltham, MA, USA) following the manufacturer's protocol. Complementary DNA (cDNA) was synthesized with the High-Capacity cDNA Reverse Transcription Kit (Thermo Fisher Scientific, Waltham, MA, USA).

qPCR was performed using either TaqMan primers and probes (Applied Biosystems, Foster City, CA, USA) for *klk1b11* (Mm00662365_g1), *klk1b27* (Mm00834759_gH), *irf7* (Mm00516788_m1), *isg15* (Mm01705338_s1), *cxcl10* (Mm00445235_m1), *mx1* (Mm00487796_m1), *hmgb1* (Mm00849805_gH), *b1r* (Mm04207315_s1), and *b2r* (Mm00437788_s1); or SYBR Green reagents and primers for genes listed in Table S2. *Gapdh* (Mm99999915_g1 for TaqMan reaction) was used as a reference gene. The reaction master mixes used for the TaqMan and SYBR Green systems were TaqMan™ Fast Advanced Master Mix and Applied Biosystems™ SYBR™ Green PCR Master Mix, respectively. ΔΔCt method was used to calculate the fold changes in gene expression by normalizing the values to the control group in each experiment.

4.6. Western Blot

Spleen and kidney tissues were homogenized and stored in the lysis buffer (Cell Lytic buffer with protease and phosphatase inhibitors added, Thermo-Fisher Scientific, Waltham, MA, USA) at −80 °C. The total protein from the samples was assayed by BCA colorimetric assay. About 30 μg of protein from each sample was loaded in a 4–20% Bis-Tris gel (Bio-Rad Laboratories, Hercules, CA, USA) after denaturation at 95 °C for 10 min. After proteins from the gel were transferred onto a nitrocellulose membrane, Ponceau staining was performed to make sure that protein transfer was even. The membrane was then blocked with a 2% blocking buffer (non-fat milk in PBS with 0.1% Tween) for 1 h and washed with PBST (PBS + 0.1% Tween). The nitrocellulose membrane was incubated overnight with the following primary anti-mouse antibodies at 4 °C in a shaking condition: anti- anti-Klk1

(Abcepta, San Diego, CA, USA, 1:1000), anti-IFNAR1 (Leinco Technologies, Fenton, MO, USA, 1:1000), anti-JAK1 (Thermo Fisher Scientific, Waltham, MA, USA, 1:1000), anti-C3 (Santacruz Biotechnology Inc, Santa Cruz, CA, USA, 1:500), anti-IgG (Abcam, Trumpington, Cambridge, UK, 1:5000), anti-B1R (Alomone Labs, Jerusalem, Israel, 1:200), anti-B2R (Alomone Labs, Jerusalem, Israel, 1:1000), and anti-β-actin (Cell Signaling, Danvers, MA, USA, 1:1000) antibodies. Membranes were washed with PBST, incubated with a secondary antibody (IR-dye-800-goat anti-rabbit antibody or IR-dye-680-goat anti-rabbit antibody, 1:10,000) for 1 h, again washed with PBST, and scanned in an Odyssey Infrared Imaging System (LI-COR Biosciences, Lincoln, NE, USA) under the 800 and 680 nm green channel for protein band visualization. ImageJ 1.54f software was used to quantify the band intensities. Band intensities were normalized to β-actin control (MW: 42 kDa).

4.7. Proinflammatory Cytokine Analysis

Proinflammatory cytokines and chemokine multiplex ELISA kits were bought from Mesoscale Discovery (MSD MULTI-SPOT Assay System, Rockville, MD, USA). Briefly, plasma samples and manufacturer-provided calibrator were diluted with Diluent 41 per the manufacturer's instructions. After washing the MSD plates with 1XMSD wash buffer, 50 μL diluted samples or calibrators were added to each well and incubated for 2 h at room temperature on a shaker at 400 rpm. The plates were washed three times. A detection antibody (25 μL) was added to each well, and the plates were incubated for 2 h at room temperature on a shaker at 400 rpm. Following the incubation, the plates were washed three times, and 150 μL Read buffer T was added to each well. The plates were immediately read using an MSD instrument.

4.8. IFNa ELISA

IFNα levels in plasma were detected using the high-sensitivity Verikine IFNα ELISA kit from PBL (PBL Assay Science, Piscataway, NJ, USA). Briefly, standards were diluted as per the manufacturer's instructions. Plasma samples and diluted standards were added to a plate, followed by 1 h incubation on a shaker at 400 rpm at room temperature. After washing the plate, the antibody solution was added, and the plate was incubated for 30 min at room temperature. After washing, the plate was incubated with HRP solution for 4 min at room temperature. Finally, the plate was washed and incubated with TMB substrate for 20 min in the dark, followed by the addition of the stop solution. The plate was immediately read at 450 nm. IFNα concentrations were determined by plotting the graph against standards.

4.9. Autoantibody Detection

Plasma was tested for anti-DNA and anti-chromatin antibodies by ELISA [82]. Briefly, polypropylene 96-well plates were coated with chicken erythrocyte-derived chromatin at 3 mg/mL or with calf thymus-derived dsDNA at 2.5 mg/mL in borate-buffered saline (BBS). Plates were coated with poly (L-lysine (1 mg/mL; Sigma-Aldrich, Allentown, PA, USA) before being coated with the antigen for anti-dsDNA ELISA. Plates were blocked with blocking buffer (3% BSA and 1% Tween 80 in BBS), and plasma samples were diluted 1:250 in BBT (0.4% Tween 80, 0.5% BSA in BBS) and added in duplicate and incubated overnight at 4 °C. Alkaline phosphatase-conjugated goat anti-mouse IgG (Fc γ specific; Jackson ImmunoResearch Laboratories, West Grove, PA, USA) was used as secondary antibody. Color was developed using 1 mg/mL para-nitrophenyl phosphate substrate (Sigma-Aldrich, Allentown, PA, USA) in 0.01 M diethanolamine (pH 9.8). Plasma from old MRL/lpr mice with high antibody titer and plasma from C57BL/6 mice were used as positive and negative controls, respectively.

4.10. Immunohistochemistry

Microscopic examination of the brain and kidneys was performed as per the standardized immunohistochemistry protocol [83]. Paraffin sections (5 μm) were used for the evaluation of microglia and Klk1 expression using the anti-IBA1 antibodies (Wako Chemicals, Richmond, VA, USA, 1:100) and the anti-Klk1 antibodies (Abcepta, San Diego, CA, USA, 1:100), respectively. Primary antibodies were detected by peroxidase using the Envision HRP or AP Labeled Polymer Kit (Vector Laboratories, Newark, CA, USA). Samples were imaged under 40× objective magnification using an Olympus BX31 microscope. For each mouse, four to six randomly selected fields were analyzed. ImageJ 1.54f software was used to measure the % area for each image.

4.11. Plasma Serotonin Analysis

Plasma serotonin levels in the plasma samples were assayed using the Serotonin ELISA Kit from Abcam (Waltham, MA, USA, cat. no. ab133053) as per the manufacturer's instructions.

4.12. TST

TST was performed as a measure of depressive-like behavior after 17 days of drug administration. The total duration of immobility induced by tail suspension was measured according to the method [38]. The time during which mice remained immobile was quantified during a test period of 6 min. Mice were considered immobile only when they hung passively and were completely motionless. The immobility was scored by two independent readers and were blinded for analysis.

4.13. Rotarod Test

The rotarod test was used in the mice to check for locomotor function. The mice were placed on a horizontally oriented, rotating cylinder (rod) suspended above a cage floor. The rotating cylinder was high enough to induce avoidance of falls but not high enough to injure the animal. Three trials were performed, with the latency and speed at fall recorded under the following parameters: duration of trial = 5 min, maximal speed = 20 RPM, and time to maximal speed = 15 s [84].

4.14. Statistical Analysis

Prism 10.3.1 software (GraphPad, San Diego, CA, USA) was used for statistical analysis. An unpaired *t*-test was used for comparison between the two groups, and the results are shown as mean ±SEM. Pearson correlation analysis was applied to measure the correlations between immobility time (Sec) and IFNα, IRGs, or serotonin-related markers. $p < 0.05$ were considered significant: * $p \leq 0.05$, ** $p \leq 0.01$, *** $p \leq 0.001$.

5. Conclusions

In all, our study shows that tissue Klk1 has the potential to ameliorate systemic as well as CNS lupus by reducing Type I IFN production and inflammatory response in the periphery and brain (Figure 10). The consequential depressive-like behavior response is also reduced. Our previous report indicated this reduction may be mediated by partially signaling via the B1/B2 receptors or PARs. In this study, we have shown that Klk1 reduced the proinflammatory B1R expression and increased B2R and PAR2 expression, which may also be protective. The mechanistic aspects of Klk1 action need to be investigated further.

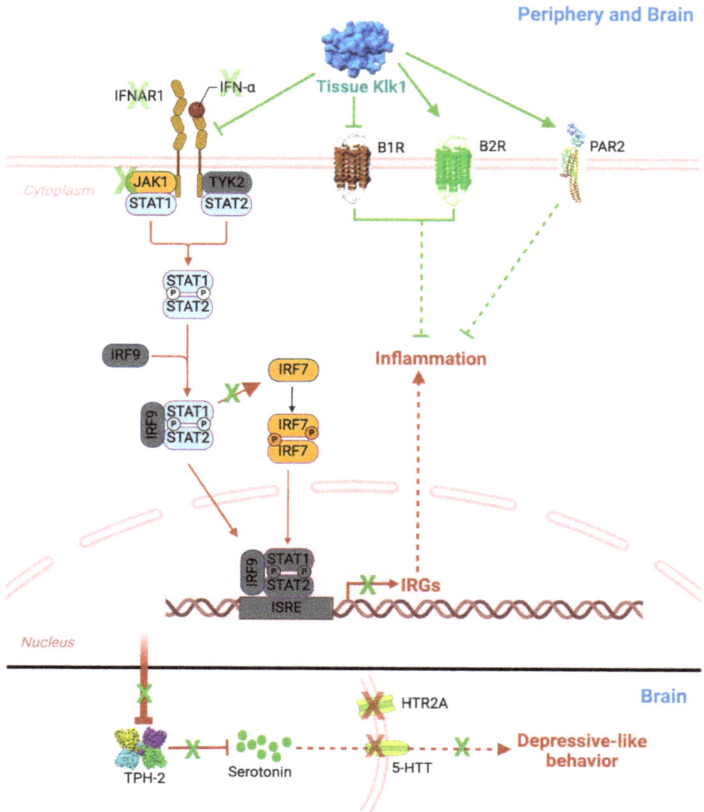

Figure 10. Tissue Klk1 suppresses Type I IFN responses through IFNAR1, BRs, and PAR2 and reduces depressive-like behavior in the MRL/lpr lupus-prone mice: The present study demonstrates that tissue Klk1 administration reduces IFNα, IFNAR1, JAK1, and IRF7, consequently suppressing IRG expression. Our previous study [11] has shown a reduction in signal transducer and activator of transcription (STAT) phosphorylation (shown in blue color) following bradykinin (BK) administration, which, along with other pathway proteins (shown in grey color), will be studied in detail in the future. We observed a consequential reduction in the levels of tryptophan hydroxylase 2 (TPH2, a rate-limiting enzyme in serotonin biosynthesis), serotonin (5-HT), serotonin transporter (5-HTT), and 5-hydroxytryptamine receptor 2A (HTR2A, a serotonin receptor). We also observed depressive-like behaviors in MRL/lpr mice. Alleviation of inflammatory and IFN responses may be mediated via the alteration in BK receptors (B1R and B2R) and protease-activated receptor-2 (PAR2) expression; the mechanisms need to be studied in detail (indicated with dashed arrows). The therapeutic effects of Klk1 are shown in green notation, and SLE and NPSLE pathogenesis are represented in red notation.

Supplementary Materials: The following supporting information can be downloaded at https://www.mdpi.com/article/10.3390/ijms251810080/s1.

Author Contributions: Conceptualization, U.S.; methodology, P.S.B., C.N., N.S.T., M.W., C.L., S.K., A.S. and N.M.; software, P.S.B.; validation, U.S., Y.P. and E.M.U.; formal analysis, P.S.B.; investigation, U.S.; resources, U.S. and Y.P.; data curation, P.S.B. and U.S.; writing—original draft preparation, U.S. and P.S.B.; writing—review and editing, U.S., P.S.B. and Y.P.; visualization, N.M. and P.S.B.; supervision, U.S.; project administration, U.S.; funding acquisition, U.S. and E.M.U. All authors have read and agreed to the published version of the manuscript.

Funding: This research was funded by NIH-NIAID grant R21AI171247 to U.S., NIH-NIDA grant P30 DA013429 to E.M.U., and funds from the Department of Pathology and Laboratory Medicine.

Institutional Review Board Statement: The animal study protocol was approved by the Institutional Review Board (or Ethics Committee) of the Institutional Animal Care and Use Committee of Temple University under a fully approved protocol (IACUC protocol number 5052 and date of approval: 18 July 2021).

Informed Consent Statement: Not applicable.

Data Availability Statement: The data that support the findings of this study are available from the corresponding author upon reasonable request.

Acknowledgments: The authors thank Sudhir Kotnala and Rebecca Hancock for their technical assistance.

Conflicts of Interest: The authors declare no conflicts of interest.

References

1. Hawro, T.; Krupinska-Kun, M.; Rabe-Jablonska, J.; Sysa-Jedrzejowska, A.; Robak, E.; Bogaczewicz, J.; Wozniacka, A. Psychiatric disorders in patients with systemic lupus erythematosus: Association of anxiety disorder with shorter disease duration. *Rheumatol. Int.* **2011**, *31*, 1387–1391. [PubMed]
2. Morrison, E.; Carpentier, S.; Shaw, E.; Doucette, S.; Hanly, J.G. Neuropsychiatric systemic lupus erythematosus: Association with global disease activity. *Lupus* **2014**, *23*, 370–377. [PubMed]
3. Govoni, M.; Hanly, J.G. The management of neuropsychiatric lupus in the 21st century: Still so many unmet needs? *Rheumatology* **2020**, *59* (Suppl. S5), v52–v62. [CrossRef]
4. Palagini, L.; Mosca, M.; Tani, C.; Gemignani, A.; Mauri, M.; Bombardieri, S. Depression and systemic lupus erythematosus: A systematic review. *Lupus* **2013**, *22*, 409–416. [CrossRef] [PubMed]
5. Obermoser, G.; Pascual, V. The interferon-alpha signature of systemic lupus erythematosus. *Lupus* **2010**, *19*, 1012–1019. [CrossRef]
6. Hagberg, N.; Ronnblom, L. Systemic Lupus Erythematosus--A Disease with A Dysregulated Type I Interferon System. *Scand. J. Immunol.* **2015**, *82*, 199–207. [CrossRef]
7. Shiozawa, S.; Kuroki, Y.; Kim, M.; Hirohata, S.; Ogino, T. Interferon-alpha in lupus psychosis. *Arthritis Rheum.* **1992**, *35*, 417–422. [CrossRef]
8. Bonaccorso, S.; Marino, V.; Biondi, M.; Grimaldi, F.; Ippoliti, F.; Maes, M. Depression induced by treatment with interferon-alpha in patients affected by hepatitis C virus. *J. Affect. Disord.* **2002**, *72*, 237–241.
9. Pavol, M.A.; Meyers, C.A.; Rexer, J.L.; Valentine, A.D.; Mattis, P.J.; Talpaz, M. Pattern of neurobehavioral deficits associated with interferon alfa therapy for leukemia. *Neurology* **1995**, *45*, 947–950.
10. Aw, E.; Zhang, Y.; Carroll, M. Microglial responses to peripheral type 1 interferon. *J. Neuroinflamm.* **2020**, *17*, 340. [CrossRef]
11. Nocito, C.; Lubinsky, C.; Hand, M.; Khan, S.; Patel, T.; Seliga, A.; Winfield, M.; Zuluaga-Ramirez, V.; Fernandes, N.; Shi, X.; et al. Centrally Acting Angiotensin-Converting Enzyme Inhibitor Suppresses Type I Interferon Responses and Decreases Inflammation in the Periphery and the CNS in Lupus-Prone Mice. *Front. Immunol.* **2020**, *11*, 573677. [CrossRef] [PubMed]
12. Seliga, A.; Lee, M.H.; Fernandes, N.C.; Zuluaga-Ramirez, V.; Didukh, M.; Persidsky, Y.; Potula, R.; Gallucci, S.; Sriram, U. Kallikrein–Kinin System Suppresses Type I Interferon Responses: A Novel Pathway of Interferon Regulation. *Front. Immunol.* **2018**, *9*, 156. [CrossRef]
13. Kalinska, M.; Meyer-Hoffert, U.; Kantyka, T.; Potempa, J. Kallikreins—The melting pot of activity and function. *Biochimie* **2016**, *122*, 270–282. [CrossRef] [PubMed]
14. Blaber, S.I.; Ciric, B.; Christophi, G.P.; Bernett, M.J.; Blaber, M.; Rodriguez, M.; Scarisbrick, I.A. Targeting kallikrein 6 proteolysis attenuates CNS inflammatory disease. *FASEB J.* **2004**, *18*, 920–922. [CrossRef] [PubMed]
15. Chao, J.; Shen, B.; Gao, L.; Xia, C.F.; Bledsoe, G.; Chao, L. Tissue kallikrein in cardiovascular, cerebrovascular and renal diseases and skin wound healing. *Biol. Chem.* **2010**, *391*, 345–355. [CrossRef] [PubMed]
16. Moreau, M.E.; Garbacki, N.; Molinaro, G.; Brown, N.J.; Marceau, F.; Adam, A. The kallikrein-kinin system: Current and future pharmacological targets. *J. Pharmacol. Sci.* **2005**, *99*, 6–38.
17. Herring, A.; Munster, Y.; Akkaya, T.; Moghaddam, S.; Deinsberger, K.; Meyer, J.; Zahel, J.; Sanchez-Mendoza, E.; Wang, Y.; Hermann, D.M.; et al. Kallikrein-8 inhibition attenuates Alzheimer's disease pathology in mice. *Alzheimers Dement.* **2016**, *12*, 1273–1287. [CrossRef]
18. Spencer, B.; Valera, E.; Rockenstein, E.; Trejo-Morales, M.; Adame, A.; Masliah, E. A brain-targeted, modified neurosin (kallikrein-6) reduces alpha-synuclein accumulation in a mouse model of multiple system atrophy. *Mol. Neurodegener.* **2015**, *10*, 48. [CrossRef]
19. Yoon, H.; Scarisbrick, I.A. Kallikrein-related peptidase 6 exacerbates disease in an autoimmune model of multiple sclerosis. *Biol. Chem.* **2016**, *397*, 1277–1286. [CrossRef]
20. Bhoola, K.D.; Figueroa, C.D.; Worthy, K. Bioregulation of kinins: Kallikreins, kininogens, and kininases. *Pharmacol. Rev.* **1992**, *44*, 1–80.

21. Avgeris, M.; Mavridis, K.; Scorilas, A. Kallikrein-related peptidase genes as promising biomarkers for prognosis and monitoring of human malignancies. *Biol. Chem.* **2010**, *391*, 505–511. [CrossRef] [PubMed]
22. Chao, J.; Chao, L. Kallikrein-kinin in stroke, cardiovascular and renal disease. *Exp. Physiol.* **2005**, *90*, 291–298. [CrossRef] [PubMed]
23. Regoli, D.; Plante, G.E.; Gobeil, F., Jr. Impact of kinins in the treatment of cardiovascular diseases. *Pharmacol. Ther.* **2012**, *135*, 94–111. [CrossRef] [PubMed]
24. Heuberger, D.M.; Schuepbach, R.A. Protease-activated receptors (PARs): Mechanisms of action and potential therapeutic modulators in PAR-driven inflammatory diseases. *Thromb. J.* **2019**, *17*, 4. [CrossRef]
25. Lewkowich, I.P.; Day, S.B.; Ledford, J.R.; Zhou, P.; Dienger, K.; Wills-Karp, M.; Page, K. Protease-activated receptor 2 activation of myeloid dendritic cells regulates allergic airway inflammation. *Respir. Res.* **2011**, *12*, 122. [CrossRef]
26. Ossovskaya, V.S.; Bunnett, N.W. Protease-activated receptors: Contribution to physiology and disease. *Physiol. Rev.* **2004**, *84*, 579–621. [CrossRef]
27. Rothmeier, A.S.; Ruf, W. Protease-activated receptor 2 signaling in inflammation. *Semin. Immunopathol.* **2012**, *34*, 133–149. [CrossRef]
28. Yamaguchi, R.; Yamamoto, T.; Sakamoto, A.; Ishimaru, Y.; Narahara, S.; Sugiuchi, H.; Yamaguchi, Y. A protease-activated receptor 2 agonist (AC-264613) suppresses interferon regulatory factor 5 and decreases interleukin-12p40 production by lipopolysaccharide-stimulated macrophages: Role of p53. *Cell Biol. Int.* **2016**, *40*, 629–641. [CrossRef]
29. Zhong, B.; Ma, S.; Wang, D.H. Protease-activated receptor 2 protects against myocardial ischemia-reperfusion injury through the lipoxygenase pathway and TRPV1 channels. *Exp. Ther. Med.* **2019**, *18*, 3636–3642. [CrossRef]
30. Ponticelli, C.; Meroni, P.L. Kallikreins and lupus nephritis. *J. Clin. Investig.* **2009**, *119*, 768–771. [CrossRef]
31. Liu, K.; Li, Q.Z.; Delgado-Vega, A.M.; Abelson, A.K.; Sanchez, E.; Kelly, J.A.; Li, L.; Liu, Y.; Zhou, J.; Yan, M.; et al. Kallikrein genes are associated with lupus and glomerular basement membrane-specific antibody-induced nephritis in mice and humans. *J. Clin. Investig.* **2009**, *119*, 911–923. [CrossRef]
32. Li, Q.Z.; Zhou, J.; Yang, R.; Yan, M.; Ye, Q.; Liu, K.; Liu, S.; Shao, X.; Li, L.; Zhou, X.J.; et al. The lupus-susceptibility gene kallikrein downmodulates antibody-mediated glomerulonephritis. *Genes. Immun.* **2009**, *10*, 503–508. [CrossRef]
33. Banchereau, J.; Pascual, V. Type I interferon in systemic lupus erythematosus and other autoimmune diseases. *Immunity* **2006**, *25*, 383–392. [CrossRef]
34. Niewold, T.B.; Clark, D.N.; Salloum, R.; Poole, B.D. Interferon alpha in systemic lupus erythematosus. *J. Biomed. Biotechnol.* **2010**, *2010*, 948364. [CrossRef]
35. Theofilopoulos, A.N.; Baccala, R.; Beutler, B.; Kono, D.H. Type I interferons (alpha/beta) in immunity and autoimmunity. *Annu. Rev. Immunol.* **2005**, *23*, 307–336. [CrossRef]
36. Figueiredo-Braga, M.; Cornaby, C.; Cortez, A.; Bernardes, M.; Terroso, G.; Figueiredo, M.; Mesquita, C.D.S.; Costa, L.; Poole, B.D. Depression and anxiety in systemic lupus erythematosus: The crosstalk between immunological, clinical, and psychosocial factors. *Medicine* **2018**, *97*, e11376. [CrossRef]
37. Gao, H.X.; Campbell, S.R.; Cui, M.H.; Zong, P.; Hee-Hwang, J.; Gulinello, M.; Putterman, C. Depression is an early disease manifestation in lupus-prone MRL/lpr mice. *J. Neuroimmunol.* **2009**, *207*, 45–56. [CrossRef]
38. Can, A.; Dao, D.T.; Terrillion, C.E.; Piantadosi, S.C.; Bhat, S.; Gould, T.D. The tail suspension test. *J. Vis. Exp.* **2012**, *59*, e3769. [CrossRef]
39. Curzon, P.; Zhang, M.; Radek, R.J.; Fox, G.B. The Behavioral Assessment of Sensorimotor Processes in the Mouse: Acoustic Startle, Sensory Gating, Locomotor Activity, Rotarod, and Beam Walking. In *Methods of Behavior Analysis in Neuroscience*, 2nd ed.; Buccafusco, J.J., Ed.; CRC Press/Taylor & Francis: Boca Raton, FL, USA, 2009.
40. Catena-Dell'Osso, M.; Rotella, F.; Dell'Osso, A.; Fagiolini, A.; Marazziti, D. Inflammation, serotonin and major depression. *Curr. Drug Targets* **2013**, *14*, 571–577. [CrossRef]
41. Paolicelli, R.C.; Sierra, A.; Stevens, B.; Tremblay, M.E.; Aguzzi, A.; Ajami, B.; Amit, I.; Audinat, E.; Bechmann, I.; Bennett, M.; et al. Microglia states and nomenclature: A field at its crossroads. *Neuron* **2022**, *110*, 3458–3483. [CrossRef]
42. Weissmann, G. Rheumatoid arthritis and systemic lupus erythematosus as immune complex diseases. *Bull. NYU Hosp. Jt. Dis.* **2009**, *67*, 251–253.
43. Qin, L.; Du, Y.; Ding, H.; Haque, A.; Hicks, J.; Pedroza, C.; Mohan, C. Bradykinin 1 receptor blockade subdues systemic autoimmunity, renal inflammation, and blood pressure in murine lupus nephritis. *Arthritis Res. Ther.* **2019**, *21*, 12. [CrossRef]
44. Shao, X.; Yang, R.; Yan, M.; Li, Y.; Du, Y.; Raman, I.; Zhang, B.; Wakeland, E.K.; Igarashi, P.; Mohan, C.; et al. Inducible expression of kallikrein in renal tubular cells protects mice against spontaneous lupus nephritis. *Arthritis Rheum.* **2013**, *65*, 780–791. [CrossRef]
45. Loncharich, M.F.; Anderson, C.W. Interferon Inhibition for Lupus with Anifrolumab: Critical Appraisal of the Evidence Leading to FDA Approval. *ACR Open Rheumatol.* **2022**, *4*, 486–491. [CrossRef]
46. Crow, M.K.; Olferiev, M.; Kirou, K.A. Targeting of type I interferon in systemic autoimmune diseases. *Transl. Res.* **2015**, *165*, 296–305. [CrossRef]
47. Sforzini, L.; Cattaneo, A.; Ferrari, C.; Turner, L.; Mariani, N.; Enache, D.; Hastings, C.; Lombardo, G.; Nettis, M.A.; Nikkheslat, N.; et al. Higher immune-related gene expression in major depression is independent of CRP levels: Results from the BIODEP study. *Transl. Psychiatry* **2023**, *13*, 185. [CrossRef]
48. Liu, T.; Son, M.; Diamond, B. HMGB1 in Systemic Lupus Erythematosus. *Front. Immunol.* **2020**, *11*, 1057. [CrossRef]

49. Xu, S.Y.; Jia, J.Q.; Sun, M.; Bao, X.Y.; Xia, S.N.; Shu, S.; Liu, P.Y.; Ji, S.L.; Ye, L.; Cao, X.; et al. QHRD106 ameliorates ischemic stroke injury as a long-acting tissue kallikrein preparation. *iScience* **2023**, *26*, 107268. [CrossRef]
50. Vital, E.M.; Merrill, J.T.; Morand, E.F.; Furie, R.A.; Bruce, I.N.; Tanaka, Y.; Manzi, S.; Kalunian, K.C.; Kalyani, R.N.; Streicher, K.; et al. Anifrolumab efficacy and safety by type I interferon gene signature and clinical subgroups in patients with SLE: Post hoc analysis of pooled data from two phase III trials. *Ann. Rheum. Dis.* **2022**, *81*, 951–961. [CrossRef]
51. Bruce, I.N.; Furie, R.A.; Morand, E.F.; Manzi, S.; Tanaka, Y.; Kalunian, K.C.; Merrill, J.T.; Puzio, P.; Maho, E.; Kleoudis, C.; et al. Concordance and discordance in SLE clinical trial outcome measures: Analysis of three anifrolumab phase 2/3 trials. *Ann. Rheum. Dis.* **2022**, *81*, 962–969. [CrossRef]
52. Fushida, N.; Horii, M.; Oishi, K.; Matsushita, T. Anifrolumab for systemic lupus erythematosus: A clinical study of Japanese patients in Kanazawa University Hospital. *J. Dermatol.* **2024**, *51*, 607–611. [CrossRef]
53. Tanaka, Y.; Luo, Y.; O'Shea, J.J.; Nakayamada, S. Janus kinase-targeting therapies in rheumatology: A mechanisms-based approach. *Nat. Rev. Rheumatol.* **2022**, *18*, 133–145. [CrossRef]
54. Gonzales, E.L.; Jeon, S.J.; Han, K.M.; Yang, S.J.; Kim, Y.; Remonde, C.G.; Ahn, T.J.; Ham, B.J.; Shin, C.Y. Correlation between immune-related genes and depression-like features in an animal model and in humans. *Brain Behav. Immun.* **2023**, *113*, 29–43. [CrossRef]
55. Fischer, C.W.; Eskelund, A.; Budac, D.P.; Tillmann, S.; Liebenberg, N.; Elfving, B.; Wegener, G. Interferon-alpha treatment induces depression-like behaviour accompanied by elevated hippocampal quinolinic acid levels in rats. *Behav. Brain Res.* **2015**, *293*, 166–172. [CrossRef]
56. Zeng, J.; Meng, X.; Zhou, P.; Yin, Z.; Xie, Q.; Zou, H.; Shen, N.; Ye, Z.; Tang, Y. Interferon-alpha exacerbates neuropsychiatric phenotypes in lupus-prone mice. *Arthritis Res. Ther.* **2019**, *21*, 205. [CrossRef]
57. Lood, C.; Tyden, H.; Gullstrand, B.; Klint, C.; Wenglen, C.; Nielsen, C.T.; Heegaard, N.H.; Jonsen, A.; Kahn, R.; Bengtsson, A.A. Type I interferon-mediated skewing of the serotonin synthesis is associated with severe disease in systemic lupus erythematosus. *PLoS ONE* **2015**, *10*, e0125109. [CrossRef]
58. Saldanha, D.; Kumar, N.; Ryali, V.; Srivastava, K.; Pawar, A.A. Serum Serotonin Abnormality in Depression. *Med. J. Armed Forces India* **2009**, *65*, 108–112. [CrossRef]
59. Wang, N.; Tian, B. Brain-derived neurotrophic factor in autoimmune inflammatory diseases (Review). *Exp. Ther. Med.* **2021**, *22*, 1292. [CrossRef]
60. Zheng, Q.; Xu, M.J.; Cheng, J.; Chen, J.M.; Zheng, L.; Li, Z.G. Serum levels of brain-derived neurotrophic factor are associated with depressive symptoms in patients with systemic lupus erythematosus. *Psychoneuroendocrinology* **2017**, *78*, 246–252. [CrossRef]
61. Quilter, M.C.; Hiraki, L.T.; Korczak, D.J. Depressive and anxiety symptom prevalence in childhood-onset systemic lupus erythematosus: A systematic review. *Lupus* **2019**, *28*, 878–887. [CrossRef]
62. Kollias, G.; Kontoyiannis, D.; Douni, E.; Kassiotis, G. The role of TNF/TNFR in organ-specific and systemic autoimmunity: Implications for the design of optimized 'anti-TNF' therapies. *Curr. Dir. Autoimmun.* **2002**, *5*, 30–50. [PubMed]
63. Godsell, J.; Rudloff, I.; Kandane-Rathnayake, R.; Hoi, A.; Nold, M.F.; Morand, E.F.; Harris, J. Clinical associations of IL-10 and IL-37 in systemic lupus erythematosus. *Sci. Rep.* **2016**, *6*, 34604. [CrossRef] [PubMed]
64. Lee, M.H.; Gallo, P.M.; Hooper, K.M.; Corradetti, C.; Ganea, D.; Caricchio, R.; Gallucci, S. The cytokine network type I IFN-IL-27-IL-10 is augmented in murine and human lupus. *J. Leukoc. Biol.* **2019**, *106*, 967–975. [CrossRef]
65. Iikuni, N.; Okamoto, H.; Yoshio, T.; Sato, E.; Kamitsuji, S.; Iwamoto, T.; Momohara, S.; Taniguchi, A.; Yamanaka, H.; Minota, S.; et al. Raised monocyte chemotactic protein-1 (MCP-1)/CCL2 in cerebrospinal fluid of patients with neuropsychiatric lupus. *Ann. Rheum. Dis.* **2006**, *65*, 253–256. [CrossRef]
66. Lee, Y.H.; Song, G.G. Urinary MCP-1 as a biomarker for lupus nephritis: A meta-analysis. *Z. Rheumatol.* **2017**, *76*, 357–363. [CrossRef] [PubMed]
67. Okamoto, H.; Iikuni, N.; Kamitsuji, S.; Yoshio, T.; Minota, S.; Kamatani, N. IP-10/MCP-1 ratio in CSF is an useful diagnostic marker of neuropsychiatric lupus patients. *Rheumatology* **2006**, *45*, 232–234. [CrossRef] [PubMed]
68. Sarrand, J.; Soyfoo, M. Involvement of IL-33 in the Pathophysiology of Systemic Lupus Erythematosus: Review. *Int. J. Mol. Sci.* **2022**, *23*, 3138. [CrossRef]
69. Sun, Y.; Wen, Y.; Wang, L.; Wen, L.; You, W.; Wei, S.; Mao, L.; Wang, H.; Chen, Z.; Yang, X. Therapeutic Opportunities of Interleukin-33 in the Central Nervous System. *Front. Immunol.* **2021**, *12*, 654626. [CrossRef]
70. Georgakis, S.; Gkirtzimanaki, K.; Papadaki, G.; Gakiopoulou, H.; Drakos, E.; Eloranta, M.L.; Makridakis, M.; Kontostathi, G.; Zoidakis, J.; Baira, E.; et al. NETs decorated with bioactive IL-33 infiltrate inflamed tissues and induce IFN-alpha production in patients with SLE. *JCI Insight* **2021**, *6*, e147671. [CrossRef]
71. Hrycek, E.; Franek, A.; Blaszczak, E.; Dworak, J.; Hrycek, A. Serum levels of selected chemokines in systemic lupus erythematosus patients. *Rheumatol. Int.* **2013**, *33*, 2423–2427. [CrossRef]
72. Carneiro, J.R.; Fuzii, H.T.; Kayser, C.; Alberto, F.L.; Soares, F.A.; Sato, E.I.; Andrade, L.E. IL-2, IL-5, TNF-alpha and IFN-gamma mRNA expression in epidermal keratinocytes of systemic lupus erythematosus skin lesions. *Clinics* **2011**, *66*, 77–82. [CrossRef] [PubMed]
73. Li, H.; Boulougoura, A.; Endo, Y.; Tsokos, G.C. Abnormalities of T cells in systemic lupus erythematosus: New insights in pathogenesis and therapeutic strategies. *J. Autoimmun.* **2022**, *132*, 102870. [CrossRef] [PubMed]

74. Nestor, J.; Arinuma, Y.; Huerta, T.S.; Kowal, C.; Nasiri, E.; Kello, N.; Fujieda, Y.; Bialas, A.; Hammond, T.; Sriram, U.; et al. Lupus antibodies induce behavioral changes mediated by microglia and blocked by ACE inhibitors. *J. Exp. Med.* **2018**, *215*, 2554–2566. [CrossRef] [PubMed]
75. Makinde, H.M.; Winter, D.R.; Procissi, D.; Mike, E.V.; Stock, A.D.; Kando, M.J.; Gadhvi, G.T.; Droho, S.; Bloomfield, C.L.; Dominguez, S.T.; et al. A Novel Microglia-Specific Transcriptional Signature Correlates with Behavioral Deficits in Neuropsychiatric Lupus. *Front. Immunol.* **2020**, *11*, 230. [CrossRef] [PubMed]
76. Vanarsa, K.; Henderson, J.; Soomro, S.; Qin, L.; Zhang, T.; Jordan, N.; Putterman, C.; Blanco, I.; Saxena, R.; Mohan, C. Upregulation of Proinflammatory Bradykinin Peptides in Systemic Lupus Erythematosus and Rheumatoid Arthritis. *J. Immunol.* **2020**, *205*, 369–376. [CrossRef]
77. Gobel, K.; Pankratz, S.; Schneider-Hohendorf, T.; Bittner, S.; Schuhmann, M.K.; Langer, H.F.; Stoll, G.; Wiendl, H.; Kleinschnitz, C.; Meuth, S.G. Blockade of the kinin receptor B1 protects from autoimmune CNS disease by reducing leukocyte trafficking. *J. Autoimmun.* **2011**, *36*, 106–114. [CrossRef]
78. Manolis, A.J.; Marketou, M.E.; Gavras, I.; Gavras, H. Cardioprotective properties of bradykinin: Role of the B(2) receptor. *Hypertens. Res.* **2010**, *33*, 772–777. [CrossRef]
79. Itto, R.; Oe, Y.; Imaruoka, K.; Sato, E.; Sekimoto, A.; Yamakage, S.; Kumakura, S.; Sato, H.; Ito, S.; Takahashi, N. Glomerular Injury Is Exacerbated in Lupus-Prone MRL/lpr Mice Treated with a Protease-Activated Receptor 2 Antagonist. *Tohoku J. Exp. Med.* **2019**, *249*, 127–133. [CrossRef]
80. Seo, Y.; Mun, C.H.; Park, S.H.; Jeon, D.; Kim, S.J.; Yoon, T.; Ko, E.; Jo, S.; Park, Y.B.; Namkung, W.; et al. Punicalagin Ameliorates Lupus Nephritis via Inhibition of PAR2. *Int. J. Mol. Sci.* **2020**, *21*, 4975. [CrossRef]
81. Iablokov, V.; Hirota, C.L.; Peplowski, M.A.; Ramachandran, R.; Mihara, K.; Hollenberg, M.D.; MacNaughton, W.K. Proteinase-activated receptor 2 (PAR2) decreases apoptosis in colonic epithelial cells. *J. Biol. Chem.* **2014**, *289*, 34366–34377. [CrossRef]
82. Sriram, U.; Varghese, L.; Bennett, H.L.; Jog, N.R.; Shivers, D.K.; Ning, Y.; Behrens, E.M.; Caricchio, R.; Gallucci, S. Myeloid dendritic cells from B6.NZM Sle1/Sle2/Sle3 lupus-prone mice express an IFN signature that precedes disease onset. *J. Immunol.* **2012**, *189*, 80–91. [CrossRef] [PubMed]
83. Rom, S.; Heldt, N.A.; Gajghate, S.; Seliga, A.; Reichenbach, N.L.; Persidsky, Y. Hyperglycemia and advanced glycation end products disrupt BBB and promote occludin and claudin-5 protein secretion on extracellular microvesicles. *Sci. Rep.* **2020**, *10*, 7274. [CrossRef]
84. Marcinko, K.; Parsons, T.; Lerch, J.P.; Sled, J.G.; Sakic, B. Effects of prolonged treatment with memantine in the MRL model of CNS lupus. *Clin. Exp. Neuroimmunol.* **2012**, *3*, 116–128. [CrossRef] [PubMed]

cells

MDPI

Article

Blocking Thromboxane-Prostanoid Receptor Signaling Attenuates Lipopolysaccharide- and Stearic Acid-Induced Inflammatory Response in Human PBMCs

Vinothkumar Rajamanickam [1,2], Cyrus V. Desouza [1,2], Romilia T. Castillo [1,2] and Viswanathan Saraswathi [1,2,*]

1 Division of Diabetes, Endocrinology and Metabolism, Department of Internal Medicine, University of Nebraska Medical Center, Omaha, NE 68198, USA; vrajamanickam@unmc.edu (V.R.); cdesouza@unmc.edu (C.V.D.); rocastillo@unmc.edu (R.T.C.)

2 Research Service, VA Nebraska-Western Iowa Health Care System, Omaha, NE 68105, USA

* Correspondence: s.viswanathan@unmc.edu

Abstract: Inflammation is implicated in the etiology of obesity-related diseases. Thromboxane-prostanoid receptor (TPR) is known to play a role in mediating an inflammatory response in a variety of cells. Gut-derived lipopolysaccharide (LPS), a TLR4 agonist, is elevated in obesity. Moreover, free fatty acids (FFAs) are important mediators of obesity-related inflammation. However, the role and mechanisms by which TPR regulates the inflammatory response in human immune cells remain unclear. We sought to determine the link between TPR and obesity and the role/mechanisms by which TPR alters LPS- or stearic acid (SA)-induced inflammatory responses in PBMCs. Cells were pre-treated with agents blocking TPR signaling, followed by treatment with LPS or stearic acid (SA). Our findings showed that TPR mRNA levels are higher in PBMCs from individuals with obesity. Blockade of TPR as well as ROCK, which acts downstream of TPR, attenuated LPS- and/or SA-induced pro-inflammatory responses. On the other hand, TPR activation using its agonist enhanced the pro-inflammatory effects of LPS and/or SA. Of note, the TPR agonist by itself elicits an inflammatory response, which was attenuated by blocking TPR or ROCK. Our data suggest that TPR plays a key role in promoting an inflammatory response in human PBMCs, and this effect is mediated via TLR4 and/or ROCK signaling.

Keywords: thromboxane A2; inflammation; lipopolysaccharide; stearic acid; PBMC; ROCK

1. Introduction

Worldwide, 537 million adults have been diagnosed with diabetes. This alarming number is expected to rise to 700 million by 2045 [1]. The obesity epidemic has increased the prevalence of diabetes, making diabetes one of the leading causes of death in the U.S. The excess adipose tissue (AT) seen in obesity disturbs cellular homeostasis and upregulates the production of inflammatory markers, including tumor necrosis factor α (TNF-α), monocyte chemoattractant protein-1 (MCP-1), and interleukin 6 (IL-6). Along with the increased production of cytokines, AT promotes the production of hormones and non-esterified fatty acids [2]. These mediators facilitate oxidative stress, a pro-inflammatory state impairing beta cell function, and insulin resistance [3]. Targeting the initiation steps of the inflammation cascade presents a therapeutic target for obesity-induced insulin resistance and hyperglycemia.

Thromboxane A2 (TXA2) is a lipid mediator in the arachidonic acid signaling system [4]. In an inflammatory state, the enzymes phospholipase A2 and cyclooxygenase (COX-1/COX-2) facilitate the cleavage of arachidonic acid and the conversion to prostaglandin H2 (PGH2). PGH2 is further metabolized into TXA2 by the enzyme thromboxane A synthase (THAS) [4]. TXA2 exerts its biological activity via the transmembrane G-protein-coupled receptor, the thromboxane-prostanoid receptor (TPR), also known as the TXA2 receptor. Although platelet activation and vasoconstriction are two major physiological functions of TPR, it has received significant attention in the past two decades for its pathophysiological role in many diseases. It has been extensively studied for its role in altering the inflammatory processes in endothelial cells [5–7]. However, little is known regarding the role of TPR in mediating the inflammatory response in immune cells. Of note, immune cells like macrophages are a significant source of TXA2 [8,9] and express TPR [10]. A study by Hartney et al. has shown that TPR signaling is required for fibronectin-induced matrix metalloproteinase 9 production by macrophages [11]. TPR antagonism inhibited the LPS-induced inflammatory response in rat peritoneal macrophages [12]. Moreover, TPR exerts a pro-inflammatory effect in microglial cells [13,14]. However, the link between immune cell TPR and obesity remains unknown. Moreover, the role and mechanisms by which immune cell TPR exerts an inflammatory response upon treatment with obesity-related factors, in particular LPS and FFA, remain unclear.

Human peripheral blood mononuclear cells (PBMCs) comprise monocytes, macrophages, and lymphocytes. PBMCs represent a clinically relevant model system to study the role of the immune system in the development of many diseases. LPS is an endotoxin found on the membrane of gram-negative bacteria. The circulating levels of gut-derived LPS are increased in obesity [15]. Moreover, obesity is characterized by an increase in AT lipolysis and a release of FFA from the AT. The LPS-induced inflammatory response is initiated by the activation of toll-like receptor 4 (TLR4), which induces the release of inflammatory cytokines from PBMCs [16]. Similarly, saturated fatty acids are reported to promote an inflammatory response via TLR4 [17]. However, the role and mechanisms by which TPR mediates the pro-inflammatory effects of these obesity-related factors, in particular LPS and FFAs, in human immune cells are still unclear.

The objectives of this study are to assess the link between PBMC TPR and human obesity and determine the role and mechanisms by which TPR mediates the pro-inflammatory effects in human immune cells, in particular PBMCs.

2. Materials and Methods

2.1. Chemicals

SQ29548 (SQ) (#19025), a TPR antagonist, Ozagrel (OZA) (#70515), a selective inhibitor of THAS, and BM567 (BM) (#10155), a dual-acting agent that inhibits both TPR and THAS, were used to block TXA2 signaling and were obtained from Cayman Chemical (Ann Arbor, MI, USA). [1S-[1α,2α(Z),3β(1E,3S*),4α]]-7-[3-[3-hydroxy-4-(4-iodophenoxy)-1-butenyl]-7-oxabicyclo [2.2.1] hept-2-yl]-5-heptenoic acid (IBOP) (#19600), a TXR agonist, was also obtained from Cayman Chemical (Ann Arbor, MI, USA). Y-27632 2HCl, a selective ROCK1 and ROCK2 inhibitor (#1293823), was obtained from Biogems (Westlake Village, CA, USA). The thromboxane B2 ELISA kit (#501020) and the LDH Cytotoxicity Assay kit (#601170) were obtained from Cayman Chemical (Ann Arbor, MI, USA). Lipopolysaccharide (#L2630) and stearic acid (#N-18A-AU27-T) were purchased from Sigma-Aldrich (St. Louis, MO, USA) and Nuchek Prep (Elysian, MN, USA), respectively.

2.2. Human Subjects

Study 1. Study Design and Patient Population. Blood samples were collected from normal subjects (BMI < 30) and individuals with obesity (BMI > 30). Peripheral blood mononuclear cells (PBMCs) were collected to detect the mRNA levels of TPR. This study was approved by the institutional review board of the VA Nebraska-Western Iowa Health Care System. Informed consent was obtained from all subjects involved in the study. The characteristics of the study subjects are shown in Table 1.

Inclusion and exclusion criteria were applied while choosing the subjects for the study. The inclusion criteria were as follows: (1) age 19 to 75; (2) lean/overweight group: BMI between 20 and 29.9 kg/m^2; obesity group: BMI 30–55 kg/m^2; (3) subjects should be on a stable dose of any medications for at least two months. The exclusion criteria were as follows: (1) patients currently taking NSAIDs more than 3/week on a prescription basis or taking a daily dose of NSAID; (2) history of diabetes and patients taking diabetes medications, as these drugs may alter AT metabolic functions; (3) history of uncontrolled hypertension defined as >160 systolic and 95 diastolic on medication; (4) history of renal disease with GFR < 60; (5) history of hepatic failure or AST/ALT > three times the normal range; (6) patients with active cancer within the last 2 years except for skin cancers; (7) patients with acute illness needing hospitalization within the last 2 months; (8) patients with acute inflammation; (9) patients with cardiovascular events such as myocardial infarction, stroke, amputation, or unstable angina within the last six months; (10) pregnancy; and (11) presence of psychosis, suicidal ideations, untreated major depression, dementia, or history of stimulant dependence/substance abuse. The study was approved by the institutional review board at the VA Nebraska-Western Iowa Health Care System (NWIHCS). All participants provided informed consent.

Table 1. Baseline characteristics.

Measurement	**Normal (n = 15)**	**Obesity (n = 14)**	**p Value**
Age (years)	40.20 ± 4.27	47.43 ± 2.22	0.1537
Weight (lbs)	168.7 ± 5.80	241.1 ± 7.15	<0.0001
Body mass index (kg/m^2)	24.24 ± 0.61	34.79 ± 0.96	<0.0001
Insulin (μIU/mL)	4.53 ± 1.02	12.85 ± 3.64	0.0275
Glucose (mg/dL)	90.00 ± 1.60	92.00 ± 2.67	0.5206
HOMA-IR	1.01 ± 0.23	2.88 ± 0.71	0.0144
Total cholesterol (mg/dL)	197.4 ± 6.66	208.3 ± 14.54	0.4922
Triglycerides (mg/dL)	114.8 ± 18.23	168.8 ± 42.18	0.2394
LDL cholesterol (mg/dL)	121.3 ± 6.92	140.5 ± 13.21	0.1941
HDL cholesterol (mg/dL)	53.13 ± 3.65	41.07 ± 2.67	0.0140
Creatinine (mg/dL)	1.05 ± 0.03	1.02 ± 0.05	0.7158
ALT (U/L)	17.80 ± 2.88	38.07 ± 13.29	0.1353
AST (U/L)	31.00 ± 2.12	34.64 ± 4.51	0.4616
HA1C (%)	5.43 ± 0.51	5.77 ± 1.85	0.0063
GFR (mL/min)	82.87 ± 4.08	82.36 ± 5.03	0.9375
CRP (mg/L)	2.69 ± 1.03	2.94 ± 0.68	0.8442
Fat mass (%)	19.53 ± 1.14	35.51 ± 1.32	<0.0001

Values are mean ± SEM. HOMA-IR, Homeostatic Model Assessment for Insulin Resistance; ALT, alkaline phosphatase; AST, acid phosphatase.

Study 2. Blood samples collected from this study were used to isolate PBMCs to perform ex vivo mechanistic studies. This study was approved by the institutional review board of the VA Nebraska-Western Iowa Health Care System and the University of Nebraska Medical Center. Informed consent was obtained from all subjects involved in the study.

2.3. PBMC Isolation and Culture

Heparinized peripheral blood was collected from all study subjects. PBMCs were isolated from whole blood by Ficoll-Paque Plus (#17144002, Cytiva, MA, USA) density gradient centrifugation at 400× g for 35 min at 20 °C. Isolated cells were treated with RBC lysis buffer (#00-4333-57, Invitrogen, CA, USA), washed with PBS, and then resuspended at 1 × 10^6 cells/mL in RPMI 1640 (Cytiva, MA, USA) medium containing 5% fetal bovine serum (R&D system, Minneapolis, MN, USA). After an overnight incubation, PBMCs were treated with various agents. Media supernatants were collected at 6 h and 24 h for further analyses.

2.4. Real-Time Quantitative Polymerase Chain Reaction

For gene expression analysis, total RNA was isolated from human PBMCs using Trizol (#15596018, Thermo Fisher Scientific, Waltham, MA USA), and cDNA was synthesized using 5X iScript reverse transcription supermix (#1708841, Bio-Rad, Hercules, CA, USA). We conducted real-time polymerase chain reaction (PCR) using iQ Supermix (#1708860,

Bio-Rad, Hercules, CA, USA) to identify the mRNA level of *TXA2R* (encoding for TPR). To quantify gene expression, we used the ΔΔCT method and normalized the values to 18s ribosomal RNA. Human *TXA2R* (#Hs00169054_m1) and 18S (#Hs99999901_s1) primers were obtained from Thermo Fisher Scientific (Waltham, MA, USA).

2.5. Enzyme-Linked Immunosorbent Assay (ELISA)

Cell culture supernatants collected at 6 h and 24 h were centrifuged at 1200 rpm at 4 °C for 3 min to remove cell debris. The protein levels of tumor necrosis factor-alpha (TNFα, #555212), interleukin-1β (IL-1β, #55753), monocyte chemoattractant protein-1 (MCP-1, #555179) (BD bioscience, San Jose, CA, USA) and macrophage inflammatory protein-1 alpha (MIP-1α, #DY270, R&D system, Minneapolis, MN, USA) were analyzed using ELISA kits. Briefly, microplates were coated with a diluted capture antibody and incubated at 4 °C overnight. Then, plates were washed 3 times using a wash buffer. Plates were blocked by adding 200 μL of assay diluent for 1 h. Then diluted samples and standards were added, sealed, and incubated for 2 h at room temperature. After 3 washes, plates were incubated with detection antibodies for 1 h and then enzyme SAv-HRP for 1 h. After washing, plates were incubated with a TMB substrate solution for 30 min. After color development, 50 μL of stop solution was added to each well, and absorbance was measured at 450 nm according to the manufacturer's instructions using the Molecular Devices SpectraMax M5 Microplate Readers (San Jose, CA, USA).

2.6. Thromboxane B2 Assay

The levels of thromboxane B2 were determined in the media collected from PBMCs using the thromboxane B2 ELISA kit (Cayman Chemical, Ann Arbor, MI, USA).

2.7. LDH Cytotoxicity Assay

The levels of LDH activity in the cell culture supernatants were determined using the LDH cytotoxicity assay kit (Cayman Chemical, Ann Arbor, MI, USA).

2.8. Statistical Analysis

All of the quantitative variables are presented as the mean ± SEM. Differences among various groups were analyzed using the Student's *t*-test to compare two groups. A one-way analysis of variance followed by Tukey's post-hoc analysis was used for multiple comparisons. Statistical analysis was performed by GraphPad Prism 10 software. A *p*-value < 0.05 was considered significant.

3. Results

3.1. TPR Expression Is Increased in PBMCs in Individuals with Obesity

We analyzed the mRNA levels of *TXA2R* (encoding TPR) in PBMCs from normal subjects and individuals with obesity (Figure 1A). The *TXA2R* mRNA level was significantly higher in PBMCs collected from subjects with obesity and positively correlated with body weight and fat mass (Figure 1B–D). These data suggest that a positive relationship exists between PBMC-TPR and obesity.

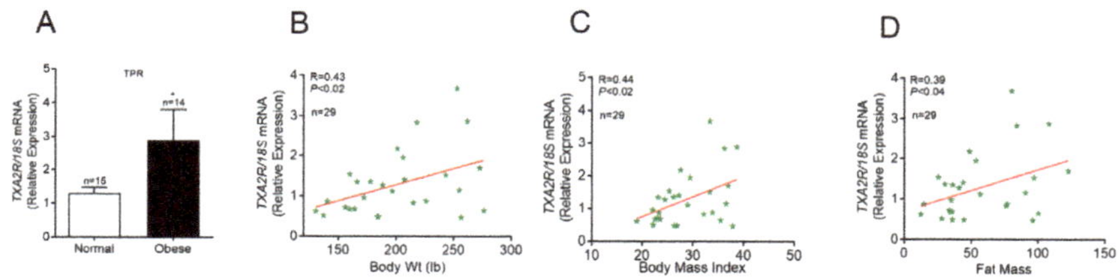

Figure 1. *TXA2R* expression levels in PBMCs from normal and obese subjects: (**A**) *TXA2R* mRNA expression in human PBMCs. Values are mean ± SEM. * $p < 0.05$ vs. Normal. Correlative analysis

performed on normal and obese subjects (n = 29) comparing *TXA2R* gene expression with (**B**) body weight, (**C**) body mass index, and (**D**) fat mass.

3.2. Blockade of TPR Signaling Reduces Lipopolysaccharide (LPS)-Induced Pro-Inflammatory Response in Human PBMCs

As mentioned, obesity is associated with an increase in circulating endotoxin levels [15]. Therefore, we sought to determine the impact of inhibiting TPR signaling on altering the LPS-induced pro-inflammatory response in PBMCs. As shown in Figure 2, our data show that LPS significantly increased the levels of TNFα, MCP-1, IL1β, and MIP-1α at 6 h (Figure 2A–D) and 24 h (Figure 2E–H). On the other hand, pretreatment with agents inhibiting TXA2 signaling, including SQ29548 (a TPR antagonist), Ozagrel (a TXA2 synthase inhibitor), and BM567 (a dual-acting agent inhibiting TXA2 synthase and TPR), attenuated the secretion of TNFα, IL1β, and MIP-1α. MCP-1 levels showed only a trend toward a decrease but not a significant decrease upon treatment with these agents (Figure 2A–H). We also measured the levels of IL6 and IL8, and we did not notice a significant difference among different groups. Next, we measured the levels of LDH, a marker of cytotoxicity, and we noted that the LDH levels did not alter among different groups, indicating that these agents did not induce cytotoxicity (Supplementary Figure S1). These findings indicate that TPR inhibitors effectively decrease the LPS-induced pro-inflammatory response in PBMCs.

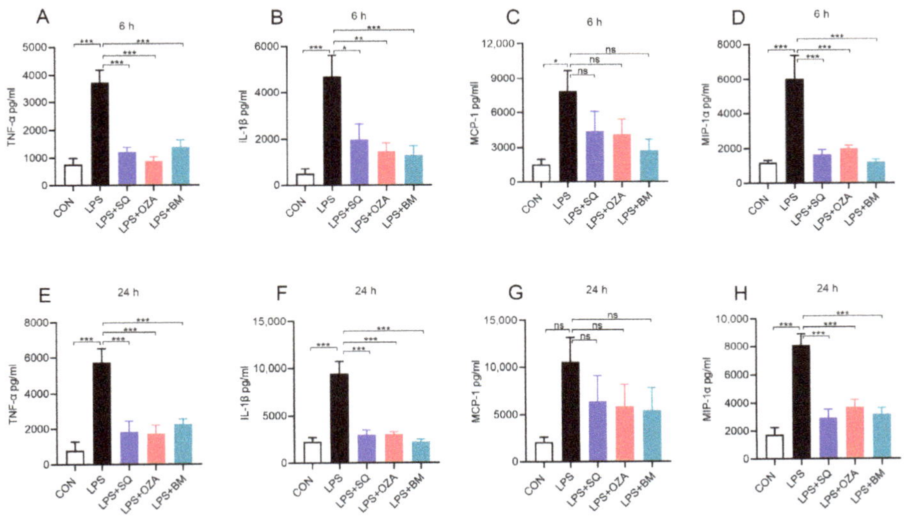

Figure 2. Inhibitors of TPR signaling reduced LPS-induced secretion of inflammatory mediators by human PBMCs. PBMCs were pre-treated with different agents inhibiting TPR signaling (10 μM) for 2 h, followed by co-incubation with LPS (10 ng/mL) for 6 h and 24 h. (**A–D**) Bar graphs show the amount of TNFα, IL-1β, MCP-1, and MIP-1α in cell culture supernatants at 6 h. (**E–H**) The levels of TNFα, IL-1β, MCP-1, and MIP-1α in cell culture supernatants after 24 h of treatment. Values are expressed as the mean ± SEM of 5 sets of experiments in duplicate (n = 10). * $p < 0.05$, ** $p < 0.01$, *** $p < 0.001$, and ns—not significant.

3.3. Inhibition of TPR Attenuates LPS-Induced TXB2 Secretion

Next, we wanted to check if LPS actually increases the formation of TXB2 in PBMCs. We analyzed the media supernatants for TXB2 levels and noted an increase in TXB2 release upon treatment with LPS. Interestingly, pre-treatment with a TPR antagonist and TXAS inhibitor, the dual-acting agent inhibiting both TPR and TXAS, inhibited LPS-induced TXB2 secretion into the media (Supplementary Figure S2).

3.4. Blockade of TPR Signaling Reduces Stearic Acid-Induced Pro-Inflammatory Response in Human PBMCs

Circulating plasma FFAs are increased in obesity and obesity-related comorbidities [18], and saturated fatty acids are known to exert an inflammatory response in obesity [19]. Therefore, we next studied the effects of TPR antagonism on SA-induced inflammatory responses in PBMCs. Our data clearly show that SA by itself led to a significant increase in the level of TNFα, IL1β, and MCP-1 at both 6 h (Figure 3A–C) and 24 h (Figure 3D–F) time points. BM567, the dual-acting agent, and SQ, a TPR antagonist, significantly reduced the SA-induced increase in TNFα, IL1β, and MCP-1, respectively. Inhibiting THAS alone using OZA showed a trend toward a decrease in these inflammatory mediators. Overall, these data suggest that the SA-induced inflammatory response can be attenuated by blocking TPR signaling. Further, we measured the levels of LDH, a marker of cytotoxicity, and noted that the LDH level did not change in any of the groups at 6 h. Although SA treatment led to an increase in LDH at 24 h, the inhibitors did not alter the LDH levels, indicating that the inhibitors block the SA-induced inflammatory response without altering cell viability (Supplementary Figure S3).

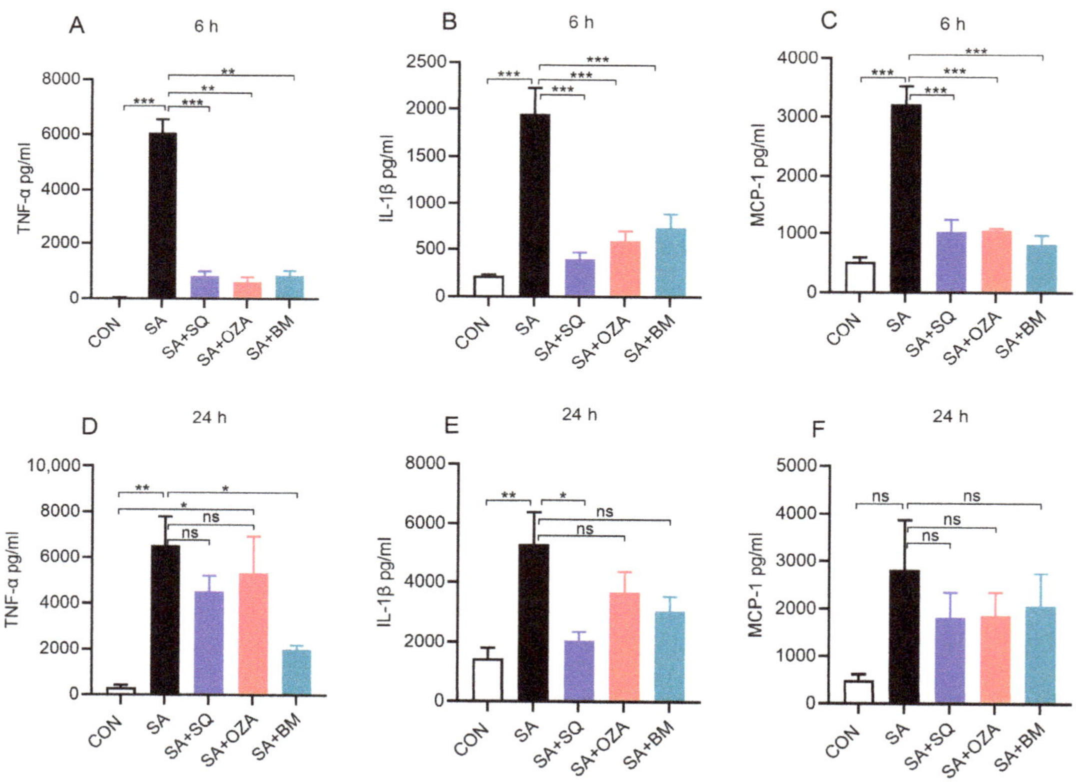

Figure 3. Inhibitors of TPR signaling reduced stearic acid (SA)-induced secretion of inflammatory mediators by human PBMCs. PBMCs were pre-treated with different agents inhibiting TPR signaling (10 μM) for 2 h, followed by co-incubation with SA (90 μM) for 6 h or 24 h. (**A–C**) Bar graphs show the amount of TNFα, IL-1β, and MCP-1 in cell culture supernatants at 6 h. (**D–F**) The levels of TNF-α, IL-1β, and MCP-1 in cell culture supernatants after 24 h of treatment. Values are expressed as the mean ± SEM of 3 sets of experiments in duplicate (n = 6). * $p < 0.05$, ** $p < 0.01$, *** $p < 0.001$, and ns—not significant.

3.5. Activation of TPR Potentiates LPS- and SA-Induced Pro-Inflammatory Response in PBMCs

PBMCs were pre-treated with IBOP, a TPR agonist, for 2 h and then stimulated with LPS or SA. We noticed that LPS or SA alone significantly increased the level of TNFα and IL1β in cultured PBMCs (Figure 4A,B). Interestingly, IBOP enhanced the pro-inflammatory effect of LPS and SA in PBMCs, as evident from the greater increase in IL1β (Figure 4B), further providing evidence that TPR activation promotes an inflammatory response in PBMCs.

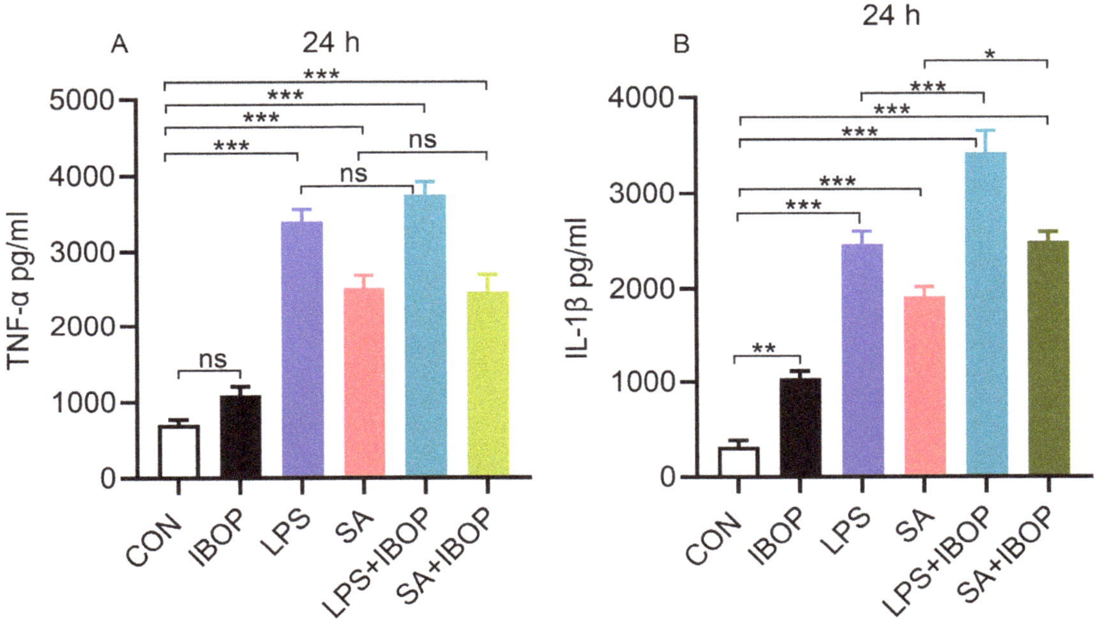

Figure 4. Thromboxane A2 receptor activation aggravates LPS- and SA-induced secretion of pro-inflammatory mediators by human PBMCs. PBMCs were pre-treated with IBOP (2 μM), a TPR agonist, for 2 h, followed by co-incubation with LPS or SA for 24 h. (**A**) Bar graphs show the level of TNFα in cell culture supernatants at 24 h. (**B**) The level of IL-1β in cell culture supernatants after 24 h of treatment. Values are expressed as the mean ± SEM of 3 sets of experiments in duplicate (n = 6). * $p < 0.05$, ** $p < 0.01$, *** $p < 0.001$, and ns—not significant.

3.6. BM567, a Dual-Inhibitor, Attenuates TPR Agonist-Mediated Inflammatory Response in PBMCs

Next, we stimulated PBMCs with IBOP alone in the presence or absence of BM567, a dual-acting agent, to determine the specific effect of TPR activation on the PBMC inflammatory response. We noted that IBOP by itself significantly increased the levels of TNFα and IL1β in the media, and this effect was attenuated by BM567 (Figure 5A–D). These data show that the direct activation of TPR using its agonist can induce an inflammatory response, which can be blocked by inhibiting TPR signaling.

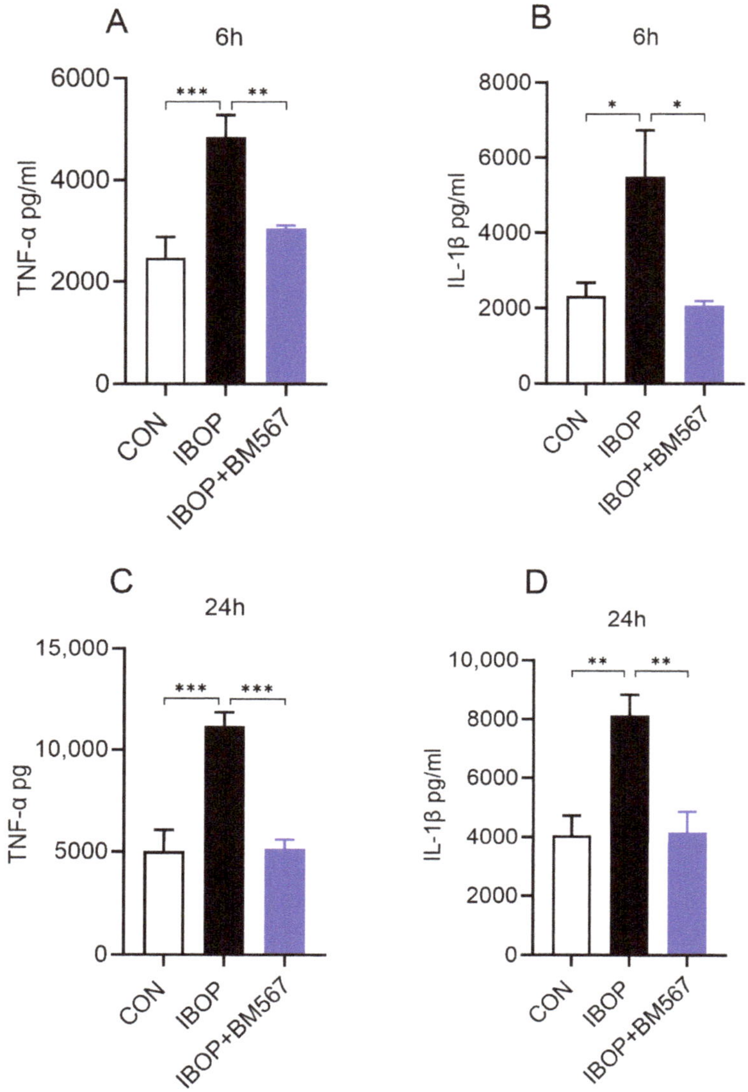

Figure 5. A dual-acting agent inhibiting TPR and TXA2 synthase inhibits IBOP-induced secretion of pro-inflammatory mediators by human PBMCs. PBMCs were pre-treated with BM567 (10 μM) for 2 h, followed by co-incubation with IBOP (2 μM) for 6 h and 24 h. (**A**,**B**) Bar graphs show the level of TNFα and IL-1β in cell culture supernatants at 6 h. (**C**,**D**) The level of TNFα and IL-1β in cell culture supernatants after 24 h of treatment. Values are expressed as the mean ± SEM of 3 sets of experiments in duplicate ($n = 6$). * $p < 0.05$, ** $p < 0.01$, and *** $p < 0.001$.

3.7. Inhibition of ROCK Activity Blocks IBOP-Induced Pro-Inflammatory Response in PBMCs

Regarding potential mechanisms, a link exists between ROCK and TPR signaling, and ROCK1 is involved in promoting an inflammatory response. Therefore, we next treated PBMCs with IBOP, a TPR agonist, in the presence or absence of Y27632, a ROCK inhibitor. As shown in Figure 6, IBOP alone increased the release of TNFα and IL1β, and this effect is blocked by the ROCK inhibitor (Figure 6A–D). These data suggest that TPR promotes an inflammatory response via ROCK.

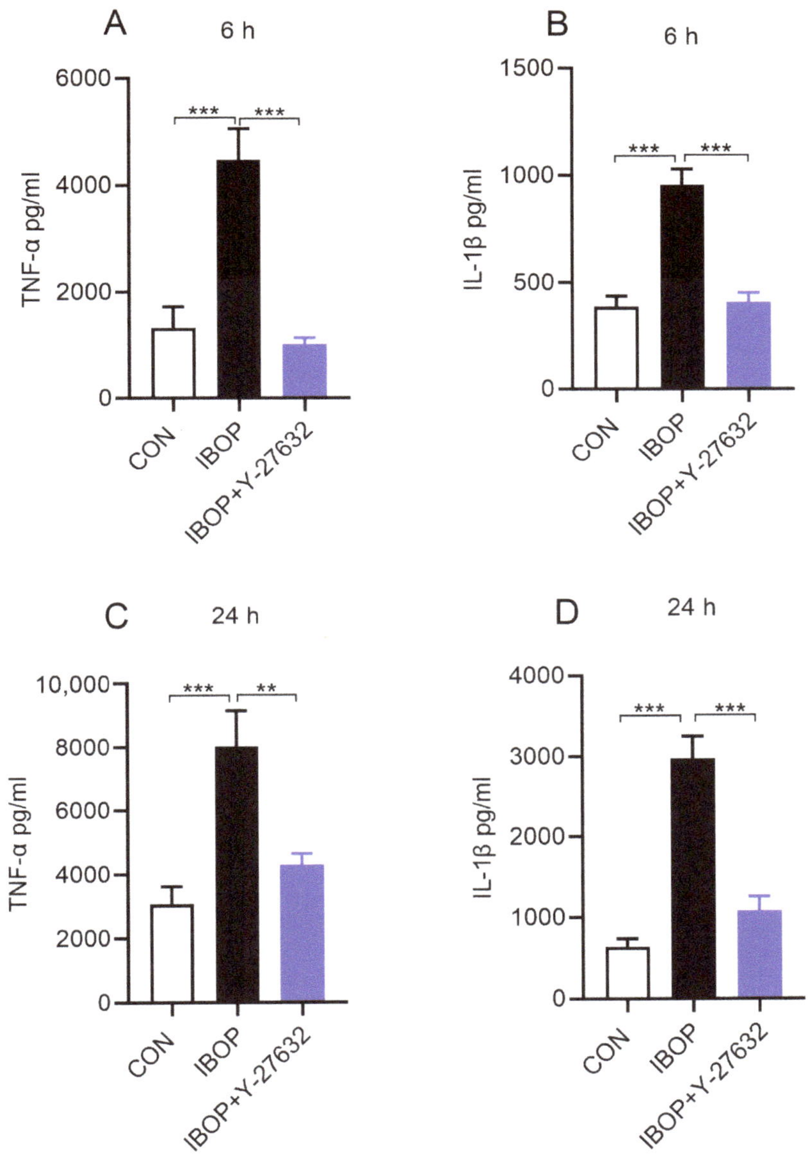

Figure 6. ROCK inhibition attenuates IBOP-induced secretion of pro-inflammatory mediators by human PBMCs. PBMCs were pre-treated with Y-27632, a ROCK inhibitor, for 2 h, followed by co-incubation with IBOP (2 μM) for 6 h and 24 h. (**A**,**B**) Bar graphs show the level of TNFα and IL-1β in cell culture supernatants at 6 h. (**C**,**D**) The level of TNFα and IL-1β in cell culture supernatants after 24 h of treatment. Values are expressed as the mean ± SEM of 4 sets of experiments (2–3 samples per group) (n = 10). ** $p < 0.01$, and *** $p < 0.001$, con vs. IBOP and IBOP vs. treatment groups.

4. Discussion

In the present study, we have demonstrated that a positive association exists between PBMC TPR and human obesity. Ex vivo studies in human PBMCs showed that LPS, a TLR4 agonist, and SA, an FFA, exerted a pro-inflammatory effect in PBMCs. Both LPS- and FFA-induced inflammatory responses are attenuated by blocking TPR signaling. Our studies show that IBOP, a TPR agonist, enhanced the LPS- or FFA-induced inflammatory response in PBMCs. Moreover, IBOP by itself induces a pro-inflammatory effect in PBMCs, which was attenuated by inhibiting TPR signaling. Interestingly, LPS-, FFA-, and IBOP-induced pro-inflammatory effects were also attenuated by inhibiting ROCK activity. Together, these data suggest that a link exists between PBMC TPR and human obesity and that TPR exerts pro-inflammatory effects in PBMCs via TLR4 and/or ROCK signaling.

Although hemostasis and vasoconstriction are important processes regulated by TPR, several lines of evidence suggest that it plays a role in promoting inflammation in endothelial cells and macrophages. Several lines of evidence support the concept that obesity-induced inflammation plays an important role in the development of insulin resistance [20–22]. Macrophages are the predominant immune cell population in human AT. The percentage of macrophages in human AT is estimated to range from 10% in lean subjects to 40% in individuals with obesity [23]. A strong link exists between obesity and inflammation [3,24,25]. Of note, an elevated TXA2 to PGI2 (an anti-inflammatory lipid mediator) ratio in urine and blood plasma has been reported in human subjects and animals exhibiting metabolic syndrome [26,27]. However, evidence for the link between PBMC TPR signaling and obesity in humans is still lacking. We provide evidence that TPR expression is increased in the PBMCs collected from individuals with obesity compared to normal subjects. In addition, PBMC TPR expression is positively correlated to body weight, body mass index, and fat mass.

The direct effects of altering TPR signaling on the inflammatory response in human PBMCs remain unknown. A great deal of emphasis has been placed on elucidating the pro-inflammatory effect of TPR in endothelial cells [5–7]. This is consistent with the well-known effects of TPR in mediating vasoconstriction. Although TPR is widely recognized as an inflammatory gene, limited studies are available on the role of TPR in altering macrophage inflammatory responses. Altavilla et al. reported that G619, a dual TXAS inhibitor and TPR antagonist, inhibits LPS-induced TNFα release in rats in vivo as well as isolated rat peritoneal macrophages [12]. In addition, TPR has been shown to promote a pro-inflammatory effect in microglia, which are resident macrophages in the brain, upon LPS treatment via the activation of MAPK and/or NFκB [13,14]. Our data are in line with these studies and provide evidence that, in addition to LPS, the SA-induced pro-inflammatory response is attenuated by blocking TPR. These data suggest that TPR plays an important role in mediating the pro-inflammatory effects of obesity-related factors, in particular LPS and SA, in human PBMCs.

Regarding potential mechanisms, the fact that LPS is a TLR4 agonist and TPR antagonism attenuates the LPS-induced inflammatory response suggests that there may be coordination between TLR4 and TPR signaling in mediating a macrophage inflammatory response. In fact, the crosstalk between TPR and TLR4 signaling in canine platelets has been reported, where inhibition of TLR4 signaling attenuated LPS-induced TXA2 production and platelet activation [28]. Our data show that the pro-inflammatory effects invoked by LPS, a well-known TLR4 agonist, are attenuated by various agents blocking TPR signaling, including the TPR antagonist, THAS inhibitor, and a dual-acting agent blocking both the enzyme and the receptor, indicating the interaction between TLR4 and TPR in mediating an inflammatory response in PBMCs.

It should also be noted that LPS- and SA-induced pro-inflammatory effects are enhanced by the TPR agonist, further supporting the notion that coordination exists between TLR4 and TPR signaling in mediating the inflammatory response. However, the involvement of other mechanisms in mediating the pro-inflammatory effects of TPR cannot be ruled out. Evidence suggests that ROCK is a key mediator of TPR, leading to endothelial cell dysfunction [29–31]. ROCK plays a role in regulating the migratory properties of bone-marrow-derived macrophages [32]. However, the role of ROCK in altering the PBMC inflammatory response remains unclear. Our data provide compelling evidence that inhibition of ROCK signaling using Y-27632 attenuates the LPS- and SA-induced inflammatory response. Moreover, Y-27932 inhibits the IBOP-induced inflammatory response, providing direct evidence for the role of ROCK in mediating the pro-inflammatory effect elicited by TPR activation.

Our study has some limitations. For example, PBMCs are a mixed population of cells that contain T lymphocytes, B lymphocytes, and monocytes. T lymphocytes are the most predominant cells in human PBMCs. About 49–77% of PBMCs are T lymphocytes. B cells and monocytes account for 6–17% and 6–12%, respectively [33]. Studies have shown that TP-R is expressed on lymphocytes, and stimulation of TP-R promotes lymphocyte activation [10,34]. It is likely that T lymphocytes may be the main source of TP-R in PBMCs, as they are the most abundant cells in a PBMC population. However, the role of TP-R in mediating a pro-inflammatory effect in B lymphocytes and monocytes cannot be ruled out. Although the contribution of individual cells in mediating the pro-inflammatory effects is unclear, PBMCs are the most commonly used immune cells, which serve as a relevant model to study the mechanisms involved in the inflammatory response in humans. Further studies are warranted to determine the role of TPR, specifically in lymphocytes or monocytes, in mediating the inflammatory response. Next, PBMCs from normal subjects and individuals with obesity and/or insulin resistance were used in ex vivo experiments. The inter-individual variability and genetic influence on cytokine responses of PBMCs to inflammatory stimuli are possible [35]. However, our data from individual experiments are derived from PBMCs collected from at least three subjects.

Taken together, our data suggest that an association exists between PBMC TPR and human obesity, and blocking TPR signaling attenuates the LPS- and/or FFA-induced inflammatory response in PBMCs. Further, our data indicate that TLR4 and ROCK1 signaling play a role in mediating the effects of TPR on inflammatory processes. Blocking TPR activity may be a therapeutic option to attenuate obesity-related inflammation and metabolic disorders. TP-R antagonists are being used to manage asthma, arterial thrombosis, and peripheral artery disease in some Asian and European countries [36,37]. Several TP-R antagonists, including Ifetroban, are being studied in various phases of preclinical and clinical investigations [36]. Our findings will be relevant to testing the effectiveness of TP-R antagonists against obesity-related comorbidities.

Supplementary Materials: The following supporting information can be downloaded at https://www.mdpi.com/article/10.3390/cells13161320/s1, Supplementary Figure S1: LDH cytotoxicity assay; Supplementary Figure S2: Thromboxane B2 (TXB2) assay; Supplementary Figure S3: LDH cytotoxicity assay.

Author Contributions: Conceptualization, V.R., V.S. and C.V.D.; methodology, V.R. and R.T.C.; formal analysis, V.R., R.T.C. and V.S.; investigation, V.R., R.T.C. and V.S.; writing—original draft preparation, V.R., R.T.C. and V.S.; writing—review and editing, V.R., C.V.D. and V.S.; supervision, C.V.D. and V.S.; project administration, C.V.D. and V.S.; funding acquisition, C.V.D. and V.S. All authors have read and agreed to the published version of the manuscript.

Funding: This work was supported by a VA-CSRD Merit Award from the Department of Veterans Affairs [1I01CX002084 to V.S. and C.V.D.] and a pilot award from the NIH-Great Plains IDeA-Clinical and Translational Research Network (U54 GM115458). V.S. is also supported by an NIH-NIAAA P50 award from the Alcohol Center of Research-Nebraska (P50AA030407-5130).

Institutional Review Board Statement: The study was conducted in accordance with the Declaration of Helsinki and approved by the VA Nebraska-Western Iowa Health Care System and the University of Nebraska Medical Center.

Informed Consent Statement: Informed consent was obtained from all subjects involved in the study.

Data Availability Statement: The raw data supporting the conclusions of this article will be made available by the authors upon request.

Acknowledgments: This paper is the result of work conducted with the resources and facilities at the VA Nebraska-Western Iowa Health Care System, Omaha.

Conflicts of Interest: The authors declare no conflicts of interest.

References

1. Saeedi, P.; Petersohn, I.; Salpea, P.; Malanda, B.; Karuranga, S.; Unwin, N.; Colagiuri, S.; Guariguata, L.; Motala, A.A.; Ogurtsova, K.; et al. Global and regional diabetes prevalence estimates for 2019 and projections for 2030 and 2045: Results from the International Diabetes Federation Diabetes Atlas, 9(th) edition. *Diabetes Res. Clin. Pract.* **2019**, *157*, 107843. [CrossRef] [PubMed]
2. Al-Goblan, A.S.; Al-Alfi, M.A.; Khan, M.Z. Mechanism linking diabetes mellitus and obesity. *Diabetes Metab. Syndr. Obes. Targets Ther.* **2014**, *7*, 587–591. [CrossRef] [PubMed]
3. Ellulu, M.S.; Patimah, I.; Khaza'ai, H.; Rahmat, A.; Abed, Y. Obesity and inflammation: The linking mechanism and the complications. *Arch. Med. Sci.* **2017**, *13*, 851–863. [CrossRef] [PubMed]
4. Rucker, D.; Dhamoon, A.S. Physiology, Thromboxane A2. In *StatPearls;* StatPearls Publishing: Treasure Island, FL, USA, 2024.
5. Cherdon, C.; Rolin, S.; Hanson, J.; Ooms, A.; de Leval, L.; Drion, P.; Michiels, C.; Pirotte, B.; Masereel, B.; Sakalihassan, N.; et al. BM-573 inhibits the development of early atherosclerotic lesions in Apo E deficient mice by blocking TP receptors and thromboxane synthase. *Prostaglandins Other Lipid Mediat.* **2011**, *94*, 124–132. [CrossRef] [PubMed]
6. Petri, M.H.; Tellier, C.; Michiels, C.; Ellertsen, I.; Dogne, J.M.; Back, M. Effects of the dual TP receptor antagonist and thromboxane synthase inhibitor EV-077 on human endothelial and vascular smooth muscle cells. *Biochem. Biophys. Res. Commun.* **2013**, *441*, 393–398. [CrossRef] [PubMed]
7. Huang, S.W.; Lien, J.C.; Kuo, S.C.; Huang, T.F. Inhibitory Effects of an Orally Active Thromboxane A2 Receptor Antagonist, nstpbp5185, on Atherosclerosis in ApoE-Deficient Mice. *Thromb. Haemost.* **2018**, *118*, 401–414. [CrossRef] [PubMed]
8. Xu, H.; Korneszczuk, K.; Karaa, A.; Lin, T.; Clemens, M.G.; Zhang, J.X. Thromboxane A2 from Kupffer cells contributes to the hyperresponsiveness of hepatic portal circulation to endothelin-1 in endotoxemic rats. *Am. J. Physiol. Gastrointest. Liver Physiol.* **2005**, *288*, G277–G283. [CrossRef] [PubMed]
9. Collins, B.J.; Blum, M.G.; Parker, R.E.; Chang, A.C.; Blair, K.S.; Zorn, G.L., 3rd; Christman, B.W.; Pierson, R.N., 3rd. Thromboxane mediates pulmonary hypertension and lung inflammation during hyperacute lung rejection. *J. Appl. Physiol.* **2001**, *90*, 2257–2268. [CrossRef] [PubMed]
10. Matsuda, H.; Ito, Y.; Hosono, K.; Tsuru, S.; Inoue, T.; Nakamoto, S.; Kurashige, C.; Hirashima, M.; Narumiya, S.; Okamoto, H.; et al. Roles of Thromboxane Receptor Signaling in Enhancement of Lipopolysaccharide-Induced Lymphangiogenesis and Lymphatic Drainage Function in Diaphragm. *Arterioscler. Thromb. Vasc. Biol.* **2021**, *41*, 1390–1407. [CrossRef]
11. Hartney, J.M.; Gustafson, C.E.; Bowler, R.P.; Pelanda, R.; Torres, R.M. Thromboxane receptor signaling is required for fibronectin-induced matrix metalloproteinase 9 production by human and murine macrophages and is attenuated by the Arhgef1 molecule. *J. Biol. Chem.* **2011**, *286*, 44521–44531. [CrossRef]
12. Altavilla, D.; Squadrito, F.; Canale, P.; Ioculano, M.; Squadrito, G.; Campo, G.M.; Serrano, M.; Sardella, A.; Urna, G.; Spignoli, G.; et al. G 619, a dual thromboxane synthase inhibitor and thromboxane A2 receptor antagonist, inhibits tumor necrosis factor-α biosynthesis. *Eur. J. Pharmacol.* **1995**, *286*, 31–39. [CrossRef]
13. Yan, A.; Cai, G.; Xia, W.; Fu, Y. Thromboxane A2 receptor antagonist SQ29548 suppresses the LPS-induced release of inflammatory cytokines in BV2 microglia cells via suppressing MAPK and NF-κB signaling pathways. *Mol. Med. Rep.* **2017**, *16*, 2491–2496. [CrossRef]
14. Yang, W.; Yan, A.; Zhang, T.; Shao, J.; Liu, T.; Yang, X.; Xia, W.; Fu, Y. Thromboxane A2 Receptor Stimulation Enhances Microglial Interleukin-1β and NO Biosynthesis Mediated by the Activation of ERK Pathway. *Front. Aging Neurosci.* **2016**, *8*, 8. [CrossRef]
15. Hersoug, L.G.; Moller, P.; Loft, S. Role of microbiota-derived lipopolysaccharide in adipose tissue inflammation, adipocyte size and pyroptosis during obesity. *Nutr. Res. Rev.* **2018**, *31*, 153–163. [CrossRef]
16. Ngkelo, A.; Meja, K.; Yeadon, M.; Adcock, I.; Kirkham, P.A. LPS induced inflammatory responses in human peripheral blood mononuclear cells is mediated through NOX4 and $G_i\alpha$ dependent PI-3kinase signalling. *J. Inflamm.* **2012**, *9*, 1. [CrossRef]
17. Rocha, D.M.; Caldas, A.P.; Oliveira, L.L.; Bressan, J.; Hermsdorff, H.H. Saturated fatty acids trigger TLR4-mediated inflammatory response. *Atherosclerosis* **2016**, *244*, 211–215. [CrossRef]
18. Henderson, G.C. Plasma Free Fatty Acid Concentration as a Modifiable Risk Factor for Metabolic Disease. *Nutrients* **2021**, *13*, 2590. [CrossRef]
19. Zhou, H.; Urso, C.J.; Jadeja, V. Saturated Fatty Acids in Obesity-Associated Inflammation. *J. Inflamm. Res.* **2020**, *13*, 1–14. [CrossRef]
20. Ueki, K.; Kondo, T.; Kahn, C.R. Suppressor of cytokine signaling 1 (SOCS-1) and SOCS-3 cause insulin resistance through inhibition of tyrosine phosphorylation of insulin receptor substrate proteins by discrete mechanisms. *Mol. Cell Biol.* **2004**, *24*, 5434–5446. [CrossRef]
21. Shi, H.; Kokoeva, M.V.; Inouye, K.; Tzameli, I.; Yin, H.; Flier, J.S. TLR4 links innate immunity and fatty acid-induced insulin resistance. *J. Clin. Investig.* **2006**, *116*, 3015–3025. [CrossRef] [PubMed]

22. Xu, H.; Barnes, G.T.; Yang, Q.; Tan, G.; Yang, D.; Chou, C.J.; Sole, J.; Nichols, A.; Ross, J.S.; Tartaglia, L.A.; et al. Chronic inflammation in fat plays a crucial role in the development of obesity-related insulin resistance. *J. Clin. Investig.* **2003**, *112*, 1821–1830. [CrossRef] [PubMed]
23. Weisberg, S.P.; McCann, D.; Desai, M.; Rosenbaum, M.; Leibel, R.L.; Ferrante, A.W., Jr. Obesity is associated with macrophage accumulation in adipose tissue. *J. Clin. Investig.* **2003**, *112*, 1796–1808. [CrossRef] [PubMed]
24. Petersen, M.C.; Smith, G.I.; Palacios, H.H.; Farabi, S.S.; Yoshino, M.; Yoshino, J.; Cho, K.; Davila-Roman, V.G.; Shankaran, M.; Barve, R.A.; et al. Cardiometabolic characteristics of people with metabolically healthy and unhealthy obesity. *Cell Metab.* **2024**, *36*, 745–761.e5. [CrossRef] [PubMed]
25. Stepien, M.; Stepien, A.; Wlazel, R.N.; Paradowski, M.; Banach, M.; Rysz, J. Obesity indices and inflammatory markers in obese non-diabetic normo- and hypertensive patients: A comparative pilot study. *Lipids Health Dis.* **2014**, *13*, 29. [CrossRef]
26. Hishinuma, T.; Tsukamoto, H.; Suzuki, K.; Mizugaki, M. Relationship between thromboxane/prostacyclin ratio and diabetic vascular complications. *Prostaglandins Leukot. Essent. Fat. Acids* **2001**, *65*, 191–196. [CrossRef]
27. Lasserre, B.; Navarro-Delmasure, C.; Pham Huu Chanh, A.; Catala, J.; Hollande, E. Modifications in the TXA(2) and PGI(2) plasma levels and some other biochemical parameters during the initiation and development of non-insulin-dependent diabetes mellitus (NIDDM) syndrome in the rabbit. *Prostaglandins Leukot. Essent. Fat. Acids* **2000**, *62*, 285–291. [CrossRef]
28. Li, R.H.L.; Nguyen, N.; Tablin, F. Canine platelets express functional Toll-like receptor-4: Lipopolysaccharide-triggered platelet activation is dependent on adenosine diphosphate and thromboxane A2 in dogs. *BMC Vet. Res.* **2019**, *15*, 245. [CrossRef]
29. Xie, X.; Sun, W.; Wang, J.; Li, X.; Liu, X.; Liu, N. Activation of thromboxane A2 receptors mediates endothelial dysfunction in diabetic mice. *Clin. Exp. Hypertens.* **2017**, *39*, 312–318. [CrossRef] [PubMed]
30. Zhao, Z.; Hu, J.; Gao, X.; Liang, H.; Yu, H.; Liu, S.; Liu, Z. Hyperglycemia via activation of thromboxane A2 receptor impairs the integrity and function of blood-brain barrier in microvascular endothelial cells. *Oncotarget* **2017**, *8*, 30030–30038. [CrossRef]
31. He, J.; Zhou, Y.; Xing, J.; Wang, Q.; Zhu, H.; Zhu, Y.; Zou, M.H. Liver kinase B1 is required for thromboxane receptor-dependent nuclear factor-κB activation and inflammatory responses. *Arterioscler. Thromb. Vasc. Biol.* **2013**, *33*, 1297–1305. [CrossRef]
32. Stinson, M.W.; Liu, S.; Laurenson, A.J.; Rotty, J.D. Macrophage migration is differentially regulated by fibronectin and laminin through altered adhesion and myosin II localization. *Mol. Biol. Cell* **2024**, *35*, ar22. [CrossRef] [PubMed]
33. Autissier, P.; Soulas, C.; Burdo, T.H.; Williams, K.C. Evaluation of a 12-color flow cytometry panel to study lymphocyte, monocyte, and dendritic cell subsets in humans. *Cytom. Part A* **2010**, *77*, 410–419. [CrossRef] [PubMed]
34. Thomas, D.W.; Rocha, P.N.; Nataraj, C.; Robinson, L.A.; Spurney, R.F.; Koller, B.H.; Coffman, T.M. Proinflammatory actions of thromboxane receptors to enhance cellular immune responses. *J. Immunol.* **2003**, *171*, 6389–6395. [CrossRef] [PubMed]
35. Li, Y.; Oosting, M.; Deelen, P.; Ricano-Ponce, I.; Smeekens, S.; Jaeger, M.; Matzaraki, V.; Swertz, M.A.; Xavier, R.J.; Franke, L.; et al. Inter-individual variability and genetic influences on cytokine responses to bacteria and fungi. *Nat. Med.* **2016**, *22*, 952–960. [CrossRef] [PubMed]
36. Capra, V.; Back, M.; Angiolillo, D.J.; Cattaneo, M.; Sakariassen, K.S. Impact of vascular thromboxane prostanoid receptor activation on hemostasis, thrombosis, oxidative stress, and inflammation. *J. Thromb. Haemost.* **2014**, *12*, 126–137. [CrossRef]
37. Dogne, J.M.; de Leval, X.; Benoit, P.; Rolin, S.; Pirotte, B.; Masereel, B. Therapeutic potential of thromboxane inhibitors in asthma. *Expert Opin. Investig. Drugs* **2002**, *11*, 275–281. [CrossRef]

healthcare

MDPI

Article

Platelet/High-Density Lipoprotein Ratio (PHR) Predicts Type 2 Diabetes in Obese Patients: A Retrospective Study

Yazeed Alshuweishi [1,*], Arwa Abudawood [2], Dalal Alfayez [2], Abdulmalik A. Almufarrih [2], Fuad Alanazi [1], Fahd A. Alshuweishi [3] and Abdulaziz M. Almuqrin [1]

[1] Department of Clinical Laboratory Sciences, College of Applied Medical Sciences, King Saud University, Riyadh 12372, Saudi Arabia; foalanazi@ksu.edu.sa (F.A.); aalmuqrin@ksu.edu.sa (A.M.A.)
[2] Department of Family and Community Medicine, Prince Sultan Military Medical City, Riyadh 11159, Saudi Arabia; aabudawood@psmmc.med.sa (A.A.); dalfayez@psmmc.med.sa (D.A.); aalmufarrih@psmmc.med.sa (A.A.A.)
[3] King Fahad Kidney Center, King Saud Medical City, Riyadh 12746, Saudi Arabia; falshuweishi@ksmc.med.sa
* Correspondence: yalshuweishi@ksu.edu.sa

Abstract: Background: Obesity and type 2 diabetes (T2D) pose global health problems that continue to rise. A chronic low-grade inflammation and activation of the immune system are well established in both conditions. The presence of these factors can predict disease development and progression. Emerging evidence suggests that platelet–high density lipoprotein ratio (PHR) is a potential inflammatory marker. The purpose of this study was to investigate the relationship between PHR and T2D among obese patients. **Methods:** 203 patients with BMI $\geq$ 30 kg/m^2 participated in the study. Patients were categorized into two groups: non-diabetic obese and diabetic obese. Comorbidities, baseline characteristics, laboratory data, as well as PHR levels of the study groups were analyzed. Medians, risk assessment, and the diagnostic performance of PHR values were examined in both groups. **Results:** In obese patients, the median PHR were significantly increased in obese patients with T2D compared to non-diabetic obese ($p < 0.0001$). Furthermore, T2D obese with high PHR had a significantly higher FBG and HbA1c ($p < 0.05$). Although PHR was weakly yet significantly correlated with glycemic markers, ROC curve analysis of the PHR indicated an AUC of 0.700 ($p < 0.0001$) in predicting T2D in obese patients, and the cutoff value was 6.96, with a sensitivity and specificity of 53.4% and 76.1%, respectively. Moreover, increased PHR (OR = 4.77, $p < 0.0001$) carried a significantly higher risk for developing T2D in obese individuals. **Conclusions:** The PHR is a convenient and cost-effective marker that can reliably predict the presence of T2D in high-risk obese population.

Keywords: obesity; T2D; platelets; HDL; hyperglycemia; inflammation

1. Introduction

Obesity is an urgent global health issue, with Saudi Arabia showing alarmingly high rates. Recent data indicate that over 50% of the Saudi population is overweight, and more than 20% are obese [1,2]. This trend is largely driven by rapid urbanization and economic growth, leading to less physical activity and higher consumption of high-calorie diets [3]. The high prevalence of obesity not only poses a significant burden on the healthcare system but also impacts the overall quality of an individual's life [3,4].

One of the significant concerns linked to obesity is the increased prevalence of type 2 diabetes (T2D), a condition closely associated with excessive body weight [5]. Obesity is known as a triggering factor for the development of T2D mainly due to the increased insulin resistance that accompanies excess body fat [6]. When BMI increases from 18.5 kg/m^2 to over 35 kg/m^2, the risk of developing T2D over the age of 18 years rises dramatically from 7% to 70% in males and from 12% to 74% in females [7]. The cellular and physiological mechanisms responsible for the link between obesity and T2D are complex and involve β cell dysfunction, alteration in adipose tissue biology, and multi-organ insulin resistance [8,9].

Although a vast majority of T2D patients are overweight or obese, not all obese individuals develop T2D, suggesting that multiple factors are involved in the development of T2D [7,10]. This includes genetics, lifestyle, and various inflammatory responses, with an increasing body of evidence supporting a key role of inflammation in obesity as well as T2D [11]. However, it is still challenging to distinguish specific inflammatory markers associated with obesity or T2D. Studies to identify distinctive inflammatory biomarkers that uniquely characterize each of the two conditions and identify diabetes risk in obese individuals are crucial for timely intervention and prevention of disease progression. Therefore, early screening for diabetes in all obese individuals is highly recommended.

During inflammatory responses, the number of neutrophils, monocytes, lymphocytes and platelets changes [12–15]. Among these, platelets, traditionally known for their role in homeostasis, play a critical role in inflammation by interacting with leukocytes and endothelial cells, and by releasing various inflammatory mediators [16–18]. It was shown that elevated platelet counts were associated with inflammation severity and treatment outcomes in patients with ankylosing spondylitis, inflammatory bowel disease, Crohn's disease, rheumatoid arthritis and systemic lupus erythematosus [19–23]. In the context of T2D, increased platelet reactivity was observed in T2D patients with significant association between HbA1c levels and platelet number [24–26]. On the other hand, high-density lipoprotein (HDL) is well known for its role in reverse cholesterol transport, but it also exhibits significant anti-inflammatory properties [27]. These anti-inflammatory actions include removing cholesterol from macrophages in atherosclerotic plaques, reducing the formation of foam cells and subsequent inflammatory responses [28]. Additionally, HDL inhibits the oxidation of low-density lipoprotein (LDL), thereby preventing the pro-inflammatory signaling triggered by oxidized LDL [29]. Consequently, reduced HDL levels were substantially associated with an increased risk of major adverse cardiovascular events in T2D obese patients [30,31].

Therefore, recent studies have utilized both platelet counts and HDL as a critical indicator of inflammatory responses in various diseases [32,33]. Jialal et al. revealed that the platelet to HDL-C ratio (PHR) is significantly increased in patients with metabolic syndrome and appears to be a valid biomarker of metabolic syndrome [34]. As metabolic syndrome is generally associated with T2D, it is possible that the PHR may be able to be used as a biomarker in predicting T2D in at-risk populations such as obese subjects. Nevertheless, the relationship between PHR level and obese patients with or without T2D remains unexplored. Therefore, this study was designed to understand the relationships between the blood-derived inflammatory marker PHR and the occurrence of T2D in obese patients. The current research also aimed to investigate the association estimate and the diagnostic accuracy of PHR for markers of glucose metabolism among diabetic and non-diabetic obese patients.

2. Methods

2.1. Study Design and Data Collection

In this study, data from a total of 203 patients were collected between 2022 and 2023 from Family Medicine Clinics at the Prince Sultan Military Medical City (PSMMC), Riyadh, Saudi Arabia. This included 103 non-diabetic obese patients from the Family Medicine Lifestyle Clinic and 100 diabetic obese patients from the Family Medicine Chronic Illnesses Clinic. Approval for this study was obtained from the Institutional Review Board (IRB) at PSMMC (IRB number: E-2165, approved on 14 September 2023). Type 2 diabetes (T2D) was confirmed by a physician and data were available from patient hospital records. According to hospital protocol, T2D was diagnosed either by a FBG level $\geq$ 126 mg/dL, a 2 h plasma glucose tolerance test of $\geq$200 mg/dL, or a HbA1c $\geq$ 6.5%, confirmed by a repeated test on a different day [35]. Obesity was defined as a body mass index (BMI) $\geq$ 30 kg/m^2 [36]. Patients were excluded if they were younger than 18 years of age, had type 1 diabetes, or were pregnant.

For further analysis, the subjects from each group were classified according to their obesity into three classes:

- Obesity Class I (BMI 30 to 34.9 kg/m^2)
- Obesity Class II (BMI 35 to 39.9 kg/m^2)
- Obesity Class III (BMI $\geq$ 40 kg/m^2)

PHR was calculated as platelet count ($\times 10^6$/mL) $\div$ HDL cholesterol (mg/dL) [34]. The optimal cut-off value for PHR value was >6.96 based on the best cutoff (i.e., highest sensitivity and specificity) as revealed by receiver operating characteristics (ROC) curve analysis. Therefore, PHR values > 6.96 were considered high. Laboratory data, including PHR levels, were then analyzed to assess the patterns of PHR among non-diabetic and diabetic obese patients.

2.2. Statistical Analysis

Since the collected data were not normally distributed, nonparametric tests were used for statistical analysis. One-way ANOVA with the Kruskal–Wallis test was used to compare between three study groups while the Mann–Whitney U test was used to compare two study groups. The analyzed data were displayed as medians ± interquartile range (IQR). The predictive power of PHR to discriminate T2D was assessed by ROC curve analysis and area under the curve (AUC). Simple linear regression analysis was utilized to assess the association between PHR and other variables. The statistical analysis was performed using GraphPad Prism v9.2.0 (GraphPad Software, Inc., 10.0.01, San Diego, CA, USA). *p*-values below 0.05 were considered statistically significant.

3. Results

3.1. Baseline Characteristics of the Studied Population

This retrospective study included 203 obese participants, 141 of whom were females. The studied population was stratified into two groups: obese with T2D (diabetic obese) group and obese without T2D group (non-diabetic obese). The average age of the diabetic obese group was 57.5 years (±51.25–64.75), whereas the average age of the non-diabetic obese group was 37 years (±29–46). The laboratory parameters showed significant differences between the diabetic obese and the non-diabetic obese groups for some parameters as illustrated in Table 1. WBC counts, neutrophils, lymphocytes, monocytes and basophils were all significantly higher in the diabetic obese group. Almost 30% of the studied subjects were hypertensive, and most of them belonged to the diabetic obese group (Table 1). The number of smokers in the studied population was 17 (16.5%) and 5 (5%) for the non-diabetic obese and diabetic obese, respectively. 77% of diabetic obese patients were dyslipidemic, whereas 18.4% of non-diabetic obese patients had dyslipidemia. As demonstrated in Table 1, Metformin was used by 93% of individuals in the diabetic obese group, while only 10.6% of subjects in the non-diabetic obese group took this medicine. In addition, 26% and 34% of the diabetic obese patients used GLP-1 agonist and SGL2 inhibitor, respectively. On the other hand, 30% of non-diabetic obese subjects used GLP-1 and no participant from the same group used SGL2 inhibitor.

3.2. PHR Is Substantially Increased in Obese T2D Patients with a Significant Diagnostic Performance in Predicting T2D in the Studied Population

The changes in the levels of PHR index in the studied groups were analyzed as illustrated in (Figure 1A). The results showed a significant increase in PHR levels in the diabetic obese (7.910 ± 6.390–9.435) compared to the non-diabetic obese group (6.050 ± 4.745–7.718). Then we evaluated the possible association between the severity of obesity and the levels of PHR within each studied group.

Table 1. Baseline characteristics of the studied subjects.

Variables	All Subjects (n = 203)	Obese (n = 103)	Obese + T2D (n = 100)	*p*-Value
Demographics				
Age (years),	48 (35–58)	37 (29–46)	58 (51–65)	<0.0001
Sex (female), n (%)	141 (69.4%)	73 (70.8%)	68 (68.0%)	-
BMI (kg/m^2),	35 (33–38)	36 (34–38)	35 (32–40)	0.4322
Lab Parameters				
RBC count ($\times 10^{12}/\mu$L)	4.88 (4.49–5.31)	4.90(4.53–5.41)	4.80 (4.40–5.10)	0.0676
Hb (g/dL)	13.0 (12.00–14.70)	13.2 (11.98–14.73)	13.0 (12–14.25)	<0.0001
Hct (L/L)	27.70 (25.60–29.00)	27.40 (25.15–29.25)	28.0 (26.0–29.0)	0.2346
WBC ($\times 10^9/\mu$L),	7.5 (6.0–7.0)	7.1 (5.5–8.3)	8.1 (6.6–9.4)	0.0002
Neutrophils ($\times 10^3/\mu$L)	3.77 (2.76–5.00)	3.49 (2.29–4.61)	4.00 (3.07–5.22)	0.0065
Lymphocytes ($\times 10^3/\mu$L)	2.75 (2.20–3.32)	2.62 (2.16–3.12)	3.00 (2.29–3.80)	0.0085
Monocytes ($\times 10^3/\mu$L)	0.55 (0.44–0.68)	0.54 (0.40–0.65)	0.57 (0.50–0.74)	0.0080
Basophils ($\times 10^3/\mu$L)	0.05 (0.03–0.07)	0.04 (0.03–0.06)	0.05 (0.04–0.07)	0.0035
Eosinophils ($\times 10^3/\mu$L)	0.18 (0.11–0.28)	0.18 (0.11–0.25)	0.20 (0.11–0.32)	0.1343
ALT (U/L)	17 (13–26)	16 (12–25)	18 (14–26)	0.1152
PLT count ($\times 10^6$/mL)	312.0 (265.3–369.8)	299.0 (255.5–363.3)	327.5 (272.3–378.3)	0.1166
FBG (mg/dL)	97.30 (90.1–140.1)	90.09 (82.9–93.7)	131.5 (97.3–162.2)	<0.0001
HbA1c (%)	6.2 (5.7–7.4)	5.7 (5.5–5.9)	7.4 (6.7–8.7)	<0.0001
TC (mg/dL)	177.9 (147.7–211.3)	196.8 (172.1–227.8)	154.7 (135.3–185.6)	<0.0001
TG (mg/dL)	115.1 (88.6–156.8)	103.6 (77.1–150.6)	124.0 (88.6–159.4)	0.0393
HDL (mg/dL)	43.7 (38.5–52.4)	47.6 (39.8–59.6)	40.8 (36.9–46.4)	<0.0001
LDL (mg/dL)	108.9 (85.1–136.8)	127.2 (106.1–152.1)	92.8 (69.6–116.0)	<0.0001
PHR	7.06 (5.71–8.785)	6.05 (4.75–7.72)	7.91 (6.39–9.44)	<0.0001
Comorbidities				
Hypertension, n (%)	60 (29.5%)	13 (12.6%)	47 (47%)	-
Hypothyroidism, n (%)	18 (8.8%)	16 (15.5%)	2 (2%)	-
DLD, n (%)	96 (47.2%)	19 (18.4%)	77 (77%)	-
Smoking, n (%)	22 (10.8%)	17 (16.5%)	5 (5%)	-
Medications				-
Metformin, n (%)	104 (51.2%)	11 (10.6%)	93 (93%)	-
GLP-1 agonist, n (%)	57 (28%)	31 (30%)	26 (26%)	-
SGL2 inhibitor, n (%)	34 (16.7%)	0 (0%)	34 (34%)	-

Abbreviations: BMI (body mass index); RBC (Red blood cells); Hb (hemoglobin); Hct (hematocrit test); WBC (white blood count); ALT (Alanine transaminase); PLT (Platelet); FBG (Fasting blood glucose); HbA1c (Glycated hemoglobin); TC (Total cholesterol); TG (Triglycerides); HDL (High-density lipoprotein); LDL (Low-density lipoprotein); PHR (Platelet/high-density lipoprotein cholesterol ratio); DLD (Dyslipidemia); GLP-1 (Glucagon-like peptide-1); SGL2 (Sodium–glucose cotransporter-2).

The obese subjects were stratified into three groups according to obesity severity: Obesity class I, Obesity class II, and Obesity class III (Supplemental Table S1). Although statistical significance was not achieved, our findings exhibited a proportional increase in PHR according to the severity of obesity in the non-diabetic obese group. (PHR; 5.93 $\pm$ 4.645–8.24 vs. 6.13 $\pm$ 4.72–7.54 vs. 6.475 $\pm$ 5.59–7.81) (Figure 1B). Interestingly, when the same analysis was performed in the diabetic obese group, we observed a significant increase in PHR levels in obesity class I subjects (8.340 $\pm$ 6.990–10.68) compared to obesity class II subjects (7.200 $\pm$ 5.710–8.485) (Figure 1C). In addition, the analysis revealed an increase in PHR levels among obesity class I subjects compared to those classified within obesity class III; however, statistical significance was not obtained (Figure 1C).

Nevertheless, when comparing PHR values between non-diabetic obese and diabetic obese patients within each obesity class (Figure 1D), PHR levels were significantly higher in diabetic obese class I and II compared to their non-diabetic obese counterparts (Class I, 8.34 $\pm$ 6.99–10.68 vs. 6.09 $\pm$ 4.69–8.48; Class II, 7.20 $\pm$ 5.71–8.49 vs. 6.13 $\pm$ 4.72–7.54). Obesity class III, despite a trend toward higher PHR levels in diabetic obese class III, did not achieve statistical significance (Figure 1D; 7.295 $\pm$ 5.918–9.085 vs. 6.48 $\pm$ 5.59–7.81). Although the reasons for the lack of significant difference in the class III group are not known, they might be related to the small size number, especially in non-diabetic obese III patients (Supplemental Table S1), who made up 12.6% of all non-diabetic obese patients.

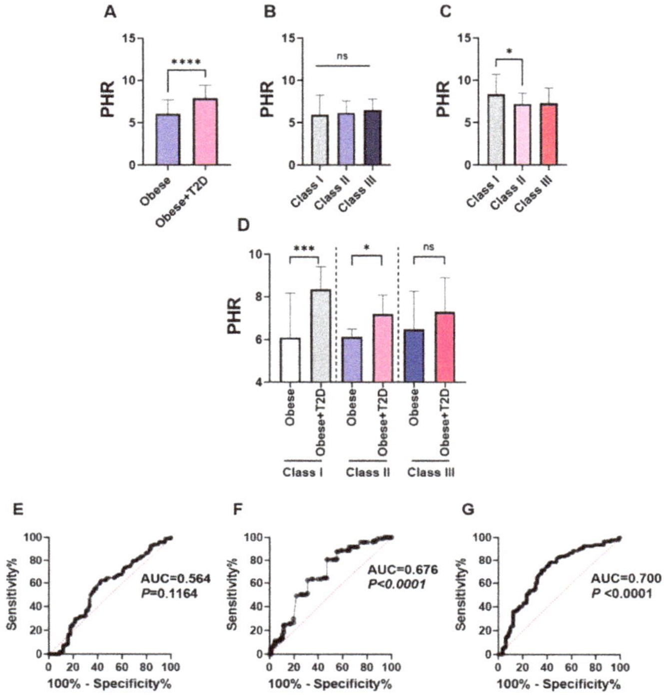

Figure 1. Comparison of PHR levels between non-diabetic and diabetic obese groups and ROC curve of PHR for T2D prediction. Changes in PHR levels between non-diabetic and diabetic obese groups are presented in (**A**). PHR values according to obesity classes for non-diabetic obese (**B**) and diabetic obese (**C**) and both groups (**D**) are shown. ROC curve analysis of PLT count (**E**), HDL levels (**F**), and PHR (**G**) to distinguish T2D among obese patients are illustrated. ns indicates not significant while * ($p < 0.05$), *** ($p < 0.001$), and **** ($p < 0.0001$).

The receiver operating characteristic (ROC) curve of PLT was performed to evaluate its predictive ability in discriminating T2D subjects in the studied population. The results demonstrated a poor predictive ability of the PLT count for T2D in the studied population (AUC = 0.564, $p = 0.116$) (Figure 1E). Following that, the diagnostic ability of the HDL marker for T2D was assessed. HDL demonstrated a markedly better predictive ability for T2D compared to the platelet count (AUC = 0.67, $p < 0.0001$) (Figure 1F). Finally, the combined predictive capability of the platelet to HDL ratio (PHR) for T2D was evaluated. This combined marker demonstrated superior performance in the ROC curve analysis for T2D prediction compared to the PLT count and HDL markers (AUC = 0.700, $p < 0.0001$) (Figure 1G).

3.3. FBG and HbA1c Were Significantly Higher in High-PHR Obese Patients with T2D

To analyse the association between BMI, FBG, and HbA1c with PHR levels in the studied population, patients within both the diabetic obese and non-diabetic obese groups were classified based on their PHR levels into three distinct tertiles (T1, T2, and T3). T1 includes subjects with the lowest values of PHR, representing the metric's minimum range. T2 encompasses the PHR values of subjects that fall within the intermediate range, while

T3 contains subjects with the highest PHR values. As shown in Figure 2A–C, no significant difference was observed in patterns of BMI, FBG, and HBA1c between the T1, T2, and T3 tertiles within the non-diabetic obese group. In contrast, we observed a significant difference between T1 and T3 in light of FBG (113.5 ± 93.69–145.9 vs. 149.5 ± 113.5–200.9) and HbA1c (7.320 ± 6.425–7.800 vs. 8.170 ± 7.200–10.20) within the diabetic obese group, while no statistically significant was observed between T1, T2, and T3 in the context of BMI (Figure 2D–F).

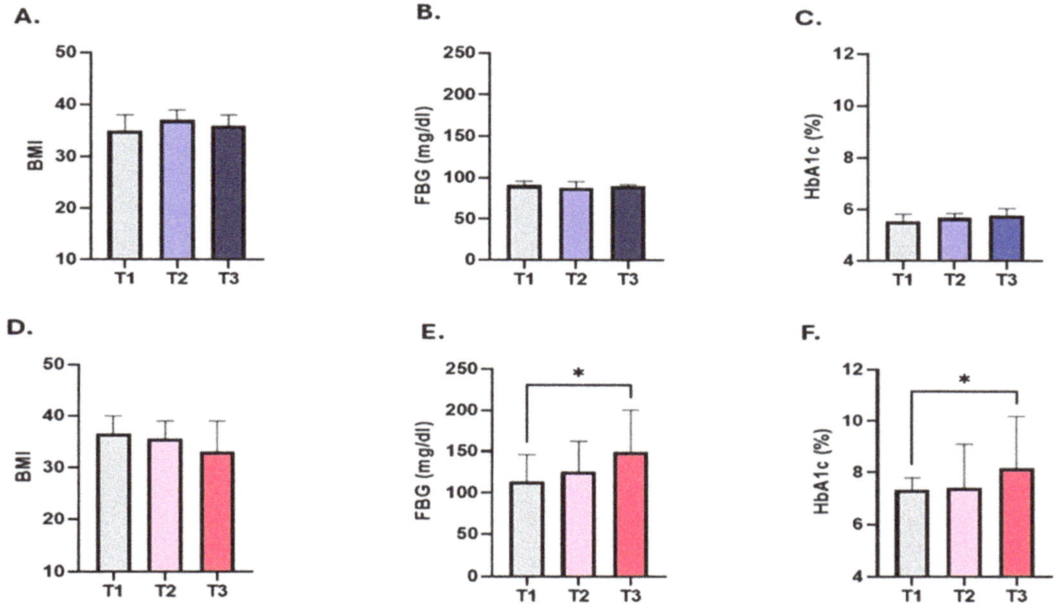

Figure 2. Evaluating the BMI, FBG, and HbA1c levels in relation to PHR in the studied population. The non-diabetic and diabetic obese groups were categorized based on their PHR levels into three distinct tertiles (T1, T2, and T3). Medians ± IQR of BMI (**A**), FBG (**B**), and HbA1c (**C**) in relation with each tertile in the non-diabetic are presented. Medians ± IQR of BMI (**D**), FBG (**E**), and HbA1c (**F**) according to each tertile in the in diabetic obese group are shown. * indicates ($p < 0.05$).

3.4. Correlation of PHR Values with BMI and Glycemic Parameters, FBG and HbA1c

Furthermore, our linear regression analysis found no significant correlation between the PHR levels and BMI, FBG, and HbA1c in the non-diabetic obese group (Figure 3A–C). In contrast, our observation revealed a significant correlation between the PHR levels and BMI ($R^2 = 0.0407$ and $p = 0.0475$), FBG ($R^2 = 0.05622$ and $p = 0.0419$), and HbA1c ($R^2 = 0.08022$ and $p = 0.0049$) in diabetic obese subjects, as shown in (Figure 3D–F).

Then, we compared the capability of elevated PHR to predict BMI, FBG, and HbA1c. In the non-diabetic obese group, PHR did not significantly differentiate patients with elevated FBG or HbA1c levels (Figure 4B,C). In contrast, in the diabetic obese group, PHR demonstrated a stronger capability to discriminate between patients with increased FBG (AUC = 0.643, $p = 0.049$) and higher HbA1c levels (AUC = 0.624, $p = 0.046$), as shown in Figure 4E,F. We acknowledge that the statistical significance ($p = 0.049$) is marginal; however, our findings indicate that PHR's predictive capacity for dysglycemia is notably better in the context of diabetic obesity compared to non-diabetic obesity.

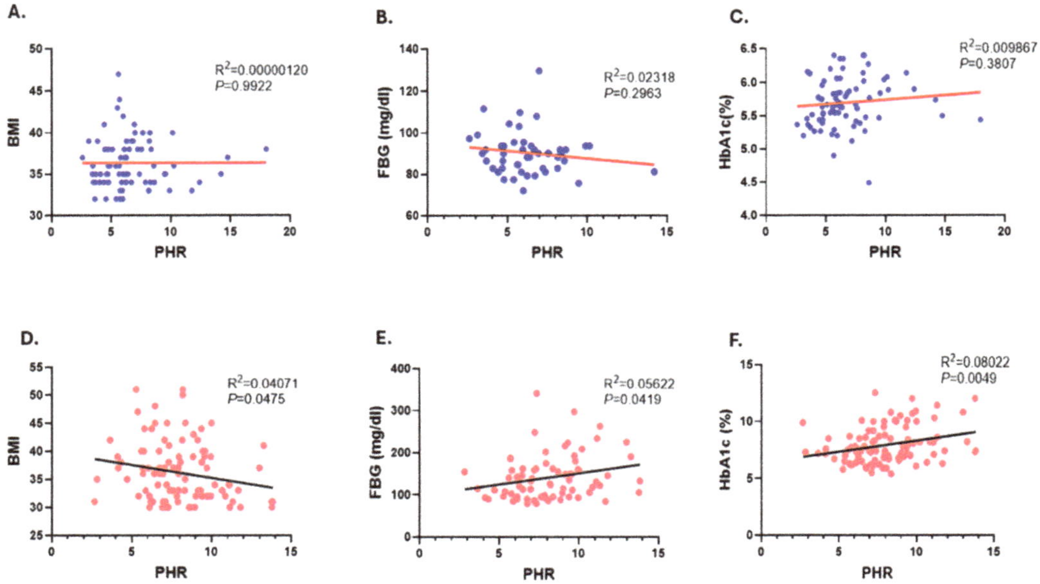

Figure 3. Association of PHR with BMI, FBG, and HbA1c in the studied subjects. Simple linear regression of the association of PHR with BMI (**A**), FBG (**B**), and HbA1c (**C**) in non-diabetic subjects. Simple linear regression of the association of PHR and BMI (**D**), FBG (**E**), and HbA1c (**F**) in diabetic obese subjects.

3.5. Elevated PHR Is Associated with an Increased Risk of T2D in Obese Patients

As demonstrated in Table 2, the prevalence of elevated PHR levels was considerably higher among the diabetic obese (70.10%) compared to the non-diabetic obese patients (32.93%). In addition, our analysis revealed that 67.07% of non-diabetic obese had normal levels of PHR. This percentage reduced to 29.90% within the diabetic obese group.

Table 2. Prevalence of normal and elevated PHR levels among the studied population.

Parameter	Non-Diabetic Obese	Diabetic Obese
N-PHR	67.07%	29.90%
H-PHR	32.93%	70.10%

The risk assessment analysis revealed an association between the elevated levels of PHR and occurrence of T2D in the overall studied population (Table 3, RR = 2.13, 95% CI: 1.52 to 2.97, $p < 0.0001$). Similar results were obtained for subjects that were classified under obesity class I (RR = 2.12, 95% CI: 1.23 to 3.67, $p = 0.0067$). The analysis showed the risk of increased PHR in developing T2D within obese class II participants was 1.60 (RR = 1.6, 95% CI: 0.86 to 2.97, $p = 0.1345$). Nonetheless, statistical significance was not obtained. On the other hand, our observation suggested that the elevation in PHR levels for those classified under obesity class III was associated with a 42% reduction in the risk of developing T2D (RR = 0.58, 95% CI: 0.41 to 0.81, $p = 0.0018$). Additionally, the results showed that increased PHR levels in the overall studied population, obesity class I subjects, and obesity class II participants were 4.77, 5.81, and 5.62 times more likely to fall into the T2D group, respectively.

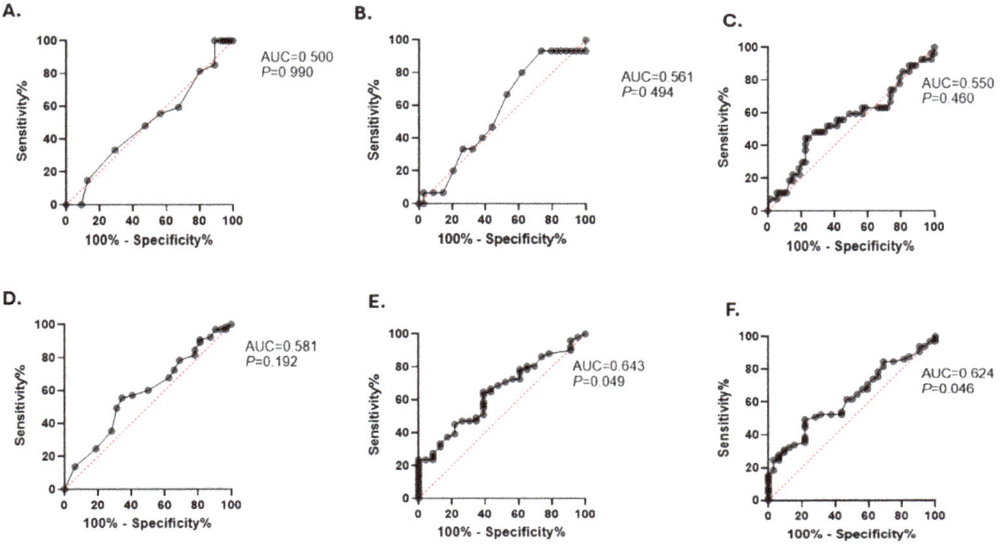

Figure 4. Evaluating the ability of elevated PHR to predict BMI, FBG, and HbA1c markers in the studied population. ROC curves of the elevated PHR and BMI (**A**), FBG concentrations (**B**), and HbA1c levels (**C**) for the non-diabetic obese participants are shown. ROC curves of the elevated PHR and BMI (**D**), FBG concentrations (**E**), and HbA1c levels (**F**) for the diabetic obese subjects are illustrated.

Table 3. Risk assessment of elevated PHR and T2D.

	Score	95% CI	Z Statistic	Significance Level
RR				
Total subjects	2.13	1.52 to 2.97	4.42	$p < 0.0001$
Obesity class I	2.12	1.23 to 3.67	2.71	$p = 0.0067$
Obesity class II	1.6	0.86 to 2.97	1.49	$p = 0.1345$
Obesity class III	0.58	0.41 to 0.81	3.12	$p = 0.0018$
OR				
Total subjects	4.77	2.53 to 8.99	4.83	$p < 0.0001$
Obesity class I	5.81	2.01 to 16.78	3.25	$p = 0.0011$
Obesity class II	5.62	1.87 to 16.83	3.08	$p = 0.002$
Obesity class III	0.15	0.0074 to 3.16	1.21	$p = 0.225$

4. Discussion

A quarter of Saudi Arabia's population suffers from diabetes mellitus (DM), a severe and common inflammatory disease that is predicted to quadruple in prevalence by 2030 [37]. Prognostic and monitoring biomarkers are highly desired in the clinical setting to predict individuals at high risk for developing T2D. The current study was undertaken to demonstrate the link between blood-derived PHR and the occurrence of T2D among obese individuals. For obese patients, including non-diabetic and diabetic obese patients, we showed for the first time that PHR was significantly elevated among diabetic obese participants compared to the non-diabetic obese group. Additionally, ROC curve analysis revealed that PHR was able to differentiate between non-diabetic obese and diabetic obese. Particularly among diabetic obese patients, FBG and HbA1c were significantly higher in the highest PHR tertile, compared with patients in the other tertiles. In line with this, PHR was significantly associated with glycemic parameters FBG and HbA1c in diabetic but not non-diabetic obese patients. These findings demonstrate differential patterns of PHR among non-diabetic and diabetic obese patients, suggesting that PHR could serve as a marker of dysglycemia.

There is a paucity of studies involving PHR and its relationship with obesity and T2D. Comparing obese patients with and without T2D showed that PHR levels were significantly elevated, with an approximately 25% increase among diabetic groups. The ability of the PHR to discriminate diabetic obese from non-diabetic obese suggests that the PHR may be a sensitive marker for predicting T2D among high-risk populations such as obese patients. However, our findings suggest that the severity of obesity does not seem to be associated with PHR, since PHR levels were not significantly altered when obese patients were stratified into class I, II, or III obesity, either in obese or diabetic obese groups. Nevertheless, when comparing PHR values between non-diabetic and diabetic obese patients within each obesity class, we observed significantly higher PHR levels in diabetic obese class I and II compared to their non-diabetic counterparts. However, this difference was not observed in class III, where we noted a trend toward higher PHR levels that did not achieve statistical significance. Moreover, the risk assessment analysis revealed that elevated levels of PHR had higher odds of T2D in the overall studied population as well as in obesity class I and II but not class III. This lack of significant effects of elevated PHR in class III may be related to a small sample size, particularly among non-diabetic obese class III patients, who constituted only 12.6% of all non-diabetic obese patients. Additionally, there are conflicting data regarding the relationship between platelet counts and body mass index (BMI), which might contribute to the observed variations in PHR levels among different obesity classes. A number of studies showed that platelet counts were altered in subjects with high BMI [38–40], while Coban et al. reported normal platelet counts in the obese individuals when compared to non-obese normal individuals [41]. Based on these findings, it appears that the observed elevation of PHR levels in T2D might not be related to obesity status; however, further longitudinal studies are certainly warranted.

One important finding in this study is the significant association of PHR with glycemic parameters among T2D patients. The potential reasons for such an association might be related to the role of individual components of PHR, platelets and HDL in light of T2D. Indeed, it was reported that patients with T2D exhibited higher platelet counts compared to non-diabetic controls [42]. Moreover, an early study by Gordon et al. followed by more recent studies have shown that diabetic patients typically exhibit lower HDL levels compared to non-diabetic controls [43–45]. This relationship might be due to the chronic inflammatory state induced by hyperglycemia, the hallmark metabolic abnormality associated with T2D. Indeed, we observed a significant increase in numbers of total leukocytes, neutrophils, lymphocytes, monocytes, and basophils in the diabetic obese group compared to the non-diabetic obese group, indicating ongoing chronic inflammation associated with T2D. Moreover, the elevated leukocyte counts observed in our study suggest a persistent immune activation, which is known to exacerbate insulin resistance and further impair glucose metabolism. The specific increase in neutrophils and monocytes may reflect an enhanced innate immune response, which has been linked to endothelial dysfunction and the development of cardiovascular diseases commonly seen in T2D patients. Elevated lymphocytes, on the other hand, indicate adaptive immune system involvement, which has been implicated in the autoimmune aspects of diabetes pathogenesis [46]. Notably, chronic hyperglycemia induces a proinflammatory state that has detrimental effects on the hematopoietic system, leading to increased megakaryocyte proliferation and platelet production [47]. The persistent high glucose levels enhance platelet turnover and activation, contributing to the observed hematological changes [48]. Moreover, Kodiatte et al. demonstrated that HbA1c levels were positively correlated with the mean platelet volume (MPV), a marker of platelet activation, suggesting that poor glycemic control leads to greater platelet activation [49]. Insulin resistance, a hallmark of T2D, also contributes to changes observed in platelet number and function [50]. Under normal conditions, insulin inhibits platelet aggregation by suppressing the $P2Y_{12}$ pathway in healthy volunteers [51]; however, such antithrombotic protection is hampered in T2DM patients due to reduced insulin sensitivity by platelets [52]. Furthermore, reactive oxygen species (ROS), commonly observed in diabetes, also play a critical role in modifying platelet function and increasing platelet counts in diabetic conditions [53,54]. Based on the above reports regarding the role of platelets on glycemic parameters, we could infer that platelet count or function might be unfavorable prognostic factors in the context of dysglycemia and diabetes.

It is well documented that individuals with T2D often have reduced levels of HDL cholesterol largely due to the altered metabolism of lipids seen in T2D conditions [55]. It was shown that insulin normally promotes the production of apolipoprotein A-I (ApoA-1), a major component of HDL [56]. This event is impaired in insulin-resistant states leading to lower HDL levels [57,58]. Additionally, the glycation process has been proposed as one of the mechanisms explaining the link between HDLs, inflammation, and diabetes. It was demonstrated that hyperglycemia causes glycation of the ApoA-1 molecule of HDL particles, leading to an increase in its degradation three times faster than in a person without diabetes [59]. Beyond the reduction in quantity, HDL functionality is also compromised in diabetes, due to oxidative modification and glycation of the HDL protein. It has been reported that glycated HDL was not able to reduce in vitro palmitate-induced inflammation in cultured adipocytes, likely due to increased serum amyloid A (SAA) concentrations in HDL following inflammation [60]. In diabetic nephropathy, increased SAA levels were directly associated with impaired HDL capacity to reduce the secretion of TNF-α from human peripheral blood mononuclear cells (PBMCs) [61]. Mechanistically, SAA enrichment causes displacement of paraoxonase 1 (PON1) and ApoA-I from HDL particles, potentially leading to HDL dysfunction [62]. A recent proteomics study comparing serum HDL from control and diabetic individuals revealed that the diabetic HDL had significantly higher glycated ApoA-I [59], suggesting that this parameter could be considered a valuable diagnostic tool to assess the metabolic state of diabetic patients. These findings clearly suggest how inflammation along with hyperglycemia might contribute to HDL perturbation in the light of T2D. Therefore, our findings showing elevated levels of PHR in diabetic patients might be a result of reduced HDL levels.

The incidence of T2D is rapidly increasing in developing countries, with varied prevalence between rural and urban areas [63]. Ethnic groups such as South Asians and Africans tend to develop T2D about a decade earlier and with a lower body mass index [64,65]. Screening services for T2D are not equally distributed between developing and developed countries. This highlights the urgent need for a simple, effective, and affordable screening method. In this study, we introduced the PHR as one of the blood-derived inflammatory indices linked to hyperglycemia and elevated HbA1c levels in diabetic patients. Unlike inflammatory cytokines like IL-6, IL-8, IL-1β, and TNF-α, the PHR ratio is easy to calculate from peripheral blood tests, which are affordable, convenient, and straightforward to interpret. Hence, PHR has the potential to be used as a universal, non-invasive, and cost-effective test to assess diabetic risk in obese patients.

The findings presented in this study showed a significant association between PHR and glycemic markers in diabetic obese patients and suggested that PHR can be used as a potential marker for dysglycemia among T2D patients to reduce its severity and mortality. Our study has a few limitations. This is a single-centered study, which restricts the generalizability of the results. Given the retrospective nature of this study, it was not possible to determine a causal relationship between elevated PHR values and disturbances in glucose metabolism in diabetes. Therefore, additional research is necessary to determine the role of the PHR in predicting T2D in obese patients.

5. Conclusions

In conclusion, PHR is elevated in obese patients when T2D is present. This observation is likely due to the significant association of PHR and dysglycemia. Our findings underscore the validity of the blood-derived inflammatory ratio such as PHR, an easily obtainable routine test, in predicting T2D in individuals with obesity. Further longitudinal studies are needed to elucidate the fundamental molecular mechanisms responsible for this association to gain insights into alternative prophylactic and therapeutic intervention strategies.

Supplementary Materials: The following supporting information can be downloaded at: https://www.mdpi.com/article/10.3390/healthcare12151540/s1, Table S1: Baseline characteristics based on obesity classes.

Author Contributions: Conceptualization, Y.A. and A.M.A.; methodology, A.A., D.A. and A.A.A.; software, A.M.A. and F.A.; validation, Y.A. and F.A.A.; formal analysis, all authors; investigation, Y.A. and A.M.A.; resources, Y.A. and A.M.A.; data curation, Y.A., A.A., D.A. and A.A.A.; writing—original draft preparation, all authors; writing—review and editing, all authors; visualization, Y.A. and A.M.A.; supervision, Y.A.; project administration, Y.A.; funding acquisition, A.M.A. All authors have read and agreed to the published version of the manuscript.

Funding: This project was funded by the Researchers Supporting Project number (RSPD2024R933), King Saud University, Riyadh, Saudi Arabia.

Institutional Review Board Statement: The Institutional Review Board (IRB) for this study was obtained from the institutional review board at PSMMC (IRB number: E-2165, approved on 14 September 2023).

Informed Consent Statement: This study was retrospective in nature and according to local ethical regulations, retrospective studies in which no patient identifier information are accessible, are exempt from the requirement of an informed consent. Therefore, subject consent was waived in this study.

Data Availability Statement: Data are contained within the article and Supplementary Materials.

Acknowledgments: The authors thank the funding from the Researchers Supporting Project number (RSPD2024R933), King Saud University, Riyadh, Saudi Arabia.

Conflicts of Interest: The authors declare no conflicts of interest.

References

1. Alqarni, S.S.M. A Review of Prevalence of Obesity in Saudi Arabia. *J. Obes. Eat. Disord.* **2016**, *2*, 1–6. [CrossRef]
2. Althumiri, N.A.; Basyouni, M.H.; AlMousa, N.; AlJuwaysim, M.F.; Almubark, R.A.; BinDhim, N.F.; Alkhamaali, Z.; Alqahtani, S.A. Obesity in Saudi Arabia in 2020: Prevalence, Distribution, and Its Current Association with Various Health Conditions. *Healthcare* **2021**, *9*, 311. [CrossRef]
3. Salem, V.; AlHusseini, N.; Razack, H.I.A.; Naoum, A.; Sims, O.T.; Alqahtani, S.A. Prevalence, risk factors, and interventions for obesity in Saudi Arabia: A systematic review. *Obes. Rev.* **2022**, *23*, e13448. [CrossRef]
4. Malkin, J.D.; Baid, D.; Alsukait, R.F.; Alghaith, T.; Alluhidan, M.; Alabdulkarim, H.; Altowaijri, A.; Almalki, Z.S.; Herbst, C.H.; Finkelstein, E.A.; et al. The economic burden of overweight and obesity in Saudi Arabia. *PLoS ONE* **2022**, *17*, e0264993. [CrossRef]
5. Ruze, R.; Liu, T.; Zou, X.; Song, J.; Chen, Y.; Xu, R.; Yin, X.; Xu, Q. Obesity and type 2 diabetes mellitus: Connections in epidemiology, pathogenesis, and treatments. *Front. Endocrinol.* **2023**, *14*, 1161521. [CrossRef]
6. Pérez, M.R.; Medina-Gómez, G. Obesity, adipogenesis and insulin resistance. *Endocrinol. Nutr. (Engl. Ed.)* **2011**, *58*, 360–369. [CrossRef]
7. Narayan, K.; Boyle, J.P.; Thompson, T.J.; Gregg, E.W.; Williamson, D.F. Effect of BMI on Lifetime Risk for Diabetes in the U.S. *Diabetes Care* **2007**, *30*, 1562–1566. [CrossRef]
8. Longo, M.; Zatterale, F.; Naderi, J.; Parrillo, L.; Formisano, P.; Raciti, G.A.; Beguinot, F.; Miele, C. Adipose Tissue Dysfunction as Determinant of Obesity-Associated Metabolic Complications. *Int. J. Mol. Sci.* **2019**, *20*, 2358. [CrossRef]
9. Klein, S.; Gastaldelli, A.; Yki-Järvinen, H.; Scherer, P.E. Why does obesity cause diabetes? *Cell Metab.* **2022**, *34*, 11–20. [CrossRef]
10. Daousi, C.; Casson, I.F.; Gill, G.V.; MacFarlane, I.A.; Wilding, J.P.H.; Pinkney, J.H. Prevalence of obesity in type 2 diabetes in secondary care: Association with cardiovascular risk factors. *Postgrad. Med. J.* **2006**, *82*, 280–284. [CrossRef]
11. Rohm, T.V.; Meier, D.T.; Olefsky, J.M.; Donath, M.Y. Inflammation in obesity, diabetes, and related disorders. *Immunity* **2022**, *55*, 31–55. [CrossRef] [PubMed]
12. Ford, E.S. Leukocyte Count, Erythrocyte Sedimentation Rate, and Diabetes Incidence in a National Sample of US Adults. *Am. J. Epidemiol.* **2002**, *155*, 57–64. [CrossRef]
13. Libby, P.; Nahrendorf, M.; Swirski, F.K. Leukocytes link local and systemic inflammation in ischemic cardiovascular disease an expanded cardiovascular continuum. *J. Am. Coll. Cardiol.* **2016**, *67*, 1091–1103. [CrossRef] [PubMed]
14. Herrero-Cervera, A.; Soehnlein, O.; Kenne, E. Neutrophils in chronic inflammatory diseases. *Cell. Mol. Immunol.* **2022**, *19*, 177–191. [CrossRef] [PubMed]

15. Akboga, M.K.; Canpolat, U.; Yuksel, M.; Yayla, C.; Yilmaz, S.; Turak, O.; Ozeke, O.; Topaloglu, S.; Aras, D. Platelet to lymphocyte ratio as a novel indicator of inflammation is correlated with the severity of metabolic syndrome: A single center large-scale study. *Platelets* **2015**, *27*, 178–183. [CrossRef] [PubMed]
16. Maurer, S.; Kopp, H.-G.; Salih, H.R.; Kropp, K.N. Modulation of Immune Responses by Platelet-Derived ADAM10. *Front. Immunol.* **2020**, *11*, 44. [CrossRef]
17. Rossaint, J.; Margraf, A.; Zarbock, A. Role of Platelets in Leukocyte Recruitment and Resolution of Inflammation. *Front. Immunol.* **2018**, *9*, 2712. [CrossRef]
18. Van der Poll, T.; Parker, R.I. Platelet Activation and Endothelial Cell Dysfunction. *Crit. Care Clin.* **2020**, *36*, 233–253. [CrossRef]
19. Qian, H.; Chen, R.; Wang, B.; Yuan, X.; Chen, S.; Liu, Y.; Shi, G. Associations of Platelet Count with Inflammation and Response to Anti-TNF-α Therapy in Patients with Ankylosing Spondylitis. *Front. Pharmacol.* **2020**, *11*, 559593. [CrossRef]
20. Gibson, P.R.; Iser, J. Inflammatory bowel disease. *Aust. Fam. Physician* **2005**, *34*, 233–237. [CrossRef]
21. Li, L.; Xu, P.; Zhang, Z.; Zhou, X.; Chen, C.; Lu, C. Platelets can reflect the severity of Crohn's disease without the effect of anemia. *Clinics* **2020**, *75*, e1596. [CrossRef]
22. Milovanovic, M.; Nilsson, E.; Järemo, P. Relationships between platelets and inflammatory markers in rheumatoid arthritis. *Clin. Chim. Acta* **2004**, *343*, 237–240. [CrossRef]
23. Jung, J.-H.; Soh, M.-S.; Ahn, Y.-H.; Um, Y.-J.; Jung, J.-Y.; Suh, C.-H.; Kim, H.-A. Thrombocytopenia in Systemic Lupus Erythematosus. *Medicine* **2016**, *95*, e2818. [CrossRef]
24. Angiolillo, D.J.; Fernandez-Ortiz, A.; Bernardo, E.; Ramírez, C.; Sabaté, M.; Jimenez-Quevedo, P.; Hernández, R.; Moreno, R.; Escaned, J.; Alfonso, F.; et al. Platelet Function Profiles in Patients With Type 2 Diabetes and Coronary Artery Disease on Combined Aspirin and Clopidogrel Treatment. *Diabetes* **2005**, *54*, 2430–2435. [CrossRef]
25. Neergaard-Petersen, S.; Hvas, A.-M.; Grove, E.L.; Larsen, S.B.; Gregersen, S.; Kristensen, S.D. The Influence of Haemoglobin A1c Levels on Platelet Aggregation and Platelet Turnover in Patients with Coronary Artery Disease Treated with Aspirin. *PLoS ONE* **2015**, *10*, e0132629. [CrossRef]
26. De Pergola, G.; Giagulli, V.; Guastamacchia, E.; Bartolomeo, N.; Tatoli, R.; Lampignano, L.; Silvestris, F.; Triggiani, V. Platelet number is positively and independently associated with glycated hemoglobin in non-diabetic overweight and obese subjects. *Nutr. Metab. Cardiovasc. Dis.* **2019**, *29*, 254–259. [CrossRef] [PubMed]
27. Barter, P.J.; Nicholls, S.; Rye, K.-A.; Anantharamaiah, G.; Navab, M.; Fogelman, A.M. Antiinflammatory Properties of HDL. *Circ. Res.* **2004**, *95*, 764–772. [CrossRef]
28. Zhang, S.; Ritter, L.R.; Ibragimov, A.I. Foam cell formation in atherosclerosis: HDL and macrophage reverse cholesterol transport. *Discret. Contin. Dyn. Syst. Ser. S* **2013**, *2013*, 825–835. [CrossRef]
29. Brites, F.; Martin, M.; Guillas, I.; Kontush, A. Antioxidative activity of high-density lipoprotein (HDL): Mechanistic insights into potential clinical benefit. *BBA Clin.* **2017**, *8*, 66–77. [CrossRef]
30. Denimal, D.; Monier, S.; Bouillet, B.; Vergès, B.; Duvillard, L. High-Density Lipoprotein Alterations in Type 2 Diabetes and Obesity. *Metabolites* **2023**, *13*, 253. [CrossRef]
31. Barter, P.J. The Causes and Consequences of Low Levels of High Density Lipoproteins in Patients with Diabetes. *Diabetes Metab. J.* **2011**, *35*, 101–106. [CrossRef] [PubMed]
32. Zhang, H.; Xu, Y.; Xu, Y. The association of the platelet/high-density lipoprotein cholesterol ratio with self-reported stroke and cardiovascular mortality: A population-based observational study. *Lipids Health Dis.* **2024**, *23*, 121. [CrossRef] [PubMed]
33. Wu, W.; Jia, C.; Xu, X.; He, Y.; Xie, Y.; Zhou, Y.; Lu, H.; Liu, J.; Chen, J.; Liu, Y. Impact of Platelet-to-HDL-Cholesterol Ratio on Long-Term Mortality in Coronary Artery Disease Patients with or Without Type 2 Diabetes: Insights from a Chinese Multicenter Cohort. *J. Inflamm. Res.* **2024**, *17*, 2731–2744. [CrossRef]
34. Jialal, I.; Jialal, G.; Adams-Huet, B. The platelet to high density lipoprotein -cholesterol ratio is a valid biomarker of nascent metabolic syndrome. *Diabetes/Metab. Res. Rev.* **2020**, *37*, e3403. [CrossRef]
35. American Diabetes Association Professional Practice Committee; ElSayed, N.A.; Aleppo, G.; Bannuru, R.R.; Bruemmer, D.; Collins, B.S.; Ekhlaspour, L.; Gaglia, J.L.; Hilliard, M.E.; Johnson, E.L.; et al. 2. Diagnosis and Classification of Diabetes: *Standards of Care in Diabetes—2024*. *Diabetes Care* **2023**, *47*, S20–S42. [CrossRef]
36. Weir, C.B.; Jan, A. *BMI Classification Percentile and Cut Off Points*; StatPearls Publishing: Treasure Island, FL, USA, 2019.
37. Robert, A.A.; Al Dawish, M.A. The Worrying Trend of Diabetes Mellitus in Saudi Arabia: An Urgent Call to Action. *Curr. Diabetes Rev.* **2019**, *16*, 204–210. [CrossRef]
38. Farhangi, M.A.; Keshavarz, S.-A.; Eshraghian, M.; Ostadrahimi, A.; Saboor-Yaraghi, A.-A. White Blood Cell Count in Women: Relation to Inflammatory Biomarkers, Haematological Profiles, Visceral Adiposity, and Other Cardiovascular Risk Factors. *J. Health Popul. Nutr.* **2013**, *31*, 58–64. [CrossRef]
39. Han, S.; Gan, D.; Wang, G.; Ru, Y.; Huang, C.; Lin, J.; Zhang, L.; Meng, Z.; Zhu, S. Associations of Platelet Indices with Body Fat Mass and Fat Distribution. *Obesity* **2018**, *26*, 1637–1643. [CrossRef]
40. Samocha-Bonet, D.; Justo, D.; Rogowski, O.; Saar, N.; Abu-Abeid, S.; Shenkerman, G.; Shapira, I.; Berliner, S.; Tomer, A. Platelet Counts and Platelet Activation Markers in Obese Subjects. *Mediat. Inflamm.* **2008**, *2008*, 834153. [CrossRef]
41. Coban, E.; Ozdogan, M.; Yazicioglu, G.; Akcit, F. The mean platelet volume in patients with obesity. *Int. J. Clin. Pract.* **2005**, *59*, 981–982. [CrossRef]

42. Vazzana, N.; Ranalli, P.; Cuccurullo, C.; Davì, G. Diabetes mellitus and thrombosis. *Thromb. Res.* **2011**, *129*, 371–377. [CrossRef] [PubMed]
43. Gordon, L.; Ragoobirsingh, D.; Morrison, E.Y.S.A.; Choo-Kang, E.; McGrowder, D.; Martorell, E. Lipid Profile of Type 2 Diabetic and Hypertensive Patients in the Jamaican Population. *J. Lab. Physicians* **2010**, *2*, 025–030. [CrossRef] [PubMed]
44. Hwang, Y.-C.; Hayashi, T.; Fujimoto, W.Y.; Kahn, S.E.; Leonetti, D.L.; McNeely, M.J.; Boyko, E.J. Differential Association Between HDL Subclasses and the Development of Type 2 Diabetes in a Prospective Study of Japanese Americans. *Diabetes Care* **2015**, *38*, 2100–2105. [CrossRef] [PubMed]
45. Tabara, Y.; Arai, H.; Hirao, Y.; Takahashi, Y.; Setoh, K.; Kawaguchi, T.; Kosugi, S.; Ito, Y.; Nakayama, T.; Matsuda, F. Different inverse association of large high-density lipoprotein subclasses with exacerbation of insulin resistance and incidence of type 2 diabetes: The Nagahama study. *Diabetes Res. Clin. Pract.* **2017**, *127*, 123–131. [CrossRef] [PubMed]
46. Zhou, T.; Hu, Z.; Yang, S.; Sun, L.; Yu, Z.; Wang, G. Role of Adaptive and Innate Immunity in Type 2 Diabetes Mellitus. *J. Diabetes Res.* **2018**, *2018*, 7457269. [CrossRef] [PubMed]
47. Lee, R.H.; Bergmeier, W. Sugar makes neutrophils RAGE: Linking diabetes-associated hyperglycemia to thrombocytosis and platelet reactivity. *J. Clin. Investig.* **2017**, *127*, 2040–2043. [CrossRef] [PubMed]
48. Keating, F.K.; Sobel, B.E.; Schneider, D.J. Effects of increased concentrations of glucose on platelet reactivity in healthy subjects and in patients with and without diabetes mellitus. *Am. J. Cardiol.* **2003**, *92*, 1362–1365. [CrossRef] [PubMed]
49. Kodiatte, T.A.; Manikyam, U.K.; Rao, S.B.; Jagadish, T.M.; Reddy, M.; Lingaiah, H.K.M.; Lakshmaiah, V. Mean Platelet Volume in Type 2 Diabetes Mellitus. *J. Lab. Physicians* **2012**, *4*, 005–009. [CrossRef] [PubMed]
50. Spectre, G.; Östenson, C.-G.; Li, N.; Hjemdahl, P. Postprandial Platelet Activation Is Related to Postprandial Plasma Insulin Rather Than Glucose in Patients with Type 2 Diabetes. *Diabetes* **2012**, *61*, 2380–2384. [CrossRef]
51. Ferreira, I.A.; Eybrechts, K.L.; Mocking, A.I.M.; Kroner, C.; Akkerman, J.-W.N. IRS-1 Mediates Inhibition of Ca2+ Mobilization by Insulin via the Inhibitory G-protein Gi. *J. Biol. Chem.* **2004**, *279*, 3254–3264. [CrossRef]
52. Ferreira, I.A.; Mocking, A.I.; Feijge, M.A.; Gorter, G.; van Haeften, T.W.; Heemskerk, J.W.; Akkerman, J.-W.N. Platelet Inhibition by Insulin Is Absent in Type 2 Diabetes Mellitus. *Arter. Thromb. Vasc. Biol.* **2006**, *26*, 417–422. [CrossRef]
53. Monnier, L.; Mas, E.; Ginet, C.; Michel, F.; Villon, L.; Cristol, J.-P.; Colette, C. Activation of oxidative stress by acute glucose fluctuations compared with sustained chronic hyperglycemia in patients with type 2 diabetes. *JAMA* **2006**, *295*, 1681–1687. [CrossRef] [PubMed]
54. Sampson, M.J.; Gopaul, N.; Davies, I.R.; Hughes, D.A.; Carrier, M.J. Plasma F2 isoprostanes: Direct evidence of increased free radical damage during acute hyperglycemia in type 2 diabetes. *Diabetes Care* **2002**, *25*, 537–541. [CrossRef]
55. Femlak, M.; Gluba-Brzózka, A.; Ciałkowska-Rysz, A.; Rysz, J. The role and function of HDL in patients with diabetes mellitus and the related cardiovascular risk. *Lipids Health Dis.* **2017**, *16*, 207. [CrossRef]
56. Lam, J.K.; Matsubara, S.; Mihara, K.; Zheng, X.-L.; Mooradian, A.D.; Wong, N.C.W. Insulin Induction of Apolipoprotein AI, Role of Sp1. *Biochemistry* **2003**, *42*, 2680–2690. [CrossRef] [PubMed]
57. Taskinen, M.-R. LDL-cholesterol, HDL-cholesterol or triglycerides—Which is the culprit? *Diabetes Res. Clin. Pract.* **2003**, *61*, S19–S26. [CrossRef] [PubMed]
58. Feng, X.; Gao, X.; Yao, Z.; Xu, Y. Low apoA-I is associated with insulin resistance in patients with impaired glucose tolerance: A cross-sectional study. *Lipids Health Dis.* **2017**, *16*, 69. [CrossRef]
59. Kashyap, S.R.; Osme, A.; Ilchenko, S.; Golizeh, M.; Lee, K.; Wang, S.; Bena, J.; Previs, S.F.; Smith, J.D.; Kasumov, T. Glycation Reduces the Stability of ApoAI and Increases HDL Dysfunction in Diet-Controlled Type 2 Diabetes. *J. Clin. Endocrinol. Metab.* **2018**, *103*, 388–396. [CrossRef]
60. Han, C.Y.; Tang, C.; Guevara, M.E.; Wei, H.; Wietecha, T.; Shao, B.; Subramanian, S.; Omer, M.; Wang, S.; O'Brien, K.D.; et al. Serum amyloid A impairs the antiinflammatory properties of HDL. *J. Clin. Investig.* **2016**, *126*, 266–281. [CrossRef]
61. Mao, J.Y.; Sun, J.T.; Yang, K.; Shen, W.F.; Lu, L.; Zhang, R.Y.; Tong, X.; Liu, Y. Serum amyloid A enrichment impairs the anti-inflammatory ability of HDL from diabetic nephropathy patients. *J. Diabetes Complicat.* **2017**, *31*, 1538–1543. [CrossRef]
62. Jayaraman, S.; Haupt, C.; Gursky, O. Paradoxical effects of SAA on lipoprotein oxidation suggest a new antioxidant function for SAA. *J. Lipid Res.* **2016**, *57*, 2138–2149. [CrossRef]
63. Animaw, W.; Seyoum, Y. Increasing prevalence of diabetes mellitus in a developing country and its related factors. *PLoS ONE* **2017**, *12*, e0187670. [CrossRef] [PubMed]
64. Hills, A.P.; Arena, R.; Khunti, K.; Yajnik, C.S.; Jayawardena, R.; Henry, C.J.; Street, S.J.; Soares, M.J.; Misra, A. Epidemiology and determinants of type 2 diabetes in south Asia. *Lancet Diabetes Endocrinol.* **2018**, *6*, 966–978. [CrossRef]
65. Ng, M.C.Y. Genetics of Type 2 Diabetes in African Americans. *Curr. Diabetes Rep.* **2015**, *15*, 74. [CrossRef] [PubMed]

cells MDPI

Article

Combinatorial Genomic Biomarkers Associated with High Response in IgE-Dependent Degranulation in Human Mast Cells

Issan Yee San Tam [1,†], Tak Hong Lee [2,‡], Hang Yung Alaster Lau [1] and See-Ying Tam [3,*]

1 School of Biomedical Sciences, Faculty of Medicine, The Chinese University of Hong Kong, Shatin, Hong Kong; iystam@hku.hk (I.Y.S.T.); hyalau@cuhk.edu.hk (H.Y.A.L.)
2 Allergy Centre, Hong Kong Sanatorium and Hospital, Happy Valley, Hong Kong; takhong.lee@hksh.com
3 Department of Pathology, Stanford University School of Medicine, Stanford, CA 94305, USA
* Correspondence: stam@stanford.edu
† Current address: Department of Paediatrics and Adolescent Medicine, The University of Hong Kong, Pok Fu Lam, Hong Kong.
‡ Deceased author.

Abstract: Mast cells are the major effector cells that mediate IgE-dependent allergic reactions. We sought to use integrated network analysis to identify genomic biomarkers associated with high response in IgE-mediated activation of primary human mast cells. Primary human mast cell cultures derived from 262 normal donors were categorized into High, Average and Low responder groups according to their activation response profiles. Transcriptome analysis was used to identify genes that were differentially expressed in different responder cultures in their baseline conditions, and the data were analyzed by constructing a personalized perturbed profile (PEEP). For upregulated genes, the construction of PEEP for each individual sample of all three responder groups revealed that High responders exhibited a higher percentage of "perturbed" samples whose PEEP values lay outside the normal range of expression. Moreover, the integration of PEEP of four selected upregulated genes into distinct sets of combinatorial profiles demonstrated that the specific pattern of upregulated expression of these four genes, in a tandem combination, was observed exclusively among the High responders. In conclusion, this combinatorial approach was useful in identifying a set of genomic biomarkers that are associated with high degranulation response in human mast cell cultures derived from the blood of a cohort of normal donors.

Keywords: inflammation; allergy; immunoglobulin E; mast cell degranulation; integrated network analysis; genomic biomarkers; precision medicine diagnostics

1. Introduction

Mast cells are the major effector cells of the immune system that mediate IgE-dependent allergic and hypersensitivity reactions, as well as innate and adaptive immunity [1–6]. High-affinity IgE receptors (FcεRI) are expressed on the surface of mast cells, and the crosslinking of FcεRI by allergen binding to the cell-bound allergen-specific IgE results in mast cell degranulation. Such FcεRI-dependent degranulation causes the immediate release of preformed granule mediators, such as histamine, followed by the synthesis and release of diverse lipid mediators and cytokines [5,7]. Mast cells reside in all tissues and are particularly abundant in barrier sites such as the skin, lung and gut; they are mostly derived from CD34+ pluripotent progenitor cells in the bone marrow, and these progenitors migrate into the blood and then reside in the tissues where they differentiate and mature under the influence of local environmental factors [8–11].

Stem cell factor (SCF), or c-kit ligand, was identified as the key mast cell growth factor and has been utilized to generate mature primary human mast cell cultures from pluripotent hematopoietic stem cells isolated from bone marrow, fetal liver, and cord blood and peripheral blood [12,13]. Specifically, many different protocols for generating human mast cells from the peripheral blood have been developed for human mast cell studies because of the readily accessibility to human donor peripheral blood. Moreover, these protocols have been widely used in many functional and mechanistic studies because the functional properties of such blood-derived human mast cells have been well characterized and validated [12–30]. This approach of using blood-derived human mast cells has been used in several recent studies that attempted to explore new technical investigative approaches for understanding human mast cell biology and to develop novel, innovative diagnostic tools for clinical allergy [27,30–36].

We have recently utilized peripheral-blood-derived mast cells generated from allergic patients for developing a patient-specific mast cell activation test (MAT) that was cross-referenced to a reference baseline database, which was originally constructed using a profile of IgE-dependent activation responses for mast cells derived from the peripheral blood of a cohort of healthy individual human donors [35]. Interestingly, the data collected for our reference baseline database revealed a high degree of functional heterogeneity in activation responses among mast cell cultures derived from our cohort. Specifically, we were able to categorize the full spectrum of activation responses into three different responder groups of High, Average and Low, which were defined by the values of mean $\pm$ standard deviation (SD) of the histamine release levels calculated for the activation responses [35].

Recent studies employing transcriptomic and epigenomic comparisons of peripheral blood-derived human mast cells with skin-derived and tonsillar mast cells have suggested that the peripheral blood-derived human mast cells recapitulate many unique functional genomic characteristics of human tissue-resident mast cells [32]. By taking advantage of these properties of the peripheral blood-derived human mast cells, we used the differential gene expression analysis to identify a set of "signature" response genes that were upregulated or downregulated in mast cells of the High responders as compared to those of the Low and Average responders. Furthermore, we employed the approach of personalized perturbation profile (PEEP) analysis, recently outlined by Menche et al. [37], to further analyze our differential gene expression data. The profiling allowed us to integrate the PEEP of a set of 4 selected genes into a distinct combinatorial gene expression pattern, or a barcode, for each individual sample. We showed that the specific pattern of upregulated expression of these 4 genes in a tandem combination was observed exclusively among the High responders. Our studies thus revealed that PEEP profiling can be used to identify genomic biomarkers that are associated with high degranulation response in mast cell cultures derived from a cohort of normal healthy human donors.

2. Materials and Methods

2.1. Normal Human Buffy Coats and Allergic Patient Peripheral Blood Samples

The protocol of using human buffy coats in our studies was approved by The Chinese University of Hong Kong Joint CUHK-NTEC Clinical Research Ethics Review Committee (CREC #2016.421). Fresh human buffy coats from unidentified healthy adult donors were obtained from the Hong Kong Red Cross within 24 h after blood donation. The studies employing human peripheral blood derived from allergic patients (SH#1, SH#5, SH#7) recruited from Hong Kong Sanatorium and Hospital were conducted as described in the Hospital Ethics Committee approved clinical trial (REC-2017-17) and registered at ClinicalTrials.Gov (Identifier NCT03406325). Written informed consent was obtained from each patient participant as stated in the protocol. For patients SH#1, SH#5 and SH#7, about 70–100 mL of peripheral venous blood from individual patients were drawn by syringes and collected in a blood-collecting tube containing EDTA, which was promptly processed within 2 h for the generation of human cultured mast cells.

2.2. Generation of Primary Human-Cultured Mast Cells

Primary human cultured mast cells with characteristics of MC_{TC} phenotypes were generated using the protocol previously described by our group [25]. Briefly, $CD34^+$ progenitors isolated from fresh adult buffy coat using MACS system (Miltenyi Biotec, Auburn,

CA, USA) were cultured in complete IMDM (Iscove's modified Dulbecco's medium with 1X insulin–transferrin–selenium, 1X penicillin–streptomycin, 50 μM 2-mercaptoethanol and 0.1% BSA) with 200 ng/mL human SCF (PeproTech, Cranbury, NJ, USA), 100 ng/mL IL-6 and 1 ng/mL IL-3 for one week. Subsequently, the spent medium was replaced by complete IMDM with 200 ng/mL SCF, 100 ng/mL IL-6 and 15 ng/mL IL-9 for another week. For these initial 2 weeks of culturing, cells were incubated in hypoxic conditions (5% CO_2, 5% O_2, 37 °C). After the first 2 weeks, the spent medium was replaced by complete IMDM with 200 ng/mL SCF and 100 ng/mL IL-6 weekly for another two weeks. In week 5, the spent medium was replaced by complete IMDM with 200 ng/mL SCF, 100 ng/mL IL-6 and 10 ng/mL IL-4. From week 6 and thereafter, cells were cultured in complete IMDM with 100 ng/mL SCF and 50 ng/mL IL-6. From week 3 onwards, these cultures were incubated at normoxic conditions (5% CO_2, 21% O_2, 37 °C). After week 6, fully mature and homogenous populations of primary human MC_{TC} mast cells were generated and ready for functional studies.

2.3. Mast Cell Activation Assay

Release of histamine from mature human cultured mast cells (cultured for 9 weeks) was measured as an index of mast cell activation, as previously described [25]. Briefly, cells were harvested, seeded and sensitized with 0.5 μg/mL human myeloma IgE overnight in complete IMDM with 100 ng/mL SCF and 50 ng/mL IL-6. Cells were then washed once in PBS and resuspended in full HEPES buffer (FHB: 137 mM NaCl, 5.56 mM glucose, 12 mM HEPES, 2.7 mM KCl, 0.4 mM NaH_2PO_4, 1 mM $CaCl_2$ at pH 7.4) with 0.03% HSA and then challenged by anti-human IgE (stock: 1 mg/mL; dilution: 1:1000) (Sigma-Aldrich, St. Louis, MO, USA) for 30 min at 37 °C. For studies using substance P (SP), compound 48/80, ionomycin, or A23187 as the stimulus, human mast cells were washed and resuspended in FHB with 0.03% HSA and then treated with each compound at the selected concentrations for 30 min. Samples of cell-free supernatant and corresponding cell pellet were then collected by centrifugation at 4 °C. Cells incubated in buffer alone served as the controls for spontaneous histamine release. Histamine contents in mast cell pellets and supernatants were measured spectrofluorometrically using Bran+Luebbe AutoAnalyzer 3 (Bran+Luebbe, Norderstedt, Germany). Histamine release was expressed as a percentage of the total cellular contents of histamine (sum of supernatant content and cell pellet content) that were released into the supernatant [histamine release (%)]. The results were corrected for the corresponding control spontaneous release of histamine in buffer alone.

2.4. Transcriptome Profiling

Assessment of levels of protein-coding and long intergenic non-coding RNA transcripts was performed using GeneChip Human Gene 2.0 ST Array (Affymetrix, Sunnyvale, CA, USA). Microarray data were analyzed using Partek Genomics Suite 6.6 software (Chesterfield, MO, USA). Affymetrix CEL files were loaded using the Robust Multi-Chip Average (RMA) method. Unsupervised sample clustering was performed using Principal Component Analysis (PCA). Group-wise differential gene expression analyses among High, Average and Low responders were performed using Mixed Model ANOVA using the Restricted Maximum Likelihood Estimation (REML) method. Lists of differentially expressed genes were created using the cutoff criteria of unadjusted p-value < 0.05 and fold-change > 1.2 or <−1.2 for a specific group comparison in the 5-way ANOVA.

2.5. Validation of Differential Gene Expression Data by Real-Time qPCR

Each individual cDNA sample derived from each donor culture of human mast cells was labeled as High, Average, or Low responder according to its activation profile. Transcripts of the target genes and reference gene (GAPDH) in each cDNA sample were quantified using TaqMan probes, TaqMan Fast Advanced Master Mix (Applied Biosystems, Foster City, CA), and Applied Biosystems QuantStudio 7 Flex Real-Time PCR System (Life Technologies, Carlsbad, CA, USA). QPCR Human Reference Total RNA (Cat.#750500,

Agilent, Santa Clara, CA, USA) was used to prepare the standard curves. Quantities of the gene transcripts were converted from Ct values and calculated according to the standard curves using QuantStudio Software v1.3 (Life Technologies, Carlsbad, CA, USA). Expression level of a target gene in an individual cDNA sample was calculated as follows:

$$\text{Expression level} = (\text{Qs}/\text{NFq})/(\text{Gs}/\text{NFg}) \tag{1}$$

where

NFq = Qc/Average of all Qc;

NFg = Gc/Average of all Gc;

Qs = Mean quantity of the triplicate for target gene of each individual sample;

Qc = Mean quantity of the triplicate for target gene of plate-to-plate reference cDNA control;

NFq = Normalization factor for a plate (ratio of Qc/Average of all Qc for that target gene);

NFg = Normalization factor for a plate (ratio of Gc/Average of all Gc);

Gs = Mean quantity of the triplicate for GAPDH of each individual sample;

Gc = Mean quantity of the triplicate for GAPDH of plate-to-plate reference cDNA control.

The normalized expression level was then Log2 converted for each sample for each target gene. Using this method, an upregulated gene expression would give a positive Log2-converted expression level, whereas a down-regulated gene expression would give a negative value.

TaqMan probes used are listed as the following: AKAP12 (Hs00374507_m1), ARHGAP15 (Hs00251227_m1), CALB2 (Hs00242372_m1), CEBPD (Hs00270931_s1), DPP4 (Hs00897386_m1), FCGR1A/B/CP (Hs02340030_m1), FOXF1 (Hs00230962_m1), GADD45B (Hs00169587_m1), GAPDH (Hs03929097_g1), IL13AR1 (Hs00609812_m1), IL1R1 (Hs00991010_m1), IRF1 (Hs00971965_m1), ITM2C (Hs00985194_g1), KCNMA1 (Hs01119504_m1), NELL2 (Hs00196254-m1), PTGDR (Hs00235003_m1), SIGLEC8 (Hs00274289_m1), SOCS2 (Hs00919620_m1), SPTLC3 (Hs00217867_m1), THEMIS (Hs01041269_m1), TMEM255B (Hs00415678_m1).

2.6. Personalized Perturbation Profile (PEEP) Analysis

In our analysis, the absolute mRNA levels for individual samples were calculated using a human reference RNA standard and then normalized with the corresponding intrinsic GAPDH expression values. The absolute values of expression levels were then transformed by Log2 conversion, and the mean and standard deviation (SD) of the combined Average and Low (Ave + Low) responders for each gene were calculated. A "normal range" of expression levels was defined as those levels whose values lay between mean + SD and mean—SD. For a particular gene of an individual sample whose expression level value was found to be outside of the "normal range" of expression levels calculated for the combined (Ave + Low) responder groups, this gene is defined as being "perturbed", as defined by the primary PEEP model outlined by Menche et al. [37]. Furthermore, the expression level of a gene was labeled as "Up" if it was higher than the upper limit of the "Normal range", whereas those labeled "Down" had levels that were lower than the lower limit of the "Normal" range. The mean Log2-converted expression level and the SD for the 8 selected genes were calculated for High responders (n = 19) and the remaining donors (Average and Low responders, n = 32). The population-specific cutoff for perturbation defined for each gene was calculated as follows:

$$\text{Up-regulation cutoff} = M_{\text{Ave\_Low}} + SD_{\text{Ave\_Low}}$$

$$\text{Down-regulation cutoff} = M_{\text{Ave\_Low}} - SD_{\text{Ave\_Low}}$$

If M_D > Up-regulation cutoff, that donor would be classified as "Up" for that gene;

If M_D < Down-regulated cutoff, that donor would be classified as "Down" for that gene.

Total number of "Perturbed" observed = number of "Up" + number of "Down";

where:

M_{Ave_Low} = Mean Log2-converted expression level for Average and Low responders;

SD_{Ave_Low} = Log2-converted expression level standard deviation for Average and Low responders;

M_D = Mean Log2-converted expression level of an individual donor.

3. Results

3.1. Construction of Reference Baseline Database of Activation Responses of Human-Cultured Mast Cells Derived from a Cohort of Normal Healthy Donors

To establish a population of primary human mast cell cultures derived from a cohort of normal healthy donors, we generated in vitro cultured mast cells from 262 normal donor buffy coats using a protocol previously reported by our group [25]. Mature mast cell cultures were subjected to functional characterization by activating them with different stimuli, such as anti-IgE (to induce the FcεRI-dependent cell activation) [5], SP (an agonist that induces MRGPRX2 receptor-dependent cell activation) [5], compound 48/80 (an agonist that induces MRGPRX2 receptor-dependent cell activation) [5], ionomycin (a calcium ionophore that induces calcium-dependent cell activation) [25], and A23187 (a calcium ionophore that induces calcium-dependent cell activation) [25], in order to present a broad functional characterization of these mast cell cultures by showing that these mast cell cultures were indeed fully functional mature and active in response to different selected stimuli (Figure 1A). When the anti-IgE-induced degranulation response was further analyzed for this cohort of donors, these mast cell cultures exhibited an unimodal distribution of histamine release response (Figure 1B): % histamine release [mean ± SD] was 24.1 ± 15.1%. We defined the range for Average responders to be between 9.0% and 39.2% (n = 161), which represents the two values that are ± one SD from the mean. Donors with responses < 9.0% release were classified as Low responders (n = 50), whereas those with responses > 39.2% were classified as High responders (n = 51) [35].

A

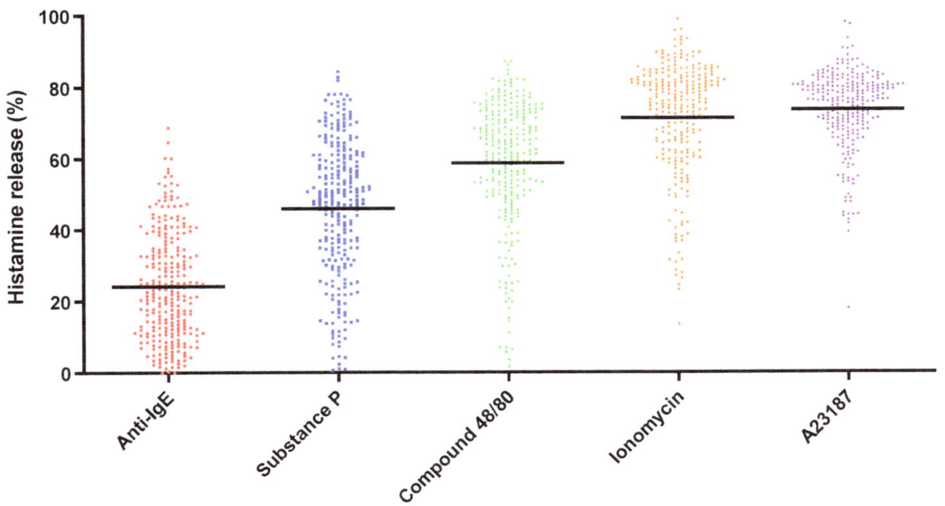

Figure 1. *Cont.*

B

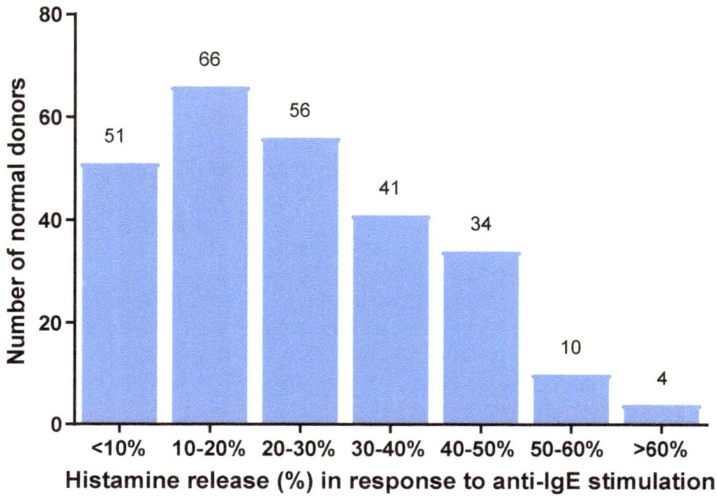

Figure 1. (**A**) Degranulation responses (histamine releases) induced by activation by different stimuli for 30 min in human mast cell cultures derived from a cohort of normal blood donors (n = 262): anti-IgE (1 µg/mL), substance P (10 µM), compound 48/80 (1 µg/mL), ionomycin (1 µM), A23187 (1 µM). Each dot of different colors shown in the figure represents a single normal individual donor. (**B**) Distribution of anti-IgE-induced degranulation responses among human mast cultures derived from a cohort of normal blood donors (n = 262). The numbers on the top of the boxes indicate the numbers of donors whose responses were within the range of % histamine release represented by each box.

3.2. Gene Expression Analysis of Human Mast Cell Cultures Derived from Selected High, Average and Low Responders under Basal Unstimulated Conditions

To identify genomic biomarkers that were associated with high response in IgE-mediated activation in human mast cells, we compared the patterns of gene expression of human mast cell cultures under basal unstimulated conditions that were derived from selected donors of each responder group. We chose to assess the gene expression of the unstimulated cultures, as we reasoned that the gene expression profiles under the basal unstimulated conditions would directly reflect the different intrinsic transcriptional genomic programs that contributed to different genomic predispositions underlying the expression of differential functional responses in mast cell cultures derived from different responder groups. RNAs were isolated from selected unstimulated mast cell cultures derived from 22 High, 17 Average and 21 Low responders and then subjected to microarray gene expression analysis (total n = 60) (Figure S1). PCA mapping of genes expressed in the 60 selected samples showed that Average responders and Low responders shared a similar gene expression pattern than that of High responders, which was represented by the blue ellipse, whose plane was tilted at a different angle than those representing the Low and Average responder groups (Figure 2A).

The heat-map analysis, as illustrated in Figure 2B, showed that the patterns of gene expression of the enriched gene list were largely clustered into two main groups under the categories of "High responders" and "Average and Low responders". These data were thus consistent with our PCA mapping results. In addition, genes differentially expressed in High responders vs. Average and Low responders were enlisted using a volcano plot. By selecting unadjusted $p < 0.05$ and fold-change > 1.2 or < -1.2 as the cutoff values, the numbers of genes enlisted in the volcano plot were narrowed down from 31,135 to 289 (Figure 2C).

3.3. Real-Time qPCR Validation of Selected Microarray Data and Identification of a Specific Gene Set Associated with Mast Cells Derived from High Responders

We initially selected 15 differentially expressed genes based on their statistical significance and physiological relevance, and TaqMan qPCR was performed using cDNA derived from 20 selected donor samples (7 High, 7 Average, 6 Low responders). As shown in Table S1, we found a highly consistent correlation in the patterns of gene expression of High responders vs. Low responders between those determined by microarray analysis and those calculated using qPCR analysis: i.e., genes that were upregulated in High responders exhibited a positive slope, whereas genes that were down-regulated in High responders showed a negative slope, suggesting that the qPCR analysis provided a consistent and accurate approach for further validation of our microarray data.

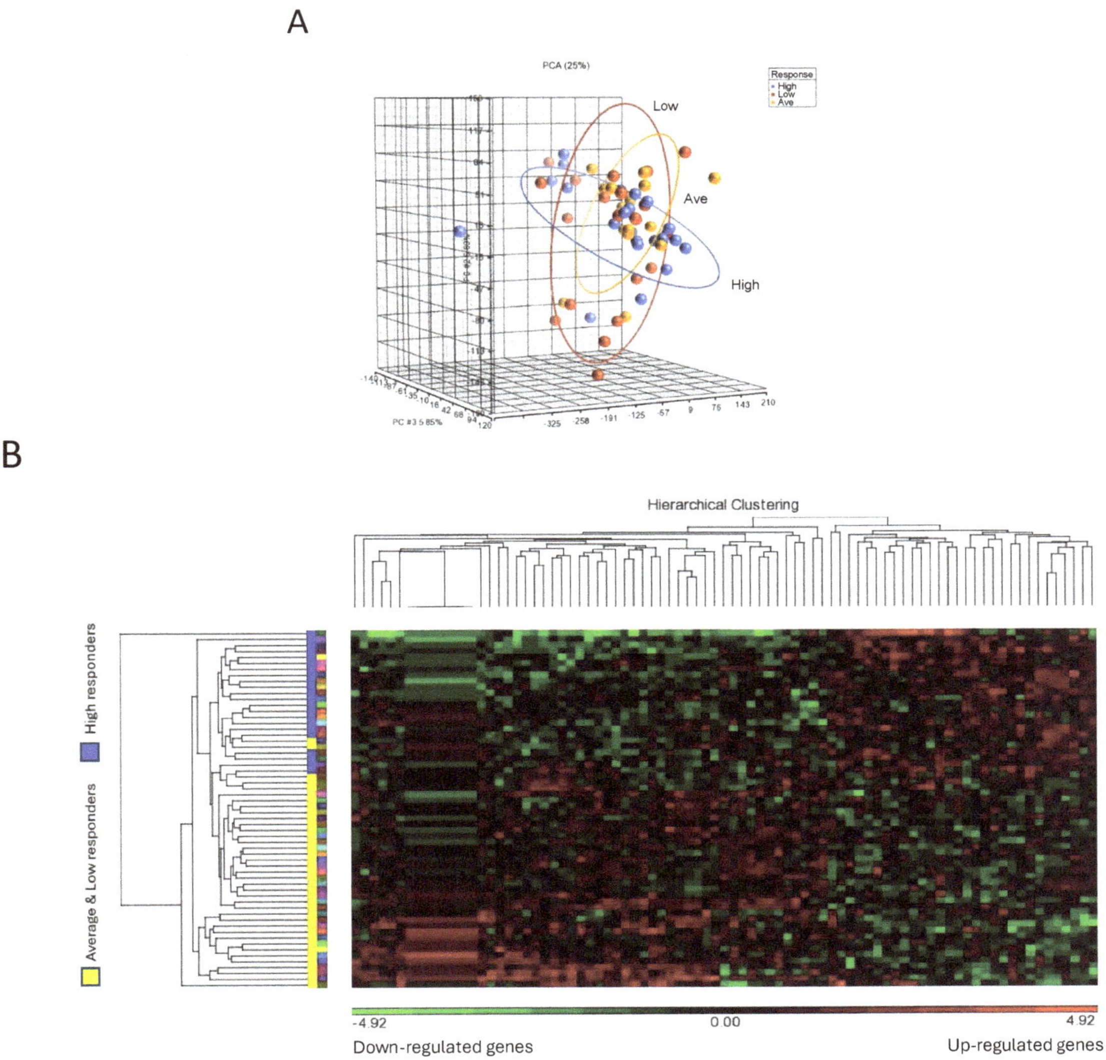

Figure 2. *Cont.*

C

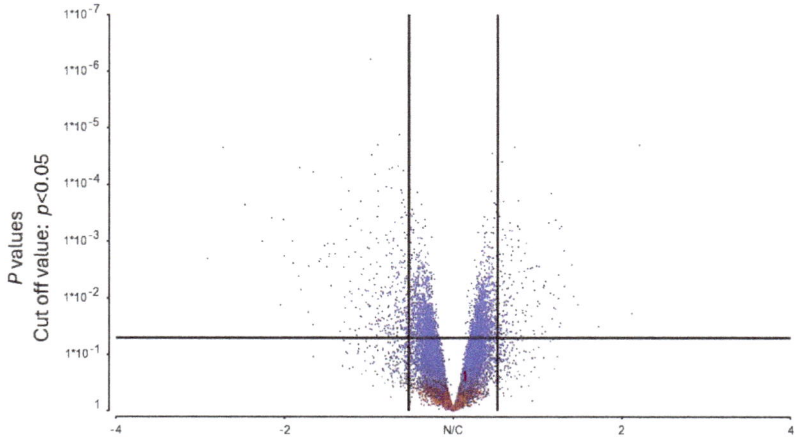

Figure 2. Microarray analysis of selected unstimulated mast cell cultures derived from High, Average and Low responder groups. (**A**) PCA mapping of genes expressed in all the selected samples showing the different gene expression patterns among unstimulated High, Average and Low responder mast cell cultures. (**B**) Heat-map analysis constructed by hierarchical clustering of the enriched gene list. Column: genes upregulated are shown in red, and genes downregulated are shown in green. Row: High responders are represented in blue; Average and Low responders are represented in yellow. (**C**) Volcano plot showing genes that were differentially expressed according to their respective responder groups. X-axis: fold-changes in gene expression by comparing High vs. Average and Low responders; cutoff values set at >1.2 or <−1.2. Y-axis: p values with a cutoff value set at $p < 0.05$.

Next, we selected 8 genes from the 15-gene list, and TaqMan qPCR analysis was performed with a larger number of samples (total n = 51). We picked these 8 genes based on the assumption that they are genes encoding signaling transduction factors and, therefore, are more likely to be involved in the IgE-receptor-mediated cell activation in human mast cells [5,33]. Figure 3 shows the expression levels of the 8 selected genes determined by TaqMan qPCR in samples that were derived from High, Average and Low responders. Statistical analysis revealed that significant differences in mRNA levels of DPP4, GADD45B, NELL2, IL13RA1, AKAP12, CALB2 and ITM2C were detected between High vs. Low responders and High vs. Average responders (Figure 3).

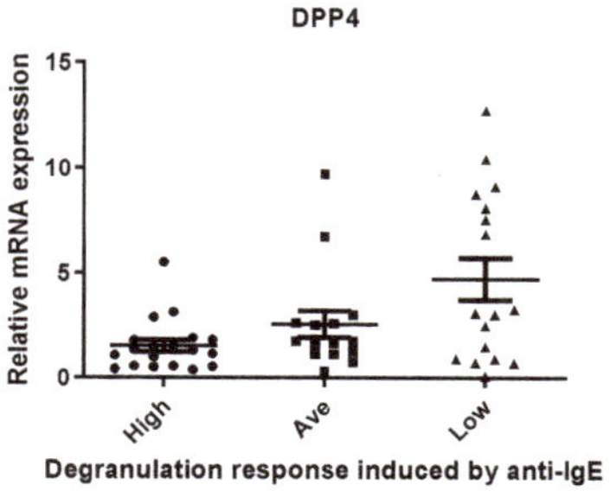

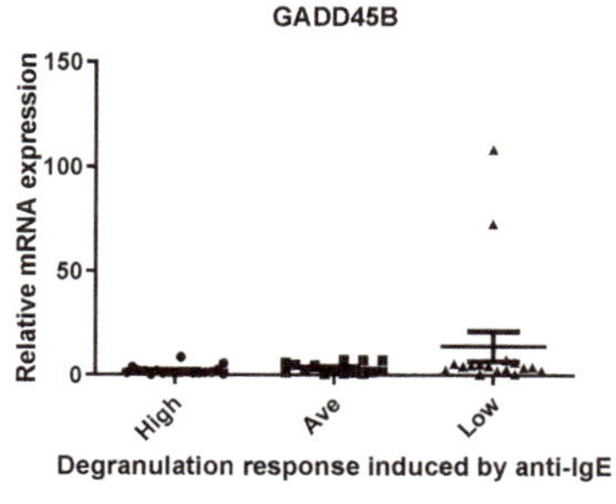

Figure 3. *Cont.*

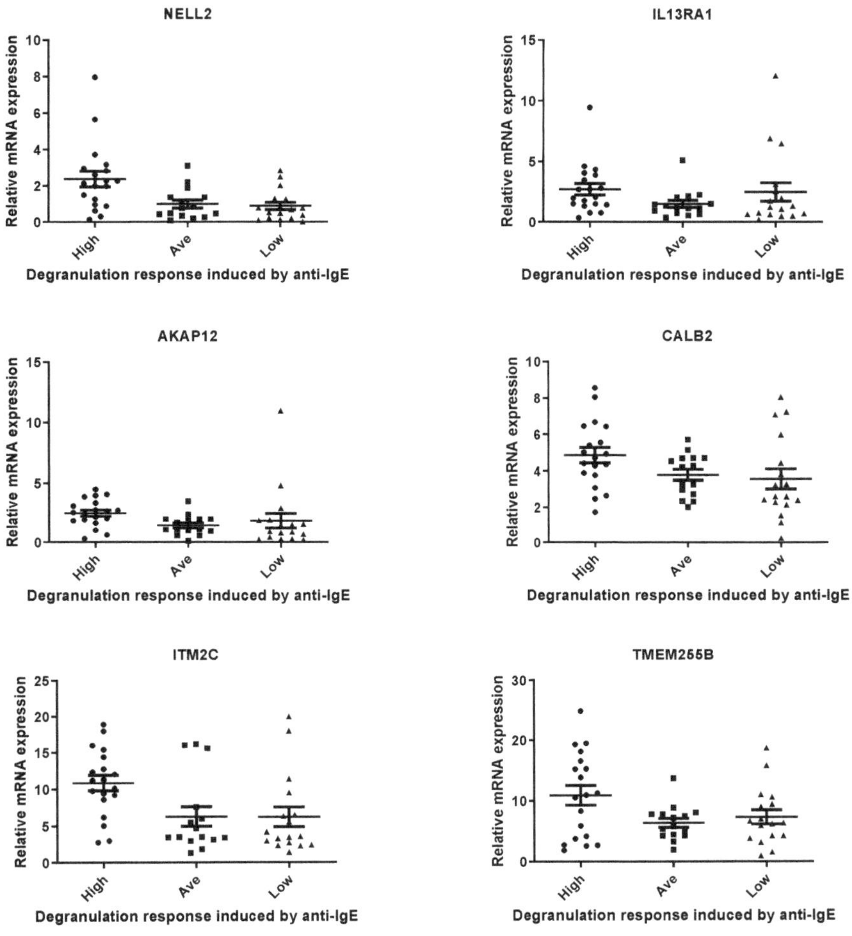

P values	DPP4	GADD45B	NELL2	IL13RA1	AKAP12	CALB2	ITM2C	TMEM255B
High vs Low	0.0161*	0.0019**	0.0019**	0.0933	0.0084**	0.0359*	0.0054**	0.2048
High vs Ave	0.1349	0.1991	0.0062**	0.0268*	0.0062**	0.0844	0.0153*	0.1017
Ave vs Low	0.2416	0.2777	0.6481	0.9703	0.4059	0.3451	0.8894	0.8450

Unpaired t-test (non-Gaussian distribution), two-tailed, using Mann–Whitney test for ranks comparison (GraphPad Prism 9.4.0); * p values = 0.01 to 0.05; **p values = 0.001 to 0.01

Figure 3. Relative expression levels of the 8 genes selected for TaqMan PCR analysis of samples from High, Average and Low responders. Statistical analysis revealed that significant differences in expression levels of DPP4, GADD45B, NELL2, IL13RA1, AKAP12, CALB2 and ITM2C were detected between High vs. Low responders and High vs. Average responders. Data calculated from the statistical analysis of the comparisons between different groups for each of the 8 genes are shown in the table beneath the figures.

3.4. Analysis of Heterogeneity of Gene Expression Patterns by Constructing Personalized Perturbation Profiles

To characterize the heterogeneity of such gene expression patterns among different responders, we employed the method of personalized perturbation profile (PEEP) outlined by Menche et al. to construct the PEEP of a particular gene for each individual sample in order to characterize and compare the patterns of expression levels among different individuals in each responder group [37]. PEEP for each of the 8 selected genes was calculated for each individual sample in each responder group, and the "% perturbed", "% up" and "% down" for each responder group were further determined (see "Materials and Methods" section for details) [37]. For genes such as AKAP12, CALB2, ITM2C, IL13RA1, NELL2 and TMEM255B, whose expression levels were upregulated in the High responders as compared to those in other groups (Figure 3), we found that their "% perturbed" and "% up" values in the High responders were higher than those calculated for other responder groups (Table 1). Similarly, for genes such as GADD45B and DPP4, whose expression levels were downregulated in the High responders as compared to those in other groups (Figure 3), we found that their "% perturbed" and "% up" values in the High responders were lower than those calculated for other responder groups (Table 1). These data thus suggest that the profiling using PEEP revealed the heterogeneity of expression levels of each of these genes in different responder groups and may provide a better assessment of how differential gene expression between the case and control groups can help to identify a set of genes as biomarkers.

Table 1. PEEP profiling revealed the heterogeneity of expression levels of each of the 8 selected genes in different responder groups. For AKAP12, CALB2, ITM2C, IL13RA1, NELL2 and TMEM255B genes, whose expression levels were upregulated in the High responders as compared to those in other groups, their "% perturbed" and "% up" values in the High responders were higher than those calculated for other responder groups. For GADD45B and DPP4 genes, whose expression levels were downregulated in the High responders as compared to those in other groups, their "% perturbed" and "% up" values in the High responders were lower than those calculated for other responder groups.

Gene Name	High	Ave	Low	Ave+Low	Total	Gene Name	High	Ave	Low	Ave+Low	Total
NELL2						CALB2					
Perturbed						Perturbed					
(N)	14	14	4	18	32	(N)	10	9	11	20	30
(%)	82.4%	22.2%	28.6%	23.4%	34.0%	(%)	58.8%	14.3%	78.6%	26.0%	31.9%
Up						Up					
(N)	14	8	2	10	24	(N)	10	7	3	10	20
(%)	82.4%	12.7%	14.3%	13.0%	25.5%	(%)	58.8%	11.1%	21.4%	13.0%	21.3%
Down						Down					
(N)	0	6	2	8	8	(N)	0	2	8	10	10
(%)	0.0%	9.5%	14.3%	10.4%	8.5%	(%)	0.0%	3.2%	57.1%	13.0%	10.6%
AKAP17						GADD45B					
Perturbed						Perturbed					
(N)	13	18	6	24	37	(N)	0	15	4	19	19
(%)	76.5%	28.6%	42.9%	31.2%	39.4%	(%)	0.0%	23.8%	28.6%	24.7%	20.2%
Up						Up					
(N)	12	9	3	12	24	(N)	0	5	3	8	8
(%)	70.6%	14.3%	21.4%	15.6%	25.5%	(%)	0.0%	7.9%	21.4%	10.4%	8.5%
Down						Down					
(N)	1	9	3	12	13	(N)	0	10	1	11	11
(%)	5.9%	14.3%	21.4%	15.6%	13.8%	(%)	0.0%	15.9%	7.1%	14.3%	11.7%
ITM2C						TMEM255B					
Perturbed						Perturbed					
(N)	13	22	3	25	38	(N)	10	12	6	18	28
(%)	76.5%	34.9%	21.4%	32.5%	40.4%	(%)	58.8%	19.0%	42.9%	23.4%	29.8%
Up						Up					
(N)	13	10	3	13	26	(N)	10	3	5	8	18
(%)	76.5%	15.9%	21.4%	16.9%	27.7%	(%)	58.8%	4.8%	35.7%	10.4%	19.1%
Down						Down					
(N)	0	12	0	12	12	(N)	0	9	1	10	10
(%)	0.0%	19.0%	0.0%	15.6%	12.8%	(%)	0.0%	14.3%	7.1%	13.0%	10.6%

Table 1. *Cont.*

Gene Name	High	Ave	Low	Ave+Low	Total	Gene Name	High	Ave	Low	Ave+Low	Total
IL13RA1						DPP4					
Perturbed						Perturbed					
(N)	10	14	4	18	28	(N)	4	18	8	26	30
(%)	58.8%	22.2%	28.6%	23.4%	29.8%	(%)	23.5%	28.6%	57.1%	33.8%	31.9%
Up						Up					
(N)	10	6	3	9	19	(N)	2	6	8	14	16
(%)	58.8%	9.5%	21.4%	11.7%	20.2%	(%)	11.8%	9.5%	57.1%	18.2%	17.0%
Down						Down					
(N)	0	8	1	9	9	(N)	2	12	0	12	14
(%)	0.0%	12.7%	7.1%	11.7%	9.6%	(%)	11.8%	19.0%	0.0%	15.6%	14.9%

Sample Profiles

	Mean	Standard Deviation
Histamine release (%)	26.96%	0.1530
Responders	Histamine release	Numbers (*n*)
High	>42.26%	17
Ave	11.66–42.26%	63
Low	<11.66%	14
Ave + Low	<42.26%	77
Total		94

3.5. Generation of Genomic Biomarkers Associated with High Mast Cell Activation Response Using a Combinatorial Model of a "Signature Gene Set" for Phenotypic Association of Human Mast Cell Cultures

We selected 4 genes from the 8-gene set and employed the PEEP data of these 4 genes as "modules" to construct a combinatorial model that would permit the association of phenotypic characteristics of human mast cells with high activation response. Specifically, we selected those 4 genes whose expressions were upregulated in High responders (AKAP12, ITM2C, IL13RA1, NELL2), and the PEEP of these 4 genes were integrated for every individual sample derived from the 3 different responder groups as "modules" to construct different combinatorial expression patterns. Such patterns were distinct for each individual sample using the perturbation criteria that were previously defined in our construction of PEEP: Expression of each gene in each individual sample was as follows: (1) within the normal range (Norm); (2) >upper limit of the normal range (Up); (3) <lower limit of the normal range (Down). Using such criteria, we would expect, in theory, 15 possible combinatorial patterns, or barcodes, each consisting of the 4 selected genes, that were represented in each individual sample (Table 2). These 15 different patterns were, in turn, classified into 6 "Categories" (Table 2).

From our normal donor cohort, we selected 3 individual mast cell samples (D#148, D#014, D#118) that belonged to each of the 3 responder groups, respectively, and assessed how the expression levels of these 4 genes in tandem combination in each sample would fall into each of the 6 "Categories". As shown in Table 3, D#148 was a High responder to anti-IgE stimulation with upregulated expression of all 4 selected genes [4U0N0D], and thus the pattern fell into the category of "4-Up". On the other hand, D#014 (Average responder) with the [0U2N2D] pattern and D#118 (Low responder) with the [0U4N0D] pattern both belonged to the category of "Others" (Table 3). In addition, we selected 3 mast cell samples (SH#1, SH#5, SH#7) from a group of allergic patients that were included in our recent study on mast cell activation test (MAT) using patient-derived mast cells [35]. We showed that [3U1N0D] ("3-Up") was the pattern associated with the SH#7 mast cell culture, which had been determined to be a High responder. Furthermore, mast cell cultures derived from SH#1 and SH#5, which were both Average responders, exhibited the patterns of [0U4N0D] ("Others") and [0U2N2D] ("Others"), respectively (Table 3). These data thus suggested that the combinatorial patterns of the expression levels of the 4 genes were highly correlated with the mast cell activation responses in both normal donors and allergic patients.

Table 2. Theoretical deduction of 15 possible combinatorial expression patterns of each individual sample derived by combining the observed expression levels of each of the 4 selected genes (AKAP12, ITM2C, IL13RA1, NELL2).

Up	Norm	Down	Combination	Category
4	0	0	4U0N0D	4-Up
3	1	0	3U1N0D	3-Up
2	2	0	2U2N0D	2-Up
1	3	0	1U3N0D	1-Up
0	4	0	0U4N0D	Others
3	0	1	3U0N1D	Others
2	1	1	2U1N1D	Others
1	2	1	1U2N1D	1-Up-1-Down
0	3	1	0U3N1D	Others
2	0	2	2U0N2D	Others
1	1	2	1U1N2D	Others
0	2	2	0U2N2D	Others
1	0	3	1U0N3D	Others
0	1	3	0U1N3D	Others
0	0	4	0U0N4D	Others

U = Up. N = Norm. D = Down.

Table 3. Combinatorial expression patterns of samples selected from the normal donor cohort (D#148, D#104, D#118) and allergic patient cohort (SH#1, SH#5, SH#7) were constructed by combining the observed expression levels (Up, Norm, Down) of each of the 4 selected genes (AKAP12, ITM2C, IL13RA1, NELL2) in tandem in each individual sample.

Sample ID	Histamine Release	Responder Group	NELL2	ITM2C	AKAP12	IL13RA1	Combination	Category
D#148	57.3%	High	Up	Up	Up	Up	4U0N0D	4-Up
D#014	20.4%	Ave	Norm	Down	Down	Norm	0U2N2D	Others
D#118	5.9%	Low	Norm	Norm	Norm	Norm	0U4U0D	Others
SH#1	11.5%	Ave	Norm	Norm	Norm	Norm	0U4N0D	Others
SH#5	36.3%	Ave	Norm	Down	Down	Norm	0U2N2D	Others
SH#7	44.2%	High	Up	Norm	Up	Up	3U1N0D	3-Up

By plotting the combinatorial patterns of the 4 signature genes in each individual sample derived from different responder groups versus the distribution frequencies of such patterns among each of the 3 responder groups, we found that the "4-Up" combinatorial pattern was associated exclusively with ~35% (6 out of 17) of the High responder group (Figure 4). Furthermore, the majority of the "3-Up" samples were found in ~30% (5 out of 17) of the High responders, whereas "2-Up" samples were found equally in all responder groups (Figure 4). On the other hand, the numbers of "1-Up" pattern samples were slightly higher in both Average and Low responders. It was of interest to note that we found only a few "1-Up-1-Down" samples, and all the other combinations ("Others"), such as those within the normal range and "4-Down", were derived predominantly from ~68% (43 out of 63) of the Average and ~57% (8 out of 14) of the Low responders (Figure 4). These data thus suggested that the distribution of the patterns of combinatorial profiles of upregulated genes in different responder groups can be used as genomic biomarkers that are associated with high mast cell activation responses exhibited by the High responders.

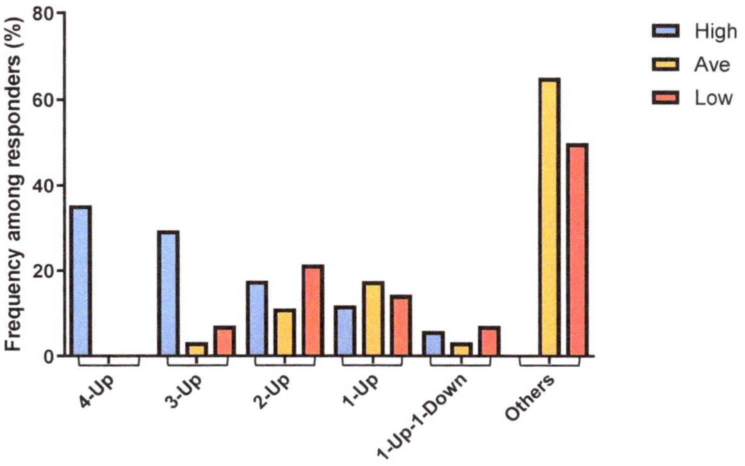

Figure 4. Different frequencies among different responders were determined for the combinatorial patterns comprising the 4 signature genes in each individual sample derived from High, Average and Low responder groups, showing the correlation of the patterns of differential numbers of upregulated genes with different mast cell activation responses among different responders.

4. Discussion

In the present study, we established a cohort of functionally characterized human mast cell cultures derived from the peripheral blood of 262 normal human donors for our transcription profiling studies. We further classified these cultures into High, Average and Low responder groups according to their anti-IgE-induced degranulation responses, and selected cultures were subjected to differential gene expression analysis. The rationale of our approach of employing a healthy human cohort dataset was consistent with that of a recent study by Bonaguro et al. [38], which used the variance of gene expression in healthy human cohorts to predict the role of individual genes or groups of genes in selected biological functions by integrating the expression, phenotypic and functional data from the cohort datasets. Using an approach designated as "*huva*" ("human variation"), this published study derived 2 experimental groups with High and Low expression of the gene of interest from a normal reference dataset, which allowed the subsequent comparisons of their transcriptional profiles and functional parameters, leading to the identification of phenotypic relevance of 16,000 genes-of-interest and stratification of genes according to their functions [38,39]. Thus, both their study and ours have demonstrated the wide applicability of using reference datasets of normal individuals for the elucidation of gene functions/phenotypes in functional genomics studies.

Many integrated network analysis tools have been developed and employed to analyze the transcriptomic data that are obtained using microarray or RNAseq techniques as the approaches to identify predictive biomarkers for patient stratification [40]. These approaches include unsupervised classification or supervised machine learning (such as Bayesian classifiers and support vector machine), differential expression gene analysis, differential network analysis, personalized perturbation profile (PEEP) analysis, and sample-specific network [40]. In this study, we identified large numbers of genes that were differentially regulated in the High responder mast cells compared to Average and Low responders, and 8 of these genes were selected for further analysis by constructing PEEP for each individual sample in each responder group. PEEP analysis is a bioinformatics tool recently introduced by Menche et al. both to address the limitations posed by the machine learning approaches and to systematically analyze the heterogeneity that is inherent in gene expression data [37]. In this approach, instead of comparing the mean of the case group vs. that of the control group, each case sample value is individually assessed on whether it lies within or outside ("perturbed") the range of values calculated for the control samples [37]. For genes such as AKAP12, CALB2, ITM2C, IL13RA1, NELL2 and TMEM255B, whose expression levels were upregulated in the High responders as compared to those in other groups, we found that their "% perturbed" in the High responders were significantly higher than those calculated for other responder groups. On the other hand, for genes GADD45B and DPP4, whose expression levels were downregulated in the High responders as compared to those in other groups, we found that their "% perturbed" values in the High responders were significantly lower than those calculated for other responder groups. Consistent with the study by Menche et al., by comparing the PEEP of each test sample against the range of values derived from the controls, the heterogeneity inherent in such data can be better revealed than the conventional method of comparing the mean of the test samples against the mean of the control samples [37]. Moreover, importantly, the profiling using PEEP allowed us to further integrate the PEEP of a set of signature genes to form a combinatorial gene expression pattern or a barcode, for each individual sample, leading to the identification of a set of genomic biomarkers that was associated with specific functional characteristics of human mast cell cultures derived from a normal population of healthy donors.

In this study, we selected 4 upregulated genes from the 8-gene list and integrated the PEEPs of these 4 genes of each individual sample of all responders into different combinatorial patterns, or barcodes, which indicated the actual numbers of upregulated genes in each sample. As shown in Table 2, there are 15 possible combinatorial expression patterns (permutations) of each individual sample derived by combining the observed expression levels of each of the 4 genes. If we had chosen to perform PEEP profiling with 8 genes, the number of possible permutations of each individual sample derived by combining the observed expression levels of each of the 8 genes would be 45. In that case, the resulting data would be far too extensive and complicated to be analyzed for a proof-of-principle study such as ours. Indeed, in this study, we assessed the distribution of such combinatorial patterns among each of the 3 responder groups and found that the specific combinatorial pattern consisted of all 4 upregulated genes ("4-Up") was found exclusively in ~35% of the High responder group (Figure 4). These data suggest that we can use the "4-Up" combinatorial pattern of the 4 selected genes as the specific genomic biomarker for the High responders of the IgE-mediated human mast cell activation, whereas the "Others" combinatorial patterns (see Table 2 for classification) can be used as the specific genomic biomarkers for the Low and Average responders of the IgE-mediated human mast cell activation. Our data are thus in line with the approach outlined by Menche et al. that the analysis using a distinct PEEP combinatorial perturbed gene expression pattern for each individual sample can be used to identify biomarkers that are associated with the functional status of that individual sample [37].

It will be of interest to determine further the regulatory mechanisms by which the coordinated upregulated expression of the 4 selected genes can confer the high activation response observed with the High responders. Indeed, both NELL2 (neural EGFL like 2) protein and AKAP12 (A-kinase anchoring protein 12) protein are known protein kinase C interacting partners [41,42], and protein kinase C has been shown to mediate IgE-dependent activation of mast cells [43,44]. Furthermore, it has been reported that IL-13 stimulation of human lung mast cells via IL13RA1 (interleukin 13 receptor subunit alpha 1) increases mast cell proliferation and FcεRI expression [45]. However, the role of ITM2C (integral membrane protein 2C) in mast cell activation has not been elucidated so far. In this context, reconstruction of gene regulatory networks (GRNs) has been proposed to address the relationship between the genes and their regulators, which is based on the rationale that every single gene may have a slight individual effect, but several genes disrupted together may have a strong, robust effect when they converge into some connected key regulatory pathways [46].

We have recently shown that peripheral-blood-derived mast cell cultures generated from different allergic patients exhibited extensive heterogeneity with differential activation/interaction of the high-affinity IgE receptors [35]. In that study, among the 7 allergic patients that were studied, we found that 5 of the mast cell cultures derived from these patients exhibited anti-IgE induced cell activation in the category of High responders by using the same criteria and the normal donor cohort that were employed in this present study [35]. Moreover, one of these High-responder patient mast cell cultures exhibited hyper-activation (>100th percentile of the cohort population) [35]. These findings thus suggest that high response in IgE-dependent mast cell activation may represent a genomic characteristic trait or signature response of mast cell cultures derived from allergic patients. Further implication can be extended to the apparently normal individuals in the general population who may be susceptible to mast cell-mediated allergic diseases because of their high mast cell activation profiles.

In the present study, as a preliminary attempt to validate our findings obtained with the PEEP analysis using our normal human cohort, we assessed whether our PEEP analysis could also be associated with the functional status of individual samples derived from an entirely different patient cohort. Indeed, with a limited sample size of 3 allergic patients that were derived from our previous allergic patient cohort [35], we were able to show that the combinatorial pattern of the expression levels of the 4 signature genes was closely correlated with the mast cell activation response observed in each of the 3 patient-derived cultures (Table 3). Further studies will be useful in identifying and developing specific genomic biomarkers that are specific for mast cells derived from different types of allergic patients as a new approach for patient stratification in the practice of personalized medicine.

5. Conclusions

A reference baseline dataset of IgE-dependent activation response of human mast cell cultures derived from a cohort of normal healthy donors was created, and the cultures were classified into 3 groups of responders: High, Average and Low. We constructed PEEP of a set of 4 genes that were differentially expressed at higher levels in the High responders and integrated such PEEP into combinatorial gene signatures that are associated with the high degranulation response in human mast cells. Our study thus represents a proof-of-principle to illustrate the concept of using both the reference baseline database and PEEP profiling as a novel approach for differential gene expression analysis and for the identification of genomic biomarkers associated with specific functional characteristics.

6. Patents

All the data presented in this report were included in a patent application filed with the U.S. Patent Office.

Supplementary Materials: The following supporting information can be downloaded at: https://www.mdpi.com/article/10.3390/cells13151237/s1, Table S1: Direct correlation between microarray data and TaqMan q-PCR data on the association between differential gene expression levels and IgE-dependent activation responses among different human mast cell responders. Human mast cell cultures derived from normal donors were classified as High, Average or Low responders according to their responses to anti-IgE stimulation. RNA samples derived from unstimulated mast cell cultures from each of the 3 responder groups, respectively, were analyzed by microarray (n = 60 for mast cell cultures) and TaqMan q-PCR (n = 20 for each selected gene); Figure S1: Anti-IgE induced degranulation responses exhibited by human mast cell cultures that were selected from High (n = 22), Average (n =17), and Low (n = 21) responder groups for microarray gene expression analysis. Each dot of different colors shown in this figure represents a single normal individual donor

Author Contributions: Conceptualization, S.-Y.T.; methodology, I.Y.S.T., H.Y.A.L. and S.-Y.T.; software, I.Y.S.T.; validation, I.Y.S.T., H.Y.A.L. and S.-Y.T.; formal analysis, I.Y.S.T.; investigation, I.Y.S.T.; resources, T.H.L., H.Y.A.L. and S.-Y.T.; data curation, I.Y.S.T.; writing—original draft preparation, I.Y.S.T., T.H.L., H.Y.A.L. and S.-Y.T.; writing—review and editing, I.Y.S.T., H.Y.A.L. and S.-Y.T.; visualization, I.Y.S.T.; supervision, H.Y.A.L. and S.-Y.T.; project administration, T.H.L., H.Y.A.L. and S.-Y.T.; funding acquisition, H.Y.A.L. and S.-Y.T. All authors have read and agreed to the published version of the manuscript.

Funding: This study was supported in part by the University-Industry Collaboration Programme Grant UIM/306 from the Innovation and Technology Fund (Innovation and Technology Commission of the Government of Hong Kong) to Hang Yung Alaster Lau.

Institutional Review Board Statement: The protocol for using human buffy coats in our studies was approved by the Chinese University of Hong Kong Joint CUHK-NTEC Clinical Research Ethics Review Committee (CREC #2016.421). The studies employing human peripheral blood derived from allergic patients (SH#1, SH#5, SH#7) recruited from Hong Kong Sanatorium and Hospital were conducted as described in the Hospital Ethics Committee-approved clinical trial (REC-2017-17) and registered at ClinicalTrials.Gov (Identifier NCT03406325).

Informed Consent Statement: Written informed consent was obtained from each patient participant as stated in the protocol.

Data Availability Statement: Restrictions apply to the availability of these data. Data were obtained from Apollonian Biosystems and are available from the corresponding author (S.-Y.T.) with permission from Apollonian Biosystems.

Acknowledgments: We wish to thank Joseph Wing-On Tam of Pangenia, Inc. (Hong Kong) for his support and encouragement throughout the course of this study.

Conflicts of Interest: T.H. Lee declared no conflict of interest. S.-Y. Tam is the founder of Apollonian Biosystems. All the data presented in this report were included in a patent application filed with the U.S. Patent Office by S.-Y. Tam, I.Y.S. Tam and H.Y. A. Lau.

References

1. Metcalfe, D.D.; Baram, D.; Mekori, Y.A. Mast cells. *Physiol. Rev.* **1997**, *77*, 1033–1079. [CrossRef]
2. Boyce, J.A. Mast cells and eicosanoid mediators: A system of reciprocal paracrine and autocrine regulation. *Immunol. Rev.* **2007**, *217*, 168–185. [CrossRef] [PubMed]
3. Abraham, S.N.; St John, A.L. Mast cell-orchestrated immunity to pathogens. *Nat. Rev. Immunol.* **2010**, *10*, 440–452. [CrossRef] [PubMed]
4. Galli, S.J.; Tsai, M. IgE and mast cells in allergic disease. *Nat. Med.* **2012**, *18*, 693–704. [CrossRef] [PubMed]
5. Galli, S.J.; Gaudenzio, N.; Tsai, M. Mast Cells in Inflammation and Disease: Recent Progress and Ongoing Concerns. *Annu. Rev. Immunol.* **2020**, *38*, 49–77. [CrossRef] [PubMed]
6. Dahlin, J.S.; Maurer, M.; Metcalfe, D.D.; Pejler, G.; Sagi-Eisenberg, R.; Nilsson, G. The ingenious mast cell: Contemporary insights into mast cell behavior and function. *Allergy* **2022**, *77*, 83–99. [CrossRef] [PubMed]
7. Mukai, K.; Tsai, M.; Saito, H.; Galli, S.J. Mast cells as sources of cytokines, chemokines, and growth factors. *Immunol. Rev.* **2018**, *282*, 121–150. [CrossRef] [PubMed]
8. Dahlin, J.S.; Hallgren, J. Mast cell progenitors: Origin, development and migration to tissues. *Mol. Immunol.* **2015**, *63*, 9–17. [CrossRef]
9. Wu, C.; Boey, D.; Bril, O.; Grootens, J.; Vijayabaskar, M.S.; Sorini, C.; Ekoff, M.; Wilson, N.K.; Ungerstedt, J.S.; Nilsson, G.; et al. Single-cell transcriptomics reveals the identity and regulators of human mast cell progenitors. *Blood Adv.* **2022**, *6*, 4439–4449. [CrossRef]
10. St John, A.L.; Rathore, A.P.S.; Ginhoux, F. New perspectives on the origins and heterogeneity of mast cells. *Nat. Rev. Immunol.* **2023**, *23*, 55–68. [CrossRef]
11. Chia, S.L.; Kapoor, S.; Carvalho, C.; Bajenoff, M.; Gentek, R. Mast cell ontogeny: From fetal development to life-long health and disease. *Immunol. Rev.* **2023**, *315*, 31–53. [CrossRef]
12. Radinger, M.; Jensen, B.M.; Kuehn, H.S.; Kirshenbaum, A.; Gilfillan, A.M. Generation, isolation, and maintenance of human mast cells and mast cell lines derived from peripheral blood or cord blood. *Curr. Protoc. Immunol.* **2010**, *90*, 7–37. [CrossRef]
13. Saito, H.; Kato, A.; Matsumoto, K.; Okayama, Y. Culture of human mast cells from peripheral blood progenitors. *Nat. Protoc.* **2006**, *1*, 2178–2183. [CrossRef]
14. Rottem, M.; Okada, T.; Goff, J.P.; Metcalfe, D.D. Mast cells cultured from the peripheral blood of normal donors and patients with mastocytosis originate from a CD34+/Fc epsilon RI- cell population. *Blood* **1994**, *84*, 2489–2496. [CrossRef]
15. Kirshenbaum, A.S.; Metcalfe, D.D. Growth of human mast cells from bone marrow and peripheral blood-derived CD34+ pluripotent progenitor cells. *Methods Mol. Biol.* **2006**, *315*, 105–112.
16. Wang, X.S.; Sam, S.W.; Yip, K.H.; Lau, H.Y. Functional characterization of human mast cells cultured from adult peripheral blood. *Int. Immunopharmacol.* **2006**, *6*, 839–847. [CrossRef]
17. Lappalainen, J.; Lindstedt, K.A.; Kovanen, P.T. A protocol for generating high numbers of mature and functional human mast cells from peripheral blood. *Clin. Exp. Allergy* **2007**, *37*, 1404–1414. [CrossRef]
18. Holm, M.; Andersen, H.B.; Hetland, T.E.; Dahl, C.; Hoffmann, H.J.; Junker, S.; Schiøtz, P.O. Seven week culture of functional human mast cells from buffy coat preparations. *J. Immunol. Methods* **2008**, *336*, 213–221. [CrossRef]

19. Frandsen, P.M.; Krohn, I.J.; Hoffmann, H.J.; Schiotz, P.O. The Influence of IgE on Cultured Human Mast Cells. *Allergy Asthma Immunol. Res.* **2013**, *5*, 409–414. [CrossRef]
20. Gaudenzio, N.; Laurent, C.; Valitutti, S.; Espinosa, E. Human mast cells drive memory CD4+ T cells toward an inflammatory IL-22+ phenotype. *J. Allergy Clin. Immunol.* **2013**, *131*, 1400–1407.e11. [CrossRef]
21. Hoffmann, H.J. Generation of a human allergic mast cell phenotype from CD133(+) stem cells. *Methods Mol. Biol.* **2014**, *1192*, 57–62.
22. Schmetzer, O.; Valentin, P.; Smorodchenko, A.; Domenis, R.; Gri, G.; Siebenhaar, F.; Metz, M.; Maurer, M. A novel method to generate and culture human mast cells: Peripheral CD34+ stem cell-derived mast cells (PSCMCs). *J. Immunol. Methods* **2014**, *413*, 62–68. [CrossRef]
23. Joulia, R.; Gaudenzio, N.; Rodrigues, M.; Lopez, J.; Blanchard, N.; Valitutti, S.; Espinosa, E. Mast cells form antibody-dependent degranulatory synapse for dedicated secretion and defence. *Nat. Commun.* **2015**, *6*, 6174. [CrossRef]
24. Cop, N.; Decuyper, I.I.; Faber, M.A.; Sabato, V.; Bridts, C.H.; Hagendorens, M.M.; De Winter, B.Y.; De Clerck, L.S.; Ebo, D.G. Phenotypic and functional characterization of in vitro cultured human mast cells. *Cytometry B Clin. Cytom.* **2017**, *92*, 348–354. [CrossRef]
25. Tam, I.Y.S.; Ng, C.W.; Tam, S.Y.; Lau, H.Y.A. Novel six-week protocol for generating functional human connective tissue-type (MC(TC)) mast cells from buffy coats. *Inflamm. Res.* **2017**, *66*, 25–37. [CrossRef]
26. Yin, Y.; Bai, Y.; Olivera, A.; Desai, A.; Metcalfe, D.D. An optimized protocol for the generation and functional analysis of human mast cells from CD34(+) enriched cell populations. *J. Immunol. Methods* **2017**, *448*, 105–111. [CrossRef]
27. Bahri, R.; Custovic, A.; Korosec, P.; Tsoumani, M.; Barron, M.; Wu, J.; Sayers, R.; Weimann, A.; Ruiz-Garcia, M.; Patel, N.; et al. Mast cell activation test in the diagnosis of allergic disease and anaphylaxis. *J. Allergy Clin. Immunol.* **2018**, *142*, 485–496 e16. [CrossRef]
28. Derakhshan, T.; Bhowmick, R.; Ritchey, J.W.; Gappa-Fahlenkamp, H. Development of Human Mast Cells from Hematopoietic Stem Cells within a 3D Collagen Matrix: Effect of Stem Cell Media on Mast Cell Generation. *Stem Cells Int.* **2018**, *2018*, 2136193. [CrossRef]
29. Luo, Y.; Frischbutter, S.; Scheffel, J.; Siebenhaar, F. Generation and Culture of Peripheral CD34(+) Stem Cell-Derived Mast Cells (PSCMCs). *Methods Mol. Biol.* **2020**, *2163*, 63–67.
30. Elst, J.; van der Poorten, M.L.; Van Gasse, A.L.; De Puysseleyr, L.; Hagendorens, M.M.; Faber, M.A.; Van Houdt, M.; Passante, E.; Bahri, R.; Walschot, M.; et al. Mast cell activation tests by flow cytometry: A new diagnostic asset? *Clin. Exp. Allergy* **2021**, *51*, 1482–1500. [CrossRef]
31. Gaudenzio, N.; Sibilano, R.; Marichal, T.; Starkl, P.; Reber, L.L.; Cenac, N.; McNeil, B.D.; Dong, X.; Hernandez, J.D.; Sagi-Eisenberg, R.; et al. Different activation signals induce distinct mast cell degranulation strategies. *J. Clin. Investig.* **2016**, *126*, 3981–3998. [CrossRef] [PubMed]
32. Cildir, G.; Toubia, J.; Yip, K.H.; Zhou, M.; Pant, H.; Hissaria, P.; Zhang, J.; Hong, W.; Robinson, N.; Grimbaldeston, M.A.; et al. Genome-wide Analyses of Chromatin State in Human Mast Cells Reveal Molecular Drivers and Mediators of Allergic and Inflammatory Diseases. *Immunity* **2019**, *51*, 949–965.e6. [CrossRef] [PubMed]
33. Folkerts, J.; Gaudenzio, N.; Maurer, M.; Hendriks, R.W.; Stadhouders, R.; Tam, S.-Y.; Galli, S.J. Rapid identification of human mast cell degranulation regulators using functional genomics coupled to high-resolution confocal microscopy. *Nat. Protoc.* **2020**, *15*, 1285–1310. [CrossRef] [PubMed]
34. Folkerts, J.; Redegeld, F.; Folkerts, G.; Blokhuis, B.; van den Berg, M.P.; de Bruijn, M.J.; van IJcken, W.F.; Junt, T.; Tam, S.Y.; Galli, S.J.; et al. Butyrate inhibits human mast cell activation via epigenetic regulation of FcepsilonRI-mediated signaling. *Allergy* **2020**, *75*, 1966–1978. [CrossRef] [PubMed]
35. Tam, I.Y.S.; Lau, H.Y.A.; Tam, S.Y.; Lee, T.H. Mast cell activation test using patient-derived mast cells exhibits distinct combinatorial phenotypic profiles among allergic patients. *Allergy* **2020**, *75*, 1796–1799. [CrossRef]
36. Fereydouni, M.; Ahani, E.; Desai, P.; Motaghed, M.; Dellinger, A.; Metcalfe, D.D.; Yin, Y.; Lee, S.H.; Kafri, T.; Bhatt, A.P.; et al. Human Tumor Targeted Cytotoxic Mast Cells for Cancer Immunotherapy. *Front. Oncol.* **2022**, *12*, 871390. [CrossRef]
37. Menche, J.; Guney, E.; Sharma, A.; Branigan, P.J.; Loza, M.J.; Baribaud, F.; Dobrin, R.; Barabási, A.-L. Integrating personalized gene expression profiles into predictive disease-associated gene pools. *NPJ Syst. Biol. Appl.* **2017**, *3*, 10. [CrossRef]
38. Bonaguro, L.; Schulte-Schrepping, J.; Carraro, C.; Sun, L.L.; Reiz, B.; Gemünd, I.; Saglam, A.; Rahmouni, S.; Georges, M.; Arts, P.; et al. Human variation in population-wide gene expression data predicts gene perturbation phenotype. *iScience* **2022**, *25*, 105328. [CrossRef] [PubMed]
39. Aschenbrenner, A.C.; Bonaguro, L. huva: A human variation analysis framework to predict gene perturbation from population-scale multi-omics data. *STAR Protoc.* **2023**, *4*, 102193. [CrossRef]
40. Delhalle, S.; Bode, S.F.N.; Balling, R.; Ollert, M.; He, F.Q. A roadmap towards personalized immunology. *NPJ Syst. Biol. Appl.* **2018**, *4*, 9. [CrossRef]
41. Kuroda, S.; Tanizawa, K. Involvement of epidermal growth factor-like domain of NELL proteins in the novel protein-protein interaction with protein kinase C. *Biochem. Biophys. Res. Commun.* **1999**, *265*, 752–757. [CrossRef]
42. Qasim, H.; McConnell, B.K. AKAP12 Signaling Complex: Impacts of Compartmentalizing cAMP-Dependent Signaling Pathways in the Heart and Various Signaling Systems. *J. Am. Heart Assoc.* **2020**, *9*, e016615. [CrossRef] [PubMed]
43. Zhang, C.; Hirasawa, N.; Beaven, M.A. Antigen activation of mitogen-activated protein kinase in mast cells through protein kinase C-dependent and independent pathways. *J. Immunol.* **1997**, *158*, 4968–4975. [CrossRef] [PubMed]

44. Liu, Y.; Graham, C.; Parravicini, V.; Brown, M.J.; Rivera, J.; Shaw, S. Protein kinase C theta is expressed in mast cells and is functionally involved in Fcepsilon receptor I signaling. *J. Leukoc. Biol.* **2001**, *69*, 831–840. [CrossRef] [PubMed]
45. Kaur, D.; Hollins, F.; Woodman, L.; Yang, W.; Monk, P.; May, R.; Bradding, P.; Brightling, C.E. Mast cells express IL-13R alpha 1: IL-13 promotes human lung mast cell proliferation and Fc epsilon RI expression. *Allergy* **2006**, *61*, 1047–1053. [CrossRef]
46. van der Wijst, M.G.P.; de Vries, D.H.; Brugge, H.; Westra, H.J.; Franke, L. An integrative approach for building personalized gene regulatory networks for precision medicine. *Genome Med.* **2018**, *10*, 96. [CrossRef]

diseases

MDPI

Article

Effects of Combustible Cigarettes and Heated Tobacco Products on Systemic Inflammatory Response in Patients with Chronic Inflammatory Diseases

Nikolina Kastratovic [1,2], Natasa Zdravkovic [1,3,4], Ivan Cekerevac [1,3,5], Vanesa Sekerus [6,7], Carl Randall Harrell [8], Violeta Mladenovic [3,4], Aleksandar Djukic [3,4], Ana Volarevic [1,9], Marija Brankovic [10,11], Tijana Gmizic [10,11], Marija Zdravkovic [11,12], Jelica Bjekic-Macut [13], Nebojsa Zdravkovic [1,14], Valentin Djonov [15] and Vladislav Volarevic [1,2,16,17,*]

1 Center for Research on Harmful Effects of Biological and Chemical Hazards, Faculty of Medical Sciences, University of Kragujevac, 69 Svetozar Markovic Street, 34000 Kragujevac, Serbia; n_kastratovic@outlook.com (N.K.); natasasilvester@gmail.com (N.Z.); icekerevac@gmail.com (I.C.); ana.volarevic@fmn.kg.ac.rs (A.V.); nzdravkovic@gmail.com (N.Z.)
2 Department of Genetics, Faculty of Medical Sciences, University of Kragujevac, 69 Svetozar Markovic Street, 34000 Kragujevac, Serbia
3 Department of Internal Medicine, Faculty of Medical Sciences, University of Kragujevac, 69 Svetozar Markovic Street, 34000 Kragujevac, Serbia; vikicam2004@gmail.com (V.M.); adjukic@fmn.kg.ac.rs (A.D.)
4 Center for Endocrinology, Diabetes and Metabolic Diseases, University Clinical Center Kragujevac, 30 Zmaj Jovina Street, 34000 Kragujevac, Serbia
5 Pulmonology Clinic, University Clinical Center Kragujevac, 30 Zmaj Jovina Street, 34000 Kragujevac, Serbia
6 Institute for Pulmonary Diseases of Vojvodina, 4 Institutski Put, 21204 Novi Sad, Serbia; vanesa.sekerus@mf.uns.ac.rs
7 Department of Biochemistry, Faculty of Medicine, University of Novi Sad, 3 Hajduk Veljkova Street, 21000 Novi Sad, Serbia
8 Regenerative Processing Plant, LLC, 34176 US Highway 19 N, Palm Harbor, FL 34684, USA; dr.harrell@regenerativeplant.org
9 Department of Psychology, Faculty of Medical Sciences, University of Kragujevac, 69 Svetozar Markovic Street, 34000 Kragujevac, Serbia
10 Department of Gastroenterology, University Medical Center "Bežanijska Kosa", Dr Zoza Matea bb, 11080 Belgrade, Serbia; brankovic.marija@bkosa.edu.rs (M.B.); tijana93@hotmail.com (T.G.)
11 Faculty of Medicine, University of Belgrade, Dr Subotica 8, 11000 Belgrade, Serbia; sekcija.kardioloska@gmail.com
12 Department of Cardiology, University Medical Center "Bežanijska Kosa", Dr Zoza Matea bb, 11080 Belgrade, Serbia
13 Department of Endocrinology, University Medical Center "Bežanijska Kosa", Dr Zoza Matea bb, 11080 Belgrade, Serbia; jbjekic@yahoo.com
14 Department of Statistics, Faculty of Medical Sciences, University of Kragujevac, 69 Svetozar Markovic Street, 34000 Kragujevac, Serbia
15 Institute of Anatomy, University of Bern, Baltzerstrasse 2, 3012 Bern, Switzerland; valentin.djonov@unibe.ch
16 Department of Microbiology and Immunology, Faculty of Medical Sciences, University of Kragujevac, 69 Svetozar Markovic Street, 34000 Kragujevac, Serbia
17 Faculty of Pharmacy Novi Sad, Trg Mladenaca 5, 21000 Novi Sad, Serbia
* Correspondence: drvolarevic@yahoo.com; Tel./Fax: +381-34306800

Abstract: Smoke derived from combustible cigarettes (CCs) contains numerous harmful chemicals that can impair the viability, proliferation, and activation of immune cells, affecting the progression of chronic inflammatory diseases. In order to avoid the detrimental effects of cigarette smoking, many CC users have replaced CCs with heated tobacco products (HTPs). Due to different methods of tobacco processing, CC-sourced smoke and HTP-derived aerosols contain different chemical constituents. With the exception of nicotine, HTP-sourced aerosols contain significantly lower amounts of harmful constituents than CC-derived smoke. Since HTP-dependent effects on immune-cell-driven inflammation are still unknown, herein we used flow cytometry analysis, intracellular staining, and an enzyme-linked immunosorbent assay to determine the impact of CCs and HTPs on systemic inflammatory response in patients suffering from ulcerative colitis (UC), diabetes mellitus (DM), and chronic obstructive pulmonary disease (COPD). Both CCs and HTPs significantly modulated cytokine production in circulating immune cells, affecting the systemic inflammatory response in COPD, DM, and UC patients. Compared to CCs, HTPs had weaker capacity to induce the synthesis of inflammatory cytokines (IFN-γ, IL-1β, IL-5, IL-6, IL-12, IL-23, IL-17, TNF-α), but more efficiently induced the production of immunosuppressive IL-10 and IL-35. Additionally, HTPs significantly enhanced the synthesis of pro-fibrotic TGF-β. The continuous use of CCs and HTPs aggravated immune-cell-driven systemic inflammation in COPD and DM patients, but not in UC patients, suggesting that the immunomodulatory effects of CC-derived smoke and HTP-sourced aerosols are disease-specific, and need to be determined for specific immune-cell-driven inflammatory diseases.

Keywords: combustible cigarettes; heated tobacco products; systemic inflammation; cytokines; chronic inflammatory diseases

1. Introduction

The systemic inflammatory response has a profound impact on the progression and exacerbation of chronic inflammatory diseases [1]. Prolonged systemic inflammation results in tissue damage and fibrosis in various organs [1,2]. The continuous activation of immune cells and the massive release of inflammatory mediators results in the destruction of parenchymal and endothelial cells (ECs) throughout the body, exacerbating the pathology of chronic inflammatory conditions [3]. Sustained inflammatory signaling is usually associated with impaired tissue repair and an excessive deposition of collagen in the vital organs, resulting in their dysfunction [2,3]. Additionally, systemic inflammation can trigger or exacerbate autoimmune response [4]. A detrimental systemic inflammatory response can disrupt the balance between pro-inflammatory and anti-inflammatory immune cells in injured tissues, leading to immune dysregulation and impaired immune tolerance [4]. A dysregulated immune response leads to the massive release of self-antigens from injured parenchymal cells, followed by the activation of autoreactive lymphocytes, resulting in the development and progression of autoimmune diseases [1,4].

Accordingly, the identification of factors that induce systemic inflammatory response and the mitigation of their detrimental effects could prevent exacerbations of inflammation-related diseases [1]. Prolonged exposure to combustible cigarette (CC)-derived smoke is considered an important risk factor for the induction of systemic inflammatory response and for the development of organ-specific immune-cell-driven diseases [5–10]. Smoke from CCs contains many harmful substances that can negatively impact the ability of immune cells to survive, proliferate, produce inflammatory cytokines, and migrate in injured tissues [11]. Neutrophils exposed to CC-sourced smoke had altered migratory characteristics and were not able to optimally produce reactive oxygen species (ROS) [12]. Similarly, CC-derived smoke favored an alternative activation of macrophages and suppressed their phagocytic ability against pathogenic bacteria [9]. A decrease in the number of M1 inflammatory macrophages was observed in healthy CC users compared to healthy non-smokers. The transition towards the M2-polarization phenotype was found to be more prominent in CC users who suffer from chronic obstructive pulmonary disease (COPD) [13]. High, but not low, levels of CC-derived smoke suppressed allergic airway inflammation in mice [14]. This suppression was achieved by inhibiting the function of T cells, reducing eosinophilia and decreasing the levels of IL-4 and IL-5 in the bronchoalveolar lavage [14]. Additionally, the smoke exposure led to a loss of ovalbumin antigen-specific proliferation and cytokine production in T cells [14]. Chronic exposure to CC-derived smoke may lead to a progression from M1 macrophage-dependent oxidative burst response to M2 macrophage-driven sensitization [14]. However, this M2 macrophage-driven immune response may be suppressed due to the loss of T-cell function and the suppression of IL-4 and IL-5 production [14]. Long-term exposure to cigarette smoking altered the production of perforins and granzymes in cytotoxic T lymphocytes (CTLs) and natural killer (NK) cells, affecting their anti-viral properties [10]. Additionally, increased expressions of E and

P selectins were observed on ECs that were exposed to CC-derived smoke, facilitating the migration of circulating leukocytes in injured and inflamed tissues [7]. Accordingly, cigarette smoking is considered the main driver of inflammatory and malignant diseases of the lungs (COPD, pulmonary fibrosis, and lung cancer) and represents one of the main risk factors for the aggravation of immune-cell-driven organ-specific and systemic diseases [15]. The frequent use of CCs increases the risk of developing heart disease, stroke, peripheral arterial disease, atherosclerosis, diabetes, osteoporosis, and rheumatoid arthritis [15].

In order to avoid the detrimental effects of cigarette smoking, many CC users have replaced CCs with heated tobacco products (HTPs), which heat tobacco instead of burning it [16,17]. HTPs consist of a stick, capsule, or cartridge of tobacco that is inserted into a device that heats the tobacco to release nicotine and flavor without producing smoke [16]. The tobacco in HTPs is heated to a specific temperature, usually between 250 and 350 °C [16,17]. This temperature is enough to release nicotine and other chemicals without generating harmful combustion byproducts [16,17]. Due to the different methods of tobacco processing, CC-sourced smoke and HTP-derived aerosols contain different chemical constituents [18]. With the exception of nicotine, HTP-derived aerosols contain different concentrations of harmful and potentially harmful constituents than CC-derived smoke [17,18]. CC-derived tar, carbon monoxide (CO), benzene, 1, 3 butadiene, acrylonitrile, and ethylene oxide are present in lower amounts in HTP-sourced aerosols, but concentrations of several bioactive substances are higher in HTP-derived emissions compared to CC-sourced smoke, indicating that cessation from CCs and HTPs is the most effective strategy in the prevention of inflammatory and malignant diseases [18]. Compared to CC-derived smoke, HTP-sourced aerosols had different impacts on the phenotypes and functions of immune cells that infiltrated the lungs of COPD mice and COPD patients [5,19]. HTP-exposed lung dendritic cells (DCs) had impaired capacity for the optimal activation of inflammatory Th1, Th2, and Th17 lymphocytes compared to DCs that were continuously exposed to CCs [5]. Similarly, a reduced activation of the NLRP3 inflammasome was observed in the neutrophils and monocytes of HTP-exposed COPD mice and COPD patients [5,19]. Despite the fact that DC:T cell crosstalk and the NLRP3-dependent activation of circulating leukocytes are crucially responsible for the development of systemic immune response in patients suffering from COPD, ulcerative colitis (UC), and diabetes mellitus (DM), the long-term effects of HTPs on immune-cell-driven systemic inflammation are still unknown [16]. Accordingly, in this study, we analyzed the effects of CCs and HTPs on cytokine production in the circulating immune cells of patients suffering from these chronic inflammatory diseases, and we compared concentrations of inflammatory and immunosuppressive cytokines in their serum samples, paving the way to a better understanding of CC- and HTP-dependent effects on the immune-cell-driven systemic inflammatory response.

2. Material and Methods

2.1. Study Population

In total, 74 patients with ulcerative colitis (UC), 78 patients with chronic obstructive pulmonary disease (COPD), and 33 patients with diabetes mellitus (DM) were recruited in this study. The diagnosis of UC was confirmed by endoscopic, histological, and clinical scores. Endoscopic disease activity was evaluated with the Mayo endoscopic subscore. The clinical score was determined using the Truelove and Witts clinical activity index. The histological score was determined using Geboes grade. The inclusion criterion for COPD patients was the diagnosis of airflow limitation that was not fully reversible. The diagnosis was confirmed by spirometry. The presence of a post-bronchodilator forced expiratory volume in 1 s (FEV_1) < 80% of the predicted value, in combination with an FEV_1/forced vital capacity (FVC) ratio < 70% confirmed the presence of airflow limitation that was not fully reversible. The inclusion criterion for DM was fasting glycaemia equal or greater than 126 mg/dL.

The patients were recruited from the Centers of Gastroenterology, Endocrinology and Pulmonology, University Clinical Center of Kragujevac, Centers of Gastroenterology and Endocrinology, University Clinical Center "Bezanijska Kosa" Belgrade, and from the Institute for Pulmonary Diseases of Vojvodina, Sremska Kamenica. UC, COPD, and DM patients who used CCs and HTPs were recruited to experimental groups (UC^{CC}, $COPD^{CC}$, DM^{CC}, UC^{HTP}, $COPD^{HTP}$, and DM^{HTP}), while UC, COPD and DM non-smokers were recruited to the UC^{AIR}, $COPD^{AIR}$, DM^{AIR} groups. Healthy volunteers who used CCs or HTPs or were non-smokers were stratified in three control groups (CCs, HTPs, and AIR). Participants from the experimental and control groups used 10–15 cigarettes or HTP heatsticks per day for at least one year. CC and HTP dual users were not included in the study. Information about the duration and frequency of CC/HTP usage was based on a self-reported questionnaire signed by each study participant. All participants from the experimental and control groups were matched according to age, gender, duration, and frequency of CC and HTP usage. An exclusion criterion for all groups was if participants had previously been diagnosed with any other disease instead of the one that was being investigated. Precisely, this included pregnancy, organ-specific autoimmune diseases (Addison's disease, autoimmune hepatitis, coeliac disease, Grave's disease, Guillain–Barre syndrome, Hashimoto's thyroiditis, Crohn's disease, multiple sclerosis, myasthenia gravis, pernicious anemia, primary biliary cholangitis, sclerosing cholangitis, etc.), systemic autoimmune diseases (systemic lupus erythematosus, polymyositis, dermatomyositis, rheumatoid arthritis, systemic sclerosis, Sjögren's syndrome, etc.), psoriasis, fatty liver disease, liver cirrhosis, hepatitis A-E, and malignant and other life-treating diseases (heart failure, arrythmias, renal insufficiency, respiratory insufficiency, fulminant liver injury, etc.).

All experiments were approved by the local Ethics Committees of University Clinical Center of Kragujevac (No. 01/22-341), University Clinical Center "Bezanijska Kosa" (No. 1711/1), and the Institute for Pulmonary Diseases of Vojvodina, Sremska Kamenica (No. 21-IV/3). The Declaration of Helsinki and *Principles of Good Clinical Practice* were always followed. Each patient provided informed consent before having their blood analyzed.

2.2. Isolation of Immune Cells

For the isolation of immune cells from the study participants, blood samples were obtained in heparinized collection tubes. Leukocytes were separated from erythrocytes and dead cells by Ficoll Paque (Amersham Biosciences, Otelfingen, Switzerland) gradient centrifugation, as previously described [20].

2.3. Intracellular Staining and Flow Cytometry Analysis of Immune Cells

Isolated immune cells (1×10^6 cells per sample) were stained for the intracellular content of TNF-α, IFN-γ, TGF-β, IL-1β, IL-4, IL-5, IL-6, IL-10, IL-12, IL-13, IL-17, IL-22, IL-23 and IL-35 by using the fixation/permeabilization kit and appropriate anti-human monoclonal antibodies conjugated with fluorescein isothiocyanate (FITC), phycoerythrin (PE), peridinin chlorophyll protein (PerCP), or allophycocyanin (APC) (BD Biosciences, San Jose, CA, USA) [21]. Flow cytometric analysis was conducted on a BD Biosciences FACSCalibur. The acquired data were analyzed using the Flowing software analysis program (version 2.5.1; Turku Bioscience Centre, Turku, Finland).

2.4. Measurement of Cytokines in Serum Samples

The concentrations of inflammatory and immunosuppressive cytokines (TNF-α, IFN-γ, TGF-β, IL-1β, IL-4, IL-5, IL-6, IL-10, IL-12, IL-13, IL-17, IL-22, IL-23, and IL-35) were determined in the serum samples previously obtained from the study participants. For this purpose, the blood samples were centrifuged for 15 min, and then the serum was removed and kept at −80 °C. Commercial enzyme-linked immunosorbent assay (ELISA) kits (R&D Systems, Minneapolis, MN, USA) were used in accordance with the manufacturer's instructions.

2.5. Statistics

Statistical analyses were performed using SPSS 21.0 for Windows software (SPSS, Inc., Chicago, IL, USA). The distribution of the data was checked by the Shapiro–Wilk or Kolmogorov–Smirnov test. Differences between mean values within groups were determined using one-way ANOVA. In cases when ANOVA identified a significant difference, individual differences were examined using two tailed Student's t tests with a Tukey correction for multiple comparisons. The normality of the data distribution was investigated by Kolmogorov–Smirnov or Shapiro–Wilk tests according to the number of patients. After testing for normality, correlations were tested with the appropriate correlation coefficient: Pearson or Spearman's. A multivariate linear regression model was used to discover deeper relations between clinical factors and measured levels of cytokines in the serum of the patients. The level of significance was $p < 0.05$. Data are expressed as the mean $\pm$ SEM for each group. All reported p values were 2-sided, and $p < 0.05$ was considered statistically significant.

3. Results

3.1. Continuous Use of Either CCs or HTPs Modulates Cytokine Production in Immune Cells of COPD Patients

Lung-infiltrated immune cells, through the production of TNF-α, IL-1β, IL-6, IL-13, IL-17, IL-22, and IL-23, induce chronic lung inflammation, mucous hypersecretion, and ciliary dysfunction, which lead to airflow obstruction and hyperinflation that are clinically diagnosed by decreased FEV1 ($COPD^{AIR}$ (74.57 $\pm$ 5.34) vs. $COPD^{CCs}$ (61.97 $\pm$ 7.12) and $COPD^{HTPs}$ (66.75 $\pm$ 4.94)) [22]. In line with these findings, we observed significantly higher numbers of inflammatory cells, as well as TNF-α-, IL-1β-, IL-13-, IL-17-, IL-22-, and IL-23-producing immune cells (Figure 1), and elevated levels of TNF-α, IL-1β, IL-13, IL-17, IL-22, and IL-23 in the serum samples of COPD patients compared to healthy individuals (Figure 2). Also, there was a positive correlation between the serum concentrations of these inflammatory cytokines and FEV1 (correlation coefficients were in the range of 0.133–0.403; $p < 0.05$), and a negative correlation between FEV1 and the serum levels of immunosuppressive IL-35 (correlation coefficients were in the range of values 0.064–0.642 with $p < 0.05$). Additionally, multivariate linear regression (adjusted R square = 28.2%, F = 7.887; $p < 0.001$) showed that the continuous use of CCs had a significant effect on FEV1 values (FEV1 values were higher than 0.728 in CC group, compared to AIR group).

By affecting cytokine production in immune cells, both HTPs and CCs altered the systemic inflammatory response in COPD patients. An increased number of immunosuppressive, IL-10-, TGF-β-, and IL-35-producing immune cells (Figure 1) and an elevated serum level of TGF-β were observed in $COPD^{HTP}$ compared to $COPD^{AIR}$ patients. The continuous use of HTPs also increased the production of Th17 cell-derived inflammatory cytokines (IL-17, IL-22) in COPD patients (Figure 1). Similarly, the long-term use of CCs increased the production of inflammatory cytokines, which importantly contributed to the development of airflow obstruction in $COPD^{CC}$ patients, affecting COPD development and progression. A significantly higher number of IL-17- and IFN-γ-producing immune cells (Figure 1) and increased serum levels of TNF-α, IL-1β, IL-17, IL-23, and IL-13 (Figure 2) were observed in $COPD^{CC}$ compared to $COPD^{AIR}$ patients.

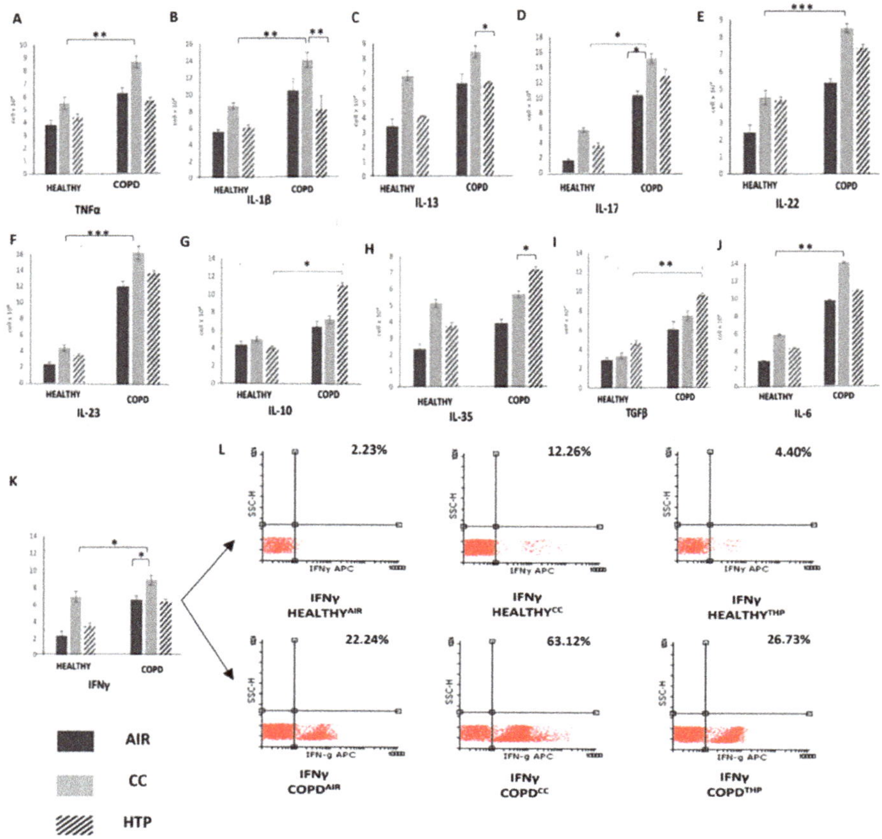

Figure 1. Continuous use of either CCs or HTPs modulates cytokine production in immune cells of COPD patients. Total numbers of TNF-α- (**A**), IL-1β- (**B**), IL-13- (**C**), IL-17- (**D**), IL-22- (**E**), IL-23- (**F**), IL-10- (**G**), IL-35- (**H**), TGF-β- (**I**), IL-6- (**J**), and IFN-γ-producing immune cells (**K**) in the blood of healthy volunteers and $COPD^{CC}$, $COPD^{HTP}$, and $COPD^{AIR}$ patients, including representative dot plots (**L**), demonstrating altered capacity for cytokine production in leukocytes of COPD patients who used CCs or HTPs. Values are presented as mean ± SEM; * $p < 0.05$, ** $p < 0.01$, *** $p < 0.001$.

Importantly, CCs and HTPs differed in their immunomodulatory properties. Higher numbers of TNF-α-, IL-1β-, IL-6-, IL-17-, and IFN-γ- producing leukocytes (Figure 1) and increased serum concentrations of TNF-α, IL-1β, IL-6, IFN-γ, IL-17, and IL-22 (Figure 2) were observed in $COPD^{CC}$ compared to $COPD^{HTP}$ patients. CCs had weaker capacity than HTPs to induce the synthesis of immunosuppressive cytokines (IL-10, IL-35) and pro-fibrotic TGF-β in COPD patients. Higher numbers of IL-10- and TGF-β-producing immune cells and remarkably higher serum levels of IL-10, IL-35, and TGF-β were observed in $COPD^{HTP}$ compared to $COPD^{CC}$ patients.

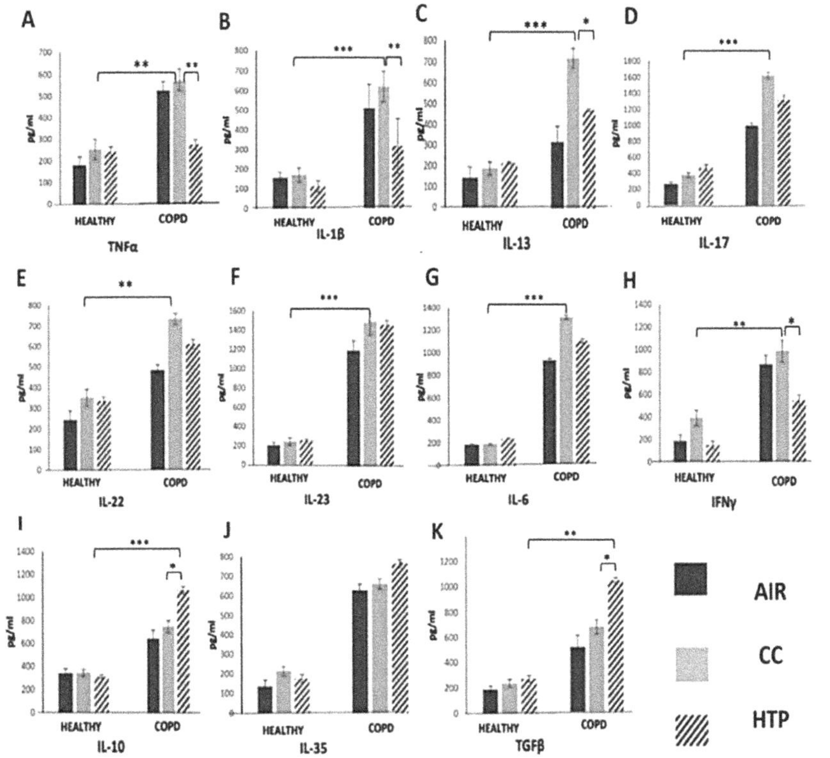

Figure 2. CC- and HTP-dependent effects on serum levels of inflammatory, pro-fibrotic, and immunosuppressive cytokines in healthy volunteers and COPD patients. Concentrations of TNF-α (**A**), IL-1β (**B**), IL-13 (**C**), IL-17 (**D**), IL-22 (**E**), IL-23 (**F**), IL-6 (**G**), IFNγ- (**H**), IL-10 (**I**), IL-35 (**J**), and TGF-β (**K**) in serum samples of healthy volunteers and $COPD^{CC}$, $COPD^{HTP}$, and $COPD^{AIR}$ patients show that both CCs and HTPs altered production of inflammatory, immunosuppressive, and pro-fibrotic cytokines in COPD patients. Values are presented as mean ± SEM; * $p < 0.05$, ** $p < 0.01$, *** $p < 0.001$.

3.2. Compared to CCs, HTPs Had Weaker Capacity to Induce Production of Th1- and Th17-Related Cytokines in Immune Cells of DM Patients

TNF-α and IL-1β are inflammatory cytokines that attract circulating leukocytes in injured pancreatic islets, importantly contributing to the aggravation of DM [23]. We observed a positive correlation between the serum concentrations of TNF-α and IL-1β and parameters of DM progression (glycemia and glycohemoglobin (HbA1c)) in DM patients who used CCs or HTPs (correlation coefficients were in the range of 0.066–0.849; $p < 0.05$). Additionally, serum levels of immunosuppressive IL-35, which attenuate the systemic inflammatory response, negatively correlated with HbA1c in DM^{CC} and DM^{HTP} patients (correlation coefficients were in the range of 0.383–0.775 with $p < 0.05$). Furthermore, multivariate linear regression (adjusted R square = 62.5%, F = 42.594; $p < 0.001$) showed that the continuous use of CCs had a significant effect on glycemia (values higher than 0.153 in CC group compared to AIR group) and HbA1c (values higher than 0.09 in CC group compared to AIR group).

Th1 and Th17 cells have an important pathogenic role in the destruction of insulin-producing pancreatic beta cells [24]. Accordingly, increased serum levels of Th1- and Th17-related inflammatory cytokines crucially contribute to the generation of systemic inflammatory response in DM patients and the development of DM-associated complications [24]. We noticed an increased number of immune cells that produced Th1- (IL-12, TNF-α, IFN-γ) and Th17-related cytokines (IL-1β, IL-6, IL-17, IL-23) (Figure 3) in the blood of DM^{CC} and DM^{HTP} compared to DM^{AIR} patients, and we observed increased concentrations of these inflammatory cytokines in the serum samples of DM^{CC} and DM^{HTP} patients (Figure 4). Compared to CCs, HTPs had a weaker capacity to induce the production of inflammatory, Th1-, and Th17-related cytokines in DM patients. Lower numbers of TNF-α-, IL-12-, IFN-γ-, IL-1β-, IL-6-, and IL-17-producing immune cells (Figure 3) and lower serum levels of TNF-α, IL-12, IFN-γ, IL-1β, IL-6, IL-17 (Figure 4) were observed in DM^{HTP} than in DM^{CC} patients.

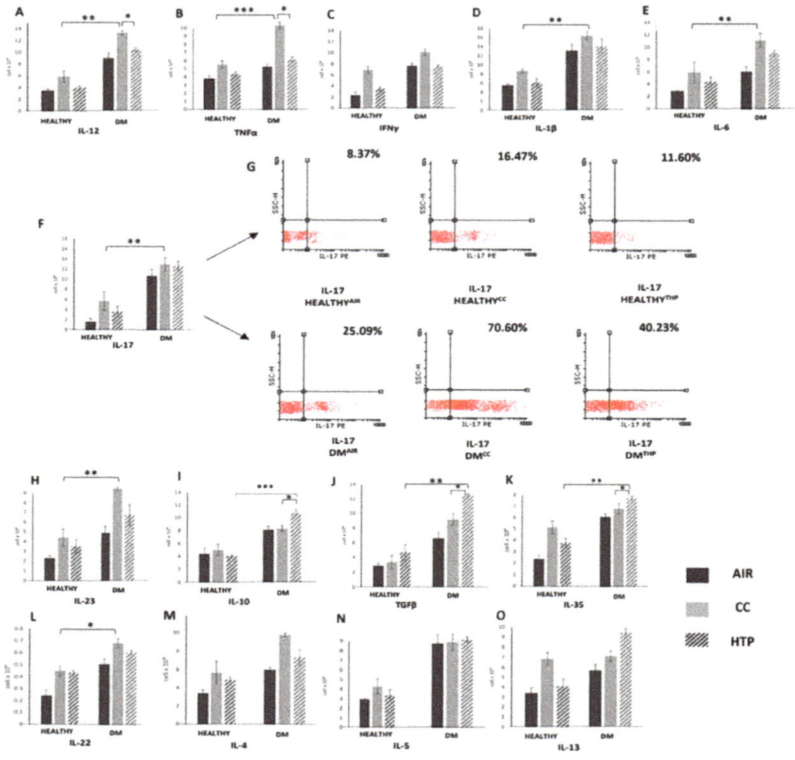

Figure 3. CC- and HTP-based modulation of cytokine production in circulating immune cells of DM patients. Total numbers of immune cells producing inflammatory, Th1-related (IL-12 (**A**), TNF-α (**B**), IFN-γ (**C**)) and Th17-related cytokines (IL-1β (**D**), IL-6 (**E**), IL-17 (**F**), IL-23 (**H**)) were lower and total numbers of immunosuppressive, IL-10- (**I**), TGF-β- (**J**), and IL-35-producing (**K**) immune cells were higher in the blood of DM^{HTP} than in the blood of DM^{CC} patients, indicating that, compared to CCs, HTPs had weaker capacity to induce the production of Th1- and Th17-related cytokines in the blood of DM patients. There was no statistical difference in the amount of IL-22 (**L**), IL-4 (**M**), IL-5 (**N**), or IL-13 (**O**) between DM^{HTP} and DM^{CC} patients. Representative dot plots show IL-17-producing cells (**G**). Values are presented as mean ± SEM; * $p < 0.05$, ** $p < 0.01$, *** $p < 0.001$.

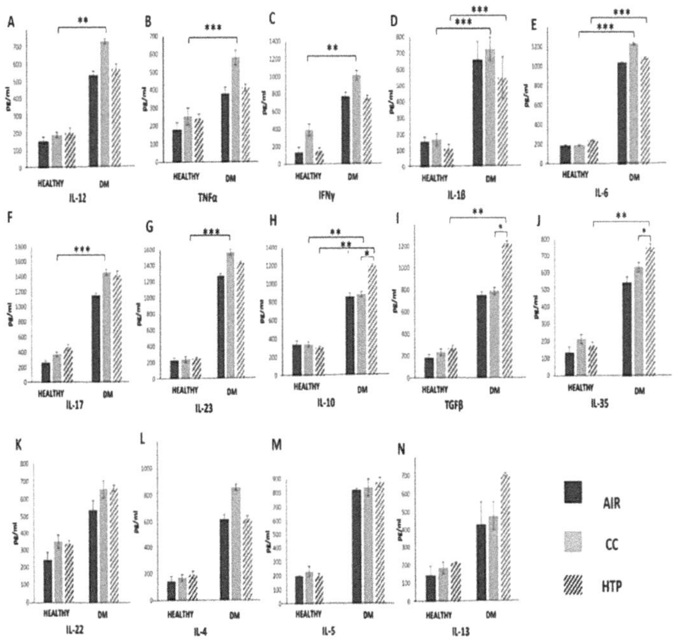

Figure 4. Effects of CCs and HTPs on serum levels of inflammatory and immunosuppressive cytokines in healthy individuals and DM patients. Concentrations of Th1-related cytokines (IL-12 (**A**), TNF-α (**B**), IFN-γ (**C**)) and Th17-related cytokines (IL-1β (**D**), IL-6 (**E**), IL-17 (**F**), IL-23 (**G**)) in serum samples of healthy volunteers and DM^{CC}, DM^{HTP}, and DM^{AIR} patients show that, in DM patients, CCs more efficiently enhanced the production of inflammatory, Th1-, and Th17-related cytokines compared to HTPs. CCs had weaker capacity than HTPs to induce the production of pro-fibrotic TGF-β (**I**) and immunosuppressive IL-10 (**H**) and IL-35 (**J**). There was no statistical difference in the concentrations of IL-22 (**K**) and Th2-related cytokines (IL-4 (**L**), IL-5 (**M**), IL-13 (**N**)) between serum samples of DM^{HTP} and DM^{CC} patients. Values are presented as mean ± SEM; * $p < 0.05$, ** $p < 0.01$, *** $p < 0.001$.

Compared to CCs, HTPs more efficiently induced the expansion of immunosuppressive, IL-10- and TGF-β-producing leukocytes, which was manifested with increased concentrations of IL-10 and TGF-β in the serum samples of DM^{HTP} compared to DM^{CC} and DM^{AIR} patients. Also, HTPs increased the serum concentration of immunosuppressive IL-35, which was higher in DM^{HTP} than in DM^{CC} patients. Both CCs and HTPs increased the synthesis of IL-22 and did not significantly alter the production of Th2-related cytokines (IL-4, IL-5, IL-13) in DM patients.

3.3. *Compared to CCs, HTPs More Efficiently Induce Production of Immunosuppressive Cytokines in Immune Cells of UC Patients*

Through the production of inflammatory and immunosuppressive cytokines, immune cells orchestrate systemic immune response, affecting UC development and progression [21,25]. Significantly increased numbers of inflammatory immune cells (Figure 5) and remarkably elevated concentrations of inflammatory cytokines (Figure 6) were observed in UC patients compared to the healthy controls. The analysis of UC patients' blood and serum samples showed that the continuous use of either CCs or HTPs modulated the secretory properties of UC patients' leukocytes, affecting UC progression. Significantly lower numbers of immune cells, which produce inflammatory cytokines that induce the systemic inflammatory response (IFN-γ, IL-1β, IL-5, IL-6, IL-12, IL-23, IL-17), and significantly lower concentrations of these cytokines were observed in the serum samples of UC^{CC} and UC^{HTP} compared to UC^{AIR} patients.

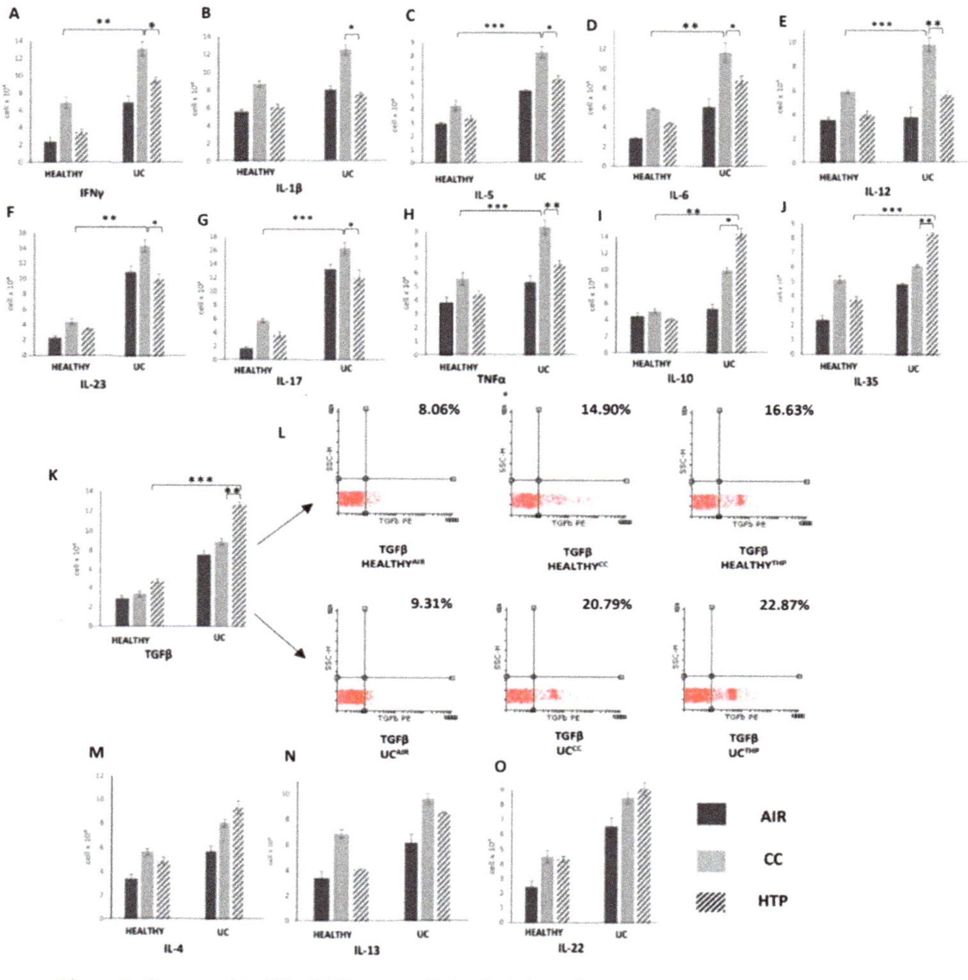

Figure 5. Compared to CCs, HTPs more efficiently induce the production of immunosuppressive cytokines in the immune cells of UC patients. Total numbers of IFN-γ- (**A**), IL-1β- (**B**), IL-5- (**C**), IL-6- (**D**), IL-12- (**E**), IL-23- (**F**), IL-17- (**G**), TNF-α- (**H**), IL-10- (**I**), IL-35- (**J**), TGF-β- (**K**), IL-4- (**M**), IL-13- (**N**), and IL-22-producing immune cells (**O**) in the blood of healthy volunteers and UC^{CC}, UC^{HTP}, and UC^{AIR} patients, including representative dot plots (**L**), demonstrate the increased presence of leukocytes producing immunosuppressive cytokines in the blood of UC^{HTP} compared to UC^{CC} patients. Values are presented as mean ± SEM; * $p < 0.05$, ** $p < 0.01$, *** $p < 0.001$.

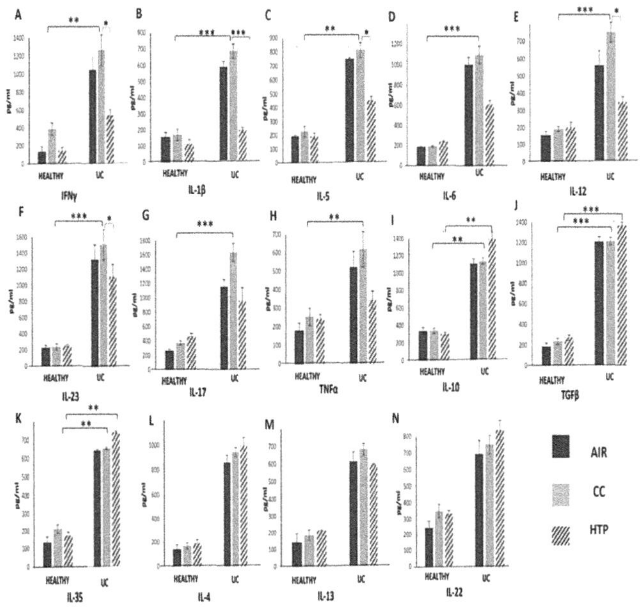

Figure 6. CC- and HTP-dependent effects on serum levels of inflammatory, pro-fibrotic, and immunosuppressive cytokines in healthy volunteers and UC patients. Concentrations of IFN-γ (**A**), IL-1β (**B**), IL-5 (**C**), IL-6 (**D**), IL-12 (**E**), IL-23 (**F**), IL-17 (**G**), TNF-α (**H**), IL-10 (**I**), IL-35 (**J**), TGF-β (**K**), IL-4 (**L**), IL-13 (**M**), and IL-22 (**N**) in serum samples of healthy volunteers and UC^{CC}, UC^{HTP} and UC^{AIR} patients show that CCs more efficiently promoted the production of inflammatory cytokines and HTPs more efficiently induced the production of immunosuppressive and pro-fibrotic cytokines in UC patients. Values are presented as mean ± SEM; * $p < 0.05$, ** $p < 0.01$, *** $p < 0.001$.

Interestingly, CCs and HTPs exhibited variances in their capacity to stimulate the production of inflammatory and immunosuppressive cytokines in UC patients. Lower numbers of IFN-γ-, IL-1β-, IL-5-, IL-6-, IL-12-, IL-23-, IL-17-, and TNF-α-producing immune cells and higher numbers of IL-10-, TGF-β- and IL-35-producing immune cells were noticed in the blood of UC^{HTP} compared to UC^{CC} patients (Figure 5). Accordingly, lower levels of IFN-γ, IL-1β, IL-5, IL-6, IL-12, IL-23, IL-17, and TNF-α and higher levels of IL-10, IL-35, and TGF-β were observed in the serum samples of UC^{HTP} compared to UC^{CC} patients (Figure 6). There were no significant differences in the concentrations of IL-4, IL-13, or IL-22 between the blood and serums samples of UC^{AIR}, UC^{CC}, and UC^{HTPs} patients.

4. Discussion

Although COPD, UC, and DM develop due to the immune-cell-driven injury of parenchymal cells in the lungs, gut, or pancreatic tissue, the systemic inflammatory response is considered crucially responsible for the aggravation and progression of these diseases [1,22–26]. Systemic inflammation can lead to increased airway inflammation and narrowing, importantly contributing to the development of acute exacerbations that can be life-threatening for patients with severe COPD [26]. In UC patients, the systemic inflammatory response can compromise the integrity of the intestinal barrier, allowing harmful substances to enter the bloodstream. This can trigger a detrimental immune response, which aggravates the inflammatory process in the colon, increasing the risk of bowel perforation [25]. In DM patients, systemic inflammation impairs insulin sensitivity, leading to poorly controlled blood sugar levels, significantly increasing the risk of stroke, diabetic nephropathy, and retinopathy [23]. In line with these findings, identifying and addressing factors that induce systemic inflammatory response in COPD, DM, and UC patients is crucially important for disease management and for improving outcomes for individuals living with these chronic conditions [1].

Herein, we have demonstrated that the continuous use of either CCs or HTPs modulates cytokine production in circulating leukocytes, affecting systemic inflammatory response in COPD, DM, and UC patients. Long-term exposure to CC-derived smoke and HTP-sourced aerosols altered immune-cell-driven inflammation, importantly contributing to the progression of these chronic inflammatory diseases.

It is well known that CC-derived smoke contains thousands of toxic chemicals that generate ROS and cause oxidative stress in alveolar epithelial cells, inducing the enhanced release of damage-associated molecular patterns (DAMPs) and alarmins into the extracellular environment [27]. These inflammatory mediators are captured by dendritic cells (DCs), initiating detrimental immune response in the lungs [28,29]. Upon binding to Toll-like receptors (TLRs) on lung DCs, DAMPs and alarmins initiate the MyD88-driven intracellular signaling pathway and induce an enhanced activation of the transcription factors NF-κβ, IRFs, and AP1, which regulate the expression of genes that elicit the production of inflammatory cytokines (TNF-α, IL-1β, IL-6, IL-17, and IFN-γ) [23,24]. Accordingly, we observed significantly higher numbers of TNF-α-, IL-1β-, IL-6-, IL-17- and IFN-γ-producing immune cells and elevated levels of these inflammatory cytokines in the blood of $COPD^{CC}$ compared to $COPD^{AIR}$ patients (Figures 1 and 2). Since TNF-α, IL-1β, and IL-6 are key mediators of systemic inflammation [1], we assume that the CC-dependent increased production of these cytokines was mainly responsible for the generation of detrimental immune response in $COPD^{CC}$ patients. TNF-α, IL-1β, and IL-6 increased the expression of adhesion molecules on the lung ECs of CC users, facilitating the recruitment of immune cells into the inflamed lungs [30]. Additionally, TNF-α and IL-1β trigger an NF-kB-driven intracellular signaling cascade in lung-infiltrated Th17 lymphocytes, enhancing the production of IL-17, which promotes the production of ROS, elastases, and matrix metalloproteinases (MMPs) in neutrophils, exacerbating tissue destruction and remodeling in the lungs of COPD patients [31]. In addition to increased serum levels of TNF-α, IL-1β, and IL-6, prolonged exposure to CC-derived smoke also increased the production of IL-13, which stimulated the goblet cells to produce and secrete mucus [32]. Excessive mucus production can aggravate airway obstruction, impair mucociliary clearance, and increase susceptibility to respiratory infections in $COPD^{CC}$ patients [33]. Additionally, the increased concentration of IL-13 could enhance collagen deposition, smooth muscle hypertrophy, and fibrosis, aggravating airway hyperresponsiveness in $COPD^{CC}$ patients [32,33]. In line with these findings, it can be concluded that the long-term use of CCs significantly increases the risk of exacerbating and aggravating COPD.

Compared to CCs, HTPs had an impaired capacity to induce the secretion of inflammatory, pro-Th1, and pro-Th17 cytokines, but managed to more efficiently enhance the production of immunosuppressive cytokines in COPD patients (Figures 1 and 2). Although these findings may indicate that the long-term use of HTPs could be less harmful to COPD patients than CCs, it has to be highlighted that continuous exposure to HTP-derived aerosols also significantly increased the presence of TGF-β-secreting immune cells in the blood of $COPD^{HTP}$ patients (Figures 1 and 2). TGF-β plays a central role in the development of pulmonary fibrosis in response to lung injury and inflammation [34,35]. It induces epithelial-to-mesenchymal transition and stimulates the differentiation of fibroblasts into myofibroblasts, enabling the massive production and deposition of collagen in inflamed lungs [34,35]. Additionally, the excessive secretion of TGF-β may result in the formation of disorganized blood vessels in inflamed lungs, further contributing to the aggravation of lung inflammation and fibrosis [34]. Since continuous exposure to HTP-derived aerosols increased the production of pro-fibrotic TGF-β in $COPD^{HTP}$ patients (Figures 1 and 2), up-coming experimental and clinical studies should focus on investigating the effects of HTP-derived aerosols on the TGF-β-dependent development and progression of lung fibrosis.

In a similar manner as was observed in COPD patients, CCs and HTPs differed in their capacity to regulate the secretion of inflammatory and immunosuppressive cytokines in the immune cells of DM patients (Figures 3 and 4). Higher numbers of leukocytes producing pro-Th1 (TNF-α, IL-12, IFN-γ) and pro-Th17 cytokines (IL-17, IL-1β, IL-6, IL-22, IL-23) were observed in the blood of DM^{CC} compared to DM^{HTP} patients (Figure 3). The NF-kB-dependent signaling pathway is activated in immune cells that are continuously exposed to CC-derived smoke [36]. By triggering an NF-kB-driven intracellular cascade in neutrophils, DCs, macrophages, and T lymphocytes, CCs enhance the secretion of inflammatory cytokines, crucially contributing to the development of systemic, Th1-, and Th17-cell-driven immune response, which aggravates on-going inflammation in the pancreatic islets [23,24,36]. In line with these findings, we noticed a positive correlation between parameters of DM progression (glycemia, HbA1c) and concentrations of Th1- and Th17-related cytokines in the serum samples of DM patients who continuously used CCs.

The total numbers of inflammatory immune cells and the serum levels of inflammatory cytokines were also higher in DM^{HTPs} compared to DM^{AIR} patients (Figures 3 and 4), suggesting that continuous exposure to HTP-derived aerosols also generated a detrimental systemic inflammatory response in DM patients. Importantly, compared to CCs, HTPs more efficiently promoted the production of immunosuppressive cytokines (IL-10 and IL-35) in the leukocytes of DM patients, and therefore, HTP-dependent systemic inflammation was weaker than the systemic immune response elicited by CC-derived smoke. In a similar manner as was observed in $COPD^{HTP}$ patients, long-term exposure to HTP-derived aerosols enhanced the synthesis of pro-fibrotic TGF-β in the immune cells of DM^{HTP} patients, increasing the risk of the development of excessive fibrosis [34]. Additionally, the increased production of TGF-β has been linked with an increased activity of osteoclasts and with the aggravation of osteoporosis in DM patients [37]. Since DM patients have lower bone mineral density and are at a higher risk of developing osteoporosis [38], the long-term consequences of the HTP-dependent activation of the TGF-β pathway in immune cells on the development and progression of osteoporosis in DM^{HTP} patients should be explored in detail in future experimental and clinical studies.

In contrast to the findings observed in COPD and DM patients, the use of CCs and HTPs did not significantly aggravate the systemic inflammatory response in UC patients (Figures 5 and 6). Continuous exposure to CC-derived smoke and HTP-derived aerosols did not increase the production of inflammatory cytokines that play a pathogenic role in the development and progression of colon injury (Figure 6). Importantly, HTPs managed to induce the expansion of IL-10- and IL-35-producing immunosuppressive immune cells in the blood of UC patients (Figure 5). Since nicotine may regulate the phenotype and function of immune cells in the gut [39], we assume that nicotine was mainly responsible for the expansion of immunosuppressive cells. By interacting with α7 nAChR on DCs and macrophages, nicotine enhances the production of anti-inflammatory IL-10, leading to the generation of immunosuppressive Tregs [40]. Furthermore, nicotine activates the α7 nAChR/PI3K/Akt/Erk1/Erk2 signaling pathway, promoting the self-renewal and proliferation of Tregs and enhancing their ability to produce immunosuppressive IL-35 [40].

Considering that nicotine concentration is approximately the same in HTP-derived aerosols and in CC-sourced smoke [18], we hypothesize that lower numbers of immunosuppressive immune cells in UC^{CC} compared to UC^{HTP} patients developed as a consequence of different CC- and HTP-dependent tobacco processing. The HTP-specific heating process occurs at lower temperatures than CC-associated combustion, resulting in the production of aerosols which have different compounds than CC-derived smoke [18]. CC-derived smoke contains carbon monoxide (CO) and tar [41]. CO- and tar-containing oxidants generate ROS, which induce oxidative stress, DNA damage, and apoptosis in rapidly proliferating immunosuppressive immune cells [42]. HTPs do not generate tar, and the level of CO in HTP-derived aerosols was found to be 1% of that contained in CC-sourced smoke [18]. Additionally, CC-derived smoke contains benzene, 1, 3 butadiene, acrylonitrile, and ethylene oxide, which negatively affect the proliferation of activated Tregs in the colons of UC patients [43,44]. Consequently, it is highly probable that the reduced number of immunosuppressive leukocytes in the blood of UC^{CC} compared to UC^{HTP} patients was primarily due to the toxic effects CC-derived smoke on their viability and proliferation.

In summary, due to different methods of tobacco processing, CC-sourced smoke and HTP-derived aerosols contain different chemical constituents and, therefore, possess different immunomodulatory characteristics. The toxic chemicals contained in CC-derived smoke (CO, benzene, 1, 3 butadiene, acrylonitrile, ethylene oxide, etc.) induce oxidative stress in immune cells, elicit an MAPK-signaling cascade, and activate transcriptional factors NF-kB and AP-1, which results in the enhanced production of inflammatory cytokines and in the generation of a potent systemic inflammatory response [11,12,41]. HTP-dependent tobacco processing does not involve combustion, and therefore the concentrations of all these combustion-associated toxic compounds are present at a value of less than 1% in HTP-derived aerosols [16,17]. Compared to CCs, HTPs have weaker capacity to induce the production of inflammatory cytokines, but they are able to more efficiently induce the activation of the PI3K/Erk-driven signaling pathway in circulating immune cells, resulting in the increased synthesis of immunosuppressive cytokines and pro-fibrotic TGF-β [16,17].

Accordingly, the long-term use of either CCs or HTPs significantly modulated cytokine production in circulating leukocytes, affecting the systemic inflammatory response in patients suffering from chronic inflammatory diseases. The continuous use of CCs and HTPs aggravated immune-cell-driven systemic inflammation in COPD and DM patients, but not in UC patients, suggesting that the immunomodulatory effects of CC-derived smoke and HTP-sourced aerosols are disease-specific. Therefore, the immunomodulatory effects of CCs and HTPs cannot be generalized, and have to be determined for particular immune-cell-driven inflammatory diseases. In this study, all members of the experimental and control groups were matched according to the frequency and duration of CC/HTP usage, as well as demographic and clinical parameters, which resulted in a relatively small number of participants in some groups, potentially affecting the statistical power of the study. Therefore, the results presented in this study should be considered as a starting point for the design and implementation of up-coming experimental and larger clinical studies, which should analyze CC- and HTP-dependent alterations in cytokine-related intracellular signaling pathways in immune cells that infiltrate particular inflamed organs in detail.

It should be also noted that, in this study, short- and mid-term effects of CCs and HTPs on immune-cell-driven systemic inflammation were determined and that samples were obtained only from Serbian patients, suggesting limited generalizability of the findings to other populations or regions. Therefore, future clinical trials should include patients from different parts of the world and should determine the long-term consequences of CC- and HTP-dependent immunomodulation on the progression of chronic inflammatory disease.

Author Contributions: Conceptualization, V.V.; methodology, I.C., V.S., V.M., A.D., A.V., M.B., T.G., M.Z. and J.B.-M.; software, N.Z. (Nebojsa Zdravkovic); formal analysis, N.K., N.Z. (Nebojsa Zdravkovic) and V.V.; resources, A.D., M.B., T.G., M.Z. and J.B.-M.; data curation, N.K., N.Z. (Natasa Zdravkovic), I.C., V.S. and V.M.; writing—original draft preparation, A.V. and V.V.; writing—review and editing, C.R.H. and V.D.; funding acquisition, V.V. All authors have read and agreed to the published version of the manuscript.

Funding: This study was funded by a grant from the Foundation for a Smoke-Free World, Inc. (FSFW) (the grant No. W3-032). Through September 2023, the Foundation received charitable gifts from PMI Global Services Inc. ("PMI"). Independent from PMI since its founding in 2017, the Foundation continues to operate in a manner that ensures its independence from any commercial entity. FSFW's mission is to end smoking in this generation. For more information about FSFW, please visit its website (https://www.smokefreeworld.org). This study was also supported by grants from the Ministry of Science Republic of Serbia (451-03-65/2024-03/200111) and the Faculty of Medical Sciences University of Kragujevac (MP01/18).

Institutional Review Board Statement: The study was conducted in accordance with the Declaration of Helsinki, and approved by the Ethics Committee of of University Clinical Center of Kragujevac

(No. 01/22-341), University Clinical Center "Bezanijska Kosa" (No. 1711/1), and the Institute for Pulmonary Diseases of Vojvodina, Sremska Kamenica (No. 21-IV/3).

Informed Consent Statement: Informed consent was obtained from all subjects involved in the study.

Data Availability Statement: The data that support the findings of this study are available from the corresponding author upon reasonable request.

Conflicts of Interest: Author Carl Randall Harrell was employed by the company Regenerative Processing Plant. The remaining authors declare that the research was conducted in the absence of any commercial or financial relationships that could be construed as a potential conflict of interest.

References

1. Chen, L.; Deng, H.; Cui, H.; Fang, J.; Zuo, Z.; Deng, J.; Li, Y.; Wang, X.; Zhao, L. Inflammatory responses and inflammation-associated diseases in organs. *Oncotarget* **2017**, *9*, 7204–7218. [CrossRef] [PubMed]
2. Antar, S.A.; Ashour, N.A.; Marawan, M.E.; Al-Karmalawy, A.A. Fibrosis: Types, Effects, Markers, Mechanisms for Disease Progression, and Its Relation with Oxidative Stress, Immunity, and Inflammation. *Int. J. Mol. Sci.* **2023**, *24*, 4004. [CrossRef] [PubMed]
3. Palomo, M.; Moreno-Castaño, A.B.; Salas, M.Q.; Escribano-Serrat, S.; Rovira, M.; Guillen-Olmos, E.; Fernandez, S.; Ventosa-Capell, H.; Youssef, L.; Crispi, F.; et al. Endothelial activation and damage as a common pathological substrate in different pathologies and cell therapy complications. *Front. Med.* **2023**, *10*, 1285898. [CrossRef] [PubMed]
4. Xiang, Y.; Zhang, M.; Jiang, D.; Su, Q.; Shi, J. The role of inflammation in autoimmune disease: A therapeutic target. *Front. Immunol.* **2023**, *14*, 1267091. [CrossRef] [PubMed]
5. Kastratovic, N.; Markovic, V.; Harrell, C.R.; Arsenijevic, A.; Stojanovic, M.D.; Djonov, V.; Volarevic, V. Effects of combustible cigarettes and electronic nicotine delivery systems on the development and progression of chronic lung inflammation in mice. *Nicotine Tob. Res.* **2023**, *26*, 704–714. [CrossRef] [PubMed]
6. Pavlovic, D.; Miloradovic, D.; Stojanovic, M.D.; Harrell, C.R.; Polosa, R.; Rust, S.; Volti, G.L.; Caruso, M.; Jakovljevic, V.; Djonov, V.; et al. Cigarette smoke attenuates mesenchymal stem cell-based suppression of immune cell-driven acute liver failure. *Toxicol. Lett.* **2023**, *385*, 12–20. [CrossRef] [PubMed]
7. Caruso, M.; Emma, R.; Distefano, A.; Rust, S.; Poulas, K.; Giordano, A.; Volarevic, V.; Mesiakaris, K.; Boffo, S.; Arsenijevic, A.; et al. Comparative assessment of electronic nicotine delivery systems aerosol and cigarette smoke on endothelial cell migration: The Replica Project. *Drug Test Anal.* **2023**, *15*, 1164–1174. [CrossRef] [PubMed]
8. Russell, A.E.; Liao, Z.; Tkach, M.; Tarwater, P.M.; Ostrowski, M.; Théry, C.; Witwer, K.W. Cigarette smoke-induced extracellular vesicles from dendritic cells alter T-cell activation and HIV replication. *Toxicol. Lett.* **2022**, *360*, 33–43. [CrossRef] [PubMed]
9. Lugg, S.T.; Scott, A.; Parekh, D.; Naidu, B.; Thickett, D.R. Cigarette smoke exposure and alveolar macrophages: Mechanisms for lung disease. *Thorax* **2022**, *77*, 94–101. [CrossRef]
10. Chen, J.; Wang, X.; Schmalen, A.; Haines, S.; Wolff, M.; Ma, H.; Zhang, H.; Stoleriu, M.G.; Nowak, J.; Nakayama, M.; et al. Antiviral CD8+ T-cell immune responses are impaired by cigarette smoke and in COPD. *Eur. Respir. J.* **2023**, *62*, 2201374. [CrossRef]
11. Qiu, F.; Liang, C.L.; Liu, H.; Zeng, Y.Q.; Hou, S.; Huang, S.; Lai, X.; Dai, Z. Impacts of cigarette smoking on immune responsiveness: Up and down or upside down? *Oncotarget* **2017**, *8*, 268–284. [CrossRef] [PubMed]
12. White, P.C.; Hirschfeld, J.; Milward, M.R.; Cooper, P.R.; Wright, H.J.; Matthews, J.B.; Chapple, I.L.C. Cigarette smoke modifies neutrophil chemotaxis, neutrophil extracellular trap formation and inflammatory response-related gene expression. *J. Periodontal Res.* **2018**, *53*, 525–535. [CrossRef] [PubMed]
13. Shaykhiev, R.; Krause, A.; Salit, J.; Strulovici-Barel, Y.; Harvey, B.G.; O'Connor, T.P.; Crystal, R.G. Smoking-dependent reprogramming of alveolar macrophage polarization: Implication for pathogenesis of chronic obstructive pulmonary disease. *J. Immunol.* **2009**, *183*, 2867–2883. [CrossRef] [PubMed]
14. Thatcher, T.H.; Benson, R.P.; Phipps, R.P.; Sime, P.J. High-dose but not low-dose mainstream cigarette smoke suppresses allergic airway inflammation by inhibiting T cell function. *Am. J. Physiol.-Lung Cell Mol. Physiol.* **2008**, *295*, L412–L421. [CrossRef]
15. Ortiz-Quintero, B.; Martínez-Espinosa, I.; Pérez-Padilla, R. Mechanisms of Lung Damage and Development of COPD Due to Household Biomass-Smoke Exposure: Inflammation, Oxidative Stress, MicroRNAs, and Gene Polymorphisms. *Cells* **2022**, *12*, 67. [CrossRef] [PubMed]
16. Simonavicius, E.; McNeill, A.; Shahab, L.; Brose, L.S. Heat-not-burn tobacco products: A systematic literature review. *Tob. Control* **2019**, *28*, 582–594. [CrossRef] [PubMed]
17. Znyk, M.; Jurewicz, J.; Kaleta, D. Exposure to Heated Tobacco Products and Adverse Health Effects, a Systematic Review. *Int. J. Environ. Res. Public Health* **2021**, *18*, 6651. [CrossRef] [PubMed]
18. St Helen, G.; Jacob Iii, P.; Nardone, N.; Benowitz, N.L. IQOS: Examination of Philip Morris International's claim of reduced exposure. *Tob. Control* **2018**, *27*, s30–s36. [CrossRef] [PubMed]
19. Kastratovic, N.; Cekerevac, I.; Sekerus, V.; Markovic, V.; Arsenijevic, A.; Volarevic, A.; Harrell, C.R.; Jakovljevic, V.; Djonov, V.; Volarevic, V. Effects of combustible cigarettes and heated tobacco products on immune cell-driven inflammation in chronic obstructive respiratory diseases. *Toxicol. Sci.* **2024**, kfae068. [CrossRef]

20. Acovic, A.; Simovic Markovic, B.; Gazdic, M.; Arsenijevic, A.; Jovicic, N.; Gajovic, N.; Jovanovic, M.; Zdravkovic, N.; Kanjevac, T.; Harrell, C.R.; et al. Indoleamine 2,3-dioxygenase-dependent expansion of T-regulatory cells maintains mucosal healing in ulcerative colitis. *Therap. Adv. Gastroenterol.* **2018**, *11*, 1756284818793558. [CrossRef]
21. Volarevic, V.; Zdravkovic, N.; Harrell, C.R.; Arsenijevic, N.; Fellabaum, C.; Djonov, V.; Lukic, M.L.; Simovic Markovic, B. Galectin-3 Regulates Indoleamine-2,3-dioxygenase-Dependent Cross-Talk between Colon-Infiltrating Dendritic Cells and T Regulatory Cells and May Represent a Valuable Biomarker for Monitoring the Progression of Ulcerative Colitis. *Cells* **2019**, *8*, 709. [CrossRef] [PubMed]
22. Rajabi, H.; Mortazavi, D.; Konyalilar, N.; Aksoy, G.T.; Erkan, S.; Korkunc, S.K.; Kayalar, O.; Bayram, H.; Rahbarghazi, R. Forthcoming complications in recovered COVID-19 patients with COPD and asthma; possible therapeutic opportunities. *Cell Commun. Signal* **2022**, *20*, 173. [CrossRef] [PubMed]
23. Rohm, T.V.; Meier, D.T.; Olefsky, J.M.; Donath, M.Y. Inflammation in obesity, diabetes, and related disorders. *Immunity* **2022**, *55*, 31–55. [CrossRef] [PubMed]
24. Solt, L.A.; Burris, T.P. Th17 cells in Type 1 diabetes: A future perspective. *Diabetes Manag.* **2015**, *5*, 247–250. [CrossRef] [PubMed]
25. Tatiya-Aphiradee, N.; Chatuphonprasert, W.; Jarukamjorn, K. Immune response and inflammatory pathway of ulcerative colitis. *J. Basic Clin. Physiol. Pharmacol.* **2018**, *30*, 1–10. [CrossRef] [PubMed]
26. Groenewegen, K.H.; Postma, D.S.; Hop, W.C.; Wielders, P.L.; Schlösser, N.J.; Wouters, E.F.; COSMIC Study Group. Increased systemic inflammation is a risk factor for COPD exacerbations. *Chest* **2008**, *133*, 350–357. [CrossRef] [PubMed]
27. Cha, S.R.; Jang, J.; Park, S.M.; Ryu, S.M.; Cho, S.J.; Yang, S.R. Cigarette Smoke-Induced Respiratory Response: Insights into Cellular Processes and Biomarkers. *Antioxidants* **2023**, *12*, 1210. [CrossRef] [PubMed]
28. Cook, P.C.; MacDonald, A.S. Dendritic cells in lung immunopathology. *Semin. Immunopathol.* **2016**, *38*, 449–460. [CrossRef]
29. Piccinini, A.M.; Midwood, K.S. Dampening inflammation by modulating TLR signalling. *Mediat. Inflamm.* **2010**, *2010*, 672395. [CrossRef] [PubMed]
30. Shyam Prasad Shetty, B.; Chaya, S.K.; Kumar, V.S.; Mahendra, M.; Jayaraj, B.S.; Lokesh, K.S.; Ganguly, K.; Mahesh, P.A. Inflammatory Biomarkers Interleukin 1 Beta (IL-1β) and Tumour Necrosis Factor Alpha (TNF-α) Are Differentially Elevated in Tobacco Smoke Associated COPD and Biomass Smoke Associated COPD. *Toxics* **2021**, *9*, 72. [CrossRef]
31. Kubysheva, N.; Boldina, M.; Eliseeva, T.; Soodaeva, S.; Klimanov, I.; Khaletskaya, A.; Bayrasheva, V.; Solovyev, V.; Villa-Vargas, L.A.; Ramírez-Salinas, M.A.; et al. Relationship of Serum Levels of IL-17, IL-18, TNF-α, and Lung Function Parameters in Patients with COPD, Asthma-COPD Overlap, and Bronchial Asthma. *Mediat. Inflamm.* **2020**, *2020*, 4652898. [CrossRef] [PubMed]
32. Cooper, P.R.; Poll, C.T.; Barnes, P.J.; Sturton, R.G. Involvement of IL-13 in tobacco smoke-induced changes in the structure and function of rat intrapulmonary airways. *Am. J. Respir. Cell Mol. Biol.* **2010**, *43*, 220–226. [CrossRef] [PubMed]
33. Choudhury, P.; Biswas, S.; Singh, G.; Pal, A.; Ghosh, N.; Ojha, A.K.; Das, S.; Dutta, G.; Chaudhury, K. Immunological profiling and development of a sensing device for detection of IL-13 in COPD and asthma. *Bioelectrochemistry* **2022**, *143*, 107971. [CrossRef] [PubMed]
34. Saito, A.; Horie, M.; Nagase, T. TGF-β Signaling in Lung Health and Disease. *Int. J. Mol. Sci.* **2018**, *19*, 2460. [CrossRef] [PubMed]
35. Fernandez, I.E.; Eickelberg, O. The impact of TGF-β on lung fibrosis: From targeting to biomarkers. *Proc. Am. Thorac. Soc.* **2012**, *9*, 111–116. [CrossRef] [PubMed]
36. Chung, S.; Sundar, I.K.; Hwang, J.W.; Yull, F.E.; Blackwell, T.S.; Kinnula, V.L.; Bulger, M.; Yao, H.; Rahman, I. NF-κB inducing kinase, NIK mediates cigarette smoke/TNFα-induced histone acetylation and inflammation through differential activation of IKKs. *PLoS ONE* **2011**, *6*, e23488. [CrossRef] [PubMed]
37. Kum, J.J.Y.; Howlett, C.J.; Khan, Z.A. Dysregulated transforming growth factor-beta mediates early bone marrow dysfunction in diabetes. *Commun. Biol.* **2022**, *5*, 1145. [CrossRef] [PubMed]
38. Wongdee, K.; Charoenphandhu, N. Osteoporosis in diabetes mellitus: Possible cellular and molecular mechanisms. *World J. Diabetes* **2011**, *2*, 41–48. [CrossRef]
39. Mahmoudzadeh, L.; Abtahi Froushani, S.M.; Ajami, M.; Mahmoudzadeh, M. Effect of Nicotine on Immune System Function. *Adv. Pharm. Bull.* **2023**, *13*, 69–78. [CrossRef]
40. Nakata, Y.; Miura, K.; Yamasaki, N.; Ogata, S.; Miura, S.; Hosomi, N.; Kaminuma, O. Expression and Function of Nicotinic Acetylcholine Receptors in Induced Regulatory T Cells. *Int. J. Mol. Sci.* **2022**, *23*, 1779. [CrossRef]
41. Talhout, R.; Schulz, T.; Florek, E.; van Benthem, J.; Wester, P.; Opperhuizen, A. Hazardous compounds in tobacco smoke. *Int. J. Environ. Res. Public Health* **2011**, *8*, 613–628. [CrossRef] [PubMed]
42. Chen, X.; Song, M.; Zhang, B.; Zhang, Y. Reactive Oxygen Species Regulate T Cell Immune Response in the Tumor Microenvironment. *Oxidative Med. Cell. Longev.* **2016**, *2016*, 1580967. [CrossRef] [PubMed]
43. Soeteman-Hernández, L.G.; Bos, P.M.; Talhout, R. Tobacco smoke-related health effects induced by 1,3-butadiene and strategies for risk reduction. *Toxicol. Sci.* **2013**, *136*, 566–580. [CrossRef] [PubMed]
44. Berkowitz, L.; Schultz, B.M.; Salazar, G.A.; Pardo-Roa, C.; Sebastián, V.P.; Álvarez-Lobos, M.M.; Bueno, S.M. Impact of Cigarette Smoking on the Gastrointestinal Tract Inflammation: Opposing Effects in Crohn's Disease and Ulcerative Colitis. *Front. Immunol.* **2018**, *9*, 74. [CrossRef]

International Journal of
Molecular Sciences

MDPI

Article

Mild Systemic Inflammation Increases Erythrocyte Fragility

Charlotte M. Stuart [1,†], Carmen Jacob [1,2,†], Aravinthan Varatharaj [1], Sarah Howard [3], Joe K. Chouhan [3], Jessica L. Teeling [3] and Ian Galea [1,2,*]

[1] Clinical Neurosciences, Clinical and Experimental Sciences, Faculty of Medicine, University of Southampton, Southampton SO16 6YD, UK
[2] Wessex Neurological Centre, University Hospital Southampton NHS Foundation Trust, Southampton SO16 6YD, UK
[3] Biological Sciences, Faculty of Life Sciences, University of Southampton, Southampton SO16 6YD, UK
* Correspondence: i.galea@soton.ac.uk
† These authors contributed substantially in this order.

Abstract: There is growing evidence that inflammation impairs erythrocyte structure and function. We assessed the impact of mild systemic inflammation on erythrocyte fragility in three different settings. In order to investigate causation, erythrocyte osmotic fragility was measured in mice challenged with a live attenuated bacterial strain to induce low-grade systemic inflammation; a significant increase in erythrocyte osmotic fragility was observed. To gather evidence that systemic inflammation is associated with erythrocyte fragility in humans, two observational studies were conducted. First, using a retrospective study design, the relationship between reticulocyte-based surrogate markers of haemolysis and high-sensitivity C-reactive protein was investigated in 9292 healthy participants of the UK Biobank project. Secondly, we prospectively assessed the relationship between systemic inflammation (measured by the urinary neopterin/creatinine ratio) and erythrocyte osmotic fragility in a mixed population (n = 54) of healthy volunteers and individuals with long-term medical conditions. Both human studies were in keeping with a relationship between inflammation and erythrocyte fragility. Taken together, we conclude that mild systemic inflammation increases erythrocyte fragility and may contribute to haemolysis. Further research is needed to assess the molecular underpinnings of this pathway and the clinical implications in inflammatory conditions.

Keywords: haemolysis; red blood cell; erythrocyte; fragility; inflammation

1. Introduction

There is growing evidence that erythrocytes may be affected by inflammatory processes. Patients with COVID-19 have been found to have smaller and less deformable erythrocytes compared to controls, with differences still detectable four to eight months following hospital discharge [1]. Changes to erythrocyte deformability have also been observed in patients with other conditions associated with inflammation, such as obesity [2], cardiovascular disease [3], sepsis [4], and vitamin D status [5,6].

Particularly in sepsis models, a number of pathways have been described through which inflammation may impact erythrocytes, such as mechanical factors, energy deficiency, and oxidative stress. Amongst mechanical factors, vascular changes during systemic inflammation can lead to microangiopathic haemolysis [7,8]. Reduced capillary flow and microvascular stasis, as seen in excessive inflammation associated with sepsis, increase erythrocyte fragility through mechanical and enzymatic cell damage [8,9]. Higher glucose consumption by immune processes during inflammation can severely restrict glucose availability [10,11]. Energy deficiency causes an increase in intracellular calcium ions, resulting in decreased deformability [12] and likely further changes, such as modulation of signals associated with erythrocyte clearance (leaflet phosphatidylserine distribution), morphology, and adhesion [4]. Most importantly, inflammation leads to oxidative stress, which, in turn, increases erythrocyte membrane rigidity and therefore reduces deformability [13]. Erythrocytes have an elaborate multi-dimensional defence system to protect themselves against oxidative stress [14], mainly because they contain a huge payload of haemoglobin which in itself is a potent oxidising agent. This defence system consists of a range of antioxidant enzymes (e.g., superoxide dismutase, glutathione peroxidase, glutathione reductase, peroxiredoxin 2, thioredoxin and its reductase, and catalase) as well as small molecules (e.g., glutathione, nicotinamide adenine dinucleotide phosphate, ascorbate, and tocopherol). As erythrocytes travel through the immediate tissue microenvironment of inflammatory foci characterised by neutrophil and/or macrophage oxidative burst activity, it is conceivable that the erythrocyte's auto-protective systems are unable to deal with the sudden oxidative load, leading to lipid and protein oxidation, damage to internal structures and membrane, a decrease in membrane fluidity and finally haemolysis. Once the erythrocyte's antioxidative defences are overwhelmed, haemoglobin may amplify this process since it is capable of auto-oxidation, a process that generates superoxide radicals that can no longer be neutralised.

Erythrocyte haemolysis is of particular interest as erythrocytes contain vast amounts of haemoglobin, which is highly toxic in its extracellular, unbound form [15]. Upon release from the erythrocyte, haemoglobin is immediately bound by haptoglobin, a very abundant plasma protein with an extremely high affinity for haemoglobin. This binding neutralizes haemoglobin toxicity, and the complex is cleared by CD163-mediated endocytosis. Damaged haemoglobin may release its toxic moiety haem, and a second-line system exists to scavenge haem by binding to haemopexin, followed by CD91-mediated clearance. If these systems are overwhelmed, free haemoglobin and haem have well-documented, dose-dependent systemic effects, most notably nitric oxide depletion, which causes platelet activation and smooth muscle contraction, leading to a variety of symptoms, including abdominal pain, dysphagia, arterial and pulmonary hypertension, and erectile dysfunction [16]. Kidney injury follows intravascular haemolysis via several pathways, such as oxidative stress, cytotoxicity, and direct and indirect pro-inflammatory signals [17]. Haem is a potent inflammatory stimulus, activating the innate immune system via multiple pathways. Administration of haem to mice resulted in increased vascular permeability, adhesion molecule expression, and leukocyte migration [18]. Also, haem acts as a danger-signalling damage-associated molecular pattern which binds to toll-like receptor 4 [19], stimulates neutrophil activation [20], leads to neutrophil extracellular trap formation [21], and activates the alternative complement pathway [22]. Haemolysis is thought to contribute to the pathogenesis of sepsis [8,23] and severe COVID-19 [24], and hence has been proposed as a new treatment target [24]. Due to its pro-inflammatory properties, extracellular haemoglobin may also be associated with atherosclerotic plaque instability [25]. Associations between extracellular haemoglobin levels and disease progression have also been demonstrated in neurological conditions such as multiple sclerosis [26].

Milder degrees of systemic inflammation may not cause haemolysis but be sufficient to induce external erythrocyte membrane damage, leading to reduced deformability. Changes to deformability and and erythrocyte morphology, such as increased red cell distribution width, have been reported in association with chronic conditions associated with systemic inflammation [2,3,27,28], but whether this is causative remains to be shown. While the effects of sepsis on erythrocytes have been studied [4], the consequences of low-grade systemic inflammation on erythrocyte fragility and haemolysis are not known.

Here, we investigate the hypothesis that mild systemic inflammation contributes to erythrocyte fragility. In a murine model, we tested the effects of a mild inflammatory challenge (with attenuated *Salmonella typhimurium*) and found that it increased erythrocyte fragility to an osmotic challenge (Study 1). Then, using retrospectively collected UK biobank data, we analysed the relationship between haemolytic and inflammatory parameters in a healthy human population and found a significant association (Study 2). Finally, we assessed the relationship between systemic inflammation and erythrocyte osmotic fragility in healthy volunteers and patients with a range of non-haematological long-term medical conditions in a prospective observational study, and confirmed an association (Study 3).

2. Results

2.1. Study 1—Murine Model

This experimental study in mice aimed to test the hypothesis that systemic inflammation leads to erythrocyte fragility. Intraperitoneal challenge with an attenuated form of *Salmonella typhimurium* was used as a model of mild systemic inflammation, which is prolonged yet short-lived [29,30]. The cytokine profile of this experimental model has been described elsewhere [30]. This model was selected over single challenges with lipopolysaccharides or cytokines since it more closely recapitulates naturally occurring mild systemic inflammation. Erythrocyte fragility was measured using an osmotic lysis assay and quantified as the median corpuscular fragility (MCF), which is the concentration of NaCl causing 50% haemolysis. Mice challenged with *Salmonella* did not become unwell but nevertheless developed weight loss at 24 h (Figure 1a; mean weight loss −7.78%, t (8) = 12.20; $p < 0.001$, r = 0.973), which they recovered within the next few days such that on day 6, their weight was not significantly different compared to baseline. Such a mild clinical picture is characteristic of the challenge with this attenuated strain of *Salmonella typhimurium* [30,31]. A one-way ANOVA was conducted to compare the erythrocyte fragility (as quantified by the MCF) of the *Salmonella*-challenged animals at each time point with that of the control mice (n = 3 per group). There was a significant difference in MCF between the bacterial challenge and control groups (F (3,8) = 10.57, p = 0.0037). Bonferroni post hoc test showed that erythrocytes from challenged mice demonstrated increased fragility at each time point compared with the control mice (24 h: mean = 5.494, p = 0.0191; 3 days: mean = 5.4650, p = 0.0370; 1 week: mean = 5.6127, p = 0.0017; Figure 1b).

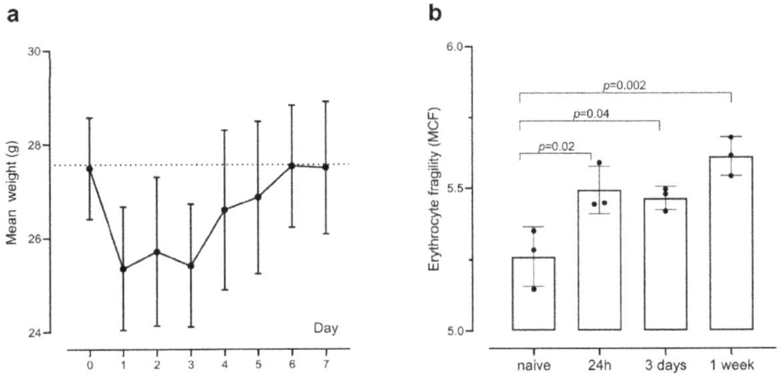

Figure 1. A mild systemic inflammatory stimulus increases erythrocyte fragility in mice. C57BL/6 mice received an intraperitoneal challenge with attenuated *Salmonella typhimurium* vaccine strain SL3261, and their erythrocyte fragility, measured in an ex vivo osmotic fragility assay, was compared at three time points (n = 3 each time point) versus naive mice (n = 3). (**a**) Daily weight of mice receiving the bacterial challenge. (**b**) Erythrocyte fragility as quantified by the median corpuscular fragility (MCF) (n = 3 each time point). Data are shown as mean ± SD.

2.2. Study 2—A Retrospective Observational Clinical Study

2.2.1. Reticulocytes Are Valid Markers of Haemolysis

Having determined that systemic inflammation leads to erythrocyte fragility, we next wanted to seek evidence for this phenomenon in humans. Short of a human experimental study, we sought observational evidence of an association between systemic inflammation and erythrocyte fragility and identified the UK Biobank as a large cohort of individuals in whom systemic inflammation was measured with a high-sensitivity C-reactive protein (hsCRP) assay with reticulocyte studies performed on the same day. The number of reticulocytes, the precursors of erythrocytes, increases in response to erythrocyte loss, which occurs during haemolysis. Three reticulocyte parameters were assessed as primary surrogate outcome measures for haemolysis: reticulocyte percentage (Ret%); high-light-scatter reticulocyte percentage (iRet%), which corresponds to the most immature reticulocytes; and the immature reticulocyte fraction (IRF) calculated by dividing the number of immature reticulocytes by the total reticulocytes. First, the three reticulocyte measures (Ret%, iRet%, and IRF) were validated as surrogate markers of haemolysis in UK Biobank participants with haemolytic anaemias (n = 1740) versus control healthy individuals (n = 9738). A main-effects ANCOVA, correcting for age and sex, showed that all three reticulocyte measures were significantly higher in people with haemolytic anaemias (Table 1).

Table 1. Validation of reticulocyte parameters as surrogate markers of haemolysis. Analysis of covariance examining reticulocyte markers between healthy participants (n = 9738) and those with haemolytic anaemias (n = 1740), adjusting for age and sex (model F (3, 11,474) = 55.467, $p < 0.001$). Abbreviations: Ret%, reticulocyte percentage; iRet%, high-light-scatter or immature reticulocyte percentage; IRF, immature reticulocyte fraction.

		Ret%	iRet%	IRF
Estimated Marginal Means	**Healthy controls**	1.274	0.356	0.276
	Haemolytic anaemia	1.647	0.568	0.330
Significance (*p*)		<0.0001	<0.0001	<0.0001
Partial eta squared		0.13	0.065	0.084

2.2.2. Reticulocytes and High-Sensitivity C-Reactive Protein

Out of the 9738 individuals with available reticulocyte data, 9292 had a hsCRP assay performed at the same time. Multivariable linear regression was carried out to determine the relationship between the three reticulocyte parameters and hsCRP in healthy participants (n = 9292). Adjustment for age and sex was performed since both of these variables may affect inflammation [32] and reticulocytes [33], and we wanted to study the effect of systemic inflammation that was independent of age and sex. The results of these analyses are summarised in Table 2. A positive association was observed between hsCRP and each reticulocyte parameter. The standardised beta coefficients show that hsCRP was more strongly predictive of the three surrogate markers of haemolysis than either age or sex.

Table 2. The association between systemic inflammation and surrogate markers of haemolysis in healthy individuals (retrospective study). The results are from three multivariable linear regression analyses showing the relationship between systemic inflammation (independent predictor variable: high-sensitivity C-reactive protein) and reticulocyte-based surrogate haemolytic markers (dependent variable in each regression: Ret%, iRet%, or IRF) while correcting for age and sex in healthy participants (n = 9292). Sex was coded as 1 for males and 0 for females. Abbreviations: Ret%, reticulocyte percentage; iRet%, high-light-scatter or immature reticulocyte percentage; IRF, immature reticulocyte fraction; hsCRP, high-sensitivity C-reactive protein; CI, confidence interval.

	Dependent Variable	Ret%	iRet%	IRF
Model	**F statistic**	13.017	55.167	51.227
	Degrees of freedom	3, 9288	3, 9288	3, 9288
	Significance (*p*)	<0.0001	<0.0001	<0.0001
	R^2 (corrected)	0.004	0.017	0.016

Table 2. *Cont.*

	Dependent Variable		Ret%	iRet%	IRF
Variables	Standardised beta coefficients	Age	−0.009	−0.030	−0.014
		Sex	0.038	0.042	−0.009
		hsCRP	0.050	0.120	0.127
	Unstandardised coefficients (95% CI)	Age	−0.001 (−0.005, 0.002)	−0.001 (−0.001, 0)	−0.0001 (0, 0)
		Sex	0.89 (0.041, 0.137)	0.018 (0.009, 0.026)	−0.001 (−0.004, 0.001)
		hsCRP	0.021 (0.013, 0.030)	0.009 (0.008, 0.011)	0.003 (0.002, 0.003)
	Significance (*p*)	Age	0.379	0.005	0.193
		Sex	<0.0001	<0.0001	0.367
		hsCRP	<0.0001	<0.0001	<0.0001

The reference range for the hsCRP assay had a lower limit of 1 mg/L, but its lower limit of quantification was 0.08 mg/L. Hence, while individuals with hsCRP < 1 mg/L are classified as having a normal CRP for clinical purposes, the assay's dynamic range extended below this level, providing quantification of subclinical degrees of systemic inflammation occurring in healthy individuals. To investigate whether the association between reticulocyte markers of haemolysis and hsCRP was also seen at these very mild degrees of systemic inflammation, a sensitivity analysis was conducted in those with hsCRP < 1 mg/L (n = 5037). This yielded similar results (Table 3).

Table 3. The association between systemic inflammation and surrogate markers of haemolysis in healthy individuals with low levels of high-sensitivity C-reactive protein (retrospective study). The results are from three multivariable linear regression analyses showing the relationship between systemic inflammation (independent predictor variable: high-sensitivity C-reactive protein) and surrogate haemolytic markers (dependent variable in each regression: Ret%, iRet%, or IRF) while correcting for age and sex in healthy participants with high-sensitivity C-reactive protein < 1 mg/L (n = 5037). Sex was coded as 1 for males and 0 for females. Abbreviations: Ret%, reticulocyte percentage; iRet%, high-light-scatter or immature reticulocyte percentage; IRF, immature reticulocyte fraction; hsCRP, high-sensitivity C-reactive protein; CI, confidence interval.

	Dependent Variable		Ret%	iRet%	IRF
Model	F statistic		20.941	52.785	24.325
	Degrees of freedom		3, 5033	3, 5033	3, 5033
	Significance (*p*)		<0.0001	<0.0001	<0.0001
	R^2 (corrected)		0.012	0.030	0.014
Variables	Standardised beta coefficients	Age	−0.052	−0.071	−0.030
		Sex	0.046	0.037	−0.010
		hsCRP	0.086	0.158	0.119

Table 3. *Cont.*

	Dependent Variable		Ret%	iRet%	IRF
Variables	Unstandardised coefficients (95% CI)	Age	−0.006 (−0.009, −0.003)	−0.002 (−0.002, −0.001)	−0.0002 (−0.0005, 0)
		Sex	0.074 (0.029, 0.118)	0.013 (0.003, 0.022)	−0.001 (−0.004, 0.002)
		hsCRP	0.290 (0.197, 0.348)	0.115 (0.095, 0.135)	0.029 (0.022, 0.036)
	Significance (p)	Age	<0.001	<0.0001	0.037
		Sex	0.0012	0.008	0.482
		hsCRP	<0.0001	<0.0001	<0.0001

2.3. Study 3—A Prospective Observational Clinical Study

2.3.1. Rationale and Study Population

Although the UK Biobank study demonstrated that systemic inflammation was associated with surrogate reticulocyte markers of haemolysis, it had severe limitations: the design was retrospective, erythrocyte fragility was not directly assessed, and a single hsCRP estimation in serum does not fully represent an individual's fluctuations in systemic inflammatory status over time. Hence, the next step was to prospectively assess erythrocyte fragility alongside an integrative marker of exposure to systemic inflammation. Resilience to osmotic stress was selected as a readout of erythrocyte fragility given its widespread and accepted use in human clinical studies [34] and to act as a parallel to the murine experimental Study 1 above. The urinary neopterin-to-creatinine ratio (UNCR) was employed to integrate the individual's exposure to systemic inflammation over the previous day [32]. Neopterin is secreted by myeloid lineage cells during any type of inflammation and rapidly enters the circulation to be excreted in the urine. Normalization of urinary neopterin to urinary creatinine removes variations due to hydration status and creatinine clearance. An early morning urine sample integrates systemic inflammation over the preceding twenty-four hours. Participants (n = 54) had a mean age of 43.3 years (SD: 13.5, range: 19–81 years), 69.8% were female, 68.2% had no comorbidities, and 71.4% were not on any regular medication.

2.3.2. Systemic Inflammation Correlates with Erythrocyte Fragility

A multivariable linear regression was performed to assess the relationship between UNCR (systemic inflammation) and MCF (erythrocyte fragility), adjusting for age and sex. The model significantly predicted MCF ($F(3,50) = 10.081$, $p < 0.0001$, $R^2 = 0.339$; Table 4) and accounted for 33.9% of the variance observed. UNCR was significantly associated with MCF. Sensitivity analyses excluding participants with comorbidities resulted in loss of statistical power but showed a similar trend (Table 4).

Table 4. The association between systemic inflammation and median corpuscular fragility (prospective study). The results are from two multivariable linear regression analyses showing the relationship between systemic inflammation (independent predictor variable: urinary neopterin-to-creatinine ratio) and median corpuscular fragility while correcting for age and sex. The first regression was a complete case analysis of all participants (n = 54); the second regression was a sensitivity analysis excluding participants with comorbidities (n = 35). Sex was coded as 1 for males and 0 for females. Abbreviations: MCF, median corpuscular fragility; UNCR, urinary neopterin-to-creatinine ratio; CI, confidence interval.

<table>
<tr><th></th><th></th><th></th><th>All Participants (n = 54)</th><th>No Comorbidities (n = 35)</th></tr>
<tr><td rowspan="4">Model</td><td colspan="2">F statistic</td><td>10.081</td><td>4.454</td></tr>
<tr><td colspan="2">Degrees of freedom</td><td>3, 50</td><td>3, 31</td></tr>
<tr><td colspan="2">Significance (p)</td><td><0.0001</td><td>0.0102</td></tr>
<tr><td colspan="2">R² (corrected)</td><td>0.339</td><td>0.234</td></tr>
<tr><td rowspan="9">Variables</td><td rowspan="3">Standardised beta coefficients</td><td>Age</td><td>0.441</td><td>0.456</td></tr>
<tr><td>Sex</td><td>−0.123</td><td>0.018</td></tr>
<tr><td>UNCR</td><td>0.353</td><td>0.296</td></tr>
<tr><td rowspan="3">Unstandardised coefficients (95% CI)</td><td>Age</td><td>0.008
(0.004, 0.012)</td><td>0.008
(0.003, 0.014)</td></tr>
<tr><td>Sex</td><td>−0.063
(−0.181, 0.055)</td><td>0.009
(−0.142, 0.159)</td></tr>
<tr><td>UNCR</td><td>0.001
(0.001, 0.002)</td><td>0.001
(0, 0.002)</td></tr>
<tr><td rowspan="3">Significance (p)</td><td>Age</td><td><0.001</td><td>0.005</td></tr>
<tr><td>Sex</td><td>0.288</td><td>0.906</td></tr>
<tr><td>UNCR</td><td>0.004</td><td>0.066</td></tr>
</table>

3. Discussion

The studies presented here support the hypothesis that mild systemic inflammatory stimuli lead to increased erythrocyte fragility. This was demonstrated in mice (Study 1) and supported by observations made in humans (Studies 2 and 3). Two remarkable observations in the human studies deserve mention. In Study 2, systemic inflammation had a larger effect size on reticulocyte parameters than age and sex, which are well-established determinants of reticulocyte turnover [33]. In Study 3, the effect size of UNCR was similar to that of age, and the combination of age and UNCR was able to together explain 33.9% of the variance in the MCF. Overall, the studies are in keeping with mild systemic inflammation leading to erythrocyte fragility. While it is well-documented that severe inflammation during sepsis affects erythrocyte morphology and function [4], the studies presented here provide new insights into the effects of mild and even subclinical levels of inflammation on erythrocyte health. We also establish a causative role for systemic inflammation in decreasing erythrocyte resilience and increasing susceptibility to haemolysis. This finding is an important contribution to the literature since it implies the possibility of positive feedback whereby inflammation can cause haemolysis and, in turn, the main products of haemolysis, namely haemoglobin and haem, can increase inflammation. As discussed in the introduction, systemic inflammation may cause erythrocyte fragility through a variety of mechanisms, but further study is required to map the underlying cellular and molecular mechanisms.

Since direct experimental interrogation to prove causation is difficult in humans, Studies 2 and 3 were aimed at gathering observational evidence that the effect of mild systemic inflammation on erythrocyte fragility is also relevant to humans. In Study 2, hsCRP was used as an indicator of systemic inflammation in healthy participants. A total of 98.4% of participants in this study had hsCRP levels not suggestive of an acute phase response (i.e., $\leq$10 mg/L; [35]). Mild to moderate increases in hsCRP (1 mg/L to 10 mg/L) have been found to be associated with increased cardiovascular risk [35] and are thought to correlate with so-called metabolic inflammation [36]. Other conditions thought to be associated with moderate elevation of C-reactive protein levels are viral infections, low-grade mucosal infections (e.g., periodontitis), obesity, insulin resistance, depression, smoking, and mild alcohol consumption [36]. Interestingly, the predictive effect of hsCRP on surrogate haemolytic markers was retained when restricting the analysis to participants with clinically "normal" levels of hsCRP (<1 mg/L). While Study 2 relied on surrogate markers of haemolysis, Study 3 was planned to directly assess erythrocyte fragility while at the same time measuring the individual's exposure to systemic inflammation using UNCR [32].

This work's major strength is that the results of all three studies support the hypothesis that erythrocyte fragility increases in the presence of mild systemic inflammation. This consistency across three different contexts, including a murine model and human observational study, and with different methodologies, demonstrates internal validity and provides an acceptable degree of confidence. We also highlight the potential utility of reticulocyte measures—these parameters are easily acquired on most commercially available automated haematology analysers used worldwide. While manual osmotic fragility testing is laborious, semi-automated instruments are now available to measure this marker using osmotic gradient ektacytometry.

There are some limitations which are highlighted here. While UNCR integrates inflammation over the preceding 24 h and is an improvement on hsCRP, which only gives information about the inflammatory status at a certain point in time, UNCR also varies from week to week [32]. However, studies on erythrocyte deformability following COVID-19 suggest that changes in erythrocyte deformability (and therefore possibly also fragility) persist over months, so the effects of inflammation on erythrocytes appear to be stable [1].

By necessity, Study 2 was restricted to employing surrogate markers of haemolysis since direct measures of haemolysis were not acquired in this retrospective study. Whilst our analyses on study participants with haemolytic anaemias supported the use of reticulocyte parameters as surrogate markers of haemolysis, it is likely that other factors apart from haemolysis influence reticulocyte parameters. For example, direct effects of inflammation on erythropoiesis as a form of stress erythropoiesis have been proposed [37]. Hence, it is possible that inflammation in Study 2 was linked to reticulocyte parameters via stress erythropoiesis rather than erythrocyte fragility. This is somewhat mitigated by the direct assessment of erythrocyte fragility in Studies 1 and 3.

Osmotic fragility testing is a widely used method to analyse erythrocyte fragility [34]. Yet osmotic stress is not encountered physiologically. While the physical and biochemical factors that cause osmotic and mechanical fragility are thought to be similar [38], future studies could utilise other more physiologically relevant methods to assess red blood cell resilience, such as ektacytometry.

Recent or regular exercise can impact erythrocyte fragility and erythropoiesis and was not controlled for in Studies 2 and 3. "Acute" exercise involves several stressors that lead to decreased deformability and mechanical rupture of erythrocytes with subsequent increases in erythropoiesis straight afterwards, whilst regular exercise leads to an overall improvement in erythrocyte integrity [39]. As we investigated a large sample of participants in Study 2, it is unlikely that different levels of exercise in individuals led to significant bias.

The present studies do not allow one to draw conclusions on how long changes in erythrocyte fragility persist following an inflammatory stimulus and whether the increase in erythrocyte fragility as assessed by MCF actually contributes to in vivo haemolysis.

However, given the relatively long lifespan of erythrocytes, it is likely that changes to erythrocyte fragility are cumulative. Longitudinal studies are needed to clarify the evolution of erythrocyte fragility alongside exposure to systemic inflammation.

When considering the potential clinical impact of low-grade intravascular haemolysis, the role of haemoglobin and haem scavenging mechanisms should not be overlooked. Haptoglobin, for example, is known to be elevated during infection as an acute phase reactant [40] and might be able to counteract the potential effects of low-grade intravascular haemolysis. Interestingly, certain haptoglobin phenotypes have been associated with an increased risk of inflammation and cardiovascular and auto-immune disease [41,42]. Future studies should measure serum haptoglobin and haemopexin, as well as haptoglobin genotype.

In the absence of inflammation, severe haemolysis overwhelming the capacity of haptoglobin/haemopexin scavenging systems may result in high serum iron and iron deposition in multiple organs, especially in the kidney [43]. Although we have not studied iron metabolism in the present work, it would be interesting to explore this in future studies. The situation would be expected to be complex during haemolysis in the context of systemic inflammation when iron metabolism is dysregulated. Typically, immune activation causes an "iron withdrawal" whereby iron absorption is reduced and shuttled away from haematopoiesis to the innate immune compartment, resulting in anaemia of inflammation [44]; besides providing macrophages and neutrophils with iron needed for respiratory chain and oxidative burst enzymes, reduced availability of iron (i.e., low serum iron) is protective during infection [44]. Hence, iron deposition in target organs during mild systemic inflammation appears unlikely, but this hypothesis requires testing. The situation would be expected to be different in the presence of focal inflammation in local tissues, which may result in local deposition of iron because of macrophage/neutrophil infiltration, microvascular damage leading to extravasation of blood, or disturbed tissue-specific iron handling. Hence, it is not uncommon to observe local tissue iron deposition in chronic disease conditions such as atherosclerosis [45], various types of arthritis [46], multiple sclerosis [47], and chronic liver diseases [48].

The clinical significance of increased erythrocyte fragility and haemolysis in people with long-term inflammatory conditions needs to be studied further. A study in people with progressive multiple sclerosis suggests an association between neurodegeneration and levels of free haemoglobin, as brain atrophy rate in patients correlated with free haemoglobin levels [26]. Our study provides a possible underlying mechanism since systemic and/or organ-specific inflammation may increase erythrocyte fragility, leading to higher levels of free haemoglobin in individuals with more rapidly progressive multiple sclerosis. It seems likely that inflammation-driven low-grade haemolysis might drive progression in neurological and other long-term conditions, but this requires further investigation.

4. Methods

4.1. Study 1—Murine Model

4.1.1. Setup

Adult male C57BL/6 mice (n = 12, 10 weeks old) were housed in groups of three in plastic cages with sawdust bedding. Food and water (standard chow, RM1, SDS, UK) were available *ad libitum*. The holding room was temperature controlled (19 to 23 °C) with a 12 h light followed by a 12 h dark cycle (light on at 07:00 h). Mice were allowed to acclimatise to the holding room for 1 week before the start of the experiment. All procedures were performed under UK Home Office project licence P4155EEE0 and in accordance with the United Kingdom Animals (Scientific Procedures) Act (1986).

4.1.2. Challenge with Salmonella typhimurium

At 10 weeks of age, mice (n = 9) were administered a single intraperitoneal injection (200 µL) of 106 colony-forming units (cfu) of attenuated *Salmonella typhimurium* vaccine strain SL3261 (generously provided by Dr. H. Atkins, DSTL, Salisbury, UK) to induce systemic inflammation. With this vaccine strain of *Salmonella*, replicative infection does not occur, and mice look outwardly well; it models a period of prolonged low-grade systemic inflammation lasting several days [29,30]. Three mice acted as negative controls. Body weight was recorded at baseline and daily after injection. Mice challenged with *Salmonella* were sacrificed at 1, 3, and 7 days after challenge (n = 3 on each day).

4.1.3. Murine Sacrifice and Blood Collection

Mice were terminally anaesthetised with an intraperitoneal injection of Avertin (2,2,2-tribromoethanol 3% *w/v* and 1.8% 2-methyl-2-butanol (Sigma Aldrich) in 7.2% alcohol diluted with 0.9% saline). After sacrifice, the thorax of the mouse was exposed, and 3 drops of heparin sodium (5000 international units per mL) were added to the cavity to prevent clotting. The left atrium was punctured, and blood was collected from the chest cavity using a 1 mL syringe and transferred to a heparin sodium-coated microcentrifuge tube. The blood was immediately used for erythrocyte osmotic fragility tests.

4.1.4. Osmotic Fragility Testing

Osmotic stress was applied using Parpart's method [49]. Briefly, 20 μL of whole blood was suspended for 30 min in 1 mL NaCl-PO_4 (Parpart's buffered saline, Clin-Tech, Guildford, UK) at increasing concentrations with total cell lysis occurring at 0 g/L. The cells were then centrifuged at 1700× *g* for 5 min at room temperature, and the haemoglobin concentration in the supernatant was determined by its optical density (OD) at 540 nm. The haemolysis level at each osmotic stress level was expressed as % of the total lysis, according to the following formula:

$$\% \text{ haemolysis} = 100 \times [(ODS - OD_0)/(ODT - OD_0)]$$

where OD_0 = OD of 9.0 g/L saline, ODS = OD of supernatant, and ODT = OD of supernatant from erythrocytes subjected to total haemolysis. A four-parameter variable slope sigmoidal model was fitted to the data in GraphPad Prism v8 and used to determine the IC50, which is the concentration of NaCl causing 50% haemolysis (also known as the median corpuscular fragility, MCF). The normal range of MCF at pH 7.4 and 20 °C is 4.0 to 4.45 g/L [49].

4.1.5. Outcome Parameters

The primary outcome was MCF. Body weight was also assessed.

4.2. Study 2—A Retrospective Observational Clinical Study

4.2.1. Participants

This project was approved by UK Biobank (approval number 61771). Between 2006 and 2010, approximately 500,000 people between the ages of 40 and 69 years were recruited to participate in the UK Biobank project (www.ukbiobank.ac.uk, accessed on 26 June 2024). Participants with available reticulocyte parameter data, who did not have any recorded diagnosis in the "First occurrence" data category number 1712 (which encodes the first occurrence of health conditions defined by their 3-character ICD10 code in any healthcare setting) and any recorded inpatient diagnosis after hospitalisation, and who did not take any regular medication, were included as healthy participants (n = 9738).

4.2.2. Outcome Parameters

We investigated the utility of reticulocyte parameters as surrogate markers of haemolysis. Reticulocytes are the immature precursors of erythrocytes, which increase in response to erythrocyte clearance. The percentage of reticulocytes to total erythrocytes in the peripheral blood indicates the rate of erythrocyte turnover, whilst the number (a raw count) of reticulocytes reflects the amount of erythropoiesis on a given day. UK Biobank participants had a full blood count, including counts of total and high-light-scatter reticulocytes.

For the purposes of the analysis here, three reticulocyte parameters were assessed as primary surrogate outcome measures for haemolysis: reticulocyte percentage (Ret%), high-light-scatter or immature reticulocyte percentage (iRet%), and immature reticulocyte fraction (IRF) calculated by dividing the number of immature reticulocytes by the total reticulocytes.

These reticulocyte parameters were first validated as surrogate markers of haemolysis in UK Biobank participants (n = 1740) with a diagnosis of haemolytic anaemia including thalassaemia (ICD-D56), sickle-cell disorders (ICD-D57), acquired haemolytic anaemia (ICD-D59), and other hereditary haemolytic anaemias (ICD-D58), versus control healthy individuals (n = 9738).

High-sensitivity C-reactive protein in serum was used as a marker of systemic inflammation.

4.2.3. Sample Collection and Analysis

Blood samples analysed at the baseline assessment were used for the present analysis since this represented the largest number of samples. Blood samples were collected in 4 mL EDTA vacutainers and analysed within 24 h. Reticulocyte parameters were acquired on an automated Beckman Coulter LH 750 Haematology Analyser. For hsCRP analysis, blood was collected in a silica clot accelerator (SST) vacutainer and allowed to clot at room temperature for 30 min. Serum aliquots were stored at −80 °C until analysed for hsCRP by immunoturbidimetry. The dynamic range of the assay was 0.08–80 mg/L. Samples above the upper limit of quantification were re-run after dilution. Reticulocyte parameters and hsCRP were available in a common dataset of 9292 healthy participants.

4.3. *Study 3—A Prospective Observational Clinical Study*

4.3.1. Participants

Adult participants were recruited and consented (national research ethics approvals 12/SC/0176 and 18/LO/2105; institutional research ethics approvals ERGO5562 and ERGO46018). Exclusion criteria for control individuals were (1) haematological disorders, (2) autoimmune or active inflammatory disorders, and (3) chronic medical conditions that were uncontrolled or active at the time of recruitment. All participants were non-smokers in the year preceding study participation.

4.3.2. Outcome Parameters

The primary outcome parameter was MCF.

4.3.3. Sample Collection

For the erythrocyte osmotic fragility tests, whole blood was collected in 6 mL K2-EDTA vacutainer tubes (BD, UK). An additional 3 mL K2-EDTA sample was collected for a full blood count, performed on a Sysmex XN10 analyser in Southampton General Hospital's haematology laboratory. Great care was taken to reduce the chance of in vitro haemolysis of the samples by careful handling and transport of samples in a padded container. Erythrocyte osmotic fragility testing was performed within 15 min of venesection.

The UNCR was measured using liquid chromatography followed by mass spectrometry; this method has been validated as a marker of systemic inflammation [32]. Participants were asked to collect the first (midstream) urine sample passed in the morning and were instructed to protect the sample from light using aluminium foil since neopterin is photosensitive. Urine specimens were centrifuged at 10 °C and 2000× *g* for five minutes and stored at −80 °C in 1 mL aliquots. The detailed protocol for UNCR measurement has been previously described [32].

4.3.4. Osmotic Fragility Testing

Osmotic fragility testing was performed as detailed in Section 4.1.4.

4.4. Statistical Analyses

SPSS v28 was used for statistical analyses, and plots were created in GraphPad Prism v9. Data distribution was determined graphically and using the Kolmogorov–Smirnov test. Parametric or non-parametric tests were used where appropriate. All hypothesis testing was two-tailed. A p-value < 0.05 was considered significant. Mean $\pm$ standard deviation (SD) is quoted unless otherwise stated.

Author Contributions: Conceptualization, I.G.; methodology, all authors; formal analysis, C.M.S. and C.J.; investigation, C.M.S., C.J., S.H., J.K.C. and J.L.T.; resources, I.G. and A.V.; data curation, C.M.S. and C.J.; writing—original draft preparation, C.M.S. and C.J.; writing—review and editing, all authors; visualisation, C.M.S. and C.J.; supervision, I.G. and J.L.T.; project administration, I.G.; funding acquisition, I.G. and A.V. All authors have read and agreed to the published version of the manuscript.

Funding: This project was funded by the Multiple Sclerosis Society (grant number 996), the UK Medical Research Council (MR/R017352/1), and the National Institute for Health and Care Research. The UK Biobank project is funded by Wellcome Trust, the UK Medical Research Council, the British Heart Foundation, Cancer Research UK, the Department of Health, the Northwest Regional Development Agency, and the Scottish Government.

Institutional Review Board Statement: The animal study protocol in Study 1 was approved by the Home Office of the UK (project licence number P4155EEE0). Study 2 was approved by UK Biobank (approval number 61771), which in turn was approved by the National Research Ethics Committee of the UK (reference number 21/NW/0157). Study 3 was conducted in accordance with the Declaration of Helsinki, and approved by the National Research Ethics Committee of the UK (reference numbers 12/SC/0176 and 18/LO/2105).

Informed Consent Statement: Informed consent was obtained from all human subjects involved in the study.

Data Availability Statement: Data are available on request subject to ethical and institutional approvals.

Acknowledgments: The authors thank Elisabeth Jarman, Connie Temple-Brown, and Sarah Cook as well as all the volunteers who took part in the human studies. This research has been conducted using data from UK Biobank, a major biomedical database (www.ukbiobank.ac.uk).

Conflicts of Interest: The authors declare no conflict of interest.

References

1. Kubánková, M.; Hohberger, B.; Hoffmanns, J.; Fürst, J.; Herrmann, M.; Guck, J.; Kräter, M. Physical phenotype of blood cells is altered in COVID-19. *Biophys. J.* **2021**, *120*, 2838–2847. [CrossRef] [PubMed]
2. Zeng, N.F.; Mancuso, J.E.; Zivkovic, A.M.; Smilowitz, J.T.; Ristenpart, W.D. Red Blood Cells from Individuals with Abdominal Obesity or Metabolic Abnormalities Exhibit Less Deformability upon Entering a Constriction. *PLoS ONE* **2016**, *11*, e0156070. [CrossRef] [PubMed]
3. Alexy, T.; Pais, E.; Wenby, R.B.; Mack, W.J.; Hodis, H.N.; Kono, N.; Wang, J.; Baskurt, O.K.; Fisher, T.C.; Meiselman, H.J. Abnormal blood rheology and chronic low grade inflammation: Possible risk factors for accelerated atherosclerosis and coronary artery disease in Lewis negative subjects. *Atherosclerosis* **2015**, *239*, 248–251. [CrossRef]
4. Bateman, R.M.; Sharpe, M.D.; Singer, M.; Ellis, C.G. The effect of sepsis on the erythrocyte. *Int. J. Mol. Sci.* **2017**, *18*, 1932. [CrossRef] [PubMed]
5. Guillot, X.; Semerano, L.; Saidenberg-Kermanac'h, N.; Falgarone, G.; Boissier, M.C. Vitamin D and inflammation. *Jt. Bone Spine* **2010**, *77*, 552–557. [CrossRef]
6. Farber, P.L.; Dias, A.; Freitas, T.; Pinho, A.C.; Viggiano, D.; Saldanha, C.; Silva-Herdade, A.S. Evaluation of hemorheological parameters as biomarkers of calcium metabolism and insulin resistance in postmenopausal women. *Clin. Hemorheol. Microcirc.* **2021**, *77*, 395–410. [CrossRef] [PubMed]
7. Heyes, H.; Köhle, W.; Slijepcevic, B. The appearance of schistocytes in the peripheral blood in correlation to the degree of disseminated intravascular coagulation. An experimental study in rats. *Haemostasis* **1976**, *5*, 66–73. [CrossRef] [PubMed]
8. Effenberger-Neidnicht, K.; Hartmann, M. Mechanisms of Hemolysis During Sepsis. *Inflammation* **2018**, *41*, 1569–1581. [CrossRef]
9. Belcher, J.D.; Chen, C.; Nguyen, J.; Milbauer, L.; Abdulla, F.; Alayash, A.I.; Smith, A.; Nath, K.A.; Hebbel, R.P.; Vercellotti, G.M. Heme triggers TLR4 signaling leading to endothelial cell activation and vaso-occlusion in murine sickle cell disease. *Blood* **2014**, *123*, 377–390. [CrossRef]

10. Jägers, J.; Brauckmann, S.; Kirsch, M.; Effenberger-Neidnicht, K. Moderate glucose supply reduces hemolysis during systemic inflammation. *J. Inflamm. Res.* **2018**, *11*, 87–94. [CrossRef]
11. Hendry, E.B. Delayed haemolysis of human erythrocytes in solutions of glucose. *J. Gen. Physiol.* **1952**, *35*, 605–616. [CrossRef]
12. Ruef, P.; Ehrhard, M.; Frommhold, D.; Koch, L.; Fritzsching, B.; Poeschl, J. Lipid A decreases human erythrocytes deformability by increasing intracellular Ca(2+): Effects of verapamil, staurosporine and the rho-kinase inhibitor Y-27632. *Clin. Hemorheol. Microcirc.* **2011**, *49*, 315–322. [CrossRef] [PubMed]
13. Maruyama, T.; Hieda, M.; Mawatari, S.; Fujino, T. Rheological Abnormalities in Human Erythrocytes Subjected to Oxidative Inflammation. *Front. Physiol.* **2022**, *13*, 837926. [CrossRef] [PubMed]
14. Orrico, F.; Laurance, S.; Lopez, A.C.; Lefevre, S.D.; Thomson, L.; Möller, M.N.; Ostuni, M.A. Oxidative Stress in Healthy and Pathological Red Blood Cells. *Biomolecules* **2023**, *13*, 1262. [CrossRef]
15. Bulters, D.; Gaastra, B.; Zolnourian, A.; Alexander, S.; Ren, D.; Blackburn, S.L.; Borsody, M.; Doré, S.; Galea, J.; Iihara, K.; et al. Haemoglobin scavenging in intracranial bleeding: Biology and clinical implications. *Nat. Rev. Neurol.* **2018**, *14*, 416–432. [CrossRef]
16. Rother, R.P.; Bell, L.; Hillmen, P.; Gladwin, M.T. The clinical sequelae of intravascular hemolysis and extracellular plasma hemoglobin: A novel mechanism of human disease. *Jama* **2005**, *293*, 1653–1662. [CrossRef]
17. Van Avondt, K.; Nur, E.; Zeerleder, S. Mechanisms of haemolysis-induced kidney injury. *Nat. Rev. Nephrol.* **2019**, *15*, 671–692. [CrossRef]
18. Wagener, F.A.D.T.G.; Eggert, A.; Boerman, O.C.; Oyen, W.J.G.; Verhofstad, A.; Abraham, N.G.; Adema, G.; van Kooyk, Y.; de Witte, T.; Figdor, C.G. Heme is a potent inducer of inflammation in mice and is counteracted by heme oxygenase. *Blood* **2001**, *98*, 1802–1811. [CrossRef] [PubMed]
19. Figueiredo, R.T.; Fernandez, P.L.; Mourao-Sa, D.S.; Porto, B.N.; Dutra, F.F.; Alves, L.S.; Oliveira, M.F.; Oliveira, P.L.; Graça-Souza, A.V.; Bozza, M.T. Characterization of Heme as Activator of Toll-like Receptor 4 *. *J. Biol. Chem.* **2007**, *282*, 20221–20229. [CrossRef]
20. Graça-Souza, A.l.V.; Arruda, M.A.B.; de Freitas, M.S.; Barja-Fidalgo, C.; Oliveira, P.L. Neutrophil activation by heme: Implications for inflammatory processes. *Blood* **2002**, *99*, 4160–4165. [CrossRef]
21. Chen, G.; Zhang, D.; Fuchs, T.A.; Manwani, D.; Wagner, D.D.; Frenette, P.S. Heme-induced neutrophil extracellular traps contribute to the pathogenesis of sickle cell disease. *Blood* **2014**, *123*, 3818–3827. [CrossRef] [PubMed]
22. Frimat, M.; Tabarin, F.; Dimitrov, J.D.; Poitou, C.; Halbwachs-Mecarelli, L.; Fremeaux-Bacchi, V.; Roumenina, L.T. Complement activation by heme as a secondary hit for atypical hemolytic uremic syndrome. *Blood* **2013**, *122*, 282–292. [CrossRef] [PubMed]
23. Larsen, R.; Gozzelino, R.; Jeney, V.; Tokaji, L.; Bozza, F.A.; Japiassú, A.M.; Bonaparte, D.; Cavalcante, M.M.; Chora, A.; Ferreira, A.; et al. A central role for free heme in the pathogenesis of severe sepsis. *Sci. Transl. Med.* **2010**, *2*, 51ra71. [CrossRef] [PubMed]
24. Ousaka, D.; Nishibori, M. Is hemolysis a novel therapeutic target in COVID-19? *Front. Immunol.* **2022**, *13*, 956671. [CrossRef] [PubMed]
25. Buttari, B.; Profumo, E.; Di Cristofano, C.; Pietraforte, D.; Lionetti, V.; Capoano, R.; Salvati, B.; Businaro, R.; Di Giammarco, G.; Riganò, R. Haemoglobin triggers chemotaxis of human monocyte-derived dendritic cells: Possible role in atherosclerotic lesion instability. *Atherosclerosis* **2011**, *215*, 316–322. [CrossRef] [PubMed]
26. Lewin, A.; Hamilton, S.; Witkover, A.; Langford, P.; Nicholas, R.; Chataway, J.; Bangham, C.R.M. Free serum haemoglobin is associated with brain atrophy in secondary progressive multiple sclerosis. *Wellcome Open Res.* **2016**, *1*, 10. [CrossRef] [PubMed]
27. Hu, Z.-D. Red blood cell distribution width: A promising index for estimating activity of autoimmune disease. *J. Lab Precis. Med.* **2016**, *1*, 4. [CrossRef]
28. Lippi, G.; Targher, G.; Montagnana, M.; Salvagno, G.L.; Zoppini, G.; Guidi, G.C. Relation between red blood cell distribution width and inflammatory biomarkers in a large cohort of unselected outpatients. *Arch. Pathol. Lab. Med.* **2009**, *133*, 628–632. [CrossRef] [PubMed]
29. Peters, S.E.; Paterson, G.K.; Bandularatne, E.S.D.; Northen, H.C.; Pleasance, S.; Willers, C.; Wang, J.; Foote, A.K.; Constantino-Casas, F.; Scase, T.J.; et al. Salmonella enterica serovar typhimurium trxA mutants are protective against virulent challenge and induce less inflammation than the live-attenuated vaccine strain SL3261. *Infect. Immun.* **2010**, *78*, 326–336. [CrossRef]
30. Püntener, U.; Booth, S.G.; Perry, V.H.; Teeling, J.L. Long-term impact of systemic bacterial infection on the cerebral vasculature and microglia. *J. Neuroinflamm.* **2012**, *9*, 146. [CrossRef]
31. Hoiseth, S.K.; Stocker, B.A. Aromatic-dependent Salmonella typhimurium are non-virulent and effective as live vaccines. *Nature* **1981**, *291*, 238–239. [CrossRef] [PubMed]
32. Stuart, C.M.; Zotova, E.; Koster, G.; Varatharaj, A.; Richardson, G.; Cornick, F.R.; Weal, M.; Newman, T.A.; Postle, A.D.; Galea, I. High-Throughput Urinary Neopterin-to-Creatinine Ratio Monitoring of Systemic Inflammation. *J. Appl. Lab. Med.* **2019**, *5*, 101–113. [CrossRef] [PubMed]
33. Tarallo, P.; Humbert, J.C.; Mahassen, P.; Fournier, B.; Henny, J. Reticulocytes: Biological variations and reference limits. *Eur. J. Haematol.* **1994**, *53*, 11–15. [CrossRef] [PubMed]
34. Walski, T.; Chludzińska, L.; Komorowska, M.; Witkiewicz, W. Individual osmotic fragility distribution: A new parameter for determination of the osmotic properties of human red blood cells. *BioMed Res. Int.* **2014**, *2014*, 162102. [CrossRef]
35. Ridker, P.M. A Test in Context. *J. Am. Coll. Cardiol.* **2016**, *67*, 712–723. [CrossRef] [PubMed]
36. Bray, C.; Bell, L.N.; Liang, H.; Haykal, R.; Kaiksow, F.; Mazza, J.J.; Yale, S.H. Erythrocyte Sedimentation Rate and C-reactive Protein Measurements and Their Relevance in Clinical Medicine. *Wmj* **2016**, *115*, 317–321. [PubMed]

37. Paulson, R.F.; Ruan, B.; Hao, S.; Chen, Y. Stress Erythropoiesis is a Key Inflammatory Response. *Cells* **2020**, *9*, 634. [CrossRef] [PubMed]
38. Orbach, A.; Zelig, O.; Yedgar, S.; Barshtein, G. Biophysical and Biochemical Markers of Red Blood Cell Fragility. *Transfus. Med. Hemotherapy* **2017**, *44*, 183–187. [CrossRef] [PubMed]
39. Mairbäurl, H. Red blood cells in sports: Effects of exercise and training on oxygen supply by red blood cells. *Front. Physiol.* **2013**, *4*, 332. [CrossRef]
40. Wassell, J. Haptoglobin: Function and polymorphism. *Clinical laboratory* **2000**, *46*, 547–552.
41. Sadrzadeh, S.M.H.; Bozorgmehr, J. Haptoglobin Phenotypes in Health and Disorders. *Pathol. Patterns Rev.* **2004**, *121*, S97–S104. [CrossRef] [PubMed]
42. Bamm, V.V.; Geist, A.M.; Harauz, G. Correlation of geographic distributions of haptoglobin alleles with prevalence of multiple sclerosis (MS)—A narrative literature review. *Metab. Brain Dis.* **2017**, *32*, 19–34. [CrossRef] [PubMed]
43. Schein, A.; Enriquez, C.; Coates, T.D.; Wood, J.C. Magnetic resonance detection of kidney iron deposition in sickle cell disease: A marker of chronic hemolysis. *J. Magn. Reson. Imaging* **2008**, *28*, 698–704. [CrossRef] [PubMed]
44. Nairz, M.; Weiss, G. Iron in infection and immunity. *Mol. Asp. Med.* **2020**, *75*, 100864. [CrossRef] [PubMed]
45. Yuan, X.M. Apoptotic macrophage-derived foam cells of human atheromas are rich in iron and ferritin, suggesting iron-catalysed reactions to be involved in apoptosis. *Free. Radic. Res.* **1999**, *30*, 221–231. [CrossRef] [PubMed]
46. Ogilvie-Harris, D.J.; Fornaiser, V.L. Synovial iron deposition in osteoarthritis and rheumatoid arthritis. *J. Rheumatol.* **1980**, *7*, 30–36. [PubMed]
47. Zierfuss, B.; Wang, Z.; Jackson, A.N.; Moezzi, D.; Yong, V.W. Iron in multiple sclerosis—Neuropathology, immunology, and real-world considerations. *Mult. Scler. Relat. Dis.* **2023**, *78*, 104934. [CrossRef] [PubMed]
48. Pinyopornpanish, K.; Tantiworawit, A.; Leerapun, A.; Soontornpun, A.; Thongsawat, S. Secondary Iron Overload and the Liver: A Comprehensive Review. *J. Clin. Transl. Hepatol.* **2023**, *11*, 932–941. [CrossRef]
49. Parpart, A.K.; Lorenz, P.B.; Parpart, E.R.; Gregg, J.R.; Chase, A.M. The osmotic resistance (fragility) of human red cells. *J. Clin. Investig.* **1947**, *26*, 636–640. [CrossRef]

cells

MDPI

Article

Ileal Crohn's Disease Exhibits Reduced Activity of Phospholipase C-β3-Dependent Wnt/β-Catenin Signaling Pathway

Tomoaki Ando [1,2,†], Ikuo Takazawa [1,†,‡], Zachary T. Spencer [3], Ryoji Ito [1,4], Yoshiaki Tomimori [1,§], Zbigniew Mikulski [5], Kenji Matsumoto [6], Tohru Ishitani [7], Lee A. Denson [8,9], Yu Kawakami [1], Yuko Kawakami [1], Jiro Kitaura [2], Yashi Ahmed [3] and Toshiaki Kawakami [1,*]

1 Laboratory of Allergic Diseases, Center for Autoimmunity and Inflammation, La Jolla, CA 92037, USA; tm-ando@juntendo.ac.jp (T.A.)
2 Atopy Research Center, Graduate School of Medicine, Juntendo University, Tokyo 113-8421, Japan
3 Department of Molecular and Systems Biology and the Dartmouth Cancer Center, Geisel School of Medicine at Dartmouth College, Hanover, NH 03755, USA; zspencer12391@gmail.com (Z.T.S.)
4 Central Institute for Experimental Animals, Kawasaki 210-0821, Kanagawa, Japan
5 Imaging Facility, La Jolla Institute for Immunology, La Jolla, CA 92037, USA
6 Department of Allergy and Clinical Immunology, National Research Institute for Child Health and Development, Tokyo 157-8535, Japan
7 Institute for Molecular and Cellular Regulation, Gunma University, Maebashi 371-0044, Gunma, Japan
8 Division of Gastroenterology, Hepatology, and Nutrition, Cincinnati Children's Hospital Medical Center, Cincinnati, OH 45229, USA
9 Department of Pediatrics, University of Cincinnati College of Medicine, Cincinnati, OH 45267, USA
* Correspondence: toshi@lji.org
† These authors contributed equally to this work.
‡ Current address: Faculty of Medicine, University of Tokyo, Tokyo 113-8654, Japan.
§ Current address: Daiichi Sankyo Company, Tokyo 103-8426, Japan.

Abstract: Crohn's disease is a chronic, debilitating, inflammatory bowel disease. Here, we report a critical role of phospholipase C-β3 (PLC-β3) in intestinal homeostasis. In PLC-β3-deficient mice, exposure to oral dextran sodium sulfate induced lethality and severe inflammation in the small intestine. The lethality was due to PLC-β3 deficiency in multiple non-hematopoietic cell types. PLC-β3 deficiency resulted in reduced Wnt/β-catenin signaling, which is essential for homeostasis and the regeneration of the intestinal epithelium. PLC-β3 regulated the Wnt/β-catenin pathway in small intestinal epithelial cells (IECs) at transcriptional, epigenetic, and, potentially, protein–protein interaction levels. PLC-β3-deficient IECs were unable to respond to stimulation by R-spondin 1, an enhancer of Wnt/β-catenin signaling. Reduced expression of PLC-β3 and its signature genes was found in biopsies of patients with ileal Crohn's disease. PLC-β regulation of Wnt signaling was evolutionally conserved in *Drosophila*. Our data indicate that a reduction in PLC-β3-mediated Wnt/β-catenin signaling contributes to the pathogenesis of ileal Crohn's disease.

Keywords: phospholipase C-β3; inflammatory bowel disease; Wnt/β-catenin signaling; KO mouse; Drosophila

1. Introduction

Inflammatory bowel disease (IBD), comprised of Crohn's disease (CD) and ulcerative colitis, is a complex disease resulting from an interaction between host genetic factors and environmental factors that leads to inflammation in the gastrointestinal tract [1,2]. Heterogeneity and chronicity clinically characterize CD. There are five different types of CD, each affecting different parts of the digestive tract: gastroduodenal CD, jejunoileitis, ileitis, ileocolitis, and Crohn's colitis. CD may present or evolve with time into more complex clinical manifestations that include strictures, fistulae, and abscesses. CD patients experience highly variable responses to therapies. Potentially related to this complexity, more than 200 genomic loci have been associated with IBD [1,3].

The Wnt family of secretory glycoproteins play important roles in various physiological and pathological processes, including embryogenesis, organ development, tissue homeostasis, metabolism, and tumorigenesis [4,5]. In the absence of Wnt stimulation, cytoplasmic β-catenin is actively phosphorylated, ubiquitinated, and targeted for proteasomal degradation by the β-catenin destruction complex, which includes the tumor suppressors Axin and adenomatous polyposis coli (APC), the Ser/Thr kinases GSK-3 and CK1, the protein phosphatase 2A (PP2A), and the E3-ubiquitin ligase β-TrCP. Wnt proteins interact with Wnt receptor complexes consisting of a member of the Frizzled (Fzd) family and the low-density lipid receptor family members LRP5 or LRP6. Wnt binding to the receptor complexes inactivates the β-catenin destruction complex. Consequently, β-catenin accumulates in the cytoplasm and nucleus and binds to members of the T-cell factor (TCF)/lymphoid enhancer factor (LEF) family transcription factors, leading to the regulation of Wnt target genes. The activation of Fzd1 leads to the activation of Wnt/β-catenin signaling in a Gαq- and Gαo-dependent manner [6], and Fzd5 stimulation by Wnt-5a activates Gαq [7]. The canonical Wnt/β-catenin pathway is essential for intestinal stem cells (ISCs) [4,5,8] and thus for the generation of all intestinal epithelial cells (IECs). Therefore, the dysregulation of this pathway may contribute to IBD pathogenesis [9].

Phospholipase C (PLC) is a family of enzymes that catalyze the hydrolysis of phosphatidylinositol 4,5-bisphosphate to generate two second messengers, i.e., diacylglycerol and inositol 1,4,5-trisphosphate [10]. Thirteen known mammalian PLC isozymes are classified into six subfamilies (PLC-β, PLC-γ, PLC-δ, PLC-ε, PLC-ζ, and PLC-η) [11]. Different PLC isozymes are activated by different receptors and mechanisms, for example, PLC-β is activated by G protein-coupled receptors (GPCRs) and PLC-γ by tyrosine kinase-linked receptors [10]. Notably, both the *PLCB3* gene and a single nucleotide polymorphism (rs792789 allele A) linked to CD and atopic dermatitis maps to human chromosome 11q13 [12,13]. Moreover, atopic dermatitis is more common in patients with IBD than in control populations [14,15]. We previously showed that reduced PLC-β3 expression is associated with a subset of atopic dermatitis [16]. As PLC-β3 is the only one among four isozymes (PLC-β1~β4) that is highly expressed in IECs (Figure S1A–C), we studied a potential role of PLC-β3 in IBD pathogenesis, using a dextran sodium sulfate (DSS)-induced colitis model [17]. Using conventional and conditional *Plcb3* knockout mice, *Plcb3*-deficient IEC lines, and human CD biopsy samples, we found that PLC-β3 positively regulates Wnt/β-catenin signaling. This regulation is conserved from Drosophila to humans. We concluded that the reduced activity of PLC-β3-dependent Wnt/β-catenin signaling contributes to the development of ileal CD.

2. Materials and Methods

2.1. Study Design

Initially, DSS model experiments were conducted, revealing the differences between WT and *Plcb3*$^{-/-}$ mice. Experiments on bone marrow chimeras and conditional KO mice were followed to show the root cause of non-hematopoietic cells for the above differences. Morphological and transcriptomic abnormalities in the intestinal epithelial cells of *Plcb3*$^{-/-}$ mice were further confirmed and extended to the discovery of PLC-β3-regulated Wnt/β-catenin signaling and microbiota using epithelial cell mutants, *Plcb3*$^{-/-}$ mice, and Crohn's disease biopsies. PLC-β-regulated Wnt/β-catenin signaling was also shown in Drosophila.

2.2. Mice

This study used 8–14-week-old age- and gender-matched mice throughout. Mice were maintained under specific pathogen-free conditions and all the procedures were approved by the Institutional Animal Care and Use Committee of the La Jolla Institute for Immunology (approved protocol AP00001048). *Plcb3 flox* mice were generated by injecting ES cells (MGI: Clone: HEPD0811_7_H11) into mouse embryos, followed by crossing with

B6;SJL-Tg(ACTFLPe)9205Dym/J to remove FLP loci and then crossing with B6 to remove Act-FLPe allele. B6.Cg-Tg(Vil1-cre)997Gum/J, STOCK Tg(Col1a2-cre/ERT,-ALPP)7Cpd/J, B6;129-Tg(Cdh5-cre)1Spe/J, B6.Cg-Tg(Itgax-cre)1-1Reiz/J, B6.FVB-Tg(Rorc-cre)1Litt/J, and B6.129P2-Lyz2tm1(cre)Ifo/J mice were obtained from The Jackson Laboratory. B6;129-Tg(Cdh5-cre)1Spe/J mice were backcrossed to B6 mice for at least 8 generations before being used for experiments. For STOCK Tg(Col1a2-cre/ERT,-ALPP)7Cpd/J mice, 75 mg/kg of tamoxifen in corn oil was administered via intraperitoneal injection for 5 consecutive days 28 days before DSS treatment. No statistical methods were used to predetermine the sample size. The genotyping primers used and estimated band sizes are listed below. For *Plcb3* flox genotyping: Forward: 5′-TCCAGATGGTGCCACTCCTT-3′, Reverse: 5′-AGAAGCCATTAGGGTCCACA-3′ (504 bp for WT, 714 bp for flox). For *Plcb3* flox recombined: R: 5′-CACTTCGTTGAGTCTCGGGT-3′ (790 bp with *Plcb3* flox genotyping F for recombined *Plcb3* flox allele).

2.3. Drosophila

RNAi lines for *Plc21C* (*Plc21C*^{i1}: Vienna Drosophila Resource Center [VDRC] #108395, *Plc21C*^{i2}: VDRC #26558, *Plc21C*^{i3}: Bloomington Drosophila Stock Center [BDSC] #31269, and *Plc21C*^{i4}: BDSC #33719) and *y* (VDRC #106068) were expressed, along with *UAS-Dcr-2* (BDSC #24648), in third instar larval wing imaginal discs using the *hh-Gal4* driver [18]. Crosses were performed at 25 °C.

2.4. Study Participants

The patient-based studies were approved by the Institutional Review Board at Cincinnati Children's Hospital Medical Center (approval number 2011-2285), and consent was obtained from parents and adult subjects and assent from pediatric subjects aged 11 and above. We prepared unstained sections from formalin-fixed, paraffin-embedded, terminal ileal biopsies obtained for clinical care from seven patients with Crohn's disease (CD) at diagnosis prior to therapy and two non-IBD controls with normal colonoscopy. The two non-IBD controls were aged 15 and 18 years and were both White, of European ancestry, and not Hispanic or Latino. The seven CD patients were mean (range) 11 (8–15) years of age. Five (71%) were female and all were White, of European ancestry, and not Hispanic or Latino. Five (71%) exhibited an inflamed ileum, with four (57%) exhibiting ileal ulcers.

2.5. DSS Treatment of Mice

A total of 1–5% (w/v) DSS was added to drinking water and mice (4–6 mice per group) were treated ad libitum for 5 days. During and after DSS treatment, mice were monitored at least once a day, the body weight was measured every day, and the mice were euthanized according to the guidelines of the US National Institutes of Health and the animal protocols approved by the Institutional Animal Care and Use Committee of La Jolla Institute for Immunology. The results of all mice were included. Stools were evaluated as follows in a genotype-blinded manner. Stool blood: no blood, 0; blood on stool, 1; gross bleeding, 2. Blood samples were analyzed by Hemavet 950 (Drew Scientific, Plantation, FL, USA) to evaluate anemia. For DSS injection experiments, 1 mg of DSS in PBS was intravenously injected once or 40 mg of DSS was orally injected twice a day for 5 days.

2.6. Crypt Isolation and Organoid Culture

Small intestines were isolated, cut open, and washed with cold PBS. Villi were removed by scraping and vigorous pipetting. The tissues were chopped into 5 mm pieces and incubated with 2 mM EDTA/PBS for 30 min on ice. After replacing the supernatant with 25 mL of fresh cold PBS, crypts were isolated by pipetting 50 times. The supernatant was filtered through a 70 μm cell strainer, washed with Advanced DMEM/F12, and resuspended in Matrigel before being seeded in culture plates. Advanced DMEM/F12 was supplemented with 100 μg/mL penicillin, 100 U/mL streptomycin, 2 mM GlutaMAX, 1x N-2 supplement, 1x B27 supplement (all from Life Technologies, Carlsbad, CA, USA),

10 mM HEPES, 1 mM N-acetylcysteine (Sigma-Aldrich, St. Louis, MO, USA) supplemented with 7.5% FCS, 100 ng/mL recombinant mouse Noggin (Peprotech, Cranbury, NJ, USA), 100 ng/mL recombinant mouse EGF (Life Technologies), 500 ng/mL recombinant mouse R-spondin 1 (Life Technologies), and Y-27632 (STEMCELL Technologies, Vancouver, BC, Canada) immediately before use. The medium was changed every 2 days and passaged every 7 or 8 days. For passage, dispase was used to dissociate the organoids.

2.7. Generation and Validation of *Plcb3*-Deficient CMT-93 Cell Lines

Three pairs of oligonucleotides (IDT) for sgRNAs targeting mouse *Plcb3* exon 1 (sgRNAs 1 and 2) or 2 (sgRNA 3) which showed high sensitivity and specificity with integrative sgRNA efficacy prediction (iSEP: http://allergy.ims.riken.jp/index.html) or a pair of oligonucleotides for scramble sgRNA were cloned into lentiCRISPRv2 plasmid as previously described [19]. lentiCRISPRv2 was a gift from Feng Zhang (Addgene plasmid # 52961; http://n2t.net/addgene:5296; RRID:Addgene_52961). Briefly, oligonucleotides were annealed and then ligated with T4 ligase (NewEngland Biolabs, Ipswich, MA, USA [NEB]) into lentiCRISPRv2 fragments (lentiCRISPRv2 plasmid was digested with BsmBI (NEB) and then the larger band was gel-purified). Ligated products were transformed into *Stbl3 E. coli* (NEB) and inoculated to LB–agar plates with ampicillin (50 μg/mL) and incubated for 16 h at 37 °C. Colonies were picked up and screened by colony-PCR (1. 98 °C for 2 min, 2. 98 °C for 5 s, 3. 50 °C for 20 s, 4. 72 °C for 30 s, repeat steps 2–4 for 30 cycles, 5. 72 °C for 3 min, 6. 4 °C. The primers are shown below). Thus, chosen plasmids were cultured in 5 mL of LB medium with ampicillin (50 μg/mL) for 16 h. Plasmids were purified with mini-prep (Zymo Research, Irvine, CA, USA) and screened with restriction enzymes (NEB) to confirm the expected band sizes. Purified plasmids were mixed with sequencing primers and sent for Sanger sequencing (GENEWIZ, South Plainfield, NJ, USA) to confirm the insertion of the correct sgRNA sequence. ABI files were analyzed with FinchTV (Geospiza, Inc., Seattle, WA, USA). A total of 100 μL of bacterial glycerol stock with correct plasmids was inoculated into 200 mL of LB medium + ampicillin (50 mg/mL) and cultured for 16 h at 37 °C, and plasmids were purified with midi-prep (MACHEREY-NAGEL, Dueren, Germany). Plasmid concentration was determined by Nanodrop (Therm o Fisher Scientific, Waltham, MA, USA) and confirmed by gel electrophoresis.

Plcb3-sgRNA-1: F: 5′-CACCGAACTTACTCCCGCGCCGCA-3′, R: 5′-AAACTGCGG CGCGGGAGTAAGTTC-3′; *Plcb3*-sgRNA-2: F: 5′-CACCGCTTAGCCATGGCGGGCGCG-3′, R: 5′-AAACCGCGCCCGCCATGGCTAAGC-3′; *Plcb3*-sgRNA-3: F: 5′-CACCGAACCTG GTGACCCTGCGTG-3′, R: 5′-AAACCACGCAGGGTCACCAGGTTC-3′; Scramble sgRNA: F: 5′-CACCGGACGCGTGGCGAATCCTACG-3′, R: 5′-AAACCGTAGGATTCGCCACGCG TCC-3′; lentiCRISPRv2 colony-PCR: F: 5′-ACGATACAAGGCTGTTAGAGAGA-3′, R: 5′-GGACTAGCCTTATTTTAACTTGCT-3′

2.8. Transfection of CMT-93 Cells and Single-Cell Sorting

CMT-93 cells (ATCC) were cultured in DMEM (Gibco, Grand Island, NY, USA) supplemented with 10% FBS, penicillin/streptomycin, and glutamine (D10 medium). Then, 10 μg of plasmids with sgRNAs were transfected into freshly seeded (before attaching to the bottom of the culture plate) 25% confluent with equivalent numbers of (about 1×10^6 cells) CMT-93 cells with 20 μL of jetPRIME (Polyplus, Illkirch-Graffenstaden, France) and 500 μL of buffer, following the manufacturer's instructions. Puromycin (6 μg/mL) was added to the culture 48 h after transfection, and cells were cultured for 21 days, changing the medium with puromycin every 3 days. Cells were washed with PBS and then stripped with 2 mL of Trypsin/EDTA by incubating for 20 min; then, 8 mL of D10 medium was added to inactivate trypsin. Cells were centrifuged at 1500 rpm for 5 min and then the supernatants were removed, washed with PBS, and resuspended with FACS sorting buffer (PBS supplemented with 1% FBS, 5 mM EDTA, and 25 mM HEPES) in 5 mL polypropylene tubes. Single cells were sorted into 96-well plates filled with 200 μL of D10 medium by

FACSAria (BD Biosciences, Franklin Lakes, NJ, USA). Cells were cultured for 14 days and passaged to 24-well plates, 6-well plates, and 10 cm dishes, in this order.

2.9. Western Blotting for PLC-β3

Cells or crushed frozen tissues from mice were lysed with 1% NP-40 buffer (20 mM Tris-HCl [pH 8.0], 0.15 M NaCl, 1 mM EDTA) mixed with protease and phosphatase inhibitors (sodium vanadate, phenylmethylsulfonyl fluoride, aprotinin, leupeptin, pepstatin, 4-nitrophenyl 4-guanidinobenzoate, sodium fluoride), homogenized by needles and syringes, resolved by 5–14% gradient acrylamide gels, and transferred to PVDF membranes. Membranes were blocked with 5% non-fat milk, cut horizontally according to the molecular weight of the target protein, incubated with individual primary antibodies (anti-PLC-β3 antibodies (Cell Signaling Technology, Danvers, MA, USA; clone D9D6S; 1/1000 dilution); anti-tubulin (1/1000 dilution)) for 16 h at 4 °C on a nutator. Blots were washed 4 times with TBS-T for 5 min with gentle agitation and then incubated with anti-rabbit-HRP (Cell Signaling Technology) or anti-mouse-HRP antibodies for 1 h at 37 °C on a nutator. Blots were washed 4 times with TBS-T for 5 min with gentle agitation and then excessive water was removed by sandwiching with paper towels. The blots were then incubated with ECL reagents for 1 min (30 s with the front side up and 30 s with the back side up). After removing excessive reagents by sandwiching them with paper towels, blots were wrapped with SARAN wrap, placed in a cassette by tapes along with auto-luminescent marker sheets, and then X-ray films were exposed to blots for 20 s and processed. While processing the first film, the second film was exposed for 2 min; 2 s and 5 s exposures were taken depending on the result of 20 s of exposure and 20 min, 40 min, 2 h, or overnight exposures were taken depending on the result of 2 min of exposure. Processed films were scanned and the brightness of the image was adjusted with Photoshop (Adobe, San Jose, CA, USA) or Powerpoint 2013 (Microsoft, Redmond, WA, USA).

2.10. Insert–Deletion Confirmation in Plcb3-Deficient CMT-93 Cells

Genomic DNAs were extracted from approximately 4×10^6 *Plcb3-deficient* (clones 3P11, 3P13, and 2P9, all from sgRNA #3 for exon 2) or WT CMT-93 cell pellets by incubation with 20 μL of Short Genotyping Buffer (2 mM NaCl, 10 mM EDTA, and 0.1% SDS in 50 mM Tris pH 8.0) mixed with 1 μL of Proteinase K (20 mg/mL) for 1 h at 55 °C. Samples were boiled at 95 °C for 5 min to inactivate Proteinase K, and 980 μL of dH_2O was added to dilute samples. PCR reactions (Indel detection primers are shown below) were performed and analyzed on agarose gels. The bands with the expected size were extracted with a gel extraction kit (QIAGEN, Hilden, Germany) and ligated into zero-blunt vectors (Invitrogen). Ligation products were transformed into *Stbl3*, and plasmids from cultured bacteria were purified by mini-prep (Zymo Research). Plasmid DNAs were sequenced by GENEWIZ.

Plcb3 Indel detection and sequencing: F: 5′-GAACTGAACCTGCAATGCCC-3′, R: 5′-TCCTTAATTGCCCCACCCAG-3′.

2.11. Antibodies

The following antibodies were used for Western blotting. Wnt4 (ab91226, Abcam, Cambridge, UK), Lgr5 (ab75780, Abcam), LRP6 (C47E12, Cell Signaling Technology), Non-phospho (Active) β-catenin (D2U8Y, Cell Signaling Technology), HNF1α (D7Z2Q, Cell Signaling Technology), NFAT1 (D43B1, Cell Signaling Technology), Olfm4 (#66479 or D6Y5A, Cell Signaling Technology), Axin2 (#6163, Prosci; ab109307, Abcam), Actin (H-196, Santa Cruz Biotechnology, Dallas, TX, USA), Dvl2 (30D2, Cell Signaling Technology), Myc-Tag (71D10, Cell Signaling Technology), Phopsho-LRP6 (Ser1490) (#2568, Cell Signaling Technology), PLC-β3 (D9D6S, Cell Signaling Technology), Tubulin (DM1A, Santa Cruz Biotechnology), LRP5 (D80F2, Cell Signaling Technology), Fzd2 (MAB1307, R&D Systems, Minneapolis, MN, USA), Fzd4 (MAB194, R&D), Fzd5 (ab75234, Abcam), Fzd7 (ab64636, Abcam), GPR177 (Wls) (PA5-42570, Invitrogen, Waltham, MA, USA), PORCN (PA5-43423, Invitrogen), Axin (C76H11, Cell Signaling Technology), β-catenin (D10A8, Cell Signaling

Technology), CK1 (#2655, Cell Signaling Technology), GSK-3β (27C10, Cell Signaling Technology), FRAT1 (ab108405, Abcam), LGR4 (C-12, Santa Cruz Biotechnology), HA-Tag (C29F4, Cell Signaling Technology), LEF1 (C12A5, Cell Signaling Technology), Anti-rabbit IgG HRP-linked (NA934, GE Healthcare Life Sciences, Chicago, IL, USA), Anti-mouse IgG HRP-linked (NA931, GE Healthcare Life Sciences), and Anti-rat IgG HRP-linked (#7077, Cell Signaling Technology).

2.12. RNA Extraction from Plcb3-Deficient CMT-93 and Microarray Data Analysis

RNAs were extracted from subconfluent CMT-93 cultured in a 10 cm dish with RNeasy (QIAGEN) an on-column DNase kit (QIAGEN) following the manufacturer's instructions. RNA integrity was assessed by 0.8% agarose gel electrophoresis. The gene expression profiles were assessed using a microarray technology with Agilent Sure Print G3 Mouse GE 8 × 60 K Ver 3.0, according to the manufacturer's instructions (Agilent, Santa Clara, CA, USA. The gMedian fluorescence of probes from individual samples was normalized by R software. Data were analyzed by IPA (QIAGEN Inc., https://www.qiagenbioinformatics.com/products/ingenuity-pathway-analysis). Canonical pathway analysis was performed with a threshold of the activation Z-score > 1.7. A heatmap was created with R software.

2.13. qRT-PCR Analysis

cDNA was synthesized from 2.2 μg of RNA with Superscript II (Invitrogen, Cat# 18064071) and Random Hexamer (Invitrogen, Cat# N8080127) following the manufacturer's protocol. Then, PCR was performed on these cDNAs using Light Cycler (Bio-Rad, Hercules, CA, USA) and following primers. Values calculated by ΔΔCT methods were normalized against housekeeping genes (HPRT or L32). The following validated primers were used.

Tjp1 (ZO-1): F: 5′-CCTGTGAAGCGTCACTGTGT-3′, R: 5′-CGCGGAGAGAGACAAGATGT-3′; *Cldn1*: F: 5′- TCTACGAGGGACTGTGGATG-3′, R: 5′- TCAGATTCAGCAAGGAGTCG-3′; *Cldn3*: F: 5′-AAGCCGAATGGACAAAGAA-3′, R: 5′-CTGGCAAGTAGCTGCAGTG-3′; *Cldn4*: F: 5′-CGCTACTCTTGCCATTACG-3′, R: 5′-ACTCAGCACACCATGACTTG-3′; *Cldn7*: F: 5′-GCTAAGAAGCCCAACACCAG-3′, R: 5′-TGCAAAATGTACGACTCGGT-3′; *Ocln*: F: 5′-CATAGTCAGATGGGGGTGGA-3′, R: 5′-ATTTATGATGAACAGCCCCC-3′; *Rpl32* (L32): F: 5′-GAAACTGGCGGAAACCCA-3′, R: 5′-GGATCTGGCCCTTGAACCTT-3′; *Wnt2*: F: 5′-ATCTCTTCAGCTGGCGTTGT-3′, R: 5′-AGCCAGCATGTCCTCAGAGT-3′; *Wnt2b*: F: 5′-CACCCGGACTGATCTTGTCT-3′, R: 5′-TGTTTCTGCACTCCTTGCAC-3′; *Wnt4*: F: 5′-AACGGAACCTTGAGGTGATG-3′, R: 5′-GGACGTCCACAAAGGACTGT-3′; *Wnt5a*: F: 5′-CACGCTATACCAACTCCTCTGC-3′, R: 5′-AATATTCCAATGGGCTTCTTCATGGC-3′; *Wls*: F: 5′-CAAATCGTTGCCTTTC-3′, R: 5′-TTGTCACACTTGTTAGGTCCC-3′; *Porcn*: F: 5′-TCCTACATGGCTTCAGTTTCCA-3′, R: 5′-GCGCTTCCGGAGGACAT-3′; *Rspo1*: F: 5′-GCAACCCCGACATGAACAAAT-3′, R: 5′-GGTGCTGTTAGCGGCTGTAG-3′; *Rspo2*: F: 5′-CCAAGGCAACCGATGGAGAC-3′, R: 5′-TCGGCTGCAACCATTGTCC-3′; *Rspo3*: F: 5′-ATGCACTTGCGACTGATTTCT-3′, R: 5′-GCAGCCTTGACTGACATTAGGAT-3′; *Fzd4*: F: 5′-GACAACTTTCACGCCGCTCATC-3′, R: 5′-CCAGGCAAACCCAAATTCTCTCAG-3′; *Fzd7*: F: 5′-ATATCGCCTACAACCAGACCATCC-3′, R: 5′-AAGGAACGGCACGGAGGAATG-3′; *Lgr5*: F: 5′-CCTACTCGAAGACTTACCCAGT-3′, R: 5′-GCATTGGGGTGAATGATAGCA-3′; *Axin2*: F: 5′-GAGTTATCCAGCGACGCACT-3′, R: 5′-CATGCGGTAAGGAGGGACTC-3′; *Olfm4*: F: 5′-GCCACTTTCCAATTTCAC-3′, R: 5′-GAGCCTCTTCTCATACAC-3′; *Ascl2*: F: 5′-CTACTCGTCGGAGGAAAG-3′, R: 5′-ACTAGACAGCATGGGTAAG-3′; *Gja1*: F: 5′-GATCGCGTGAAGGGAAGAAG-3′, R: 5′-CAGCCATTGAAGTAAGCATATTTTG-3′; *Hnf1a*: F: 5′-AGAGCCCCTTCATGGCAACC-3′, R: 5′-TGAAGACCTGCTTGGTGGGTG-3′; *Nfat1*: F: 5′-GTGCAGCTCCACGGCTACAT-3′, R: 5′-GCGGCTTAAGGATCCTCTCA-3′; and *Hprt*: F: 5′-AAGCTTGCTGGTGAAAAGGA-3′, R: 5′-TTGCGCTCATCTTAGGCTTT-3′

2.14. Gene Set Enrichment Analysis (GSEA)

The β-catenin-regulated gene set and Lgr4/5 signature gene set were obtained from the previous publications [20–24], and the original KEGG WNT signaling pathway was used. GSEA was performed as described [25,26].

2.15. Reanalysis of Publicly Available Single-Cell RNA-Seq Data

Single-cell RNA-seq data for human terminal ileum of childhood-onset Crohn's disease and matched healthy controls [27] were obtained from https://www.gutcellatlas.org/ as an H5AD file. The data were analyzed using Scanpy 1.8.1 [28]. Mouse intestine datasets [29,30] were analyzed at https://portals.broadinstitute.org/single_cell/study/fasi-immune-mouse-small-intestine and https://singlecell.broadinstitute.org/single_cell/study/SCP44/small-intestinal-epithelium.

2.16. ATAC-Seq Analysis

Subconfluent *Plcb3-deficient* (clones 3P11, 3P13, and 2P9) or control (clones Scr1, Scr2, and Scr4) CMT-93 cells were dissociated with Trypsin/EDTA (in 1x PBS pH 7.4) and the numbers of cells were counted. Cells were resuspended with PBS at 1×10^6/mL and 5×10^4 cells were aliquoted and centrifuged at 2000 rpm (500 rcf) for 5 min. The supernatant was removed and cells were resuspended with 50 μL of cold lysis buffer (10 mM Tris-Hcl, pH 7.4, 10 mM NaCl, 3 mM $MgCl_2$, 0.1% NP40) [31] in 1.5 mL Eppendorf tubes. Tubes were vortexed for 1 min and centrifuged at 2000 rpm (500 rcf) for 10 min at 4 °C. The supernatant was carefully removed and pellets were resuspended with 20 μL of Tagment DNA (TD) buffer (Illumina, San Diego, CA, USA), and 3 μL of QXT transposase was added to the samples on ice. Samples were incubated at 37 °C for 60 min and then placed on ice for 1 min to cool. A total of 2 μL of 1% SDS (final concentration 0.1%) was added and incubated at RT for 2 min to stop reactions. Then, 30 μL of AMpure beads (Thermo Fisher Scientific, Cat # NC9959336) was added to each sample, which was pipetted 10 times to mix and then incubated for 5 min at RT. Samples were placed on the magnetic stand for 2 min and then the supernatant was removed. Samples were washed with 200 μL of freshly prepared 80% ethanol twice and then air-dried for 10 min after complete removal of the residual ethanol. Pellets were resuspended with 11 μL of nuclease-free water and incubated for 2 min. Samples were placed on the magnet and incubated for 2 min. Then, 10 μL of the samples were transferred to new tubes. A total of 10 μL of the samples was mixed with Kapa-Hifi 2× master mix 25 μL, H_2O 13 μL, QXT custom 5XX primer 1 μL, and QXT custom 7XX primer 1 μL. A PCR reaction was conducted with the following protocol: 1. 68 °C for 2 min, 2. 98 °C for 2 min, 3. 98 °C for 30 s, 4. 57 °C for 30 s, 5. 72 °C for 1 min, 6. repeat steps 3 to 5 (12 cycles in total), 7. 72 °C 5 min, 8. 4 °C hold. Then, 20 μL of AMpure beads was added to the samples, which were incubated for 5 min and placed on a magnet; then, the supernatants were transferred to other tubes. A total of 30 μL of AMpure beads was added to the samples, which were incubated for 5 min, placed on a magnet, washed twice, and eluted with 13 μL of nuclease-free water. The quality of the library was checked by Tapestation HS 1000 (Agilent) and the amount of usable library was further quantified by qPCR. Samples were pooled for sequencing with HiSeq (Illumina). Sequencing data generated were uploaded to the Galaxy web platform, and the public server at usegalaxy.org was used to analyze the data. Paired-end FASTQ reads were mapped to the mouse genome (mm10) by Bowtie2 [32] with the default setting of Galaxy and then triplicated libraries were merged. Then, files were converted to bigwig files by bamtobigwig. The peaks were named with MACS2 [33]. The mapped reads were visualized with an integrative genome viewer (Broad Institute, Cambridge, MA, USA).

2.17. Co-Immunoprecipitation

A total of 25% confluent 293T cells (about 3×10^6 cells) cultured in DMEM (Gibco) supplemented with 10% FBS, penicillin/streptomycin, and glutamine was transfected with a vector control or untagged, N-terminally myc-tagged, or C-terminally myc-tagged human PLC-β3 expression vectors together with expression vectors for a test protein. Plasmids for test proteins including those coding for Tcf4, Lef1, β-catenin, GSK-3β, Axin, and NLK were provided by Dr. Tohru Ishitani. Plasmids for NFAT1 were gifts from Dr. Anjana Rao. Plasmids expressing Gαq were gifts from Dr. Shinya Tsukiji. Constitutively active Gαq mutant (Q209L) was generated using Gibson assembly (NEB) after PCR amplification with primers F: 5′-GGGGCCTGAGGTCAGAGAGAAGAAAATGGA-3′ and R: 5′-CTGACCTCAGGCCCCCTACATCGAC-3′. cDNAs for LGR4 (BC033039), LGR5 (BC096324), LRP6 (BC117136), WLS (BC110826), Dvl2 (BC014844), Frat1 (BC034476), Fzd5 (BC117723), and LRP5 (BC011374) were obtained through transOMIC technologies (Huntsville, AL, USA).

Then, 48 h after transfection, cells were washed twice with PBS and lysed with 1% NP-40 buffer mixed with protease and phosphatase inhibitors. A total of 10 μL of Dynabeads (Thermo Fisher Scientific, Cat. #10003D) was used to preincubate with 1 μg of control mouse IgG1 (MG1-45, BioLegend, San Diego, CA, USA), anti-c-Myc (MC045, Nacalai Tesque, Kyoto, Japan) anti-HA (HA124, Nacalai Tesque), anti-Flag (M2, Sigma-Aldrich), control rabbit IgG (DA1E, Cell Signaling Technology), anti-Dvl2 (30D2, Cell Signaling Technology), anti-TCF4/TCF7L2 (C48H11, Cell Signaling Technology), anti-NFAT1 (D43B1, Cell Signaling Technology), or anti-GSK-3β (27C10, Cell Signaling Technology) antibodies for 30 min at RT and then washed with lysis buffer. Beads were incubated with 100 μg of lysate in 200 μL for 10 min at RT and then washed with 200 μL of lysis buffer 3 times. Beads were resuspended with 40 μL of 1x SDS sample buffer and boiled at 95 °C for 5 min. Co-immunoprecipitated proteins were assessed by Western blotting with the following antibodies: LRP6 (C47E12, Cell Signaling Technology, 1/1000, Lot:3), LRP5 (D80F2, Cell Signaling Technology, 1:1000, Lot:2), Lgr5 (ab75780, Abcam, 1:1000, Lot:GR131564-18), Fzd5 (ab75234, Abcam, 1:1000, GR62870-20), Dvl2 (30D2, Cell Signaling Technology, 1:1000, Lot:4), β-catenin (D10A8, Cell Signaling Technology, 1:1000, Lot:5), Axin (C76H11, Cell Signaling Technology, 1:1000, Lot:4), CK1 (#2655, Cell Signaling Technology, 1:1000, Lot:2), GSK-3β (27C10, Cell Signaling Technology, 1:1000, Lot:14), Frat1 (ab108405, Abcam, 1:1000, Lot:GR49498-3), NFAT1 (D43B1, Cell Signaling Technology, 1:1000, Lot:4), GPR177 (Wls) (PA5-42570, Invitrogen, 1:1000, Lot:PK2296133), NLK (D9X3C, Cell Signaling Technology, 1:1000), Lef1 (C12A5, Cell Signaling Technology, 1:1000, Lot:5), TCF4/TCF7L2 (C48H11, Cell Signaling Technology), 1D4-tag (sc-57432, Santa Cruz Biotechnology, 1:500), and Pan-Gα (3992S, Cell Signaling Technology, 1:1000).

The presence of immunoprecipitated proteins was confirmed by re-probing of the blots after mild stripping with the following antibodies: Myc-Tag (71D10, Cell Signaling Technology, 1:1000, Lot:5), Dvl2 (30D2, Cell Signaling Technology, 1:1000, Lot:4), and TCF4/TCF7L2 (C48H11, Cell Signaling Technology).

2.18. 16S rRNA DNA Sequencing

Fecal pellets were collected from mice before and after DSS treatment. DNA was extracted from approximately 20 mg of feces with the QIAamp DNA Stool Mini Kit (QIAGEN), following the manufacturer's protocol. Libraries were prepared following a 16S metagenomic sequencing library preparation guide (Illunina) and run with Miseq v3 (Illumina). Generated FASTQ reads were processed with Illumina 16S metagenomics 1.0.1 pipeline (Illumina; basespace application). The reads classified to the individual genus and species were divided by the total number of classified reads to calculate the proportion.

2.19. Animal Experiments

FITC injection experiment. Mice were treated with water or 3% DSS ad libitum for 24 h and orally gavaged with FITC-Dextran (70 kDa). Then, 6 h later, blood was collected from the mesenteric vein and the fluorescence of FITC-Dextran in sera was measured by SpectramaxM2.

Citrobacter infection experiment. Next, 1×10^9 CFU of chloramphenicol-resistant *Citrobacter rodentium* [34] was orally injected and tissues were harvested 6 days later. The burden of bacteria in liver, spleen, and fecal samples from the colons was assessed with chloramphenicol plates by inoculating serially diluted tissue homogenates.

Antibiotics treatment. Mice were treated with a cocktail of antibiotics (ampicillin 1 mg/mL, neomycin 1 mg/mL, vancomycin 0.5 mg/mL, and metronidazole 1 mg/mL) with a sweetener (Splenda; 10 mg (*w*/*v*)) for 4 weeks before DSS treatment.

Human R-spondin1 treatment. Mice were intravenously injected with PBS or 100 μg or 200 μg of human R-spondin1 (a gift from Kyowa-Kirin, Tokyo, Japan) in 200 μL of PBS every 24 h. For Western blotting and qRT-PCR, tissues were harvested 6 h after the last i.v. injection.

Bone marrow chimera experiment. Next, 1.0×10^6 cells were collected from donor WT or *Plcb3*$^{-/-}$ mice and intravenously injected into X-ray-irradiated (480 rad × 2; 960 rad in total) recipient WT or *Plcb3*$^{-/-}$ mice. Chimeric bone marrow was confirmed by blood genotyping and mice were orally treated with 3% DSS 9 weeks after the bone marrow transfer.

Histological analysis. Mouse intestines from the stomach to the colon were harvested at days 2, 4, or 7 of DSS treatment. After measuring the length of the intestines and taking photos, the intestines were cut open longitudinally, washed, rolled up, and fixed with 4% zinc formalin for 24 h. Then, formalin was replaced with 70% isopropanol (*v*/*v*) and tissues were kept in the solution for at least 24 h. The samples were further dehydrated with 70% ethanol, 80% ethanol, 90% ethanol, 100% ethanol, and Pro-Per; then, the samples were embedded in paraffin and sectioned with microtome at a 5 μm thickness. Slides were stained with H&E, PAS, or Alcian blue and scanned by Axioscan Z1 (ZEISS). Histological scores were calculated in a blinded manner as previously described [35]. Colons were separated into 3 areas and the extent of inflammation and crypt damage was assessed for each area.

Whole mount staining of ileum. A total of 10 cm of ileum harvested from water or DSS-treated mice was washed and fixed with 4% paraformaldehyde (PFA) for 1 h, washed, and placed in Magic buffer (2% FBS, 0.5% Saponin, 0.1% Sodium Azide in PBS). Muscles were carefully scraped with forceps under a stereoscope and tissues were cut into 2 mm × 2 mm pieces; permeabilized with Magic buffer for 2 h; incubated with anti-Olfm4 (#66479, Cell signaling Technology) or Ki-67 (D3B5, Cell Signaling Technology) for 16 h at RT; incubated with Hoechst 33342 (H3570, Invitrogen), anti-rabbit IgG DyLight™ 488 (#406404, BioLegend), and Alexa Fluor™ 647 Phalloidin (A22287, Invitrogen) for 2 h at RT; and mounted on the slides with Prolong gold. For UEA-1-FITC staining or the analysis of *Lgr5-EGFP-IRES-CreERT2*$^+$ mice, the incubation step with the primary antibody was skipped. Images were taken by SP5 (Zeiss, Jena, Germany), Fluoview 10i (Olympus, Tokyo, Japan), or LSM880 airyscan (Zeiss) and processed with the Leica Application Suite (for SP5) or Bitplane-Imaris (SciTech, Preston, Australia) for 3D reconstruction. Videos of 3D reconstructed images were generated and exported through Imaris and saved in MP4 format. The numbers of bifurcated crypt lumen and non-bifurcated crypt lumen were counted.

Frozen-/paraffin-embedded-section immuno-fluorescent staining. A total of 10 cm of jejunum or ileum was harvested, washed with 4% PFA by flashing, cut open longitudinally, and fixed with 4% PFA for 1.5 h on ice. Tissues were washed with PBS 3 times and incubated with 15% or 30% sucrose–PBS for 15 or 45 min, respectively, for cryoprotection. Tissues were embedded in OCT compound (Sakura Finetek, USA, Torrance, CA, USA) and sectioned at 10 μm thicknesses. Slides were washed with PBS; permeabilized with 0.3% Triton X for 10 min; blocked with 10% normal donkey serum for 1 h; incubated with anti-ZO-1 (H-300, Santa Cruz Biotechnology), claudin4 (ZMD.306, Invitrogen), and anti-lysozyme (C-19, Santa Cruz Biotechnology) for 16 h at 4 °C; incubated with secondary antibodies for 1 h at RT; and mounted with Prolong gold (Fisher Scientific Cat. # P36390). Images were taken with FluoView FV10i (Olympus), Nikon 80i, or Axioscan Z1 and processed with Zen blue (Zeiss). For both samples and corresponding controls, the same microscopy with the same laser intensity was used for each experiment and images were processed in the same way throughout the study. For paraffin-embedded human samples, antigen retrieval was performed by heating for 10 min at 95 °C in 10 mM sodium citrate solution (pH 6.0) before permeabilization. Anti-PLC-β3 (D9D6S, Cell Signaling Technology) antibody or a rabbit IgG isotype control (DA1E, Cell Signaling Technology) was used as the primary antibody. Axioscan Z1 was used for initial quantitative analysis and FluoView FV10i was used for conformation and taking representative images.

2.20. *Drosophila Immunohistochemistry*

Third instar larval wing imaginal discs were dissected in PBS and fixed in 4% paraformaldehyde in PBS for 20 min. After fixation, discs were washed with PBS with 0.1% Triton X-100, followed by incubation in PBS with 0.1% Triton X-100 and 10% BSA for 1 h at RT. Wing discs were incubated with rabbit anti-dsRed (Clontech/TaKaRa, Cat. no. 632496, 1:500) to detect the *senseless* transcriptional reporter *mScar:T2A:sens* [36], mouse anti-Wg (4D4, Developmental Studies Hybridoma bank [DSHB], 1:500), and mouse anti-Engrailed (En) (4D9, DSHB, 1:20) at 4 °C overnight in PBS with 0.5% Triton X-100, followed by incubation with secondary antibodies (anti-mouse and anti-rabbit Alexa Fluor 488 and 555 conjugates; Thermo Fisher Scientific, 1:500) for 2 h at RT. Specimens were stained with DAPI (2 μg/mL) and mounted in Prolong Gold (Invitrogen). Images were captured using a Nikon CSU-W1 spinning disk confocal microscope and processed with Adobe Photoshop/Illustrator software. Quantitation was performed using Prism 8 software (Graphpad, Boston, MA, USA).

2.21. *Drosophila Abdomens*

Adult abdomens from crosses between the *B119-Gal4* driver and denoted RNAi lines were dissected and mounted onto glass slides and covered with glass coverslips. Images were acquired using a Leica MZ10F modular stereo microscope and a Zeiss Axiocam 208 camera. Images were processed with Zen Blue 3.0 and Adobe Photoshop/Illustrator software. Quantitation was performed using Prism 8 software (Graphpad).

2.22. *Statistical Analysis*

No statistical test was performed to pre-determine sample sizes. A log-rank test, two-tailed Student's *t*-test, paired *t*-test, Mann–Whitney U test, one-way ANOVA, or Kruskal–Wallis and Dunn's multiple comparison tests were performed through Prism (Graphpad) where applicable. p values smaller than 0.05 were considered statistically significant.

3. Results

3.1. *PLC-β3 KO Mice Exhibit DSS-Induced Lethality with Severe Inflammation in the Small Intestine and Anemia*

All *Plcb3*$^{-/-}$ mice exposed to 3% DSS in drinking water lost body weight (Figure S1D) and died within 6 days, while WT mice survived (Figure 1A). DSS-treated *Plcb3*$^{-/-}$ mice exhibited bloody stool (Figure 1B) and severe anemia (Figure 1C). *Plcb3*$^{-/-}$ mice exhibited increased intestinal permeability with or without DSS exposure, as demonstrated by FITC-dextran (70 kDa) gavage (Figure 1D) and *Citrobacter rodentium* infection (Figure S1E). These findings were consistent with DSS-induced morphological abnormalities including rough and disrupted villus tips of the jejunum and ileum (Figure 1E) and reduced expression and/or aberrant distribution of several tight junction proteins including ZO-1, occludin, and claudins 1/3/4/7, even without DSS treatment (Figure 1F,G). Similar to their expression in the IECs, crypt organoids from the small intestine of *Plcb3*$^{-/-}$ mice exhibited decreased mRNA expression of several tight junction proteins including ZO-1, occludin, and claudins 1/3/4/5/8/9/10/11 (Figure S2A,B). Some of these and other proteins were confirmed by Western blotting, immunofluorescence confocal microscopy, and qRT-PCR (Figure S2C,D). Therefore, the increased intestinal permeability in *Plcb3*$^{-/-}$ mice was likely due to IEC-intrinsic impairment. The differences in DSS-induced injury between WT and *Plcb3*$^{-/-}$ mice were limited to the small intestine, as the injury scores in the colons of DSS-exposed *Plcb3*$^{-/-}$ mice were comparable to those of WT mice (Figure S1F,G). No abnormalities were observed in heterozygous *Plcb3*$^{+/-}$ mice.

Analysis of IECs by fluorescence microscopy and 3D reconstitution revealed that the numbers of Olfm4^{+} crypt base columnar cells, which were Lgr5^{+} ISCs [37] (Figures 1H and S1H,I and Videos S1 and S2), and Ki-67^{+} proliferative cells (Figure 1I and Videos S3 and S4) were significantly reduced in the ilea of untreated and DSS-treated *Plcb3*$^{-/-}$ mice. Reduced numbers of Lgr5^{+} ISCs were also observed in DSS-treated *Plcb3*$^{-/-}$;*Lgr5-EGFP-IRES-CreERT2* reporter mice compared with control *Plcb3*$^{+/-}$;*Lgr5-EGFP-IRES-CreERT2* mice (Figure S1J,K). Consistent with the reduction in proliferative cells, crypt fissions were drastically reduced in *Plcb3*$^{-/-}$ mice (Figure S3A,B). In addition, increases in crypt goblet cells (Figures 1J and S3C,D) and mucin (Figure S3E) were observed. Furthermore, reduced expression of *lyz1*, *Reg3a*, *Reg3g*, and lysozyme protein (Figure S3F,G) and reduced α(1,2)fucosylation (Figures 1K and S3H and Videos S5 and S6) indicated abnormalities in Paneth cells [38].

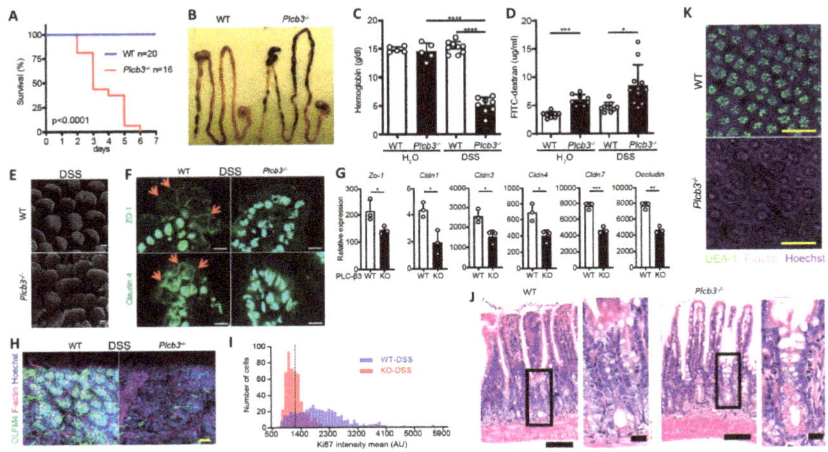

Figure 1. *Plcb3*$^{-/-}$ mice exhibited a DSS-induced lethal phenotype with severe inflammation in the small intestine and anemia. (**A**) Survival curves of mice exposed to 3% DSS for 5 days. (**B**) Gastrointestinal tracts of WT and *Plcb3*$^{-/-}$ mice after 1 day of exposure to 3% DSS. Note bloody stools in *Plcb3*$^{-/-}$ mice. (**C**) Hemoglobin concentrations in serum. **** $p < 0.0001$. (**D**) FITC-dextran was orally injected into mice pretreated with 3% DSS or H_2O for 24 h; 6 h later, FITC-dextran in serum was quantified. The graph shows mean ± SD. * $p < 0.05$; *** $p < 0.001$, determined by Kruskal–Wallis test and Dunn's multiple comparison test. (**E**) Whole mount staining of distal ilea of 2-day DSS-treated WT and *Plcb3*$^{-/-}$ mice were analyzed by confocal microscopy. Villi stained for F-actin by phalloidin, scale bar 50 μm. (**F**) Jejunal villi of WT and *Plcb3*$^{-/-}$ mice treated with DSS for 2 days were analyzed by confocal microscopy for ZO-1 (top) and claudin4 (bottom) expression. Arrows indicate staining at the cell–cell borders. Scale bar 10 μm. (**G**) qRT-PCR analysis of tight junction proteins in small intestines of DSS-untreated mice. * $p < 0.05$; ** $p < 0.01$ vs. WT by Student's *t*-test. (**H**) Ileal crypts from mice treated with DSS for 2 days were stained by Hoechst (nuclei), anti-Olfm4 (ISCs), and phalloidin (F-actin). Scale bar 20 μm. (**I**) Histograms of Ki-67 mean fluorescence intensity (MFI) per crypt cells. In total, 500 ileal epithelial cells in DSS-treated mice were measured using sections stained for Ki-67. (**J**) H&E staining of ilea of WT or *Plcb3*$^{-/-}$ mice exposed to 3% DSS for 2 days. Portions indicated by rectangles are enlarged on the right. Scale bars 100 and 10 μm. (**K**) Whole mount ilea from mice treated with DSS for 2 days were stained by Hoechst, UEA-1, and phalloidin. Scale bar 100 μm.

3.2. Multiple Non-Hematopoietic Cell Types Contribute to the DSS-Induced Lethality of *Plcb3*$^{-/-}$ Mice

Single-cell RNA sequencing data of human [27,39] and mouse [29] intestinal cells indicate that *PLCB3/Plcb3* mRNA is expressed most highly in IECs, other non-hematopoietic cells including fibroblasts and endothelial cells, and hematopoietic cells (Figure S4). Furthermore, *PLCB3/Plcb3* expression is high in the early stages of epithelial cell development and in enterocytes, whereas enteroendocrine cells and goblet cells tend to lose this expression (Figure S4C,E). Thus, abnormalities in IECs likely contribute to the DSS-induced lethality in *Plcb3*$^{-/-}$ mice. The involvement of IECs and other cell types in this phenotype was tested initially with bone marrow chimeras. Irrespective of the donor genotype, the recipient *Plcb3*$^{-/-}$ mice, but not the recipient WT mice, died upon DSS exposure (Figure 2A). This result suggests that non-hematopoietic cells are responsible for the lethal phenotype of *Plcb3*$^{-/-}$ mice. To further identify the cell type(s) responsible for the DSS-induced lethality, we made *Plcb3*$^{fl/fl}$ mice to generate conditional knock-out (cKO) mice (Figure S5A). IEC-specific deletion of the *Plcb3* gene was achieved by crossing *Villin-Cre* mice with *Plcb3*$^{fl/fl}$ mice (termed *Plcb3*$^{\Delta IEC}$ mice, Figure S5B–D). *Plcb3*$^{\Delta IEC}$ mice exhibited severe anemia when fed 5% DSS (Figure S5E) but not when fed 3% DSS (data not shown) and slightly increased intestinal permeability (Figure S5F,G). In comparison to *Plcb3*$^{fl/fl}$ mice, *Plc3*$^{\Delta IEC}$ mice were more susceptible to DSS when pretreated with antibiotics (Figure S5H), but did not display the early lethal phenotype without antibiotic treatment (Figure 2B). Furthermore, we generated fibroblast (FB)- (using Col1a2-CreERT2), endothelial cell (EC)- (using Cdh5-Cre), myeloid cell (MC)- (using LysM-Cre), dendritic cell (DC)- (using Cd11c-Cre), and type 3 innate lymphoid cell (ILC3)- (using Rorc-Cre) specific cKO mice. As expected from our results with bone marrow chimeras, the resistance of MC-, DC-, and ILC3-specific cKO mice to DSS was similar to that of WT mice (Figure 2C). No single cKO mouse showed the early lethal phenotype (Figure 2C). Interestingly, *Plcb3*$^{\Delta FB}$ mice exhibited goblet cell hyperplasia (Figure S5I), similar to *Plcb3*$^{-/-}$ mice. We then intercrossed single cKO strains to make double cKO strains and found that only *Plcb3*$^{\Delta IEC;EC}$ showed early intestinal bleeding following treatment with 3% DSS (Figure S5J). Finally, we crossed *Plcb3*$^{\Delta FB}$ and *Plcb3*$^{\Delta IEC;EC}$ to generate triple cKO mice, which exhibited increased DSS susceptibility (Figure 2D,E). Thus, these results suggest that PLC-β3-regulated signaling pathways in IECs, FBs, and ECs work together to protect from DSS-induced injury and/or promote repair.

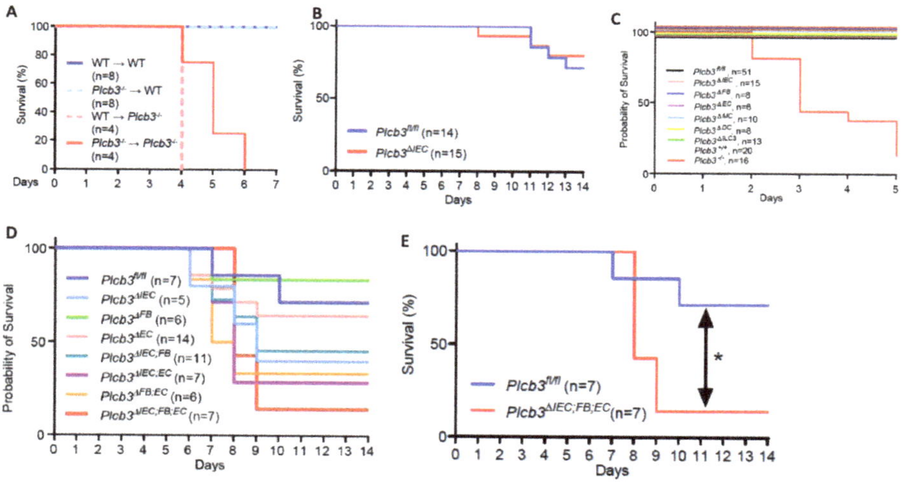

Figure 2. Multiple non-hematopoietic cell types contribute to the DSS-induced lethality of *Plcb3*$^{-/-}$ mice. (**A**) Survival curves of the recipient WT or *Plcb3*$^{-/-}$ mice that were orally treated with 3% DSS for 5 days 9 weeks after the bone marrow transfer. (**B**) Survival curves of *Plcb3*$^{fl/fl}$ and *Plcb3*$^{fl/fl}$*;villin-Cre* (*Plcb3*$^{\Delta IEC}$) mice exposed to 3% DSS. (**C**,**D**) Survival curves of multiple conditional KO strains treated with 3% DSS. IEC: intestinal epithelial cell; FB: fibroblast; EC: endothelial cell; MC: myeloid cell; DC: dendritic cell; ILC3: type 3 innate lymphoid cell. (**E**) Survival curves of *Plcb3*$^{\Delta IEC;FB;EC}$ mice or littermate *Plcb3*$^{fl/fl}$ control mice treated with 3% DSS. * $p < 0.05$ by log-rank test.

3.3. Small Intestinal Epithelial Cells from $Plcb3^{-/-}$ Mice Exhibit Decreased Wnt/β-Catenin Signaling

To gain insight into the molecular mechanisms by which *Plcb3* deficiency increases DSS susceptibility, gene expression in isolated small intestinal IECs was analyzed using DNA microarray. Consistent with reduced proliferative IECs (Figure 1I), gene set enrichment analysis (GSEA) showed that cell cycle-related E2F target genes, G2/M checkpoint genes, and Myc-regulated genes were downregulated in IECs of $Plcb3^{-/-}$ and $Plcb3^{\Delta IEC}$ mice vs. their respective controls under homeostatic conditions (Figure S6A). Importantly, GSEA also revealed reduced expression of Wnt/β-catenin signature genes [20] including *Wls, Fzd7, Axin2, Lgr5,* and *Olfm4* (Figure 3A,B) and the Lgr4-, $Lgr4^+/Lgr5^+$-, and $Ascl2^+$-stem/progenitor signature genes [21] in small intestinal IECs of $Plcb3^{-/-}$ mice under homeostatic (Figure 3A). Similarly, small intestinal IECs from $Plcb3^{\Delta IEC}$ mice under homeostatic conditions exhibited reduced expression of Wnt/β-catenin signature genes and $Lgr4^+$-, $Lgr4^+/Lgr5^+$-, and $Ascl2^+$-stem/progenitor signature genes in comparison to $Plcb3^{fl/fl}$ mice (Figure 3C). Lgr4 and Lgr5 bind to R-spondins, which bridge and internalize the negative regulators Rnf43 and Znrf3 with Lgr4/Lgr5 to promote the activation of Wnt/β-catenin signaling [40]. Lgr4 hypomorphic mice exhibit a lethal inflammatory phenotype with reduced ISCs and Paneth cells upon DSS exposure [41], similar to $Plcb3^{-/-}$ mice. Moreover, Ingenuity Pathway Analysis (IPA) [42] indicated the downregulation of Wnt/β-catenin signaling in $Plcb3^{-/-}$ mice (Figure S6B) and the opposite regulation of β-catenin-regulated genes (Figure S6C). Consistent with the involvement of mesenchymal cells in the DSS-induced lethality of $Plcb3^{-/-}$ mice, small intestinal mesenchymal cells in $Plcb3^{-/-}$ mice exhibited reduced mRNA expression of several Wnt ligands, as well as factors essential for Wnt secretion (Wls, Porcn) and Wnt signal enhancers (R-spondins 1/2/3) (Figures 3D and S6D). Reduced mRNA expression of the Wnt target genes *Wls, Fzd7, Axin2, Lgr5, Olfm4,* and *Ascl2* in $Plcb3^{-/-}$ IECs was found, several of which were confirmed by qRT-PCR (Figure 3B). Furthermore, reduced levels of Wls, Wnt-4, LRP6, Fzd2, Axin2, β-catenin, GATA6, and Olfm4 proteins in $Plcb3^{-/-}$ IECs were confirmed by Western blotting (Figure 3E). By contrast, SPDEF, which antagonizes the expression of Wnt/β-catenin target genes [43], was increased in $Plcb3^{-/-}$ IECs. These results collectively show that PLC-β3 regulates expression of the Wnt/β-catenin signaling pathway at numerous levels, including the Wnt ligands, regulators of Wnt secretion (Wls, Porcn), Wnt signal enhancers (R-spondin 1/3), Wnt co-receptors (Fzd2, Fzd7, Lgr5, LRP6), the negative feedback regulator (Axin2), and transcription factors (Ascl2, GATA6, SPDEF).

3.4. PLC-β3 Regulates the Wnt/β-Catenin Signaling Pathway in IECs at Multiple Regulatory Levels

To further explore the function of PLC-β3 in IECs, *Plcb3*-deficient CMT-93 mouse IEC lines were generated using the CRISPR/Cas9 method (Figure 4A). GSEA and IPA canonical pathway analysis of transcriptomes in three *Plcb3*-deficient clones with different mutations vs. three *Plcb3*-sufficient controls showed reduced Wnt/β-catenin signaling (Figure 4B,C), which was ranked as one of the most affected among the *Plcb3*-affected pathways (Figure S7A). The reduced expression of several Wnt/β-catenin signaling molecules was confirmed by qRT-PCR and Western blotting (Figure 4D,E). Consistent with these observations, the transcriptional activity of TCF/LEF was markedly reduced in *Plcb3*-deficient cells (Figure 4F). Moreover, ATAC-seq analysis [44] followed by pathway analysis using clusterProfiler [45] revealed that the Wnt signaling pathway, inflammatory bowel disease pathway, calcium signaling pathway, and tight junction pathway were in the top 30 pathways that were different between WT and $Plcb3^{-/-}$ cells (Figure S7B). Among them, Wnt/β-catenin pathway gene loci, including *Dkk2, Fzd7, Axin2,* and *Lgr5,* were identified (Figure 4G). Additionally, numerous other loci near *Gja1* (*Cx43*), *Ttc9, Arhgap26,* and *Robo1* were identified as chromatin accessibility sites regulated by PLC-β3 (Figure S7C). Gja1 plays a role in the innate immune control of commensal-mediated wound repair of IECs [46], although enteric glial Gja1 does not affect acute DSS-induced colitis [47].

Robo1, the receptor for the secreted glycoprotein Slit2, mediates DSS-induced colitis by activating the autophagy of Lgr5⁺ ISCs [48]. The above results collectively suggest that the expression of numerous Wnt/β-catenin pathway genes is controlled by PLC-β3 in IECs at the transcriptional and epigenetic levels.

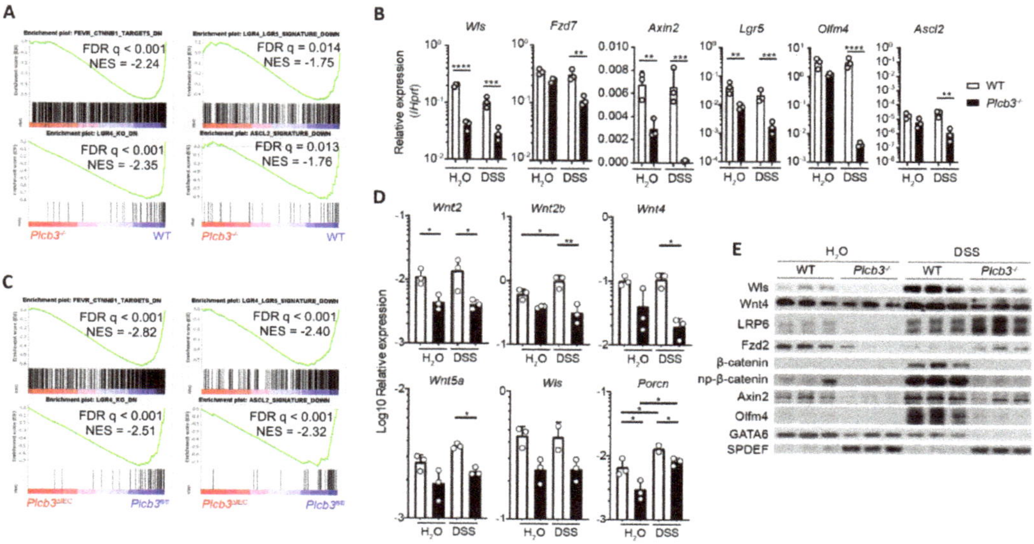

Figure 3. Small intestinal epithelial cells of *Plcb3*$^{-/-}$ mice exhibit downregulation of the Wnt/β-catenin signaling pathway. (**A**) GSEA indicates that the gene expression pattern in isolated IECs from *Plcb3*$^{-/-}$ mice correlates with the reduced expression of Wnt/β-catenin signature genes (upper left), Lgr4 regulated signature genes (lower left), Lgr4/Lgr5 regulated signature genes (upper right), and Ascl2 signature genes (lower right). NES: normalized enrichment score. $n = 3$ biological replicates. (**B**) qRT-PCR analysis of isolated IECs from WT and *Plcb3*$^{-/-}$ mice exposed to sterilized water or 3% DSS for 2 days. Normalized against *Hprt* mRNA. * $p < 0.05$; ** $p < 0.01$; *** $p < 0.001$; **** $p < 0.0001$, determined by two-tailed Student's *t*-test. (**C**) GSEA with isolated IECs from *Plcb3* $^{\Delta IEC}$ mice indicated the reduced expression of Wnt/β-catenin (upper left), Lgr4 (lower left), Lgr4/Lgr5 (upper right), and Ascl2 (lower right) signature genes at the homeostatic condition. (**D**) Small intestines of WT and *Plcb3*$^{-/-}$ mice exposed to sterilized water or 3% DSS for 2 days were separated into mesenchymal tissues. RNAs isolated were subjected to qRT-PCR analysis. mRNA amounts for several Wnt ligands and Wnt secretion enablers (*Wls* and *Porcn*) were normalized against *Hprt*. * $p < 0.05$; ** $p < 0.01$, determined by Student's *t*-test. (**E**) Western blot analysis of Wnt/β-catenin signaling proteins from WT and *Plcb3*$^{-/-}$ mice (3 mice each) under H_2O and 2-day DSS treatments.

PLC-β3, composed of several protein-interacting domains (Figure S1A), directly interacts with several proteins, such as GTP-bound Gαq subunit [49], and is activated by GPCRs. Some Fzd proteins act as Gαq-coupled receptors, similar to prototypical GPCRs, raising the possibility that an Fzd protein(s) and Gαq interact with PLC-β3. Thus, we next examined the possibility that PLC-β3 regulates the Wnt/β-catenin signaling pathway by protein–protein interactions. For this purpose, three methods were employed: first, co-immunoprecipitation experiments were performed using lysates from HEK293T cells expressing untagged or myc-tagged PLC-β3 and Wnt/β-catenin signaling proteins (Figures 4H–J and S8A,B); second, GST fusion pulldown experiments were performed using PLC-β3 domains (Figure S8C); and third, proximity ligation assays (PLAs) were applied to HEK293T transfectants (Figure 4K). Co-immunoprecipitation experiments using anti-Myc antibodies revealed that myc-tagged PLC-β3 can interact with several Wnt signaling proteins including Fzd1 (but not Fzd4/5/7/8) (Figure S8A), as well as Wls, Dvl2, NLK (which phosphorylates and activates Lef-1, downstream of Dvl2 [50]), GSK3β, Tcf-4, and Lef-1 (Figure 4H). C-myc-tagged PLC-β3 was co-immunoprecipitated with constitutively active Gαq regardless of the presence of different Fzd proteins (Fzd1/4/5/7/8), but only Fzd1 co-immunoprecipitated with WT Gαq. The interaction of Fzd1 with C-myc-tagged PLC-β3 was reduced by constitutively active Gαq (Figure S8A), and Fzd1 seemed to be stabilized by PLC-β3 (Figure S8B). PLC-β3′s co-immunoprecipitation with anti-Dvl2 was robust (Figure 4I), whereas its co-immunoprecipitation with anti-Tcf-4 antibodies was weak (Figure 4J). Strong co-immunoprecipitation of PLC-β3 with Dvl2, a scaffold protein that interacts with Fzd and LRP5/6 at the plasma membrane [51], suggests that PLC-β3 may participate in the signaling complex composed of these proteins. Dvl2 and GSK3β were pulled down with PH-EF and split catalytic domains of PLC-β3. Fzd1 was pulled down with the C-terminal portion of PLC-β3, while β-catenin and Lgr5 were pulled down with the PH-EF domain of PLC-β3 (Figure S8C). The interaction between PLC-β3 and Lef-1 was confirmed by PLA (Figure 4K). These results raise the possibility that PLC-β3 promotes Wnt/β-catenin signaling by interacting not only with the Wnt receptor complex but also with other Wnt signaling proteins, in addition to the transcriptional and epigenetic regulation of the pathway proteins.

To assess the effect of persistent Wnt/β-catenin signaling on IECs in vivo, mice were intravenously treated with R-spondin 1 and, 24 h later, Wnt/β-catenin signaling molecules were examined. Protein and/or mRNA expression of LRP6, Axin2, β-catenin, Lgr5, Olfm4, and Ascl2 was more robustly increased in the small intestinal IECs of WT mice than in those of $Plcb3^{-/-}$ mice (Figure 4L,M). Furthermore, the phosphorylation of LRP6 at Ser1490, which is an indicator of the activation of Wnt/β-catenin signaling [52–54], was strongly induced in response to R-spondin 1 in WT, but not in $Plcb3^{-/-}$ mice (Figure 4M). These results indicate that PLC-β3 promotes Wnt/β-catenin signaling in IECs.

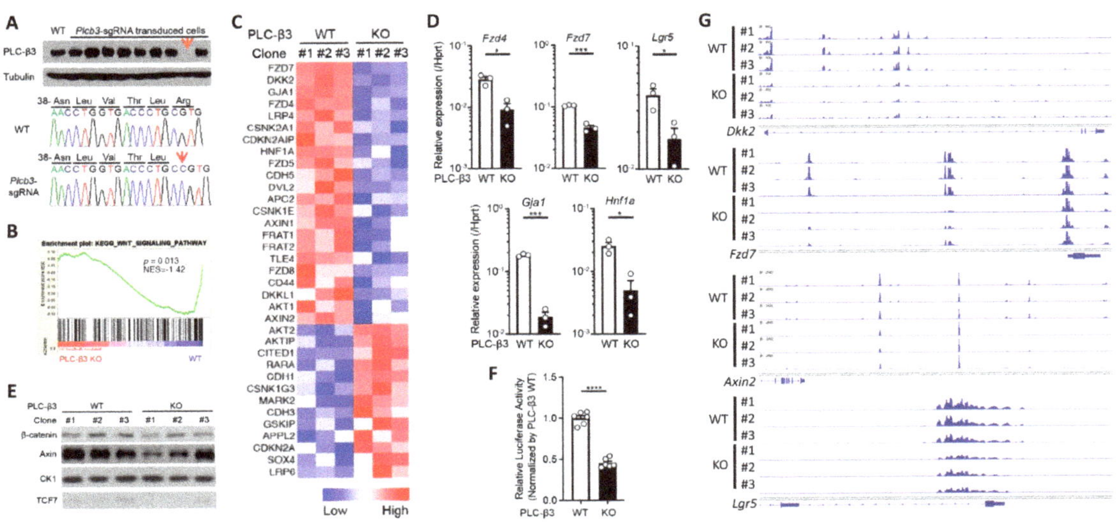

Figure 4. *Cont.*

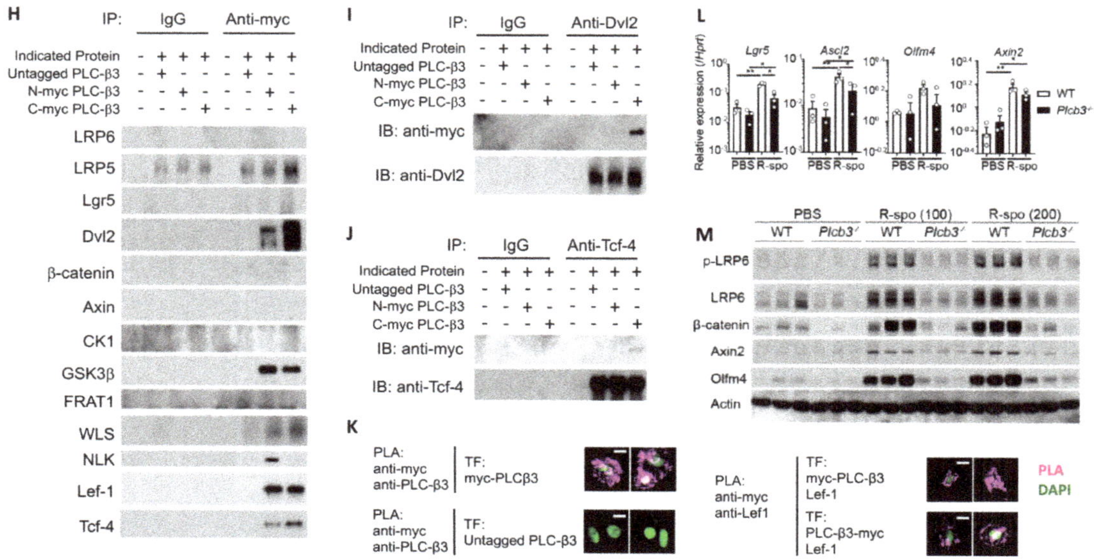

Figure 4. PLC-β3 regulates Wnt/β-catenin signaling at transcriptional, epigenetic, and protein–protein interaction levels in murine intestinal epithelial cells. (**A**) Western blot screening for *Plcb3*-deficient CMT-93 cells generated by CRISPR/Cas9. Only a small fraction of puromycin-selected lentivirus-transduced cells lacked PLC-β3 protein, probably due to the polyploidy of the cells. In clones #1 (shown) and #3 (not shown), a one-base insertion (indicated by an arrow) after Leu42-coding nucleotides in the *Plcb3* gene was confirmed by Sanger sequencing. Clone #2 (not shown) had a G insertion at the same position. The loss of PLC-β3 protein in the 3 clones was confirmed by Western blotting. (**B**) GSEA on *Plcb3*-deficient and -sufficient CMT93 cells. (**C**) Genes whose expression was most drastically altered by *Plcb3*-deficiency (22 down- and 13 up-regulated) found by IPA are listed. The order of listing is according to p values. (**D**) qRT-PCR analyses of several mRNAs in *Plcb3*-deficient and -sufficient CMT93 cells. (**E**) Western blot analysis of several Wnt/β-catenin signaling proteins. (**F**) TCF/LEF activity was analyzed by TOPFLASH luciferase assay using FOPFLASH as a negative control. **** $p < 0.0001$, determined by two-tailed Student's t-test. (**G**) ATAC-seq analysis of *Plcb3*-deficient and -sufficient CMT-93 cells. (**H–J**) Co-immunoprecipitation of PLC-β3 with the indicated proteins. Mammalian expression vector with the indicated proteins as an insert or empty vector and PLC-β3 constructs or control plasmids were transfected to HEK293T cells. Anti-myc (**H**), anti-Dvl2 (**I**), or anti-Tcf-4 (**J**) antibodies were used for immunoprecipitation. IP: immunoprecipitation; IB: immunoblotting; IgG: control antibody. (**K**) CHO Chinese hamster ovary cells were co-transfected (TF) with vectors to express indicated proteins. The proximity of expressed proteins was visualized by proximity ligation assays (PLAs) using indicated pairs of primary antibodies. (**L**,**M**) WT and *Plcb3*$^{-/-}$ mice were treated with 0, 100, or 200 µg of R-spondin 1 for 24 h. IECs from these mice were analyzed by qRT-PCR (**L**) and Western blotting (**M**) for Wnt/β catenin signaling molecules and stem cell markers. mRNA expression was normalized against *Hprt*. * $p < 0.05$; ** $p < 0.01$; *** $p < 0.001$, determined by two-tailed Student's t-test.

3.5. Dysbiosis May Also Contribute to DSS Susceptibility in Plcb3$^{-/-}$ *Mice*

As antibiotic-treated *Plc3*$^{\Delta IEC}$ mice were susceptible to DSS (Figure S5H), we further evaluated the possible effect of intestinal microbiota on DSS susceptibility. DSS treatment of co-housed WT and *Plcb3*$^{-/-}$ mice (Figure 5A), littermates from the same *Plcb3*$^{+/-}$ breeding pairs (Figure 5B), or antibiotic-treated mice (Figure 5C) indicated that the lethality of *Plcb3*$^{-/-}$ mice was largely independent of microbiota. However, microbiota-mediated protection was lost to some degree in *Plcb3*$^{-/-}$ mice, as these mice had an increased number of crypt abscesses in the small intestine (Figure 5D,E), and *Plcb3*$^{-/-}$ and *Plc3*$^{\Delta IEC}$ mice exhibited reduced expression of commensal microbe-induced genes compared with their controls (Figure 5F). 16S rRNA sequencing revealed the existence of pathogenic *Escherichia albertii* and *Escherichia coli* in *Plcb3*$^{-/-}$ mice (Figure 5G), and a dramatic increase of these pathogenic species was present after DSS treatment (Figure 5H,I). To further address the effect of microbiota on DSS susceptibility, WT mice were fostered by *Plcb3*$^{-/-}$ mice at the date of birth. Fostered WT mice showed an increased number of the *Escherichia* species (Figure 5G–I) and earlier body weight loss upon DSS treatment compared to WT mice raised by WT mice (Figure 5J). These results suggest that dysbiosis caused by PLC-β3 deficiency contributes to increased susceptibility to DSS.

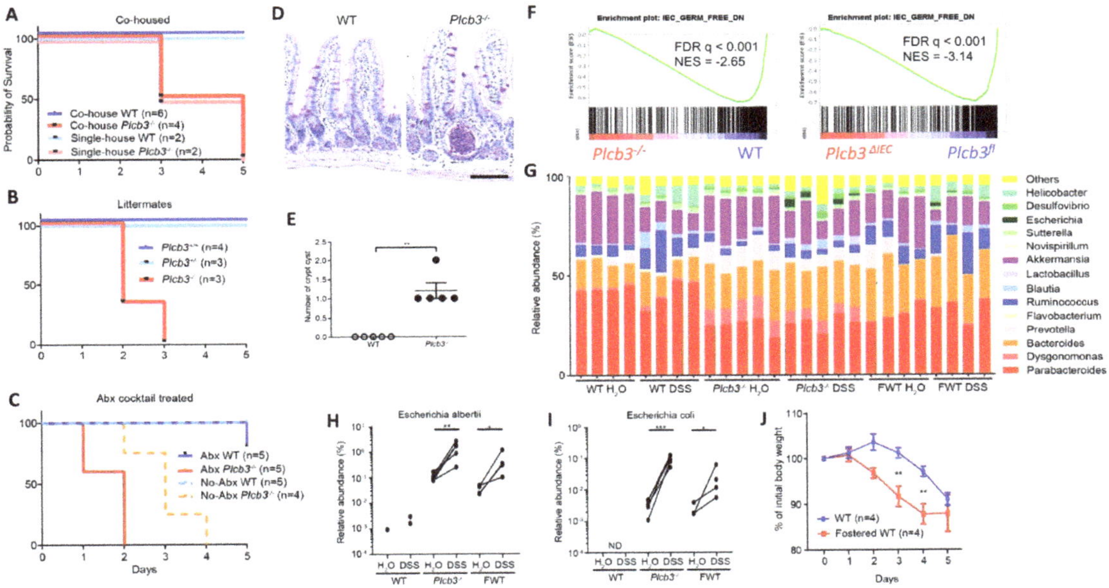

Figure 5. Dysbiosis contributes to the DSS susceptibility of PLC-β3 KO mice. (**A–C**) Survival curves of co-housed mice (**A**), littermates (**B**), or antibiotics cocktail (Abx)-treated (**C**) WT or *Plcb3*$^{-/-}$ mice. Mice were exposed to 3% DSS for 5 days. (**D**) PAS staining of ileum from WT or *Plcb3*$^{-/-}$ mice. Scale bar 100 μm. (**E**) Numbers of crypt abscesses in the whole intestine Swiss roll sections. ** $p < 0.01$, determined by Mann–Whitney test. (**F**) GSEA on isolated IECs from *Plcb3*$^{-/-}$ and *Plcb3*$^{\Delta IEC}$ mice vs. their control mice with microbiota-induced genes. (**G–I**) 16S rRNA sequencing analysis of fecal pellets from WT, *Plcb3*$^{-/-}$, and WT mice fostered by *Plcb3*$^{-/-}$ mice (FWT) before and after exposure to 3% DSS for 2 days. Genus-level data are shown (**G**). Relative abundance of *Escherichia albertii* (**H**) and *Escherichia coli* (**I**) are shown. * $p < 0.05$; ** $p < 0.01$; *** $p < 0.001$, determined by paired *t*-test. ND: not detected. (**J**) Body weight change in FWT and WT mice during exposure to 3% DSS for 5 days. FWT: WT mice fostered by *Plcb3*$^{-/-}$ mice. ** $p < 0.01$, determined by Sidak's multiple comparison test.

3.6. Reduced Expression of PLC-β3 and Altered Expression of PLC-β3-Regulated Genes in Ileal Crohn's Disease

To validate the clinical relevance of PLC-β3 levels in human IBD patients, transcriptome data from published studies were analyzed. In the GSE57945 dataset [55], *PLCB3* mRNA expression in ileal biopsy samples was lower in pediatric CD patients, especially those with deep ulcers, but not in patients with ulcerative colitis (Figures 6A and S9A). Data in GSE83448 [56] also showed reduced *PLCB3* mRNA expression in adult ileal CD patients (Figure S9B) and data in GSE179285 [57] showed reduced *PLCB3* mRNA more strongly in inflamed than in uninflamed terminal ileum of adult CD, but not in colonic CD or ulcerative colitis patients (Figure S9C). Pediatric colon biopsies also showed no reduction in *PLCB3* expression in the GSE126124 dataset [58] (Figure S9D). Despite the cellular heterogeneity of biopsy samples, reduced PLC-β3 protein in three out of seven ileal CD patients compared to healthy controls was confirmed by immunofluorescent staining (Figure 6B,C). The expression of ileal CD signature genes [55] was similarly altered in *Plcb3*$^{-/-}$ mice (Figure 6D). For example, the expression of *PLCB3* mRNA in CD patients showed an inverse correlation with that of *DUOX2*, an upregulated CD signature gene, and a positive correlation with that of *APOA1*, a lipoprotein downregulated in CD (Figure S9E). Conversely, the expression of PLC-β3 signature genes as defined by ≥2-fold changes and false discovery rate (FDR) q-values < 0.01 in *Plcb3*$^{-/-}$ vs. WT mice (Supplementary Tables S1 and S2) was similarly altered in CD biopsy specimens, especially those with deep ulcers (Figure 6E). Together with data from *Plcb3*-deficient mice and IECs, these results suggest that the reduced expression of PLC-β3 is causally linked to ileal CD.

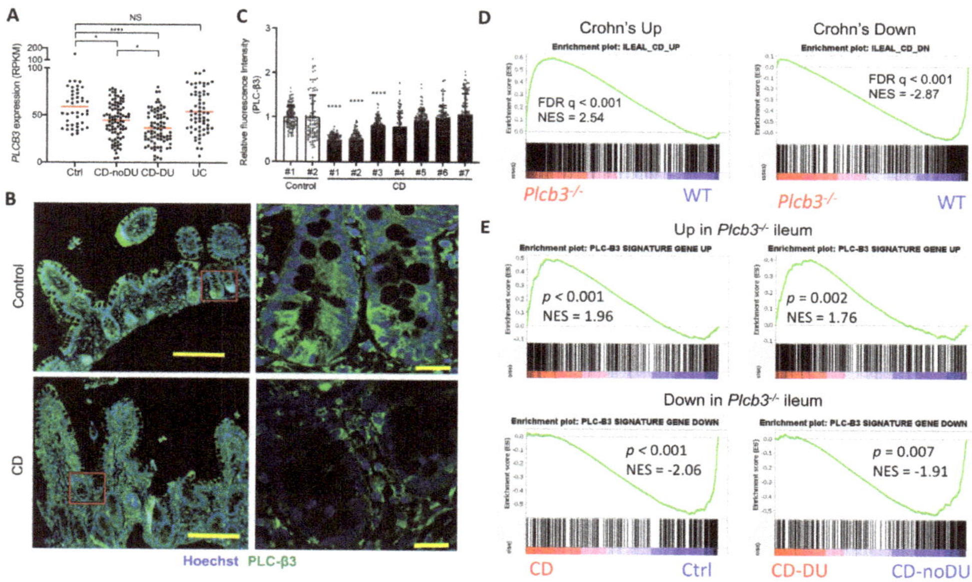

Figure 6. Reduced expression of PLC-β3 and altered expression of PLC-β3-regulated genes in ileal Crohn's disease. (**A**) RNA-seq data on ileum biopsy samples from pediatric CD patients (GSE57945) were analyzed for *PLCB3* expression. Ctrl: control; CD: Crohn's disease; DU: deep ulcer; UC: ulcerative colitis. (**B**,**C**) Biopsy samples from CD patients were stained for PLC-β3. (**B**) Representative images from 2 independent experiments. Scale bars 200 µm (left) and 20 µm (right). (**C**) Mean fluorescence intensity (MFI) for PLC-β3 from 100 epithelial cells was measured. MFI was normalized against control samples. * $p < 0.05$, **** $p < 0.0001$, determined by Kruskal–Wallis test and Dunn's multiple comparison test. (**D**,**E**) Expression profiles of ilea from *Plcb3*$^{-/-}$ mice were analyzed by microarray. Then, 359 (upregulated) and 285 (downregulated) PLC-β3 signature genes were defined by ≥2-fold changes in expression and FDR q-values < 0.01 in *Plcb3*$^{-/-}$ mice. (**D**) GSEA was performed using RNA-seq data from the CD signature gene (GSE57945) and PLC-β3 signature gene sets. (**E**) GSEA was performed using RNA-seq data from CD patients (GSE57945) and the PLC-β3 signature gene set. A comparison between control and CD (left panels) or CD-No DU and CD-DU (right panels). NES: normalized enrichment score.

3.7. PLC-β Promotes Wnt/Wingless Signaling in Drosophila

The Wnt signaling pathway is evolutionally conserved [59]. In *Drosophila melanogaster*, the only PLC-β isozyme is encoded by the gene *Plc21C*. Wingless (a Drosophila Wnt) specifies the fate of cells that form sensory bristles at the adult wing margin, in part through the expression of the Wingless target gene *senseless* (*sens*) [60]. RNAi-mediated knockdown of *Plc21C* in the posterior compartment of the wing disc using the *hedgehog (hh)-Gal4* driver decreased Sens levels solely in the posterior compartment in more than 90% of discs (marked by Engrailed, Figure 7A,B). Multiple independent RNAi constructs that target different regions of *Plc21C* reduced Sens specifically in the posterior compartment, showing a robust effect. By contrast, RNAi-mediated knockdown of a control gene *yellow (y)* resulted in minimal Sens reduction (Figure 7A,B), supporting the specificity of the *Plc21C* RNAi results. Moreover, RNAi knockdown of *Plc21C* did not inhibit *wingless* expression (Figure 7C), indicating that the reduction in Sens was not due to decreased Wingless levels but instead resulted from downstream defects in the Wingless signaling pathway.

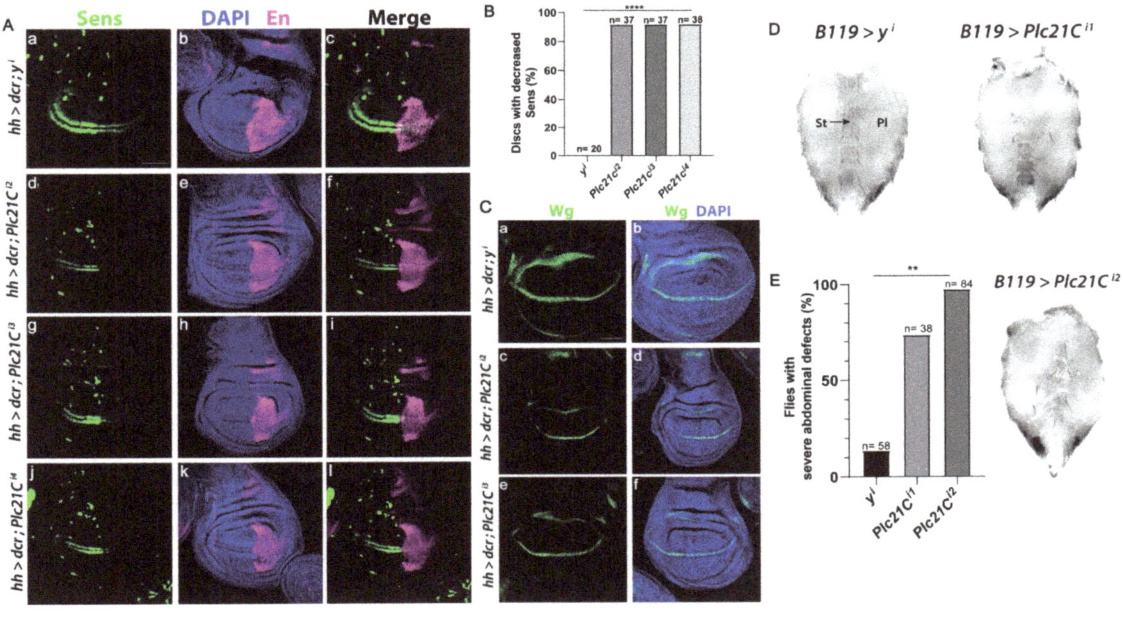

Figure 7. Plc21C is required for the expression of the Wingless target gene *Sens* in the Drosophila wing imaginal disc. (**A–C**) RNAi constructs targeting *Plc21C* or the *yellow (y)* negative control were expressed in the posterior compartment (marked by Engrailed (En)) of the third instar wing discs using the *hedgehog (hh)-Gal4* driver. A transcriptional reporter for *sens* expression, *mScar:T2A:Sens* (green), was analyzed. Scale bar (**a–l**) 20 µm. Dorsal, top and posterior, right. (**B**) Quantification is shown as a percentage of discs of each genotype with decreased Sens. N is the number of discs analyzed. (**C**) RNAi-mediated knockdown of Plc21C in the posterior compartment of third instar wing imaginal discs does not affect the expression of the *wingless* gene (green). Scale bar (**a–f**) 20 µm. Dorsal, top and posterior, right. (**D**,**E**) Loss of Plc21C in the Drosophila abdomen results in decreased Wingless signaling. Ventral abdomens of females expressing control RNAi targeting *y* using the *B119-Gal4* driver (top left) or those expressing RNAi constructs targeting *Plc21C* (top right and bottom right). Sternites and overlying sternal bristles (St, arrow) and pleura (Pl) are indicated. (**E**) At least 70% of all abdomens observed exhibited a severe phenotype. These abdomens were quantified as a percentage of total progeny. N is total number of abdomens of each genotype that were analyzed. ** $p < 0.01$; **** $p < 0.0001$.

Inactivation of core Wingless signaling pathway components, including Wingless, Armadillo/β-catenin, and Armadillo's transcriptional co-activators dTCF/Pangolin and Legless results in the loss of bristle-bearing cuticular plates known as sternites and sternal bristles in the ventral abdomen [61–63]. When two independent RNAi constructs targeting *Plc21C* were expressed using the *B119-Gal4* driver, we observed a marked loss of sternites and sternal bristles, as well as an expansion of pleura (Figure 7D,E). A severe phenotype occurred in at least 70% of the flies analyzed. This reduction in abdominal sternites was rarely observed with RNAi targeting of the control *y* gene (Figure 7D,E). These results suggest that PLC-β-mediated regulation of the Wnt signaling pathway is conserved from *Drosophila* to mice and humans.

4. Discussion

Based on mouse IBD models, molecular analyses of IECs, and ileal biopsy specimens from human CD patients as well as extensive transcriptomic and epigenetic datasets, our study suggests that PLC-β3 promotes intestinal homeostasis and repair after injury through the activation of the Wnt/β-catenin signaling pathway. Wnt/β-catenin signaling drives the cell cycle and, conversely, the cell cycle influences Wnt signaling. During the cell cycle, the expression of β-catenin oscillates, and the maximal activation of β-catenin and *Axin2* expression occurs at the G2/M transition [64–66]. Moreover, the mitosis-specific Cdk14-cyclin Y kinase complex phosphorylates LRP6 at Ser-1490 during G2/M, which promotes the activation of signaling [64]. Surprisingly, PLC-β3 regulates Wnt/β-catenin signaling through multiple regulatory mechanisms, including transcriptional, epigenetic, and, potentially, protein–protein interaction levels. Such multi-level regulatory mechanisms underlie the important role of PLC-β3 in IECs of the mouse and human small intestine. Furthermore, PLC-β regulates Wnt/Wingless signaling in *Drosophila*. Thus, we conclude that the newly identified PLC-β-mediated regulation of Wnt/β-catenin signaling is evolutionally conserved from *Drosophila* to humans.

As PLC-β3 deficiency leads to reduced β-catenin expression in IECs, PLC-β3 functions upstream of this protein within the Wnt/β-catenin pathway. One of the ten Frizzled receptors and LRP5/LRP6 act as Wnt receptor complexes [67]. Fzd is a seven-transmembrane domain receptor, like conventional GPCRs. Since PLC-β isozymes are linked to GPCRs [10], PLC-β3 likely functions similarly in the Wnt/β-catenin pathway. Consistent with this notion, Fzd1 was co-immunoprecipitated with PLC-β3. Moreover, Dvl2, which works as an oligomerizable scaffold to interact with an Fzd at the plasma membrane [51], was robustly co-immunoprecipitated with PLC-β3. R-spondins bind to their receptors Lgr4/5/6 and bridge the negative regulators Rnf43 and Znrf3 with these Lgr receptors to promote the activation of Wnt/β-catenin signaling [40]. It is known that Wnt-3a mediates the production of phosphatidylinositol 4,5-bisphoshate, the PLC substrate, to regulate LRP6 phosphorylation [68]. All these results along with those of other studies strongly support that PLC-β3 promotes Wnt/β-catenin signaling by interacting not only with the Wnt receptor complex but also with other Wnt signaling proteins.

Downstream of Wnt binding to Fzd, a PLC is thought to generate two messengers: diacylglycerol and inositol 1,4,5-trisphosphate in the Wnt/Ca^{2+} pathway [69]. PLC-β3 may play this role in IECs, as suggested by the IPA of the transcriptomes of PLC-β3-deficient CMT-93 cells (Figure S7A). If this is the case, PLC-β3 may be shared by both the Wnt/β-catenin and Wnt/Ca^{2+} signaling pathways.

Our study identified a PLC-β3-dependent Wnt/β-catenin pathway in mouse small intestinal IECs. As PLC-β3 is expressed broadly, it is likely that this pathway functions in other cell types such as fibroblasts and endothelial cells. Changes in the connective tissue are well known in Crohn's disease, including fat-wrapping due to adipocyte hyperplasia, fibrosis, muscularization, and neuronal and vascular changes [70]. Of note, we showed increased goblet cells in *Plcb3*$^{\Delta FB}$ mice and DSS-induced early intestinal bleeding in *Plcb3*$^{\Delta IEC;EC}$ mice, implying the role of fibroblasts and epithelial–endothelial cell interactions in goblet cell differentiation and the blood vessel barrier, respectively. Wnt/β-catenin signaling is implicated in fibrogenesis in a variety of tissues. It was shown that the Wnt/β-catenin signaling pathway is necessary for TGF-β-mediated fibrosis, and the interaction of both pathways is important in the pathogenesis of fibrotic diseases [71]. Wnt signaling stimulated the differentiation of resting fibroblasts into myofibroblasts, increased the release of extracellular matrix components, and induced fibrosis. The expression of Smad6, an inhibitory Smad that negatively regulates signaling downstream of TGF-β, was reduced in the ileum of *Plcb3*$^{-/-}$ mice (Table S2). On the other hand, PLC-β3 works as a negative regulator of VEGF-mediated vascular permeability by regulating intracellular Ca^{2+} release [72]. The ETS transcription factor Erg drives the expression of VE-cadherin and controls junctional integrity in endothelial cells. Birdsey et al. showed that the constitutive endothelial deletion of Erg in mice causes embryonic lethality with vascular defects [73]. Erg controls the Wnt/β-catenin pathway by promoting β-catenin stability. Thus, Erg is an essential regulator of angiogenesis and vascular stability through Wnt signaling. However, Erg expression in the ileum was not significantly affected by PLC-β3 deficiency. Despite these observations showing nonredundant roles of PLC-β3 among different non-hematopoietic cells, triple *Plcb3* cKO mice lacking *Plcb3* in IECs, fibroblasts, and endothelial cells were less susceptible to DSS than *Plcb3*$^{-/-}$ mice, suggesting that this pathway also operates in other mesenchymal cells and/or IEC–mesenchymal cell interactions. Results of single-cell RNA sequencing (Figure S4) support this possibility.

Studies of gene expression and chromatin accessibility divided CD into two classes: colon and ileal subtypes [74]. Characteristic features of ileal CD include the reduced expression of α-defensins HD-5 and HD-6, which are expressed by Paneth cells [75], and low Wnt/β-catenin signaling, as exemplified by low expression or genetic variants of TCF-4 [76,77], TCF-1 [78], and LRP6 [79]. Consistent with these previous studies and our current data with *Plcb3*$^{-/-}$ mice, we found reduced expression of *PLCB3* and altered expression of *PLCB3*-regulated signature genes in ileal CD, but not in other CD subtypes or ulcerative colitis. This is consistent with our observations that *Plcb3*$^{-/-}$ mice exhibited normal histology of the colon under homeostatic conditions and the DSS-induced severe pathology was restricted largely to the small intestine. Therefore, the pathogenic mechanism of ileal CD characterized as a "Paneth cell disease" is likely different from that of colonic CD.

In addition to the reduced Wnt signaling in IECs of ileal CD, macrophages and monocytes are known to play critical roles in IBD pathogenesis [80,81] through the production of inflammatory cytokines such as TNF, IL-1β, IL-6, and IL-23. The upregulation of a set of inflammatory response genes that include these cytokine genes was found in monocytes from IBD patients, and the expression of these genes was inversely correlated with miR-374a-5p expression [82]. Increased expression of miR-374a-5p can suppress monocyte-/macrophage-driven inflammation in all subtypes of IBD. Interestingly, Martin et al. found a pathogenic cellular module termed GIMATS, comprised of inflammatory macrophages, activated DCs, highly activated T cells, IgG^+ plasma cells, activated fibroblasts, and $ACKR1^+$-activated endothelial cells, and a $GIMATS^{high}$ subset of ileal CD patients showed resistance to anti-TNF therapies [39]. Another single-cell analysis of colonic mucosae from pediatric colitis and IBD suggested a defective cAMP response and colonic mucosal platelet aggregates as underlying pathologies, which were ameliorated by dipyridamole, a phosphodiesterase inhibitor, in a pilot clinical trial [83]. These systems biology approaches suggest the involvement of both hematopoietic and non-hematopoietic cells in mucosal inflammation as key IBD pathogenic processes. Although our study showed increased expression of IL-1β and IL-6 mRNAs in the ilea of *Plcb3*$^{-/-}$ and *Plcb3*$^{\Delta IEC}$ mice compared with control mice, the miR-374a-5p-related monocyte's inflammatory module was not significantly related to the *Plcb3*$^{-/-}$ phenotype (data not shown). However, future studies should address the relationship between GIMATS, the monocyte's inflammatory response module, and PLC-β3-dependent Wnt/β-catenin signaling. Further refinement of our understanding of the pathogenesis of the CD subtypes will help predict responses to therapeutics. Furthermore, it may be worth testing Wnt agonists [8,84] as a potential therapy for ileal CD unless *PLCB3* is totally absent.

The effect of small intestinal microbiota on DSS susceptibility as well as the effect of PLC-β3 deficiency on small intestinal microbiota were rather subtle in *Plcb3*$^{-/-}$ mice. By contrast, the protective effect of small intestinal microbiota was robust in *Plcb3*$^{\Delta IEC}$ mice compared with *Plcb3*$^{fl/fl}$ mice (Figure S4H). These results suggest the significant role of PLC-β3 in IECs for interactions with microbiota and the more subtle roles played by PLC-β3 in other cell types. Interestingly, pathogenic *Escherichia albertii* and *Escherichia coli* were found in *Plcb3*$^{-/-}$ mice, and these pathogenic species increased after DSS treatment. Thus, assuming the clinical relevance of our mouse data in ileal CD, precision editing of the gut microbiota [85] could be beneficial for ileal CD patients. Further understanding of the PLC-β3-Wnt/β-catenin pathway will likely contribute to an appropriate selection of treatment for these patients.

5. Conclusions

In summary, we demonstrated that PLC-β3 in mammals and PLC-β in *Drosophila* regulate the Wnt/β-catenin signaling pathway at transcriptional, epigenetic, and, potentially, protein–protein interaction levels. A Wnt ligand binds to Fzd1 and then Fzd1/Gαq-bound PLC-β3 is activated, leading to the inactivation of the β-catenin destruction complex, followed by increased nuclear β-catenin, which activates the TCF/LEF transcription factors. Our data collectively suggest that the reduced activity of this evolutionally conserved PLC-β3-mediated Wnt/β-catenin signaling pathway contributes to the pathogenesis of ileal Crohn's disease.

Limitations of This Study

Our data suggest that PLC-β3 regulates the Wnt/β-catenin signaling pathway in the small intestine at transcriptional, epigenetic, and, probably, protein–protein interaction levels. We are aware of the weaknesses of this study. For example, some data were obtained with CMT-93 cells, which may be a less-than-ideal model as they express PLC-β3 more than normal cell counterparts. There are still gaps in our understanding of how Wnt/β-catenin signaling is controlled by PLC-β3, which is linked to the inactivation of β-catenin destruction complexes. Future studies will be needed to determine whether and how G proteins are involved in Wnt/β-catenin signaling, whether the enzymatic activity of PLC-β3 is required for Wnt/β-catenin signaling, and whether PLC-β3 regulates both Wnt/β-catenin and Wnt/Ca^{2+} signaling pathways. Furthermore, numerous protein–protein interactions detected by overexpression experiments need to be tested in more detail.

Supplementary Materials: The following supporting information can be downloaded at https://www.mdpi.com/article/10.3390/cells13110986/s1.

Author Contributions: Conceptualization, T.A. and T.K.; Methodology, L.A.D., Z.M., T.A., I.T., T.I., Y.A., Y.K. (Yuko Kawakami) and T.K.; Investigation, T.A., I.T., Z.T.S., R.I., Y.T., K.M., Y.K. (Yu Kawakami), Y.A. and Y.K. (Yuko Kawakami); Analysis, T.A., I.T., K.M., J.K., Y.K. (Yuko Kawakami) and T.K.; Writing, T.A., I.T., Y.K. (Yu Kawakami), J.K. and T.K. All authors have read and agreed to the published version of the manuscript.

Funding: This study was supported in part by the National Institutes of Health grants R01 AR064418 (T.K.), R01 AI146042 (T.K.), and R35 GM136233 (Y.A.).

Institutional Review Board Statement: The patient-based studies were approved by the Institutional Review Board at Cincinnati Children's Hospital Medical Center (approval number 2011-2285).

Informed Consent Statement: Informed consent was obtained from parents and adult subjects and assent from pediatric subjects aged 11 and above.

Data Availability Statement: All unique/stable reagents generated in this study are available from the lead contact with a completed materials transfer agreement.

Acknowledgments: We are thankful for technical help by Minato Baba, Kenichiro Motomura, Motohiro Kuriyama, Rachel Sielski, Lulu Chea, Jeremy Day, and Steven Wlodychak and for the advice of our colleagues at La Jolla Institute for Immunology, particularly Mitchell Kronenberg,

Anjana Rao, Patrick Hogan, John Chang, and Gooyoung Seo. Kyowa Kirin provided human R-spondin 1 for this study.

Conflicts of Interest: T.K. and Y.K. served as consultants for Escient Pharma. The other authors declare no other competing interests.

References

1. Jostins, L.; Ripke, S.; Weersma, R.K.; Duerr, R.H.; McGovern, D.P.; Hui, K.Y.; Lee, J.C.; Schumm, L.P.; Sharma, Y.; Anderson, C.A.; et al. Host-microbe interactions have shaped the genetic architecture of inflammatory bowel disease. *Nature* **2012**, *491*, 119–124. [CrossRef] [PubMed]
2. Khor, B.; Gardet, A.; Xavier, R.J. Genetics and pathogenesis of inflammatory bowel disease. *Nature* **2011**, *474*, 307–317. [CrossRef] [PubMed]
3. Liu, J.Z.; van Sommeren, S.; Huang, H.; Ng, S.C.; Alberts, R.; Takahashi, A.; Ripke, S.; Lee, J.C.; Jostins, L.; Shah, T.; et al. Association analyses identify 38 susceptibility loci for inflammatory bowel disease and highlight shared genetic risk across populations. *Nat. Genet.* **2015**, *47*, 979–986. [CrossRef] [PubMed]
4. Clevers, H.; Loh, K.M.; Nusse, R. Stem cell signaling. An integral program for tissue renewal and regeneration: Wnt signaling and stem cell control. *Science* **2014**, *346*, 1248012. [CrossRef] [PubMed]
5. Clevers, H.; Nusse, R. Wnt/beta-catenin signaling and disease. *Cell* **2012**, *149*, 1192–1205. [CrossRef] [PubMed]
6. Liu, T.; DeCostanzo, A.J.; Liu, X.; Wang, H.; Hallagan, S.; Moon, R.T.; Malbon, C.C. G protein signaling from activated rat frizzled-1 to the beta-catenin-Lef-Tcf pathway. *Science* **2001**, *292*, 1718–1722. [CrossRef] [PubMed]
7. Wright, S.C.; Canizal, M.C.A.; Benkel, T.; Simon, K.; Le Gouill, C.; Matricon, P.; Namkung, Y.; Lukasheva, V.; Konig, G.M.; Laporte, S.A.; et al. FZD(5) is a Galpha(q)-coupled receptor that exhibits the functional hallmarks of prototypical GPCRs. *Sci. Signal.* **2018**, *11*, eaar5536. [CrossRef] [PubMed]
8. Nusse, R.; Clevers, H. Wnt/beta-Catenin Signaling, Disease, and Emerging Therapeutic Modalities. *Cell* **2017**, *169*, 985–999. [CrossRef] [PubMed]
9. Armbruster, N.S.; Stange, E.F.; Wehkamp, J. In the Wnt of Paneth Cells: Immune-Epithelial Crosstalk in Small Intestinal Crohn's Disease. *Front. Immunol.* **2017**, *8*, 1204. [CrossRef]
10. Rhee, S.G. Regulation of phosphoinositide-specific phospholipase C. *Annu. Rev. Biochem.* **2001**, *70*, 281–312. [CrossRef]
11. Suh, P.G.; Park, J.I.; Manzoli, L.; Cocco, L.; Peak, J.C.; Katan, M.; Fukami, K.; Kataoka, T.; Yun, S.; Ryu, S.H. Multiple roles of phosphoinositide-specific phospholipase C isozymes. *BMB Rep.* **2008**, *41*, 415–434. [CrossRef] [PubMed]
12. Barrett, J.C.; Hansoul, S.; Nicolae, D.L.; Cho, J.H.; Duerr, R.H.; Rioux, J.D.; Brant, S.R.; Silverberg, M.S.; Taylor, K.D.; Barmada, M.M.; et al. Genome-wide association defines more than 30 distinct susceptibility loci for Crohn's disease. *Nat. Genet.* **2008**, *40*, 955–962. [CrossRef] [PubMed]
13. Esparza-Gordillo, J.; Weidinger, S.; Folster-Holst, R.; Bauerfeind, A.; Ruschendorf, F.; Patone, G.; Rohde, K.; Marenholz, I.; Schulz, F.; Kerscher, T.; et al. A common variant on chromosome 11q13 is associated with atopic dermatitis. *Nat. Genet.* **2009**, *41*, 596–601. [CrossRef] [PubMed]
14. Hammer, B.; Ashurst, P.; Naish, J. Diseases associated with ulcerative colitis and Crohn's disease. *Gut* **1968**, *9*, 17–21. [CrossRef] [PubMed]
15. Pugh, S.M.; Rhodes, J.; Mayberry, J.F.; Roberts, D.L.; Heatley, R.V.; Newcombe, R.G. Atopic disease in ulcerative colitis and Crohn's disease. *Clin. Allergy* **1979**, *9*, 221–223. [CrossRef] [PubMed]
16. Ando, T.; Xiao, W.; Gao, P.; Namiranian, S.; Matsumoto, K.; Tomimori, Y.; Hong, H.; Yamashita, H.; Kimura, M.; Kashiwakura, J.; et al. Critical role for mast cell Stat5 activity in skin inflammation. *Cell Rep.* **2014**, *6*, 366–376. [CrossRef] [PubMed]
17. Eichele, D.D.; Kharbanda, K.K. Dextran sodium sulfate colitis murine model: An indispensable tool for advancing our understanding of inflammatory bowel diseases pathogenesis. *World J. Gastroenterol.* **2017**, *23*, 6016–6029. [CrossRef] [PubMed]
18. Tanimoto, H.; Itoh, S.; ten Dijke, P.; Tabata, T. Hedgehog creates a gradient of DPP activity in Drosophila wing imaginal discs. *Mol. Cell* **2000**, *5*, 59–71. [CrossRef] [PubMed]
19. Sanjana, N.E.; Shalem, O.; Zhang, F. Improved vectors and genome-wide libraries for CRISPR screening. *Nat. Methods* **2014**, *11*, 783–784. [CrossRef]
20. Fevr, T.; Robine, S.; Louvard, D.; Huelsken, J. Wnt/beta-catenin is essential for intestinal homeostasis and maintenance of intestinal stem cells. *Mol. Cell. Biol.* **2007**, *27*, 7551–7559. [CrossRef]
21. de Lau, W.; Barker, N.; Low, T.Y.; Koo, B.K.; Li, V.S.; Teunissen, H.; Kujala, P.; Haegebarth, A.; Peters, P.J.; van de Wetering, M.; et al. Lgr5 homologues associate with Wnt receptors and mediate R-spondin signalling. *Nature* **2011**, *476*, 293–297. [CrossRef] [PubMed]
22. Mustata, R.C.; Van Loy, T.; Lefort, A.; Libert, F.; Strollo, S.; Vassart, G.; Garcia, M.I. Lgr4 is required for Paneth cell differentiation and maintenance of intestinal stem cells ex vivo. *EMBO Rep.* **2011**, *12*, 558–564. [CrossRef]
23. Camp, J.G.; Frank, C.L.; Lickwar, C.R.; Guturu, H.; Rube, T.; Wenger, A.M.; Chen, J.; Bejerano, G.; Crawford, G.E.; Rawls, J.F. Microbiota modulate transcription in the intestinal epithelium without remodeling the accessible chromatin landscape. *Genome Res.* **2014**, *24*, 1504–1516. [CrossRef]

24. Liu, X.; Chen, X.; Zhong, B.; Wang, A.; Wang, X.; Chu, F.; Nurieva, R.I.; Yan, X.; Chen, P.; van der Flier, L.G.; et al. Transcription factor achaete-scute homologue 2 initiates follicular T-helper-cell development. *Nature* **2014**, *507*, 513–518. [CrossRef]
25. Mootha, V.K.; Lindgren, C.M.; Eriksson, K.F.; Subramanian, A.; Sihag, S.; Lehar, J.; Puigserver, P.; Carlsson, E.; Ridderstrale, M.; Laurila, E.; et al. PGC-1alpha-responsive genes involved in oxidative phosphorylation are coordinately downregulated in human diabetes. *Nat. Genet.* **2003**, *34*, 267–273. [CrossRef]
26. Subramanian, A.; Tamayo, P.; Mootha, V.K.; Mukherjee, S.; Ebert, B.L.; Gillette, M.A.; Paulovich, A.; Pomeroy, S.L.; Golub, T.R.; Lander, E.S.; et al. Gene set enrichment analysis: A knowledge-based approach for interpreting genome-wide expression profiles. *Proc. Natl. Acad. Sci. USA* **2005**, *102*, 15545–15550. [CrossRef]
27. Elmentaite, R.; Ross, A.D.B.; Roberts, K.; James, K.R.; Ortmann, D.; Gomes, T.; Nayak, K.; Tuck, L.; Pritchard, S.; Bayraktar, O.A.; et al. Single-Cell Sequencing of Developing Human Gut Reveals Transcriptional Links to Childhood Crohn's Disease. *Dev. Cell* **2020**, *55*, 771–783.e5. [CrossRef]
28. Wolf, F.A.; Angerer, P.; Theis, F.J. SCANPY: Large-scale single-cell gene expression data analysis. *Genome Biol.* **2018**, *19*, 15. [CrossRef]
29. Xu, H.; Ding, J.; Porter, C.B.M.; Wallrapp, A.; Tabaka, M.; Ma, S.; Fu, S.; Guo, X.; Riesenfeld, S.J.; Su, C.; et al. Transcriptional Atlas of Intestinal Immune Cells Reveals that Neuropeptide alpha-CGRP Modulates Group 2 Innate Lymphoid Cell Responses. *Immunity* **2019**, *51*, 696–708.e9. [CrossRef]
30. Haber, A.L.; Biton, M.; Rogel, N.; Herbst, R.H.; Shekhar, K.; Smillie, C.; Burgin, G.; Delorey, T.M.; Howitt, M.R.; Katz, Y.; et al. A single-cell survey of the small intestinal epithelium. *Nature* **2017**, *551*, 333–339. [CrossRef]
31. Buenrostro, J.D.; Wu, B.; Chang, H.Y.; Greenleaf, W.J. ATAC-seq: A Method for Assaying Chromatin Accessibility Genome-Wide. *Curr. Protoc. Mol. Biol.* **2015**, *109*, 21.29.1–21.29.9. [CrossRef] [PubMed]
32. Langmead, B.; Salzberg, S.L. Fast gapped-read alignment with Bowtie 2. *Nat. Methods* **2012**, *9*, 357–359. [CrossRef] [PubMed]
33. Zhang, Y.; Liu, T.; Meyer, C.A.; Eeckhoute, J.; Johnson, D.S.; Bernstein, B.E.; Nusbaum, C.; Myers, R.M.; Brown, M.; Li, W.; et al. Model-based analysis of ChIP-Seq (MACS). *Genome Biol.* **2008**, *9*, R137. [CrossRef] [PubMed]
34. LeBlanc, P.M.; Yeretssian, G.; Rutherford, N.; Doiron, K.; Nadiri, A.; Zhu, L.; Green, D.R.; Gruenheid, S.; Saleh, M. Caspase-12 modulates NOD signaling and regulates antimicrobial peptide production and mucosal immunity. *Cell Host Microbe* **2008**, *3*, 146–157. [CrossRef] [PubMed]
35. Kabashima, K.; Saji, T.; Murata, T.; Nagamachi, M.; Matsuoka, T.; Segi, E.; Tsuboi, K.; Sugimoto, Y.; Kobayashi, T.; Miyachi, Y.; et al. The prostaglandin receptor EP4 suppresses colitis, mucosal damage and CD4 cell activation in the gut. *J. Clin. Investig.* **2002**, *109*, 883–893. [CrossRef] [PubMed]
36. Kassel, S.; Hanson, A.J.; Benchabane, H.; Saito-Diaz, K.; Cabel, C.R.; Goldsmith, L.; Taha, M.; Kanuganti, A.; Ng, V.H.; Xu, G.; et al. USP47 deubiquitylates Groucho/TLE to promote Wnt-beta-catenin signaling. *Sci. Signal.* **2023**, *16*, eabn8372. [CrossRef] [PubMed]
37. Sato, T.; Vries, R.G.; Snippert, H.J.; van de Wetering, M.; Barker, N.; Stange, D.E.; van Es, J.H.; Abo, A.; Kujala, P.; Peters, P.J.; et al. Single Lgr5 stem cells build crypt-villus structures in vitro without a mesenchymal niche. *Nature* **2009**, *459*, 262–265. [CrossRef] [PubMed]
38. Kamioka, M.; Goto, Y.; Nakamura, K.; Yokoi, Y.; Sugimoto, R.; Ohira, S.; Kurashima, Y.; Umemoto, S.; Sato, S.; Kunisawa, J.; et al. Intestinal commensal microbiota and cytokines regulate Fut2$^+$ Paneth cells for gut defense. *Proc. Natl. Acad. Sci. USA* **2022**, *119*, e2115230119. [CrossRef] [PubMed]
39. Martin, J.C.; Chang, C.; Boschetti, G.; Ungaro, R.; Giri, M.; Grout, J.A.; Gettler, K.; Chuang, L.S.; Nayar, S.; Greenstein, A.J.; et al. Single-Cell Analysis of Crohn's Disease Lesions Identifies a Pathogenic Cellular Module Associated with Resistance to Anti-TNF Therapy. *Cell* **2019**, *178*, 1493–1508.e20. [CrossRef]
40. de Lau, W.; Peng, W.C.; Gros, P.; Clevers, H. The R-spondin/Lgr5/Rnf43 module: Regulator of Wnt signal strength. *Genes Dev.* **2014**, *28*, 305–316. [CrossRef]
41. Liu, S.; Qian, Y.; Li, L.; Wei, G.; Guan, Y.; Pan, H.; Guan, X.; Zhang, L.; Lu, X.; Zhao, Y.; et al. Lgr4 gene deficiency increases susceptibility and severity of dextran sodium sulfate-induced inflammatory bowel disease in mice. *J. Biol. Chem.* **2013**, *288*, 8794–8803, discussion 8804. [CrossRef] [PubMed]
42. Kramer, A.; Green, J.; Pollard, J., Jr.; Tugendreich, S. Causal analysis approaches in Ingenuity Pathway Analysis. *Bioinformatics* **2014**, *30*, 523–530. [CrossRef] [PubMed]
43. Noah, T.K.; Lo, Y.H.; Price, A.; Chen, G.; King, E.; Washington, M.K.; Aronow, B.J.; Shroyer, N.F. SPDEF functions as a colorectal tumor suppressor by inhibiting beta-catenin activity. *Gastroenterology* **2013**, *144*, 1012–1023.e6. [CrossRef] [PubMed]
44. Buenrostro, J.D.; Giresi, P.G.; Zaba, L.C.; Chang, H.Y.; Greenleaf, W.J. Transposition of native chromatin for fast and sensitive epigenomic profiling of open chromatin, DNA-binding proteins and nucleosome position. *Nat. Methods* **2013**, *10*, 1213–1218. [CrossRef] [PubMed]
45. Wu, T.; Hu, E.; Xu, S.; Chen, M.; Guo, P.; Dai, Z.; Feng, T.; Zhou, L.; Tang, W.; Zhan, L.; et al. clusterProfiler 4.0: A universal enrichment tool for interpreting omics data. *Innovation* **2021**, *2*, 100141. [CrossRef] [PubMed]
46. Ey, B.; Eyking, A.; Gerken, G.; Podolsky, D.K.; Cario, E. TLR2 mediates gap junctional intercellular communication through connexin-43 in intestinal epithelial barrier injury. *J. Biol. Chem.* **2009**, *284*, 22332–22343. [CrossRef] [PubMed]

47. Grubisic, V.; McClain, J.L.; Fried, D.E.; Grants, I.; Rajasekhar, P.; Csizmadia, E.; Ajijola, O.A.; Watson, R.E.; Poole, D.P.; Robson, S.C.; et al. Enteric Glia Modulate Macrophage Phenotype and Visceral Sensitivity following Inflammation. *Cell Rep.* **2020**, *32*, 108100. [CrossRef] [PubMed]
48. Xie, J.; Li, L.; Deng, S.; Chen, J.; Gu, Q.; Su, H.; Wen, L.; Wang, S.; Lin, C.; Qi, C.; et al. Slit2/Robo1 Mitigates DSS-induced Ulcerative Colitis by Activating Autophagy in Intestinal Stem Cell. *Int. J. Biol. Sci.* **2020**, *16*, 1876–1887. [CrossRef] [PubMed]
49. Waldo, G.L.; Ricks, T.K.; Hicks, S.N.; Cheever, M.L.; Kawano, T.; Tsuboi, K.; Wang, X.; Montell, C.; Kozasa, T.; Sondek, J.; et al. Kinetic scaffolding mediated by a phospholipase C-beta and Gq signaling complex. *Science* **2010**, *330*, 974–980. [CrossRef]
50. Ota, S.; Ishitani, S.; Shimizu, N.; Matsumoto, K.; Itoh, M.; Ishitani, T. NLK positively regulates Wnt/beta-catenin signalling by phosphorylating LEF1 in neural progenitor cells. *EMBO J.* **2012**, *31*, 1904–1915. [CrossRef]
51. Ma, W.; Chen, M.; Kang, H.; Steinhart, Z.; Angers, S.; He, X.; Kirschner, M.W. Single-molecule dynamics of Dishevelled at the plasma membrane and Wnt pathway activation. *Proc. Natl. Acad. Sci. USA* **2020**, *117*, 16690–16701. [CrossRef] [PubMed]
52. Bilic, J.; Huang, Y.L.; Davidson, G.; Zimmermann, T.; Cruciat, C.M.; Bienz, M.; Niehrs, C. Wnt induces LRP6 signalosomes and promotes dishevelled-dependent LRP6 phosphorylation. *Science* **2007**, *316*, 1619–1622. [CrossRef]
53. Zeng, X.; Huang, H.; Tamai, K.; Zhang, X.; Harada, Y.; Yokota, C.; Almeida, K.; Wang, J.; Doble, B.; Woodgett, J.; et al. Initiation of Wnt signaling: Control of Wnt coreceptor Lrp6 phosphorylation/activation via frizzled, dishevelled and axin functions. *Development* **2008**, *135*, 367–375. [CrossRef] [PubMed]
54. Zeng, X.; Tamai, K.; Doble, B.; Li, S.; Huang, H.; Habas, R.; Okamura, H.; Woodgett, J.; He, X. A dual-kinase mechanism for Wnt co-receptor phosphorylation and activation. *Nature* **2005**, *438*, 873–877. [CrossRef] [PubMed]
55. Haberman, Y.; Tickle, T.L.; Dexheimer, P.J.; Kim, M.O.; Tang, D.; Karns, R.; Baldassano, R.N.; Noe, J.D.; Rosh, J.; Markowitz, J.; et al. Pediatric Crohn disease patients exhibit specific ileal transcriptome and microbiome signature. *J. Clin. Investig.* **2014**, *124*, 3617–3633. [CrossRef] [PubMed]
56. Zabana, Y.; Loren, V.; Domenech, E.; Aterido, A.; Garcia-Jaraquemada, A.; Julia, A.; Vicario, M.; Pedrosa, E.; Ferreiro, M.; Troya, J.; et al. Transcriptomic identification of TMIGD1 and its relationship with the ileal epithelial cell differentiation in Crohn's disease. *Am. J. Physiol. Gastrointest. Liver Physiol.* **2020**, *319*, G109–G120. [CrossRef] [PubMed]
57. Keir, M.E.; Fuh, F.; Ichikawa, R.; Acres, M.; Hackney, J.A.; Hulme, G.; Carey, C.D.; Palmer, J.; Jones, C.J.; Long, A.K.; et al. Regulation and Role of alphaE Integrin and Gut Homing Integrins in Migration and Retention of Intestinal Lymphocytes during Inflammatory Bowel Disease. *J. Immunol.* **2021**, *207*, 2245–2254. [CrossRef]
58. Palmer, N.P.; Silvester, J.A.; Lee, J.J.; Beam, A.L.; Fried, I.; Valtchinov, V.I.; Rahimov, F.; Kong, S.W.; Ghodoussipour, S.; Hood, H.C.; et al. Concordance between gene expression in peripheral whole blood and colonic tissue in children with inflammatory bowel disease. *PLoS ONE* **2019**, *14*, e0222952. [CrossRef] [PubMed]
59. Swarup, S.; Verheyen, E.M. Wnt/Wingless signaling in Drosophila. *Cold Spring Harb. Perspect. Biol* **2012**, *4*, a007930. [CrossRef]
60. Nolo, R.; Abbott, L.A.; Bellen, H.J. Senseless, a Zn finger transcription factor, is necessary and sufficient for sensory organ development in Drosophila. *Cell* **2000**, *102*, 349–362. [CrossRef]
61. Kramps, T.; Peter, O.; Brunner, E.; Nellen, D.; Froesch, B.; Chatterjee, S.; Murone, M.; Zullig, S.; Basler, K. Wnt/wingless signaling requires BCL9/legless-mediated recruitment of pygopus to the nuclear beta-catenin-TCF complex. *Cell* **2002**, *109*, 47–60. [CrossRef] [PubMed]
62. Baker, N.E. Transcription of the segment-polarity gene wingless in the imaginal discs of Drosophila, and the phenotype of a pupal-lethal wg mutation. *Development* **1988**, *102*, 489–497. [CrossRef] [PubMed]
63. Brunner, E.; Peter, O.; Schweizer, L.; Basler, K. pangolin encodes a Lef-1 homologue that acts downstream of Armadillo to transduce the Wingless signal in Drosophila. *Nature* **1997**, *385*, 829–833. [CrossRef] [PubMed]
64. Davidson, G.; Shen, J.; Huang, Y.L.; Su, Y.; Karaulanov, E.; Bartscherer, K.; Hassler, C.; Stannek, P.; Boutros, M.; Niehrs, C. Cell cycle control of wnt receptor activation. *Dev. Cell* **2009**, *17*, 788–799. [CrossRef] [PubMed]
65. Hadjihannas, M.V.; Bernkopf, D.B.; Bruckner, M.; Behrens, J. Cell cycle control of Wnt/beta-catenin signalling by conductin/axin2 through CDC20. *EMBO Rep.* **2012**, *13*, 347–354. [CrossRef]
66. Olmeda, D.; Castel, S.; Vilaro, S.; Cano, A. Beta-catenin regulation during the cell cycle: Implications in G2/M and apoptosis. *Mol. Biol. Cell* **2003**, *14*, 2844–2860. [CrossRef]
67. Huang, H.C.; Klein, P.S. The Frizzled family: Receptors for multiple signal transduction pathways. *Genome Biol.* **2004**, *5*, 234. [CrossRef]
68. Pan, W.J.; Choi, S.C.; Wang, H.; Qin, Y.B.; Volpicelli-Daley, L.; Swan, L.; Lucast, L.; Khoo, C.; Zhang, X.W.; Li, L.; et al. Wnt3a-mediated formation of phosphatidylinositol 4,5-bisphosphate regulates LRP6 phosphorylation. *Science* **2008**, *321*, 1350–1353. [CrossRef]
69. De, A. Wnt/Ca^{2+} signaling pathway: A brief overview. *Acta Biochim. Biophys. Sin.* **2011**, *43*, 745–756. [CrossRef]
70. Shelley-Fraser, G.; Borley, N.R.; Warren, B.F.; Shepherd, N.A. The connective tissue changes of Crohn's disease. *Histopathology* **2012**, *60*, 1034–1044. [CrossRef]
71. Akhmetshina, A.; Palumbo, K.; Dees, C.; Bergmann, C.; Venalis, P.; Zerr, P.; Horn, A.; Kireva, T.; Beyer, C.; Zwerina, J.; et al. Activation of canonical Wnt signalling is required for TGF-beta-mediated fibrosis. *Nat. Commun.* **2012**, *3*, 735. [CrossRef]
72. Hoeppner, L.H.; Phoenix, K.N.; Clark, K.J.; Bhattacharya, R.; Gong, X.; Sciuto, T.E.; Vohra, P.; Suresh, S.; Bhattacharya, S.; Dvorak, A.M.; et al. Revealing the role of phospholipase Cbeta3 in the regulation of VEGF-induced vascular permeability. *Blood* **2012**, *120*, 2167–2173. [CrossRef] [PubMed]

73. Birdsey, G.M.; Shah, A.V.; Dufton, N.; Reynolds, L.E.; Osuna Almagro, L.; Yang, Y.; Aspalter, I.M.; Khan, S.T.; Mason, J.C.; Dejana, E.; et al. The endothelial transcription factor ERG promotes vascular stability and growth through Wnt/beta-catenin signaling. *Dev. Cell* **2015**, *32*, 82–96. [CrossRef] [PubMed]
74. Weiser, M.; Simon, J.M.; Kochar, B.; Tovar, A.; Israel, J.W.; Robinson, A.; Gipson, G.R.; Schaner, M.S.; Herfarth, H.H.; Sartor, R.B.; et al. Molecular classification of Crohn's disease reveals two clinically relevant subtypes. *Gut* **2018**, *67*, 36–42. [CrossRef] [PubMed]
75. Wehkamp, J.; Salzman, N.H.; Porter, E.; Nuding, S.; Weichenthal, M.; Petras, R.E.; Shen, B.; Schaeffeler, E.; Schwab, M.; Linzmeier, R.; et al. Reduced Paneth cell alpha-defensins in ileal Crohn's disease. *Proc. Natl. Acad. Sci. USA* **2005**, *102*, 18129–18134. [CrossRef] [PubMed]
76. Koslowski, M.J.; Kubler, I.; Chamaillard, M.; Schaeffeler, E.; Reinisch, W.; Wang, G.; Beisner, J.; Teml, A.; Peyrin-Biroulet, L.; Winter, S.; et al. Genetic variants of Wnt transcription factor TCF-4 (TCF7L2) putative promoter region are associated with small intestinal Crohn's disease. *PLoS ONE* **2009**, *4*, e4496. [CrossRef] [PubMed]
77. Wehkamp, J.; Wang, G.; Kubler, I.; Nuding, S.; Gregorieff, A.; Schnabel, A.; Kays, R.J.; Fellermann, K.; Burk, O.; Schwab, M.; et al. The Paneth cell alpha-defensin deficiency of ileal Crohn's disease is linked to Wnt/Tcf-4. *J. Immunol.* **2007**, *179*, 3109–3118. [CrossRef]
78. Beisner, J.; Teltschik, Z.; Ostaff, M.J.; Tiemessen, M.M.; Staal, F.J.; Wang, G.; Gersemann, M.; Perminow, G.; Vatn, M.H.; Schwab, M.; et al. TCF-1-mediated Wnt signaling regulates Paneth cell innate immune defense effectors HD-5 and -6: Implications for Crohn's disease. *Am. J. Physiol. Gastrointest. Liver Physiol.* **2014**, *307*, G487–G498. [CrossRef]
79. Koslowski, M.J.; Teltschik, Z.; Beisner, J.; Schaeffeler, E.; Wang, G.; Kubler, I.; Gersemann, M.; Cooney, R.; Jewell, D.; Reinisch, W.; et al. Association of a functional variant in the Wnt co-receptor LRP6 with early onset ileal Crohn's disease. *PLoS Genet.* **2012**, *8*, e1002523. [CrossRef]
80. Baillie, J.K.; Arner, E.; Daub, C.; De Hoon, M.; Itoh, M.; Kawaji, H.; Lassmann, T.; Carninci, P.; Forrest, A.R.; Hayashizaki, Y.; et al. Analysis of the human monocyte-derived macrophage transcriptome and response to lipopolysaccharide provides new insights into genetic aetiology of inflammatory bowel disease. *PLoS Genet.* **2017**, *13*, e1006641. [CrossRef]
81. Na, Y.R.; Stakenborg, M.; Seok, S.H.; Matteoli, G. Macrophages in intestinal inflammation and resolution: A potential therapeutic target in IBD. *Nat. Rev. Gastroenterol. Hepatol.* **2019**, *16*, 531–543. [CrossRef] [PubMed]
82. Perez-Sanchez, C.; Barbera Betancourt, A.; Lyons, P.A.; Zhang, Z.; Suo, C.; Lee, J.C.; McKinney, E.F.; Modis, L.K.; Ellson, C.; Smith, K.G.C. miR-374a-5p regulates inflammatory genes and monocyte function in patients with inflammatory bowel disease. *J. Exp. Med.* **2022**, *219*, e20211366. [CrossRef] [PubMed]
83. Huang, B.; Chen, Z.; Geng, L.; Wang, J.; Liang, H.; Cao, Y.; Chen, H.; Huang, W.; Su, M.; Wang, H.; et al. Mucosal Profiling of Pediatric-Onset Colitis and IBD Reveals Common Pathogenics and Therapeutic Pathways. *Cell* **2019**, *179*, 1160–1176.e24. [CrossRef] [PubMed]
84. Janda, C.Y.; Dang, L.T.; You, C.; Chang, J.; de Lau, W.; Zhong, Z.A.; Yan, K.S.; Marecic, O.; Siepe, D.; Li, X.; et al. Surrogate Wnt agonists that phenocopy canonical Wnt and beta-catenin signalling. *Nature* **2017**, *545*, 234–237. [CrossRef]
85. Zhu, W.; Winter, M.G.; Byndloss, M.X.; Spiga, L.; Duerkop, B.A.; Hughes, E.R.; Buttner, L.; de Lima Romao, E.; Behrendt, C.L.; Lopez, C.A.; et al. Precision editing of the gut microbiota ameliorates colitis. *Nature* **2018**, *553*, 208–211. [CrossRef]

diseases

MDPI

Review

Wernicke Encephalopathy Caused by Avoidance-Restrictive Food Intake Disorder in a Child: A Case-Based Review

Ida Turrini [1,†], Clotilde Guidetti [1,†], Ilaria Contaldo [1], Silvia Pulitanò [2,3], Donato Rigante [3,4,*] and Chiara Veredice [1]

1 Pediatric Neurology Unit, Policlinico Universitario A. Gemelli IRCCS, 00168 Rome, Italy; ida.turrini@guest.policlinicogemelli.it (I.T.); chiara.veredice@policlinicogemelli.it (C.V.)
2 Pediatric Intensive Care Unit, Policlinico Universitario A. Gemelli IRCCS, 00168 Rome, Italy
3 Università Cattolica Sacro Cuore, 00168 Rome, Italy
4 Department of Life Sciences and Public Health, Policlinico Universitario A. Gemelli IRCCS, 00168 Rome, Italy
* Correspondence: donato.rigante@unicatt.it; Tel.: +39-06-30155210
† These authors contributed equally to this work.

Abstract: Background: Wernicke encephalopathy (WE) is an acute and potentially fatal neuropsychiatric disorder resulting from thiamine deficiency: its etiology and clinical presentation can be heterogeneous and arduously recognized, especially in children and adolescents. Case presentation: An 8-year-old girl arrived to the emergency room with ataxic gait, nystagmus, and mental confusion after a 10-day history of repeated severe vomiting; her recent clinical history was characterized by restricted nutrition due to a choking phobia, which caused substantial *weight loss*. Brain magnetic resonance imaging revealed a bilaterally increased T2 signal in the medial areas of the thalami and cerebral periaqueductal region. Diagnosis of WE based on clinical and neuroradiological findings was established and confirmed after labwork showing low serum thiamine. Following psychiatric evaluation, the patient was also diagnosed with avoidance-restrictive food intake disorder (ARFID), which required starting cognitive behavioral therapy and introducing aripiprazole. The patient displayed improvement of the radiological findings after one month and complete resolution of her neurological symptoms and signs. Conclusions: Eating disorders like ARFID might forerun acute signs of WE; this possibility should be considered even in pediatric patients, especially when atypical neurological pictures or feeding issues come out.

Keywords: Wernicke encephalopathy; avoidance-restrictive food intake disorder; thiamine; personalized medicine; cognitive behavioral therapy; aripiprazole; child

1. Introduction

Deficiency in several micronutrients such as vitamins and minerals has been described in many patients with an eating disorder (ED) [1], and in particular, a severe deficiency in thiamine (vitamin B1) can be associated with a peculiar neuropsychiatric syndrome named Wernicke encephalopathy (WE). This is a rare neurologic emergency due to a single vitamin deficiency, thiamine, which might have a poor outcome if brain thiamine deficiency is left uncorrected: the vast majority of patients with WE are adult patients who are alcoholics. Indeed, many clinicians might miss recognizing WE in nonalcoholic individuals or in patients at risk for developing thiamine deficiency [2]. WE was first described in 1881 by Carl Wernicke, a German psychiatrist, in association with autopsy findings of punctate hemorrhages in close proximity to the third and fourth ventricles and cerebral aqueduct. Such a diagnosis is clinically based on the typical "triad" of ophthalmoplegia, gait ataxia, and cognitive impairment, consisting of confusion, delirium, and memory disturbance with body temperature dysregulation and hypotension. The majority of affected patients may have a history of chronic alcohol abuse, but they might simply display undernutrition caused by famine, malabsorption, and increased metabolic requirement or inadequate intake of vitamins, including thiamine [1,2].

Thiamine is one of the water-soluble B vitamins, naturally present in foods such as whole grains, cereals, legumes and meat, which can be added to some nutritional products, being available as a dietary supplement. It is crucial in different biochemical pathways related to energy metabolism and, therefore, decisive for growth, development, and regular function of cells. Without thiamine, glucose is metabolized through less efficient anaerobic pathways that produce lactic acid. Acidosis caused by thiamine deficiency can profoundly affect the central nervous system, mostly the thalami, mammillary bodies, oculomotor nuclei, and cerebellar vermis, resulting in severe neuropsychiatric morbidities [3,4]. Humans have the power to store thiamine primarily in the liver; however, a continuous thiamine supply from the diet is necessary, as thiamine body storage can be depleted in as little as 4 weeks, warranting central nervous system vulnerability related to thiamine critical contribution to numerous brain metabolic activities [5].

In 2013, avoidant/restrictive food intake disorder (ARFID) was first introduced as a new ED in the Diagnostic and Statistical Manual of Mental Disorders (DSM)-5 [6]. This feeding disturbance is characterized by either avoidant or restrictive nutritional habits, leading to abstaining from eating foods, which usually results in one or more of the following: progressive weight loss or failure to achieve an expected weight gain, nutritional deficiencies, dependence on either enteral feeding or oral nutritional supplements, and interference with regular and normal psychosocial functions [7]. The DSM-5 describes three core ARFID presentations: (a) food avoidance based on the sensory characteristics of foods, (b) lack of interest in different foods or in eating specific foods, and (c) fear of the adverse consequences associated with food intake, mostly after any traumatic events associated with eating, e.g., choking or uncontainable vomiting. Unlike anorexia nervosa and bulimia nervosa, ARFID is neither characterized by any preoccupation about self-body shape and body weight, nor by "intentional" behaviors aimed at achieving weight loss [8,9].

So far, the association of WE and thiamine deficiency in relationship with EDs has been mainly reported for patients with anorexia nervosa [10–14]. Our report is related to a young girl presenting with WE and a history of ARFID, who showed improvement after starting thiamine supplementation combined with cognitive behavioral therapy (CBT) and aripiprazole. A revision of the medical literature on this peculiar disease occurring in childhood has been provided herein.

2. Case Presentation

An 8-year-old girl was admitted to the Pediatric Intensive Care Unit in the Policlinico A. Gemelli IRCCS, Rome (Italy), due to mental confusion, ataxic gait, nystagmus, and uncontrollable vomiting. When first evaluated, the child had a weight of 30 kg (64th percentile), her height was 130 cm (39th percentile), and her body mass index was 17.8 kg/m^2. The patient's diet had been out of control and largely based on high-carbohydrate foods before this hospitalization. In particular, two months before, she presented with accidental choking while eating a solid meal. After this episode, the girl started to progressively restrict her diet in terms of both quantity and number of meals, developing a weight loss of 12 kg over that period of time; in addition, her parents reported that ten days earlier, she had presented with recurrent severe vomiting, but outpatient esophagogastroduodenoscopy had showed no abnormalities.

During this hospitalization, the patient's condition actually deteriorated, requiring endotracheal intubation and intermittent positive pressure ventilation. The results of routine hematologic and biochemical measurements, including glucose, sodium, potassium, calcium, urea, creatinine, amylase, lipase, alanine aminotransferase, aspartate aminotransferase, gamma-glutamyl transpeptidase, alkaline phosphatase, and blood coagulation parameters, were all within normal limits. Cerebrospinal fluid analysis was also normal. The search for infectious agents, including human immunodeficiency virus and different neurotropic viruses, was completely negative. To rule out the autoimmune nature of such conditions, anti-nuclear, anti-DNAds, anti-onconeural, anti-aquaporine-4, anti-myelin oligodendrocyte glycoprotein, anti-myelin associated glycoprotein, and anti-ganglioside antibodies were also measured, with all being negative. An expanded screening for metabolic diseases and endocrinopathies was performed, with negative results. Brain computed tomography (CT) scan revealed low-density signal abnormalities in the paraventricular thalamic regions, while brain magnetic resonance imaging (MRI, Figure 1A,B) showed slight bilateral symmetrical T2 hyperintensity in the medial thalamic nuclei, along the walls of the third ventricle and in the periaqueductal region. Neuroradiological and clinical signs were consistent with WE. Intravenous therapy with thiamine was subsequently started (600 mg twice daily). The patient's clinical condition improved four days after starting treatment. Therefore, the girl was extubated, and two days after, she was transferred to the Child Neuropsychiatry ward. At that time, the girl had both horizontal and vertical nystagmus, eyelid ptosis, and mild ataxic gait; she was also receiving enteral nutrition via nasogastric tube (900 kcal daily). The serum thiamine level was obtained 14 days after admission to the Pediatric Intensive Care Unit and confirmed to be low: 23 ng/mL (tested using Electro-ChemiLuminescence ImmunoAssay; normal reference: 32–95). Then, thiamine was administered per os (100 mg/day), as agreed upon with the nutritional counseling team.

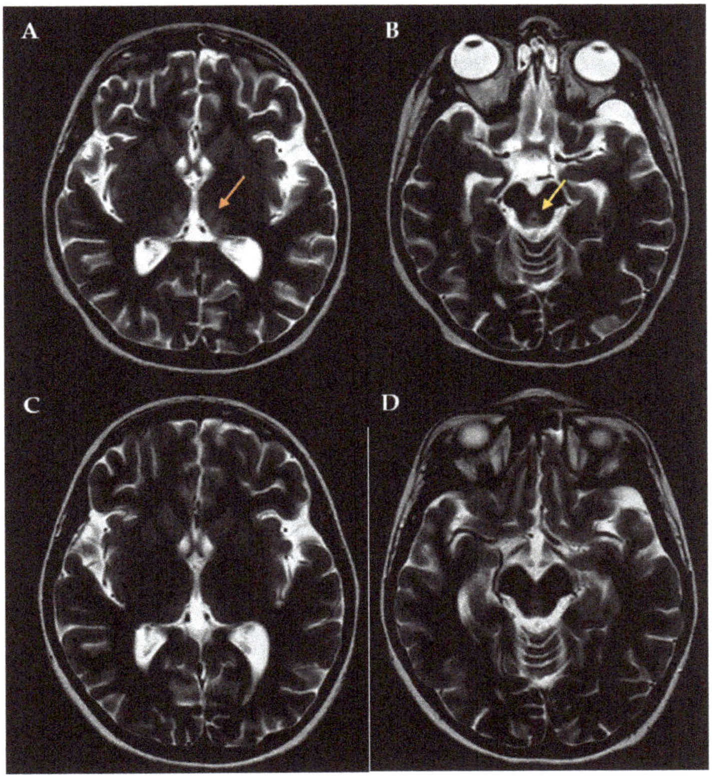

Figure 1. Brain MRI with contrast showing T2 signal hyperintensity involving the medial thalami (orange arrow in **A**) and the periaqueductal region (yellow arrow in **B**). The patient was initially treated with high-dose intravenous thiamine, then with oral thiamine on a daily basis. A new brain MRI showing a significant improvement in lesions was assessed one month after disease onset (**C**,**D**).

Video-EEG examination showed diffuse slowing of the background electric activity. The Wechsler Intelligence Scale for Children 4th Edition (WISC-IV) revealed normal intellectual functioning with a QIT result of 87; the other results were 92 for the verbal comprehension index, 91 for the perceptual reasoning index, 74 for the processing speed index, and 103 for the working memory index. The Schedule for Affective Disorders and Schizophrenia for School-Aged Children Present and Lifetime Version (K-SADS-PL), a semi-structured interview, was separately administered to both the patient and her mother, along with a non-structured interview. During the interview, the girl confirmed that in the previous two months she had been afraid of choking when swallowing different solid foods, so she felt anxious, troubled, and scared of eating normally. There was no evidence of body image or body weight concerns and no previous history of panic attacks. Through observation of the patient during her hospital stay and through the mother's report, it was established that the restricted food intake was caused by the primitive fear of swallowing food; the patient met the criteria for diagnosis of ARFID, as defined by the DSM-5, and for subthreshold anxiety symptoms (phobia type). Therefore, 2.5 mg of aripiprazole given orally once daily was started. During the second week at the ward, the patient turned out to be fully able to tolerate oral foods, and enteral feeding was discontinued. In addition, at this time, serum thiamine reached a normal level (41.3 ng/mL).

The patient had an almost complete resolution of her neurological symptoms, with persistence of mild nystagmus occurring only in extreme positions of the gaze and slight instability in static and dynamic equilibrium tests; the video-EEG revealed a normal organization of the patient's cerebral electrical activity. She was discharged on 100 mg of oral thiamine and oral aripiprazole (increased to 2.5 mg twice a day), while outpatient CBT was also arranged. After approximately 1 month of thiamine therapy, a brain MRI showed a full resolution of the previously reported altered signals in the thalami along the walls of the third ventricle and periaqueductal areas (Figure 1C,D).

While staying at home, the girl suffered from sporadic episodes of esophageal food bolus impaction followed by vomiting, and the choking phobia was sporadically reported in spite of regular CBT sessions. The patient's family was supported by community social services with lifestyle education programs targeting the child's diet quality improvement. Oral thiamine supplementation was maintained for an overall period of 14 months. Treatment with aripiprazole is still ongoing, and neuropsychiatric monitoring is performed on a biannual basis. Nevertheless, the more recent issue in this girl has been characterized by overnutrition with high-calorie nutrients, revealing a persistent conflict between the patient and food: her last weight (at 10 years) was 53 kg (99th percentile), her height was 139.5 cm (80th percentile), and her body mass index was 27.2 kg/m^2.

3. Discussion and Case-Based Review of the Medical Literature

WE is an acute but reversible brain disorder induced by thiamine deficiency, traditionally related to chronic alcoholism. However, chronic alcohol consumption does not necessarily result in WE if dietary thiamine intake is adequate: in fact, thiamine deficiency may be induced by several additional potential mechanisms, such as genetic predisposition, impaired absorption of thiamine from the gut, impairment of storage in the liver or in other tissues, thiamine transport abnormalities, decreased phosphorylation to thiamine pyrophosphate, or excessive requirements for the metabolism of alcohol. In addition, multiple clinical sceneries can exacerbate WE, such as diet imbalance, prolonged intravenous nutrition, anorexia nervosa, and malabsorption. Diagnosis of thiamine deficiency may be delayed in nonalcoholic patients as a result, and the early stages of deficiency may be heralded by gastrointestinal abnormalities such as slow gastric emptying. Many clinicians may underestimate the risk of nonalcoholic WE, in which sudden and severe weight loss or vomiting can be precociously encountered [15]. The traditional triad of WE includes ophthalmoplegia, ataxic gait, and impaired mental status, though these three signs are uncommonly found together [13]. Even if diagnosis of WE is made at a clinical level, systematic reviews suggest that Caine's criteria, using one symptom of the triad in combination with malnutrition, might have a higher sensitivity than the complete triad for the recognition of WE [14], requiring that dietary deficiencies are combined with oculomotor abnormalities, cerebellar dysfunction, or cognitive impairment. Even if thiamine absolute deficiency may directly cause WE, diagnosis may sometimes require the support of brain imaging, revealing symmetric signal abnormalities with diffusion restriction and lack of normal enhancement in the bilateral thalami or changes in the mammillary bodies. However, though imaging studies and labwork with low serum thiamine levels may support the diagnosis of WE, these findings alone are not diagnostic. Furthermore, if cases of WE are not identified, patients' neurologic status may worsen, even leading to death. One of the major barriers to early diagnosis of WE is the low index of suspicion in nonalcoholic patients, mostly if young patients with anorexia nervosa, patients on dialysis, or patients undergoing a long-lasting parenteral nutrition [4].

Foods rich in thiamine include whole grains, fortified or enriched grains, brown rice, soybean seeds, dried beans or peas, infant formulas, and meats; thiamine is physiologically absorbed from the duodenum into the blood stream, but small amounts of thiamine can be stored in the liver, though for a limited period of time [4]. In particular, thiamine diphosphate acts as a cofactor for a number of thiamine-dependent enzymes, and different metabolic pathways are involved, including production of adenosine triphosphate and oxidative degradation of carbohydrates, fatty acids, and amino acids. Without thiamine, pyruvate is unable to enter the tricarboxylic acid cycle, which leads to conversion of pyruvate into lactic acid; in addition, thiamine acts as a coenzyme for transketolase in the pentose phosphate pathway. Because thiamine-dependent enzymes have an irreplaceable role in cerebral energy utilization, thiamine deficiency may propagate brain tissue injury by inhibiting metabolism in further regions with higher metabolic demands or higher thiamine turnover, with decreased energy resources and selective neuronal death. In the end, the reduced production of succinate involved in gamma-aminobutyric acid metabolism might also impact neuronal excitability [4].

A multitude of complications may follow thiamine deficiency, including cardiomyopathy ("wet beriberi"), distal neuropathy ("dry beriberi"), central pontine myelinolysis, and a large spectrum of disorders, including WE and Wernicke–Korsakoff syndrome. The administration of thiamine can naturally lead to improvement of ocular dysfunction, gait abnormality, and disrupted state of consciousness, as well as more complex signs such as bradypsychia and bradylalia, which are openly referred to WE [16]. The Wernicke–Korsakoff syndrome is characterized by chronic neuropsychiatric symptoms occurring as a consequence of WE: its detection is pivotal to halt the progression of WE. Other causes of WE in adults may be related to hyperemesis gravidarum, intestinal obstruction malignancy, or bariatric surgery (Roux-en-Y gastric bypass, sleeve gastrectomy, duodenal switch, etc.), while the conditions associated with WE in childhood are nutrient deprivation, primitive gastrointestinal disorders, prolonged infectious illnesses including tuberculosis, acquired immunodeficiency syndrome, nephrotic syndrome, and end-stage renal diseases requiring dialysis and prolonged parenteral nutrition without a proper supplementation of thiamine [17].

The recognition of symmetrical hypodense lesions in the basal ganglia and medial thalami/hypothalamic/subthalamic areas on CT scans of the brain is a clue to consider WE in at-risk young patients [18]. Common brain MRI findings encompass symmetric T2 hyperintensities in the thalamus, mammillary bodies, and periaqueductal gray matter with restricted diffusion and prominent lactate peak, all findings that may suggest WE, though these findings cannot be evocative for diagnosis without an appropriate clinical scenery [19]. There are few data about children with WE, with most cases being misdiagnosed; identifying neurologic signs, combined with imaging studies such as brain CT or MRI, should be essential for a precocious suggestion of WE. It is important to highlight that blurred vision and nystagmus may predominate over further manifestations in children with WE, in combination with vomiting, poor appetite, lethargy, and weight loss [20]. A brain MRI can help diagnose WE in children, following hyperintense signal in specific districts that are more prone to display sensitivity to thiamine deficiency, such as the thalamus, mammillary bodies, cerebral aqueduct, and midline cerebellum [21].

The presence of a nutritional deficiency including thiamine should always be assessed in patients displaying poor nutritional intake or intractable vomiting, and pediatric patients being excluded for having metabolic derangements should be considered for WE. Nutritional deficiencies related to EDs derive from starvation in anorexia nervosa and other psychiatric disorders [22], but a persistent disturbance leading to avoidance of foods might result in significant weight loss, giving rise to the picture of ARFID. Currently, to the best of our knowledge, only four pediatric cases of WE have been related to ARFID [23–26].

A 4-year-old boy with a history of food aversion, difficulty in swallowing, and decreased appetite was hospitalized with intractable vomiting and weakness of four days' duration. The vomiting was ondansetron-resistant, and the child developed severe dehydration and weight loss, as well as ophthalmoplegia and gait ataxia. Extensive metabolic testing was negative. After three days, the patient became more lethargic, with bilateral ptosis, upgaze palsy, and abnormal walking. The brain MRI demonstrated that the thalamus, mammillary bodies, and periaqueductal regions were hyperintense in the diffusion-weighted images, while the serum thiamine level was severely decreased. He was ultimately found to have WE secondary to ARFID and was started on high-dose intravenous thiamine, showing an excellent response after only three days [23].

A 12-year-old girl was hospitalized for rehydration secondary to decreased oral intake in the previous three weeks due to crampy epigastric pain and post-prandial emesis. In particular, the girl had lost over 40 kg of her body weight in the past year due to self-imposed dietary restrictions, eliminating sugary foods. The patient denied inducing vomiting and binging. Her metabolic profile was within normal limits, and many radiological investigations ruled out acute abdomen and superior mesenteric artery syndrome. Ondansetron was initially given, but post-prandial vomiting persisted, while double vision was noted in combination with blurred vision, nystagmus, and unsteady gait. The brain MRI was normal, but the pediatric gastroenterologist empirically recommended thiamine supplementation as a trial for WE. She was ultimately confirmed to have severe thiamine deficiency with ARFID-related WE [24].

A 10-year-old girl had a two-month history of food refusal, vomiting, and lethargy; two months before, she had begun to reject many foods and drink only soft beverages. The neurological examination revealed confusion, bemusement, short-term memory impairment, and bilateral complete lateral and upgaze palsy. The brain MRI identified abnormally bright signals in the dorsomedial thalamic nuclei and in the posterior putamina. Treatment with thiamine was started and led to a considerable neurologic improvement after only 48 h [25].

A 10-year-old boy was hospitalized after a two-month history of food refusal and weight loss, following a choking episode caused by raisin ingestion. Diplopia was the reason for requiring medical assistance. In particular, he was unable to fully abduct his eyes beyond the mid position, but he also presented nystagmus and ataxia. The presumptive diagnosis was a conversion disorder, but serum thiamine concentration was low, suggesting the diagnosis of WE which urgently required thiamine supplementation. Within 12 h an improvement was noted, and within 48 h he was able to abduct each eye. One month later he showed a near-complete recovery of all neurological signs [26].

None of these patients had received a psychiatric diagnosis prior to the onset of WE, and no psychological treatment had been suggested for their previous ED. All these observations highlight the importance of a complete familiar history, including eating habits, in order to evaluate the possibility of malnutrition, even with overweight patients.

ARFID should be considered in patients with weight loss who do not meet the criteria for anorexia or disordered eating behaviors and distorted attitudes towards food, while the Caine criteria could be employed for testing the possibility of WE and immediately starting treatment with thiamine. Based on the DSM-V, ARFID may be disclosed by significant weight loss, nutritional flaws, requirement of enteral feeding, and unwieldy psychosocial dysfunction [22–27]. Due to the broad differences in age, developmental stage, gender, underpinning mechanisms, and clinical presentation, individuals with ARFID require different specialist skills and various interventions from a range of clinical services and professions, including pediatrics, pediatric emergency care, pediatric endocrinology, dietetics, pediatric gastroenterology, child and adolescent psychiatry, general mental health services, social welfare, and occupational therapy. Patients with ARFID who need hospitalization often have significant mental health comorbidities which might combine with adverse parental feeding styles [28]. Also, pediatricians should take into account WE in children with ARFID, who show neurological symptoms deriving from thiamine deficiency related to loss of interest for food and/or fear of adverse consequences after eating. Unfortunately, there is no consensus about the most exact dosage, frequency, and overall duration of thiamine administration in these patients. Many experts suggest treating WE with high parenteral doses of thiamine and gradually reducing them after both clinical and radiological improvement, as any accumulated damage in the central nervous system makes the use of oral thiamine therapeutically inadequate. Thiamine supplementation should be initiated at the earliest suspicion of thiamine depletion, even before laboratory confirmation is available [29].

Our present report is related to an 8-year-old girl with a rapidly deteriorating neurological syndrome consistent with WE caused by new-onset ARFID: this patient did not present the classic triad of WE, but otherwise, she met all the criteria suggested by Caine. Without a doubt, the most reliable method to establish thiamine deficiency is measuring erythrocyte transketolase activity (at baseline and after addition of thiamine pyrophosphate). Fortunately, the timely administration of thiamine allowed for the resolution of the patient's neurological signs, while CBT associated with aripiprazole allowed a progressively adequate control of the patient's symptoms. In recent years, clinicians' awareness of ARFID has enabled advocacy for more research and specific development of treatments for this condition. The medical literature about treatment of ARFID in adults consists of single patient case studies and small case series [30]. Due to the recent development of ARFID diagnostic criteria and due to the considerable variability in presentation, a wide array of management approaches have been proposed, including CBT, psychotherapy, and psychotropic medications. These approaches have been tested in outpatient settings, but findings related to efficacy are limited in consideration of the small number of studies available.

Our patient was treated with aripiprazole, an atypical antipsychotic drug acting as a dopaminergic antagonist or stabilizer with serotonergic activities, which is largely used for the treatment of schizophrenia and bipolar disorders, but also as an off-label tool for attention-deficit hyperactivity disorder, insomnia, obsessive-compulsive disorders, personality disorders, post-traumatic stress disorders, substance abuse disorders, Tourette's syndrome, and EDs [31]. Common side effects of atypical antipsychotics are akathisia, hyperphagia, weight gain, and diabetes mellitus, but—among all atypical antipsychotics—aripiprazole is generally thought to have fewer effects on body weight gain [32].

4. Conclusions

Thiamine deficiency is a potential risk in any chronically malnourished individual, but it is rather rare in children, in whom it may represent the foundation of acute neurological signs, which might herald WE. The presence of nutritional deficiencies, including thiamine, should always be considered in patients with a history of nutritional issues and intractable vomiting. Pediatric patients ruled out for metabolic derangements should be considered for a diagnosis of WE. Both early recognition and treatment of thiamine deficiency may slow down the progression to WE and allow a better outcome for the neurological signs. Specifically, ARFID should be recognized for its potential to cause deficiencies in vitamins, and WE should be considered if a pediatric patient shows a rapidly deteriorating neurological syndrome. Our report confirms that thiamine deficiency caused by ARFID in a child may lead to WE and that thiamine supplementation is crucial for recovery.

Author Contributions: Conceptualization, I.T. and C.G.; methodology, I.C. and S.P.; investigation, I.C. and C.V.; data curation, I.T. and C.V.; writing—original draft preparation, I.T. and C.G.;

writing—review and editing, I.C. and C.V.; supervision, D.R. All authors have read and agreed to the published version of the manuscript.

Funding: This research received no external funding.

Institutional Review Board Statement: Not applicable.

Informed Consent Statement: Written informed consent was obtained from the patient's parents.

Data Availability Statement: No new data were created.

Conflicts of Interest: The authors declare no conflicts of interest.

References

1. Gibson, D.; Workman, C.; Mehler, P.S. Medical complications of anorexia nervosa and bulimia nervosa. *Psychiatr. Clin. N. Am.* **2019**, *42*, 263–274. [CrossRef]
2. Peebles, R.; Sieke, E.H. Medical complications of eating disorders in youth. *Child. Adolesc. Psychiatr. Clin. N. Am.* **2019**, *28*, 593–615. [CrossRef]
3. Dhir, S.; Tarasenko, M.; Napoli, E.; Giulivi, C. Neurological, psychiatric, and biochemical aspects of thiamine deficiency in children and adults. *Front. Psychiatry* **2019**, *10*, 207. [CrossRef]
4. Hershkowitz, E.; Markel, A. Thiamine: The road experience of the vitamin as a manifestation of deficiency in a world of abundance. *Harefuah* **2015**, *154*, 661–664, 674.
5. Oudman, E.; Wijnia, J.W.; van Dam, M.; Biter, L.U.; Postma, A. Preventing Wernicke encephalopathy after bariatric surgery. *Obes. Surg.* **2018**, *28*, 2060–2068. [CrossRef]
6. American Psychiatric Association. *Diagnostic and Statistical Manual of Mental Disorders*, 5th ed.; American Psychiatric Association: Washington, DC, USA, 2013.
7. Fisher, M.M.; Rosen, D.S.; Ornstein, R.M.; Mammel, K.A.; Katzman, D.K.; Rome, E.S.; Callahan, S.T.; Malizio, J.; Kearney, S.; Walsh, B.T. Characteristics of avoidant/restrictive food intake disorder in children and adolescents: A "new disorder" in DSM-5. *J. Adolesc. Health* **2014**, *55*, 49–52. [CrossRef]
8. Kams, P.E.; Kuhnle, M.C.; Wons, O.B.; Jo, J.H.; Keshishian, A.C.; Hauser, K.; Becker, K.R.; Franko, D.L.; Misra, M.; Micali, N.; et al. Prevalence and correlates of psychiatric comorbidities in children and adolescents with full and subthreshold avoidant/restrictive food intake disorder. *Int. J. Eat. Disord.* **2020**, *53*, 256–265.
9. Thomas, J.J.; Lawson, E.A.; Micali, N.; Misra, M.; Deckersbach, T.; Eddy, K.T. Avoidant/restrictive food intake disorder: A three-dimensional model of neurobiology with implications for etiology and treatment. *Curr. Psychiatry Rep.* **2017**, *19*, 54. [CrossRef]
10. Saad, L.; Silva, L.F.; Banzato, C.E.; Dantas, C.R.; Garcia, C., Jr. Anorexia nervosa and Wernicke-Korsakoff syndrome: A case report. *J. Med. Case Rep.* **2010**, *4*, 217. [CrossRef]
11. Peters, T.E.; Parvin, M.; Petersen, C.; Faircloth, V.C.; Levine, R.L. A case report of Wernicke's encephalopathy in a pediatric patient with anorexia nervosa-restricting type. *J. Adolesc. Health* **2007**, *40*, 376–383. [CrossRef]
12. Brown, K.; Everwine, M.; Nieves, J. A case of Wernicke encephalopathy secondary to anorexia nervosa complicated by refeeding syndrome and Takotsubo cardiomyopathy. *Am. J. Case Rep.* **2021**, *22*, e929891. [CrossRef]
13. Mantero, V.; Rifino, N.; Costantino, G.; Farina, A.; Pozzetti, U.; Sciacco, M.; Ripolone, M.; Bianchi, G.; Salmaggi, A.; Rigamonti, A. Non-alcoholic beriberi, Wernicke encephalopathy and long-term eating disorder: Case report and a mini-review. *Eat. Weight Disord.* **2021**, *26*, 729–732. [CrossRef]
14. Watanabe, S.; Yamakura, S.; Hirano, K.; Okumura, Y.; Aiba, H. Case of infantile autism with pediatric Wernicke's encephalopathy due to severe eating disorder. *No Hattatsu* **2009**, *41*, 43–46.
15. Oudman, E.; Wijnia, J.W.; Oey, M.J.; van Dam, M.; Postma, A. Wernicke-Korsakoff syndrome despite no alcohol abuse: A summary of systematic reports. *J. Neurol. Sci.* **2021**, *426*, 117482. [CrossRef]
16. Smith, T.J.; Johnson, C.R.; Koshy, R.; Hess, S.Y.; Qureshi, U.A.; Mynak, M.L.; Fischer, P.R. Thiamine deficiency disorders: A clinical perspective. *Ann. N. Y. Acad. Sci.* **2021**, *1498*, 9–28. [CrossRef]
17. Lallas, M.; Desai, J. Wernicke encephalopathy in children and adolescents. *World J. Pediatr.* **2014**, *10*, 293–298. [CrossRef]
18. Qureshi, U.A.; Wani, N.A.; Ahmad, K.; Irshad, M.; Ali, I. Infantile Wernicke's encephalopathy. *Arch. Dis. Child.* **2015**, *100*, 648. [CrossRef]
19. Wani, N.A.; Qureshi, U.A.; Jehangir, M.; Ahmad, K.; Ahmad, W. Infantile encephalitic beriberi: Magnetic resonance imaging findings. *Pediatr. Radiol.* **2016**, *46*, 96–103. [CrossRef]
20. Cooke, C.A.; Hicks, E.; Page, A.B.; Mc Kinstry, S. An atypical presentation of Wernicke's encephalopathy in an 11-year-old child. *Eye* **2006**, *20*, 1418–1420. [CrossRef]
21. Patel, S.; Topiwala, K.; Hudson, L. Wernicke's encephalopathy. *Cureus* **2018**, *10*, e3187. [CrossRef]
22. Smith, C.M.; Komisar, J.R.; Wasserman, B.R.; Kincaid, B.R. Got 2 good eyes but you still can't see: An atypical case of Wernicke's encephalopathy. *Prim. Care Companion CNS Disord.* **2021**, *23*, 20l02780. [CrossRef]

23. Nwaobi, S.O.; Thomas, D.N.; Ugoh, A.C. An unusual case of Wernicke's encephalopathy in a child. *Cureus* **2022**, *14*, e27260. [CrossRef]
24. Basouny, N.; Spigos, J.; Khvolis, D.; McFarlane-Ferreira, Y.; Lee, A. Wernicke encephalopathy in a pediatric patient with avoidant restrictive food intake disorder: A rare presentation of thiamine deficiency. *Am. J. Case Rep.* **2023**, *24*, e940717. [CrossRef]
25. Coe, M.; Carfagnini, F.; Tani, G.; Ambrosetto, P. Wernicke's encephalopathy in a child: Case report and MR findings. *Pediatr. Radiol.* **2001**, *31*, 167–168. [CrossRef]
26. Gropman, A.L.; Gaillard, W.D.; Campbell, P.; Charya, S.V. Wernicke's encephalopathy due to self starvation in a child. *Lancet* **1998**, *351*, 1704–1705. [CrossRef]
27. Caine, D.; Halliday, G.M.; Kril, J.J.; Harper, C.G. Operational criteria for the classification of chronic alcoholics: Identification of Wernicke's encephalopathy. *J. Neurol. Neurosurg. Psychiatry* **1997**, *62*, 51–60. [CrossRef]
28. Milliren, C.E.; Crowley, M.; Carmody, J.K.; Bern, E.M.; Eldredge, O.; Richmond, T.K. Pediatric hospital utilization for patients with avoidant restrictive food intake disorder. *J. Eat. Disord.* **2024**, *12*, 42. [CrossRef]
29. Infante, M.T.; Fancellu, R.; Murialdo, A.; Barletta, L.; Castellan, L.; Serrati, C. Challenges in diagnosis and treatment of Wernicke encephalopathy: Report of 2 cases. *Nutr. Clin. Pract.* **2016**, *31*, 186–190. [CrossRef]
30. Wang, P.; Si, T. Use of antipsychotics in the treatment of depressive disorders. *Shanghai Arch. Psychiatry* **2013**, *25*, 134–140.
31. Frank, G.K.; Shott, M.E.; Hagman, J.O.; Schiel, M.A.; DeGuzman, M.C.; Rossi, B. The partial dopamine D2 receptor agonist aripiprazole is associated with weight gain in adolescent anorexia nervosa. *Int. J. Eat. Disord.* **2017**, *50*, 447–450. [CrossRef]
32. MacDonald, D.E.; Liebman, R.; Trottier, K. Clinical characteristics, treatment course and outcome of adults treated for avoidant/restrictive food intake disorder (ARFID) at a tertiary care eating disorders program. *J. Eat. Disord.* **2024**, *12*, 15. [CrossRef]

cells

MDPI

Article

NADH Intraperitoneal Injection Prevents Lung Inflammation in a BALB/C Mice Model of Cigarette Smoke-Induced Chronic Obstructive Pulmonary Disease

Nada Slama [1], Amina Abdellatif [1], Karima Bahria [1], Sara Gasmi [1], Maamar Khames [1], Abderrahmene Hadji [1], George Birkmayer [2,3,†], Mustapha Oumouna [1], Yassine Amrani [4] and Karine Benachour [1,*]

1 Laboratory of Experimental Biology and Pharmacology, Faculty of Sciences, Dr. Yahia Fares University, Medea 26000, Algeria; nadaslama94@gmail.com (N.S.); amina.abdellatif.bio@gmail.com (A.A.); karima_bhr@hotmail.com (K.B.); sarah_gasmi@yahoo.fr (S.G.); drmammar@hotmail.fr (M.K.); abdouchiwa@hotmail.fr (A.H.); oumouna@gmail.com (M.O.)

2 Department of Medical Chemistry, University of Graz, 8020 Graz, Austria

3 Birkmayer Laboratories, 1090 Vienna, Austria

4 Department of Respiratory Sciences, Institute of Lung Health and NIHR Leicester BRC-Respiratory, Glenfield Hospital, University of Leicester, Leicester LE1 7RH, UK; ya26@leicester.ac.uk

* Correspondence: benachourkarine1@gmail.com

† Died on 28 August 2022.

Abstract: Cigarette smoke is one of the main factors in Chronic Obstructive Pulmonary Disease (COPD), a respiratory syndrome marked by persistent respiratory symptoms and increasing airway obstruction. Perturbed NAD+/NADH levels may play a role in various diseases, including lung disorders like COPD. In our study, we investigated the preventive effect of NADH supplementation in an experimental model of COPD induced by cigarette smoke extract (CSE). N = 64 mice randomly distributed in eight groups were injected with NADH (two doses of 100 mg/kg or 200 mg/kg) or dexamethasone (2 mg/kg) before being exposed to CSE for up to 9 weeks. Additionally, NADH supplementation preserved lung antioxidant defenses by preventing the functional loss of key enzymes such as superoxide dismutase (SOD), glutathione peroxidase (GPX), catalase, and the expression levels of glutathione (GSH) ($n = 4$, $p < 0.001$). It also reduced oxidative damage markers, such as malondialdehyde (MDA) and nitrites ($n = 4$, $p < 0.001$). A marked increase in tissue myeloperoxidase activity was assessed (MPO), confirming neutrophils implication in the inflammatory process. The latter was significantly ameliorated in the NADH-treated groups ($p < 0.001$). Finally, NADH prevented the CSE-induced secretion of cytokines such as Tumor Necrosis Factor alpha (TNF-α), IL-17, and IFN-y ($n = 4$, $p < 0.001$). Our study shows, for the first time, the clinical potential of NADH supplementation in preventing key features of COPD via its unique anti-inflammatory and antioxidant properties.

Keywords: cigarette smoke; animal model; NADH; oxidative stress; inflammation

1. Introduction

Chronic obstructive pulmonary disease (COPD), a condition that affects 328 million people worldwide, is one of the most frequent and life-threatening non-communicable, preventable, and irreversible chronic lung diseases. The Global Burden of Disease report states that COPD is the third leading cause of death in the world [1,2]. COPD is characterized by chronic inflammation that causes damages to the airways, alveoli, and pulmonary vessels, ultimately leading to airflow limitation [3]. COPD is mainly the result of harmful environmental stimuli, including cigarette smoke, which leads to excessive inflammatory responses in the lung, abnormal tissue repair, and the destruction of lung tissue [4]. Cigarette smoking has a well-known negative health impact; it comprises around 4500 components in its gaseous and particle phases. These substances include direct carcinogens, poisons, and oxidants [5].

The mechanisms by which cigarette smoke plays a role in COPD pathogenesis are likely to be complex, but accumulating evidence suggests a potential role of mitochondrial dysfunction [6]. Mitochondria has significant functions in the lung during homeostasis. Various key functions in epithelial cells, such as surfactant synthesis, cellular senescence, mucociliary activity, and mucus secretion, can all be controlled by mitochondria [7]. Mitochondrial structural and functional perturbations have been involved in the pathogenesis of various lung diseases, including COPD. These disturbances alter cell energy as well as different essential cellular homeostatic functions in which mitochondria are known to be implicated, such as mucus secretion, surfactant production regulation, and immunologic defenses [7,8]. Nicotinamide adenine dinucleotide (NAD) is a ubiquitous intracellular electron transporter that has been involved in the majority of aging and neurodegenerative processes. NAD may be present in cells in both its oxidized (NAD+) and reduced forms (NADH) [9]. Their ratio controls the intracellular redox environment, antioxidant capability, and cell signaling and it is known to upregulate anti-inflammatory molecules in various chronic diseases [10]. In this context, an altered mitochondrial metabolism can reduce NADH production, raising the NAD+/NADH ratio, and impairing antioxidant activity, leading to increased oxidative stress and cell dysfunction [11]. Indeed, it has been reported that the intracellular NAD+/NADH level was decreased in various chronic diseases associated with an increased oxidant burden, such as diabetes [12], neurodegenerative diseases [13], and idiopathic lung fibrosis [14]. This downregulation has been linked to the hyperexpression of the NAD+-consuming poly-(ADP-ribose) polymerase 1 (PARP-1), an enzyme with numerous cellular functions, such as cell death and DNA repair function. However, in pathological states associated with intense DNA damage, PARP-1 has been described as one of the main mechanisms driving the cellular loss of NAD+ and ATP, resulting in cell death [13]. Manipulating NADH levels using pharmacological agents has the potential to restore mitochondrial respiration and has shown promising results in the treatment of diabetes and multiple disorders [12,15], chronic fatigue syndrome [16], and neurodegenerative diseases such as Parkinson's disease [17] and Alzheimer's [18], but this has not yet been studied in the context of COPD.

Accordingly, the present work was designed to evaluate the effects of NADH treatment in an experimental model of cigarette smoke extract (CSE)-induced COPD in *BALB/C* mice.

2. Materials and Methods

Animals: Female *BALB/C* mice weighing 20–23 g were obtained from the Institute Pasteur of Algiers, Algeria. Before exposure, mice spent a week getting used to the environment. Throughout the duration of the trial, mice were given free access to water and conventional rodent food (ONAB, El-Kseur, Medea district, Algeria). This study was performed according to the guidelines established by the Institutional Animal Care and Use Committee (IACUC) at the University of Medea (no. IACUC-CEEA-02).

Reagents: NADH was provided by Birkmayer NADH GmbH (Vienna, Austria); Ellman's reagent (DTNB), Pyrogallol, and other solvents and chemicals were bought from Sigma Chemicals (St. Louis, MO, USA). Acetic acid, ethanol, and other reagents were purchased from Biochem Chemopharma (Cosne-Cours-sur-Loire, France).

Preparation of Cigarette Smoke Extract (CSE): CSE was prepared by a modification of the technique described in previous studies [19]. Briefly, commercial cigarettes (Nassim) were used in this study. Three cigarettes (0.8 mg nicotine, 12 mg tar) were burned and bubbled into 3 mL of PBS. The mainstream of smoke, including tars and nicotine, was almost completely removed using a force-feeding syringe (60 mL). The CSE extracts were prepared fresh prior to each experiment and used for administration after adjusting the pH to between 7.00 and 7.40 and filtering through a 0.2 μm pore filter. CSE preparation was standardized by measuring the absorbance at a wavelength of 320 nm.

Experimental design: The animals were randomly divided into eight groups, each with its own set of conditions: the control group, CSE group, Dex (2 mg/kg/2 days) group + CSE, NADH (100 mg/kg/11 days) + CSE group, NADH (100 mg/kg/5 days) group, NADH (200 mg/kg/5 days) + CSE group, NADH (100 mg/kg/5 days) alone group, and Dex (2 mg/kg/2 days) alone group. NADH was administered by intraperitoneal injection every 11 days (11-day regimen) or 5 days (5-day regimen). All mice except those in the control group were intraperitoneally injected with NADH/dexamethasone (0.2 mL/kg) 30 min before CSE/saline (0.3 mL). Body weights were noted every 11 days, and all mice were sacrificed on day 60 after the initial CSE treatment.

Complete blood count in whole blood: EDTA-coated microcentrifuge tubes were used to collect blood from the tail at the end of each experiment. An initial sample volume of 50 µL of whole blood was required for analysis using RaytoRT7600S (Shenzhen, China), hematology analyzer which counts total white blood cells, lymphocytes, granulocytes (neutrophils, eosinophils, or basophils), and MID (monocytes and all non-granulocytes or lymphocytes blood cells).

Assessment of oxidative stress and antioxidant defense in lung homogenates: Isolated lung lobes were homogenized in 1 mL of cold PBS using a homogenizer (IKA ultraturrax, IKA, Wilmington, NC, USA) and centrifuged for 15 min at 6000 rpm to collect tissue supernatants. Protein concentration in the supernatants was calculated according to the Bradford method [20]. To determine the antioxidant effect of NADH in our COPD animal model, we measured antioxidant enzymes and oxidative biomarkers in lung homogenates using a spectrophotometer (SP-300nano) as described below.

Determination of oxidative biomarkers: Malondialdehyde (MDA) peroxidation is one of the most valid indicators to estimate lipid peroxidation. Levels of lung MDA were determined based on the method described by Ohkhawa et al. (1979), which is based on the reaction of 2-thiobarbituric acid (TBA) with MDA to form a pink chromogen, which can be measured at 532 nm [21]. MDA peroxidation was expressed as µmol/mg of total lung protein. Nitrite levels (expressed as µM) were measured in lung homogenates using the modified Griess method [22]. Myeloperoxidase (MPO) activity was measured to estimate neutrophil accumulation in lung tissue following the protocol used by Ruyssers et al., 2009 [23] and expressed as units per gram of tissue, with 1 unit equaling the amount of MPO necessary to convert 1 µmol of H_2O_2 to H_2O per minute.

Determination of the activities of antioxidant enzymes: Superoxide dismutase (SOD) activity was measured according to the Marklund and Marklund method [24] based on the enzyme's ability to inhibit pyrogallolauto-oxidation by the superoxide radical. The samples were read at 570 nm using a spectrophotometer reader. SOD was expressed as µmol/mg of total lung protein. Glutathione peroxidase (GPx) activity was measured using Flohe and Gunzler's method [25] and expressed as µmol/mg of protein. Glutathione (GSH) levels were measured by spectrophotometry according to Weckbecker and Cory's method [26] based on its ability to react with 5,5′-dithio-bis(2-nitrobenzoic acid) (DTNB), and expressed as µmol/mg of total lung protein [26]. Finally, catalase activity was determined according to the method by Aebi et al. and expressed as mmol/mg of total lung protein [27].

Measurement of inflammatory biomarkers in lung tissues: Lung tissues were homogenized in PBS on ice using a homogenizer (IKA ultra turrax) and centrifuged for 15 min at 6000 rpm to collect tissues' supernatants. The supernatants were used to determine the levels of TNF-α, IFN-γ, and IL-17 using a DuoSet ELISA Development kit (R&D system, Minneapolis, MN, USA) following the manufacturer's instructions.

Histopathological examination: The lung tissues were fixed by intratracheal instillation of 10% formalin, and then dehydrated, paraffin-embedded, and cut into 4 µm sections. Hematoxylin and eosin (H&E) staining was used for general histological examination, and trichrome coloration was used to detect the presence of collagen and fibrosis. The slides were examined under an optical light microscope (Carl ZEISS Primo Star, Oberkochen, Germany). The mean linear intercept was used to calculate alveolar enlargement as described previously [28]. The lines were briefly drawn on each lung segment, the intercepts that crossed them were counted, and the mean linear intercept was determined. Image Jv1.54j was utilized to quantify both collagen and bronchial wall thickness [29].

Statistical analysis: All data were expressed as mean ± SD. Statistics were performed using Prism 8.4.2 (GraphPad Software, San Diego, CA, USA) and one-way ANOVA with Bonferroni's correction for multiple comparisons. Differences were considered significant when $p < 0.05$.

3. Results

The results of the white blood cell count, oxidative and anti-oxidative markers, and histological evaluations all indicate that NADH treatment led to significant decreases in systemic inflammation and oxidative stress and provided protection against pulmonary damage and lung fibrosis.

3.1. Effect of NADH Treatment on Body Weights of Mice

As demonstrated in Figure 1, there was no significant difference in the mice's body weights between the control group, CSE group, and NADH-treated group ($p > 0.05$). In contrast, the mice in the dexamethasone + CSE group had weights that were significantly less than those in the respective CSE group ($p = 0.0006$).

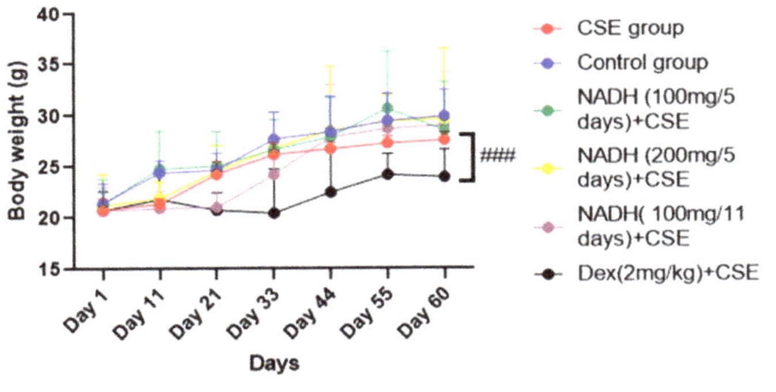

Figure 1. NADH effects on mice body weights. Mice were weighed every 11 days; ### $p < 0.001$ compared with CSE group (n = 8/per group).

3.2. Effect of NADH on CSE-Induced Changes in Total White Blood Cell Count

As revealed in Figure 2, CSE injection significantly increased the total WBC count by 2.55-fold compared with the control group ($p < 0.0001$). Irrespective of the dose (100 and 200 mg) and length of treatment (5- and 11-day regimen), NADH treatment was able to prevent all blood changes induced by CSE. NADH significantly reduced the CSE-induced increase in total WBC with a reduction average of 45.35% (Figure 2a, $n = 4$, $p < 0.001$). Dexamethasone (Dex), used as a positive control intervention for its anti-inflammatory action, resulted in a significant 41% reduction in the blood WBC count when compared to the CSE group ($n = 4$, $p < 0.001$).

The CSE group also exhibited a significant reduction (1.35-fold) in the number of lymphocytes in the blood compared to the control group (Figure 2b, $n = 4$, $p < 0.0001$). NADH and dexamethasone treatment completely prevented a CSE-induced drop in the lymphocyte number in the blood ($n = 4$, $p < 0.0001$).

CSE was also able to stimulate a significant increase in the number of total granulocytes that included neutrophils, eosinophils, and basophils from 7.22 ± 1.28 to 25.2 ± 2.7 (Figure 2c, $n = 4$, $p = 0.0002$). This significant increase was abrogated by NADH treatment with no efficacy difference between the groups ($n = 4$, $p < 0.0001$). Dexamethasone treatment also significantly decreased the granulocyte count by 77.5% when compared with the CSE group (Figure 2c, $p < 0.0001$).

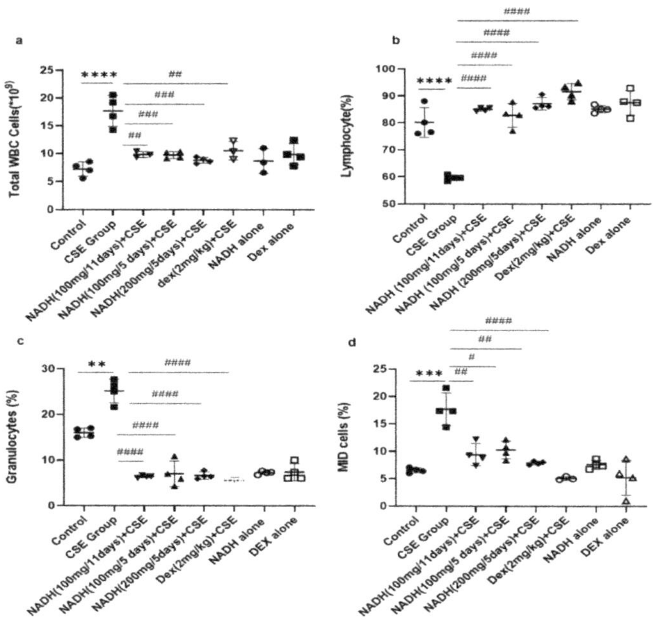

Figure 2. NADH, irrespective to the dose and treatment regimen, prevented blood inflammatory changes in mice exposed to CSE. Blood was collected at the end of the experiment from the control groups (diluent, dexamethasone alone, and NADH alone) and the groups treated with CSE alone or with NADH in a5-day or 11-day regimen. The numbers of total white blood cells (**a**), lymphocytes (**b**), granulocytes (neutrophils, eosinophils, or basophils) (**c**), and MID (monocyte and all non-granulocyte or lymphocyte blood cells) (**d**) were then determined as described in the Section 2. ** $p < 0.05$, *** $p < 0.001$, and **** $p < 0.0001$ compared with the control group; # $p < 0.05$, ## $p < 0.01$, ### $p < 0.001$, and #### $p < 0.0001$ compared with CSE group ($n = 4$/per group).

CSE significantly increased blood MID cells (which reflect the white blood cells not classified as lymphocytes or granulocytes) by 2.17-fold compared to those in the control group (Figure 2d, $n = 4$, $p = 0.008$). In contrast, in all treated groups, NADH treatment led to a decrease in MID cells induced by CSE exposure ($n = 4$, 54.7% decrease). The same results were observed among the dexamethasone-treated groups, which significantly prevented a CSE-induced increase in the MID cell count by 70% when compared to the CSE group; $p < 0.0001$ (Figure 2d, $n = 4$).

We also reported that groups treated with NADH or dexamethasone alone did not exhibit any changes in the number of inflammatory cells when compared to the control group ($p > 0.05$, Figure 2).

3.3. *Effect of NADH on CSE-Induced Lung Changes in Oxidative Stress and Antioxidant Defense Biomarkers*

We found that the CSE-induced COPD model was associated with a significant increase in MDA levels (6.14-fold) when compared to the control group ($p < 0.0005$, Figure 3a).

Treatment with 100 mg of NADH led to a marked reduction in the MDA levels in both treatment regimens (i.e., given every 11 and 5 days), although the effect was more pronounced when NADH was given every 5 days with 35 and 65% inhibition, respectively ($p < 0.0001$, $n = 4$/condition) or at a higher concentration of 200 mg given on a 5-day regime ($p < 0.0001$, $n = 4$/condition). The decrease in CSE-induced lung MDA levels was also inhibited by 41% by dexamethasone ($p = 0.0188$, Figure 3a).

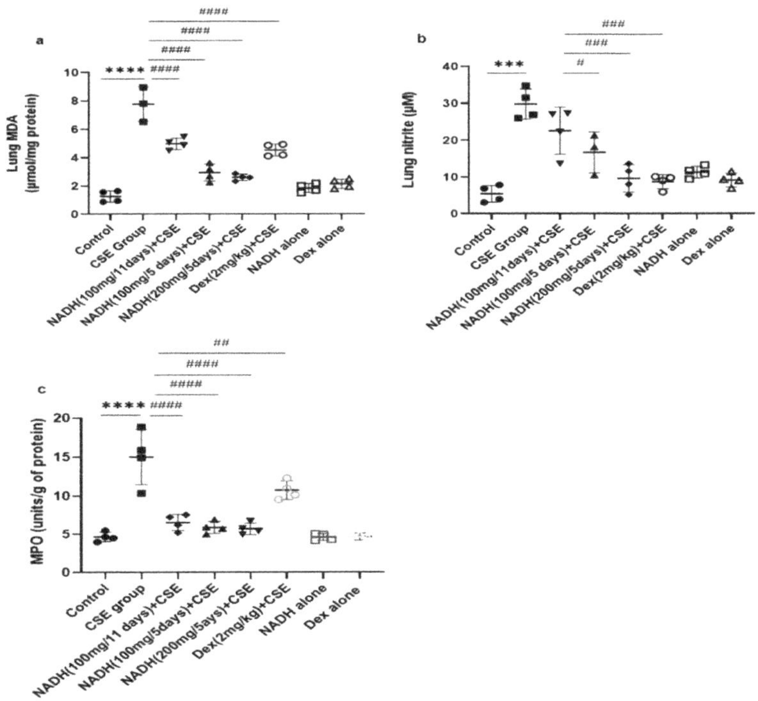

Figure 3. NADH reduced markers of oxidative stress in the lungs of mice exposed to CSE. The levels of malondialdehyde (MDA) (**a**), nitrites (**b**), and MPO (c) were assessed as described in the Section 2 in lung homogenates from the control groups (diluent, dexamethasone alone, and NADH alone) or the groups treated with CSE alone or with NADH every 5 or 11 days. *** $p < 0.001$ and **** $p < 0.0001$ versus the control group; # $p < 0.05$, ## $p < 0.01$, ### $p < 0.001$, and #### $p < 0.0001$ compared with the CSE group ($n = 4$ animals/condition).

The CSE model also led to a significant 4.7-fold increase in lung nitrite levels when compared to the control group, ($p < 0.0001$, Figure 3b). Interestingly, only the mice treated with NADH at a 100 or 200 mg dose in the 5-day regimen led to a significant reduction in nitrite levels, leading to 44% ($p = 0.006$) and 70% ($p < 0.0001$) inhibition, respectively. In contrast, 100 mg of NADH did not affect CSE-induced nitrite production in the 11-day regimen ($p = 0.0749$).

As shown in Figure 3c, CSE increased MPO activity by 3.23-fold when compared with the control group ($n = 4$, $p < 0.0001$). Interestingly, NADH treatment, irrespective of the regimen and the dose, prevented this increase by 50 to 60% ($p < 0.0001$, $n = 4$/condition). We also found that dexamethasone inhibited the CSE-induced increased MPO activity by 29% ($p = 0.009$).

We also looked at the impact of CSE on the antioxidant pathways in the lungs. As demonstrated in Figure 4a, CSE caused a marked reduction (77.73%) in SOD activity in the lung ($p = 0.0052$). Interestingly, NADH, irrespective of the dose (100 and 200 mg) or treatment plan (5-day or 11-day regimen), completely prevented the loss in SOD antioxidant activity induced by CSE ($p < 0.0001$). In contrast, dexamethasone treatment failed to prevent the decrease in lung SOD activity induced by CSE ($p = 0.1080$).

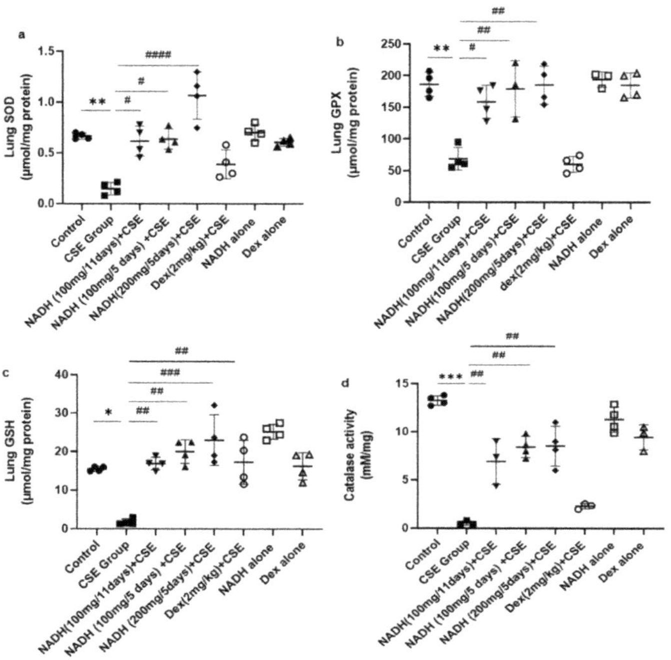

Figure 4. NADH prevented the reduced antioxidant response in the lungs of mice exposed to CSE. The activities of key detoxifying enzymes, including superoxide dismutase (SOD) (**a**), glutathione peroxidase (GPX) (**b**), glutathione (GSH) (**c**), and catalase (**d**), were assessed in lung homogenates from the control groups (diluent, dexamethasone alone, and NADH alone) or the groups treated with CSE alone or with NADH in the 5-day or 11-day regimen as described in the Section 2. * $p < 0.05$, ** $p < 0.01$ and *** $p < 0.001$ compared with the control group; # $p < 0.05$, ## $p < 0.01$, ### $p < 0.001$ and #### $p < 0.0001$ compared with the CSE group (n = 4/per group).

NADH also exerted a similar protective effect on glutathione peroxidase (GPX), whereby the 62.98% (p = 0.0026) decrease in lung GPX activity induced by CSE could be completely prevented by NADH on a 5-day regimen at a 100 mg (p = 0.0015) or 200 mg dose (p = 0.0014) or 11-day regimen at 100 mg (p = 0.0124). In contrast, dexamethasone treatment failed to prevent the decrease in lung GPX activity induced by CSE (p = 0.9995) (Figure 4b).

We also assessed the impact of NADH on the levels of glutathione (GSH), one of the essential antioxidant defense pathways. The 8-fold drop in GSH levels induced by CSE (p = 0.0186) could be completely prevented by NADH on a 5-day regimen at 100 mg (p = 0.0013) and 200 mg (p = 0.0003) doses or on an 11-day regimen at 100 mg (p = 0.004). In addition, dexamethasone treatment also prevented the decrease in lung GSH activity induced by CSE ($p < 0.05$) (Figure 4c). Interestingly, NADH treatment alone appeared to augment the lung level of GSH when compared to the levels seen in the control group ($p < 0.05$) (Figure 4c).

Finally, we looked at the changes in lung catalase activity following CSE exposure and the effect of NADH. Catalase has been described as a vital antioxidant mechanism in the lungs via its ability to convert hydrogen peroxide to oxygen and water [30]. As depicted in Figure 4d, CSE reduced lung catalase activity by 95.84% ($p < 0.0001$). All NADH-treated groups, irrespective of the treatment regimen (5-day or 11-day regimen) or doses (100 or 200 mg), showed a substantial 50–60% restoration in lung catalase activity ($p < 0.05$). In contrast, dexamethasone treatment failed to prevent the decrease in lung catalase activity induced by CSE (p = 0.7113)

3.4. Effect of NADH on CSE-Induced Changes in Inflammatory Cytokines

As demonstrated in Figure 5a, we found that CSE induced a significant increase in the TNF-alpha level in the lung homogenates (3.9-fold) when compared with the control group ($p < 0.0001$). Treatment with 100 mg of NADH significantly reduced CSE-induced increases in TNF-alpha in all treated groups. The reduction was more pronounced among the groups that were treated every 5 days with 100 mg and 200 mg of NADH, respectively (47% vs. 40% inhibition; $n = 4$/per group). Additionally, NADH showed a better anti-inflammatory effect when compared to the positive control drug dexamethasone, which inhibited CSE-induced TNF-alpha only by 30% ($p = 0.0004$).

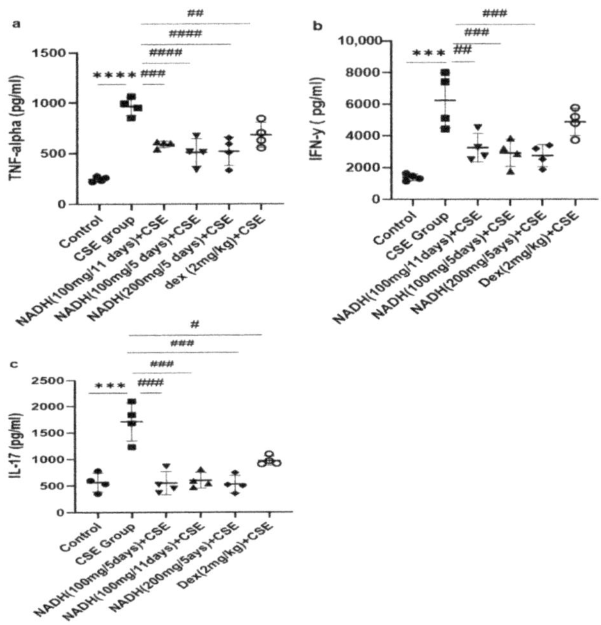

Figure 5. The effects of NADH on levels of TNF-alpha, IFN-γ, and IL-17 in the lungs of mice exposed to CSE. The levels of cytokines, including TNF-alpha (**a**), IFN-γ (**b**), and IL-17 (**c**), were assessed in lung homogenates from the control group or the groups treated with CSE alone or with NADH in the 5-day or 11-day regimen as described in the Section 2. *** $p < 0.001$ and **** $p < 0.0001$ compared with the control group; # $p < 0.05$ ## $p < 0.01$, ### $p < 0.001$, and #### $p < 0.0001$ compared with the CSE group ($n = 4$/per group).

We also investigated the impact of NADH on CSE-induced IFN-γ production. The model led to a 4.5-fold increase in the IFN-γ level when compared to the control group ($p < 0.001$), as shown in Figure 5. All NADH-treated groups exhibited a marked decrease of 40–50% in the levels of IFN-γ ($p < 0.001$), while no effect was seen in the dexamethasone-treated group ($p = 0.2874$) (Figure 5b).

As depicted in Figure 5, CSE led to a three-fold increase in the IL-17 levels in the lungs when compared with the control groups ($p < 0.0001$). All groups treated with NADH, regardless of the treatment regimen (5-day or 11-day regimen) or dosage (100 or 200 mg), revealed a significant ~70% diminution of IL-17 ($p < 0.001$, $n = 4$). Conversely, dexamethasone only reduced by 40% the increased levels of lungIL-17 induced by CSE ($p = 0.0194$, $n = 4$) (Figure 5c).

3.5. Effect of NADH on CSE-Induced Inflammatory Changes in Lungs

CSE exposure was also associated with typical emphysematous changes in the lungs, characterized by an enlarged alveolar space with a very thin alveolar septum (Figure 6D) when compared with the control group (Figure 6B). In addition, CSE caused a well-defined arteriolar congestion with a moderate inflammatory infiltrate (Figure 6C). This inflammatory cluster was observed in the perivascular region with the well-defined alveolar changes mimicking emphysematous lesions (Figure 6C,D).

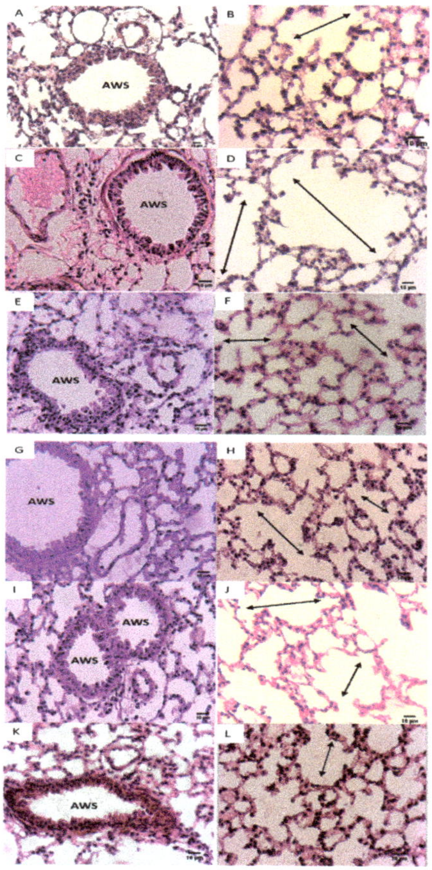

Figure 6. NADH ameliorated CSE-induced air space enlargement. Representative lung tissue sections (airways and parenchyma) stained with hematoxylin–eosin (H&E), taken at 400× magnification. (**A**,**B**) Control group; (**C**,**D**) CSE group. (**E**,**F**) NADH (100 mg/11 days) + CSE group. (**G**,**H**) NADH (100 mg/5 days) + CSE group. (**I**,**J**) NADH (200 mg/5 days) + CSE group. (**K**,**L**) Dexamethasone (2 mg/kg) + CSE group. Images are representative of $n = 4$ animals per condition. AWS = airways; double headed arrow = alveolar space enlargement.

It is worth mentioning that these lung inflammatory changes coupled to emphysematous injuries were not observed in the NADH-treated groups (Figure 6C,E–J), further supporting the anti-inflammatory effect of NADH supplementation in this animal model of COPD.

The 1.9-fold increase in MLI induced by CSE was equally reduced in the groups that were treated with 100 mg of NADH in the 5-day and 11-day regimens ($p = 0.0014$) and the group treated with 200 mg of NADH in the 5-day regimen ($p = 0.0007$, Figure 7).

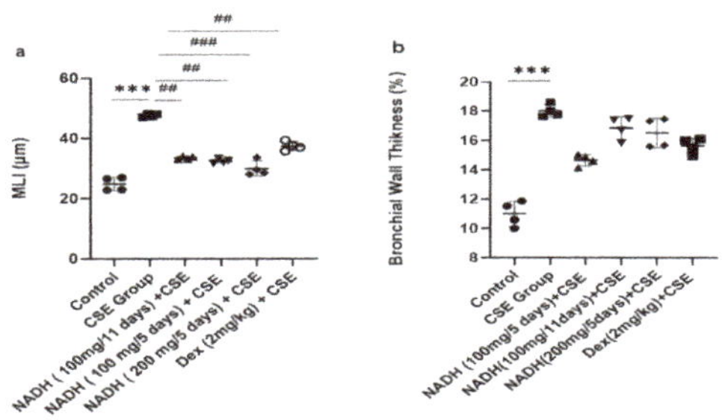

Figure 7. Lung morphometric analysis following CSE exposure in different treatment groups. Mean linear intercept (MLI) (**a**) and bronchial wall thickening (**b**) were calculated using Image J-v1.54j software. *** $p < 0.001$ versus control group, ## $p < 0.01$ and ### $p < 0.001$ vs. CSE group ($n = 4$/condition).

Dexamethasone treatment induced a moderate protection from CSE-induced emphysema when compared with the control group with a 21% reduction in the MLI ($p = 0.0098$, Figure 7a). In addition, CSE also induced a marked increase in airway wall thickening (63% increase, $p < 0.012$, Figure 7b), which was not affected by NADH or dexamethasone treatment.

NADH was also found to protect against CSE-induced lung fibrosis in the 5-day treatment regimen at both doses of 100 mg and 200 mg ($p < 0.0001$), leading to respective 58% and 82.5% decreases in lung fibrosis. In contrast, the 11-day regimen at a 100 mg dose did not provide any protection ($p = 0.6888$, Figure 8B), while dexamethasone protected against CSE-induced fibrosis by 43% compared with the CSE group, with $p = 0.0006$ (Figure 8B).

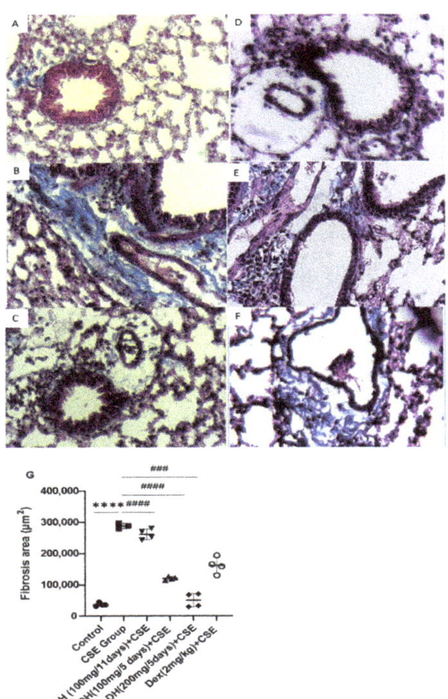

Figure 8. NADH protected against CSE-induced airway fibrosis. Representative lung tissue sections stained with Masson's trichrome, taken at 400× magnification. Top panel: (**A**) control group, (**B**) CSE

group, (C) NADH (200 mg/5 days) + CSE, (D) NADH (100 mg/5-day regimen) + CSE, (E) NADH (100 mg/11-day regimen) + CSE, (F) dexamethasone (2 mg/kg) + CSE, (G) assessment of collagen content. Bottom panel: comparison of extent of airway fibrosis (μm^2) in lungs of different experimental groups compared to control group. **** $p < 0.05$ versus control group, ### $p < 0.01$ and #### $p < 0.0001$ versus CSE group, $n = 4$/per group.

4. Discussion

There is no cure for patients with COPD, and the current available therapies (i.e., bronchodilators and steroids) do not treat the root of the problem nor do they reduce disease progression [31]. There is therefore an unmet need for novel therapies. We provide the first evidence that NADH therapy is effective in preventing the development of key pathological features associated with COPD, including airway emphysema, markers of oxidative stress, inflammation, and pulmonary fibrosis.

With cigarette smoke being the greatest risk factor for the development of COPD and emphysema, several models to mimic the disease have been developed by exposing animals to cigarette smoke (CS) either via the nose or via whole-body exposure [32,33]. Initial studies with such models have relied on various exposure protocols based on smoking apparatus involving different administration regimens, numbers of cigarettes, exposure routes (nose-only or whole-body exposure), and treatment duration (from weeks to several months) [34,35]. For example, notable differences were seen between nose-only and whole-body exposure in terms of the degree of lung inflammation and airway remodeling when side-by-side comparisons were made [36]. This suggests that the choice of animal models of COPD should really depend on the research question being asked. Additional models relying on intraperitoneal injection (IP) of cigarette smoke extracts (CSEs) have been also developed, with animals not only exhibiting lung manifestations of COPD such as inflammation, emphysema, and mucus hypersecretion, but also the systemic features of the disease such as heart and skeletal muscle dysfunction [37]. The IP injection model can also be established without the requirement of a longer treatment time (usually 3–6 weeks) [38,39]. Recent studies comparing CS exposure with IP injection models demonstrated comparable preclinical outcomes when looking at key COPD features, including the extent of lung damages (emphysema) and lung inflammatory changes [19,40–42]. Nonetheless, mice exposed to CSE represent one of the most commonly used models of COPD [34,35,39]. Here, our CSE-injection-based model of COPD given over the course of two months was able to generate clinical features of COPD, including emphysematous abnormalities, airway inflammation, and bronchial remodeling with marked lung fibrosis, as previously reported [43,44]. We relied on a combination of different parameters, such as WBC counting, oxidative stress evaluation, as well as lung morphological examination to confirm the validity of this inducible model of COPD. The choice of the treatment regimen (CSE injected every 11th day) was mostly based on previous reports showing the success of this exposure protocol to create COPD pathological features in the lung, including emphysema (94% of lung destruction) and lung inflammation [19,38,45].

Our overall finding was to investigate the potential clinical value of NADH supplementation as a preventive option in our murine model of COPD (Figure 9). This study was mostly fueled by the emerging evidence showing that an imbalanced NAD+/NADH ratio led to cellular homeostasis destabilization, which could be a driving factor for a number of chronic diseases such as diabetes [12], neurodegenerative diseases [13], and idiopathic lung fibrosis [14]. To our knowledge, no study has yet investigated the effect of NADH supplementation in any lung disease models. Here, we found that NADH supplementation at two different doses (100 and 200 mg given 30 min prior to CSE) almost completely prevented the key characteristics of COPD, including airway fibrosis (>82.5% reduction, Figure 8) as well as the structural features of emphysematous damages (>37% reduction, Figure 7) and inflammation ($p < 0.001$) that were seen in the lungs of CSE-exposed animals. Our study is in line with growing pre-clinical reports searching for novel compounds capable of reversing these CSE-induced COPD lung features. Some compounds have recently been uncovered to successfully prevent CSE-induced lung damage, including astaxanthin (AXT), a keto-carotenoid derived from the oxidation of β-carotene [46]; YPL-001, a drug candidate mixture isolated from *P. rotundum* var. Subintegrum [47]; aurintricarboxylic acid (ATA), a polyanionic aromatic compound [48]; and Retinoid X receptor agonists (RXRs) [49], all via multiple mechanisms. We believe that the protective action of NADH in our CSE model is derived from its ability to prevent mitochondrial dysfunction, which is often associated with high ROS production and oxidative stress. Indeed, we found that NADH at 100 mg and 200 mg doses in the 5-day regimen was highly effective in preventing the development of oxidative stress in the lungs by CSE, as evidenced by the marked drop in the levels of MDA and nitrites. In addition, NADH also completely prevented the loss of protective antioxidant mechanisms induced by CSE with the restoration of basal activities of SOD, GPX, GSH, and catalase.

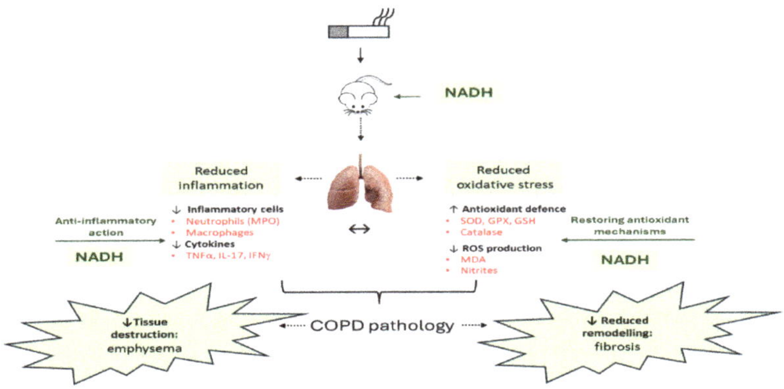

Figure 9. An overview of the therapeutic effect of NADH in the murine COPD model induced by systemic CSE exposure. The NADH-treated groups presented with a significant reduction in COPD key features, such as emphysema and airway remodeling (fibrosis). The therapeutic benefit of NADH is believed to result from blunted inflammatory pathways, as evidenced by the marked reductions in systemic granulocytes and lung neutrophils (reflected by decreased MPO levels). A significant decrease in the key COPD inflammatory cytokines (TNF-a, IFN-g, and IL-17) in the lungs may, in part, explain NADH's beneficial action. These cytokines and other growth factors (TGF-b and CTGF) are known to play central roles in the chemoattraction and activation of macrophages/monocytes and neutrophils, thereby contributing to the amplification/perpetuation of inflammation/oxidative stress/remodeling processes in lung tissues. NADH supplementation was also found to markedly reduce CSE-induced oxidative damage, as shown by the diminution of typical biomarkers (MDA and nitrites) and the prevention of CSE-associated depletion of multiple antioxidant defense mechanisms (GPX, SOD, GSH, and catalase). ↔: Indicates the impact of NADH on both airway inflammation and oxidative stress may explain its beneficial action in COPD. GPX: glutathione peroxidase, GSH: glutathione, MDA: malondialdehyde, MPO: myeloperoxidase, SOD: superoxide dismutase. The image of the lung is from Pixabay.

Our current data show that NADH exerts strong antioxidant activities. The restoration of these defense barriers by NADH is believed to explain its beneficial effects in our CSE model of COPD. This hypothesis is supported by the marked reduction in key biomarkers of oxidative stress in the lungs of NADH-treated CSE-exposed animals, such as MDA, the end-product of lipid peroxidation. The mechanisms by which NADH supplementation prevented the loss of antioxidant pathways have not clearly been defined but could be related to the mono-ADP-ribosyltransferases, sirtuins, and PPAR-γ co-activator1α (SIRT/PGC-1α) pathways. Indeed, SIRT1 has been shown to exert several beneficial effects, including promoting mitochondrial biogenesis, preventing cell apoptosis, and restoring metabolic balance [50]. Interestingly, dexamethasone, used as our anti-inflammatory control drug, failed to reverse the loss of catalase and GPX, showing the superior clinical potential of NADH in our model (Figure 4).

We believe that NADH supplementation may impact inflammation and associated lung injury by preventing CSE-induced mitochondrial dysfunction reported as an important source of ROS and proinflammatory factors in COPD, such as TNFα/IL-1β, which led to the recruitment of neutrophils [51]. Several lines of evidence from our report support this assumption. First, NADH blunted the expression of oxidative stress markers and markedly reduced the increased levels of TNF-α, IFN-γ, and IL-17 in the lungs of CSE-exposed mice. TNF-α and IFN-γ, which are predominantly produced by activated macrophages and lymphocytes, can trigger the release of CXCL10, a chemokine attracting monocytes, neutrophils, and T-cells, notably Th1 cells, thereby contributing to pulmonary emphysema [48]. In addition, all of these cytokines are involved in COPD pathogenesis via their contributions to both lung structural abnormalities and the recruitment/activation of inflammatory cells [49]. For example, a recent systemic review and meta-analysis study conducted with $n = 2268$ patients confirmed a critical role of IL-17 in driving neutrophilic inflammation and exacerbation in COPD [52]. It is not surprising to see that reducing lung levels of IL-17 by NADH was associated with a parallel decrease in lung MPO activity, an heme-containing peroxidase mainly expressed neutrophils [53]. Although we did not measure the neutrophil count in the lungs, we saw a complete drop in the total number of granulocytes recruited by CSE in the blood via NADH treatment. This again suggests that NADH therapy is a strong modulator of neutrophilic inflammation in lungs exposed to cigarette smoke. Other investigations encompassing both animal and clinical studies have emphasized the role of IL-17, primarily originating from CD4+ Th17 cells, in regulating the recruitment of macrophages and neutrophils, as well as modulating chemokine activity. Moreover, IL-17 has been closely associated with the development and progression of COPD [3,52].

Our study supports the conclusion from previous reports suggesting the implication of mitochondrial dysregulation in the pathogenesis of COPD/emphysema [54] and a pivotal role of cigarette smoke in inducing oxidative damage in the lungs as a result of perturbating mitochondrial function [8]. Manipulating NADH levels by pharmacological agents has the potential to restore mitochondrial respiration and showed promising results in the treatment of diabetes and multiple disorders [15], chronic fatigue syndrome [16], and neurodegenerative diseases [17,18]. NAD treatment reduced the activation of circulating immune cells through the blockage of NLRP/3 inflammasome formation and inflammatory cytokine production. Furthermore, NAD supplementation leads to the activation of sirtuins 1 and 2, which inhibit the transcription factor NF-κB [55,56] resulting in a decrease in the gene expression of pro-inflammatory cytokines [57]. As the reduced form of NAD, NADH can act as the major source of its intracellular regeneration [58,59]. The relationship between lung fibrosis and oxidative stress in COPD has not been clearly established. The profibrotic responses occurring in the lungs of CSE-treated animals may result from the abnormal production/activation of growth factors, such as TGFβ/CTGF, which are reported to be increased in the lungs of patients with COPD [60]. Indeed, in addition to promoting oxidative stress and the proliferation of lung fibroblasts/myofibroblasts [61], TGFβ has been reported to interfere with the activity of Nrf2, a central transcription factor in the induction of endogenous antioxidant proteins, further enhancing oxidative stress [62]. Our model of experimental COPD showed that lung fibrosis was closely associated with reduced levels of many Nrf2-inducible antioxidant proteins (i.e., SOD, catalase, and GSH) in the lungs of CSE-treated animals, and whether this was due to the action of growth factors remains an interesting hypothesis to be examined in future studies. However, lung fibrosis in COPD is believed to be a complex mechanism resulting from the chronic inflammatory environment as well as self-perpetuating oxidative microenvironment due to an oxidative stress imbalance [63].

The concept that either NAD+ or NADH cannot cross the plasma membrane has to be revisited based on some evidence demonstrating that extracellular NADH can be transported across the plasma membrane via a P2X7R-dependent mechanism in astrocytes to generate NAD+. The authors used the P2X7 receptor blocking strategy (antagonism and knockdown) to demonstrate that the receptor was essential in the NADH-induced accumulation of NAD+ inside the cells [64]. Interestingly, P2X7R is known to be expressed in several cells involved in lung diseases; it is not surprising to see that P2X7R antagonists have been suggested for the treatment of various respiratory conditions associated with lung inflammation and fibrosis [65]. In fact, the P2X7 receptor was shown to be essential in cigarette smoke-induced lung inflammation and emphysema in mice [66]. Because the P2X7 receptor was increased by cigarette smoke exposure in key inflammatory cells such as airway neutrophils, alveolar macrophages, and in whole lung tissues, it is tempting to speculate that this would be associated with an increased uptake of NADH levels in the lungs, thus potentially explaining its local therapeutic effects. Additional studies are needed to confirm this interesting hypothesis. Similarly, extracellular NAD+ was also reported to induce different cellular effects, such as nucleotide metabolism and genomic DNA replication, when exposed to cultured cell models [67]. Similar to NADH, NAD+ has been shown to be transported across the plasma membrane via different transporter proteins, with one being connexin 43 hemichannels [68,69]. These studies strongly suggest that both extracellular NAD+ and NADH have the capacity to cross the plasma membrane via mechanisms that remain to be further explored.

Our present study opens a completely new area of investigation, namely the study of the supplementation of NADH and NAD+ precursors, including nicotinamide (NAM), nicotinamide riboside (NR), and nicotinamide mononucleotide (NMN), as potential therapies in the treatment and/or prevention of COPD features. It would also be important to investigate the cellular and molecular mechanisms underlying the protective effect of NADH by looking at the factors mediating its antioxidant and anti-fibrotic actions. To further support the hypothesis that COPD is indeed associated with the dysregulation of NAD+ pathways, it would be important to determine whether the levels of NAD+ are reduced in patients with COPD and/or whether reduced levels correlate with disease severity or the rate of exacerbations. It would also be essential to determine the impact of NADH supplementation when given therapeutically, i.e., once the disease is already established, rather than preventively, as given in the present study. Lastly, testing a strategy that combines NADH/NAD precursors and current therapies (LABA, long-acting β2-agonists, or steroids, for example) in preclinical models of COPD may reveal a superior therapeutic effect that can be exploited in clinics. This is a clinically relevant area worth pursuing as different cohort studies have reported perturbed NAD pathways in aging and age-related conditions coupled to the strong preclinical evidence showing the effectiveness of NAD+ precursor supplementation in numerous animal models of human conditions. In addition, there are various ongoing clinical trials testing the supplementation of NAD+ precursors in various healthy and disease states [57]. Our studies support the use of the NAD+/NADH replenishing strategy in the management of patients with COPD.

5. Conclusions

Our study provides the first evidence of a protective role of NADH in preventing the development of key pathological features associated with COPD, including airway emphysema, markers of oxidative stress, inflammation, and pulmonary fibrosis.

Author Contributions: Conceptualization, M.O. and K.B. (Karine Benachour); Methodology, N.S., A.A., K.B. (Karima Bahria), S.G., M.K., A.H., M.O., Y.A. and K.B. (Karine Benachour); Validation, Y.A. and K.B. (Karine Benachour); Formal Analysis, K.B. (Karine Benachour); Resources, G.B.; Writing—Original Draft, N.S.; Writing—Review and Editing, Y.A. and K.B. (Karine Benachour); Supervision, Y.A. and K.B. (Karine Benachour). All authors have read and agreed to the published version of the manuscript.

Funding: This study received no specific grant from any private funding agency. All funding has been provided by the Directorate-General for Scientific Research and Technological Development (DGRSDT, Algiers, Algeria). The authors declare that they have no financial interests, and none of the authors received any financial or project funding support.

Institutional Review Board Statement: This study was performed according to the guidelines established by the Institutional Animal Care and Use Committee (IACUC) at the University of Medea. All animal procedures were approved by the Ethics Committee of Animal Experimentation at the Yahia Fares University of Medea (no. IACUC-CEEA-02).

Informed Consent Statement: Not applicable.

Data Availability Statement: The data presented in this study will be made available upon request from the corresponding author.

Acknowledgments: The authors would like to thank Douaoui Sanaa and Nadir Benahfri for their advice and technical support.

Conflicts of Interest: All authors (except for Birkmayer) declare no competing interests. The NADH used in the present study was a gift from the late Birkmayer, the founder of the Birkmayer NADH Company, who tragically died on 28 August 2022. The Birkmayer NADH Company was not involved in the study conception and design, data collection, analysis and interpretation of results, or manuscript preparation. None of the authors received any financial or project funding support from the Birkmayer NADH Company.

References

1. Dorababu, A.; Maraswami, M. Recent Advances (2015–2020) in Drug Discovery for Attenuation of Pulmonary Fibrosis and COPD. *Molecules* **2023**, *28*, 3674. [CrossRef] [PubMed]
2. Gomes, F.; Cheng, S.-L. Pathophysiology, Therapeutic Targets, and Future Therapeutic Alternatives in COPD: Focus on the Importance of the Cholinergic System. *Biomolecules* **2023**, *13*, 476. [CrossRef] [PubMed]
3. Barnes, P.J. Inflammatory Mechanisms in Patients with Chronic Obstructive Pulmonary Disease. *J. Allergy Clin. Immunol.* **2016**, *138*, 16–27. [CrossRef] [PubMed]
4. Sidhaye, V.K.; Koval, M. *Lung Epithelial Biology in the Pathogenesis of Pulmonary Disease*; Academic Press: Cambridge, MA, USA, 2017.
5. Strzelak, A.; Ratajczak, A.; Adamiec, A.; Feleszko, W. Tobacco Smoke Induces and Alters Immune Responses in the Lung Triggering Inflammation, Allergy, Asthma and Other Lung Diseases: A Mechanistic Review. *Int. J. Environ. Res. Public Health* **2018**, *15*, 1033. [CrossRef] [PubMed]
6. Nam, H.-S.; Izumchenko, E.; Dasgupta, S.; Hoque, M.O. Mitochondria in Chronic Obstructive Pulmonary Disease and Lung Cancer: Where Are We Now? *Biomark. Med.* **2017**, *11*, 475–489. [CrossRef] [PubMed]
7. Caldeira, D.D.A.F.; Weiss, D.J.; Rocco, P.R.M.; Silva, P.L.; Cruz, F.F. Mitochondria in Focus: From Function to Therapeutic Strategies in Chronic Lung Diseases. *Front. Immunol.* **2021**, *12*, 782074. [CrossRef] [PubMed]
8. Sagar, S.; Kapoor, H.; Chaudhary, N.; Roy, S.S. Cellular and Mitochondrial Calcium Communication in Obstructive Lung Disorders. *Mitochondrion* **2021**, *58*, 184–199. [CrossRef]
9. Ying, W. NAD^+/NADH and $NADP^+$/NADPH in Cellular Functions and Cell Death: Regulation and Biological Consequences. *Antioxid. Redox Signal.* **2008**, *10*, 179–206. [CrossRef] [PubMed]
10. Hu, Q.; Wu, D.; Walker, M.; Wang, P.; Tian, R.; Wang, W. Genetically Encoded Biosensors for Evaluating NAD^+/NADH Ratio in Cytosolic and Mitochondrial Compartments. *Cell Rep. Methods* **2021**, *1*, 100116. [CrossRef] [PubMed]
11. O'Rourke, B.; Ashok, D.; Liu, T. Mitochondrial Ca^{2+} in Heart Failure: Not Enough or Too Much? *J. Mol. Cell. Cardiol.* **2021**, *151*, 126–134. [CrossRef] [PubMed]
12. Abdellatif, A.; Bahria, K.; Slama, N.; Oukrif, D.; Shalaby, A.; Birkmayer, G.; Oumouna, M.; Benachour, K. NADH Intraperitoneal Injection Prevents Massive Pancreatic Beta Cell Destruction in a Streptozotocin-Induced Diabetes in Rats. *Histochem. Cell Biol.* **2024**, *161*, 239–253. [CrossRef] [PubMed]
13. Salech, F.; Ponce, D.P.; Paula-Lima, A.C.; SanMartin, C.D.; Behrens, M.I. Nicotinamide, a Poly [ADP-Ribose] Polymerase 1 (PARP-1) Inhibitor, as an Adjunctive Therapy for the Treatment of Alzheimer's Disease. *Front. Aging Neurosci.* **2020**, *12*, 255. [CrossRef] [PubMed]
14. Zhang, Y.; Huang, W.; Zheng, Z.; Wang, W.; Yuan, Y.; Hong, Q.; Lin, J.; Li, X.; Meng, Y. Cigarette Smoke-Inactivated SIRT1 Promotes Autophagy-Dependent Senescence of Alveolar Epithelial Type 2 Cells to Induce Pulmonary Fibrosis. *Free Radic. Biol. Med.* **2021**, *166*, 116–127. [CrossRef] [PubMed]
15. Guo, C.; Huang, Q.; Wang, Y.; Yao, Y.; Li, J.; Chen, J.; Wu, M.; Zhang, Z.; E, M.; Qi, H.; et al. Therapeutic Application of Natural Products: NAD^+ Metabolism as Potential Target. *Phytomedicine* **2023**, *114*, 154768. [CrossRef] [PubMed]
16. Alegre, J.; Rosés, J.M.; Javierre, C.; Ruiz-Baqués, A.; Segundo, M.J.; de Sevilla, T.F. Nicotinamide adenine dinucleotide (NADH) in patients with chronic fatigue syndrome. *Rev. Clínica Española* **2010**, *210*, 284–288. [CrossRef] [PubMed]

117. Nicotinamide Adenine Dinucleotide (NADH)—A New Therapeutic Approach to Parkinson's Disease. Comparison of Oral and Parenteral Application. Available online: https://pubmed.ncbi.nlm.nih.gov/8101414/ (accessed on 9 March 2024).
118. Birkmayer, J. Coenzyme Nicotinamide Adenine Dinucleotide: New Therapeutic Approach for Improving Dementia of the Alzheimer Type. *Ann. Clin. Lab. Sci.* **1996**, *26*, 1–9.
119. He, Z.H.; Chen, P.; Chen, Y.; He, S.D.; Ye, J.R.; Zhang, H.L.; Cao, J. Comparison between Cigarette Smoke-Induced Emphysema and Cigarette Smoke Extract-Induced Emphysema. *Tob. Induc. Dis.* **2015**, *13*, 6. [CrossRef]
120. Bradford, M.M. A Rapid and Sensitive Method for the Quantitation of Microgram Quantities of Protein Utilizing the Principle of Protein-Dye Binding. *Anal. Biochem.* **1976**, *72*, 248–254. [CrossRef] [PubMed]
121. Ohkawa, H.; Ohishi, N.; Yagi, K. Assay for Lipid Peroxides in Animal Tissues by Thiobarbituric Acid Reaction. *Anal. Biochem.* **1979**, *95*, 351–358. [CrossRef]
122. Arias-Dìaz, J.; Vara, E.; Torres-Melero, J.; García, C.; Baki, W.; Ramσrez-Armengol, J.A.; Balibrea, J.L. Nitrite/nitrate and cytokine levels in bronchoalvelar lavage fluid of lung cancer patients. *Cancer* **2014**, *74*, 1546–1551. [CrossRef]
123. Ruyssers, N.E.; De Winter, B.Y.; De Man, J.G.; Loukas, A.; Pearson, M.S.; Weinstock, J.V.; Van den Bossche, R.M.; Martinet, W.; Pelckmans, P.A.; Moreels, T.G. Therapeutic Potential of Helminth Soluble Proteins in TNBS-Induced Colitis in Mice. *Inflamm. Bowel Dis.* **2009**, *15*, 491–500. [CrossRef]
124. Marklund, S.; Marklund, G. Involvement of the Superoxide Anion Radical in the Autoxidation of Pyrogallol and a Convenient Assay for Superoxide Dismutase. *Eur. J. Biochem.* **1974**, *47*, 469–474. [CrossRef]
125. Flohé, L.; Günzler, W.A. Assays of Glutathione Peroxidase. *Methods Enzymol.* **1984**, *105*, 114–120. [CrossRef]
126. Friedberg, T.; Milbert, U.; Bentley, P.; Guenther, T.M.; Oesch, F. Purification and Characterization of a New Cytosolic Glutathione S-Transferase (Glutathione S-Transferase X) from Rat Liver. *Biochem. J.* **1983**, *215*, 617–625. [CrossRef]
127. Aebi, H. Catalase In Vitro. *Methods Enzymol.* **1984**, *105*, 121–126. [CrossRef]
128. Salaets, T.; Tack, B.; Gie, A.; Pavie, B.; Sindhwani, N.; Jimenez, J.; Regin, Y.; Allegaert, K.; Deprest, J.; Toelen, J. A Semi-Automated Method for Unbiased Alveolar Morphometry: Validation in a Bronchopulmonary Dysplasia Model. *PLoS ONE* **2020**, *15*, e0239562. [CrossRef]
129. Lin, W.; Jianbo, S.; Wanzhong, L.; Yanna, L.; Weiwei, S.; Gang, W.; Chunzhen, Z. Protective Effect of Eucalyptus Oil on Pulmonary Destruction and Inflammation in Chronic Obstructive Pulmonary Disease (COPD) in Rats. *J. Med. Plants Res.* **2017**, *11*, 129–136. [CrossRef]
130. Heck, D.E.; Shakarjian, M.; Kim, H.D.; Laskin, J.D.; Vetrano, A.M. Mechanisms of Oxidant Generation by Catalase. *Ann. N. Y. Acad. Sci.* **2010**, *1203*, 120–125. [CrossRef]
131. Adcock, I.M.; Marwick, J.; Casolari, P.; Contoli, M.; Fan Chung, K.; Kirkham, P.; Papi, A.; Caramori, G. Mechanisms of corticosteroid resistance in severe asthma and chronic obstructive pulmonary disease (COPD). *Curr. Pharm. Des.* **2010**, *16*, 3554–3573. [CrossRef]
132. Shu, J.; Li, D.; Ouyang, H.; Huang, J.; Long, Z.; Liang, Z.; Chen, Y.; Chen, Y.; Zheng, Q.; Kuang, M.; et al. Comparison and Evaluation of Two Different Methods to Establish the Cigarette Smoke Exposure Mouse Model of COPD. *Sci. Rep.* **2017**, *7*, 15454. [CrossRef]
133. Vlahos, R.; Bozinovski, S. Recent Advances in Pre-Clinical Mouse Models of COPD. *Clin. Sci.* **2014**, *126*, 253–265. [CrossRef]
134. Yang, Y.; Di, T.; Zhang, Z.; Liu, J.; Fu, C.; Wu, Y.; Bian, T. Dynamic Evolution of Emphysema and Airway Remodeling in Two Mouse Models of COPD. *BMC Pulm. Med.* **2021**, *21*, 134. [CrossRef]
135. Ghorani, V.; Boskabady, M.H.; Khazdair, M.R.; Kianmeher, M. Experimental Animal Models for COPD: A Methodological Review. *Tob. Induc. Dis.* **2017**, *15*, 25. [CrossRef]
136. Serré, J.; Tanjeko, A.T.; Mathyssen, C.; Vanherwegen, A.-S.; Heigl, T.; Janssen, R.; Verbeken, E.; Maes, K.; Vanaudenaerde, B.; Janssens, W.; et al. Enhanced Lung Inflammatory Response in Whole-Body Compared to Nose-Only Cigarette Smoke-Exposed Mice. *Respir. Res.* **2021**, *22*, 86. [CrossRef]
137. Zhang, Y.; Cao, J.; Chen, Y.; Chen, P.; Peng, H.; Cai, S.; Luo, H.; Wu, S.-J. Intraperitoneal Injection of Cigarette Smoke Extract Induced Emphysema, and Injury of Cardiac and Skeletal Muscles in BALB/C Mice. *Exp. Lung Res.* **2013**, *39*, 18–31. [CrossRef]
138. Zhang, H.; Chen, P.; Zeng, H.; Zhang, Y.; Peng, H.; Chen, Y.; He, Z. Protective Effect of Demethylation Treatment on Cigarette Smoke Extract-Induced Mouse Emphysema Model. *J. Pharmacol. Sci.* **2013**, *123*, 159–166. [CrossRef]
139. Li, A.; Liu, Y.; Zhu, X.; Sun, X.; Feng, X.; Li, D.; Zhang, J.; Zhu, M.; Zhao, Z. Methylallyl Sulfone Attenuates Inflammation, Oxidative Stress and Lung Injury Induced by Cigarette Smoke Extract in Mice and RAW264.7 Cells. *Int. Immunopharmacol.* **2018**, *59*, 369–374. [CrossRef]
140. Kettawan, A.; Ruangklai, S.; Rungruang, T.; Thongam, J.; Kettawan, A.K.; Nirmal, N.; Srisuma, S. Rice Bran Oil Improves Emphysema in Cigarette Smoke Extract-Induced Mice through Anti-Inflammatory and Antioxidative Effects. *Nutrients* **2024**, *16*, 433. [CrossRef]
141. Campos, K.K.D.; Araújo, G.R.; Martins, T.L.; Bandeira, A.C.B.; de Paula Costa, G.; Talvani, A.; Garcia, C.C.M.; Oliveira, L.A.M.; Costa, D.C.; Bezerra, F.S. The Antioxidant and Anti-Inflammatory Properties of Lycopene in Mice Lungs Exposed to Cigarette Smoke. *J. Nutr. Biochem.* **2017**, *48*, 9–20. [CrossRef]
142. Wang, S.; He, N.; Xing, H.; Sun, Y.; Ding, J.; Liu, L. Function of Hesperidin Alleviating Inflammation and Oxidative Stress Responses in COPD Mice Might Be Related to SIRT1/PGC-1α/NF-κB Signaling Axis. *J. Recept. Signal Transduct.* **2020**, *40*, 388–394. [CrossRef]

43. Sørensen, A.K.; Holmgaard, D.B.; Mygind, L.H.; Johansen, J.; Pedersen, C. Neutrophil-to-lymphocyte ratio, calprotectin and YKL-40 in patients with chronic obstructive pulmonary disease: Correlations and 5-year mortality—A cohort study. *J. Inflamm* **2015**, *12*, 20. [CrossRef]
44. Turato, G.; Zuin, R.; Saetta, M. Pathogenesis and pathology of COPD. *Respiration* **2001**, *68*, 117–128. [CrossRef]
45. Wang, W.; Zha, G.; Zou, J.j.; Wang, X.; Li, C.n.; Wu, X.j. Berberine Attenuates Cigarette Smoke Extract-Induced Airway Inflammation in Mice: Involvement of TGF-B1/Smads Signaling Pathway. *Curr. Med. Sci.* **2019**, *39*, 748–753. [CrossRef]
46. Deng, M.; Tong, R.; Bian, Y.; Hou, G. Astaxanthin Attenuates Cigarette Smoking-Induced Oxidative Stress and Inflammation in a Sirtuin 1-Dependent Manner. *Biomed. Pharmacother.* **2023**, *159*, 114230. [CrossRef]
47. Lee, K.H.; Woo, J.; Kim, J.; Lee, C.H.; Yoo, C.G. YPL-001 Shows Various Beneficial Effects against Cigarette Smoke Extract-Induced Emphysema Formation: Anti-Inflammatory, Anti-Oxidative, and Anti-Apoptotic Effects. *Antioxidants* **2023**, *12*, 15. [CrossRef]
48. Rovina, N.; Koutsoukou, A.; Koulouris, N.G. Inflammation and immune response in COPD: Where do we stand? *Mediat. Inflamm* **2013**, *2013*, 413735. [CrossRef]
49. Guo, P.; Li, R.; Piao, T.H.; Wang, C.L.; Wu, X.L.; Cai, H.Y. Pathological mechanism and targeted drugs of COPD. *Int. J. Chronic Obstr. Pulm. Dis.* **2022**, *17*, 1565–1575. [CrossRef]
50. Sharma, A.; Chabloz, S.; Lapides, R.A.; Roider, E.; Ewald, C.Y. Potential Synergistic Supplementation of NAD^+ Promoting Compounds as a Strategy for Increasing Healthspan. *Nutrients* **2023**, *15*, 445. [CrossRef]
51. Marchi, S.; Guilbaud, E.; Tait, S.W.; Yamazaki, T.; Galluzzi, L. Mitochondrial control of inflammation. *Nat. Rev. Immunol.* **2023** *23*, 159–173. [CrossRef]
52. Ma, R.; Su, H.; Jiao, K.; Liu, J. Association Between IL-17 and Chronic Obstructive Pulmonary Disease: A Systematic Review and Meta-Analysis. *Int. J. Chronic Obstr. Pulm. Dis.* **2023**, *18*, 1681–1690. [CrossRef]
53. Aratani, Y. Myeloperoxidase: Its Role for Host Defense, Inflammation, and Neutrophil Function. *Arch. Biochem. Biophys.* **2018** *640*, 47–52. [CrossRef]
54. Zhou, W.C.; Qu, J.; Xie, S.Y.; Sun, Y.; Yao, H.W. Mitochondrial dysfunction in chronic respiratory diseases: Implications for the pathogenesis and potential therapeutics. *Oxid. Med. Cell. Longev.* **2021**, *2021*, 10245–10288. [CrossRef]
55. Mahalanobish, S.; Dutta, S.; Saha, S.; Sil, P.C. Melatonin Induced Suppression of ER Stress and Mitochondrial Dysfunction Inhibited NLRP3 Inflammasome Activation in COPD Mice. *Food Chem. Toxicol.* **2020**, *144*, 111588. [CrossRef]
56. Lee, H.J.; Hong, Y.S.; Jun, W.; Yang, S.J. Nicotinamide riboside ameliorates hepatic metaflammation by modulating NLRP3 inflammasome in a rodent model of type 2 diabetes. *J. Med. Food* **2015**, *18*, 1207–1213. [CrossRef]
57. Fang, E.F.; Lautrup, S.; Hou, Y.; Demarest, T.G.; Croteau, D.L.; Mattson, M.P.; Bohr, V.A. NAD^+ in Aging: Molecular Mechanisms and Translational Implications. *Trends Mol. Med.* **2017**, *23*, 899–916. [CrossRef]
58. Eto, K.; Suga, S.; Wakui, M.; Tsubamoto, Y.; Terauchi, Y.; Taka, J.; Kadowaki, T. NADH Shuttle System Regulates KATPChannel dependent Pathway and Steps Distal to Cytosolic Ca^{2+} Concentration Elevation in Glucose-induced Insulin Secretion. *J. Biol Chem.* **1999**, *274*, 25386–25392. [CrossRef]
59. Eto, K.; Tsubamoto, Y.; Terauchi, Y.; Sugiyama, T.; Kishimoto, T.; Takahashi, N.; Yamauchi, N.; Kubota, N.; Murayama, S. Aizawa, T.; et al. Role of NADH shuttle system in glucose-induced activation of mitochondrial metabolism and insulin secretion *Science* **1999**, *283*, 981–985. [CrossRef]
60. Ning, W.; Li, C.J.; Kaminski, N.; Feghali-Bostwick, C.A.; Alber, S.M.; Di, Y.P.; Choi, A.M. Comprehensive gene expression profiles reveal pathways related to the pathogenesis of chronic obstructive pulmonary disease. *Proc. Natl. Acad. Sci. USA* **2004** *101*, 14895–14900. [CrossRef]
61. Kang, H.-R.; Lee, J.-Y.; Lee, C.G. TGF-B1 as a Therapeutic Target for Pulmonary Fibrosis and COPD. *Expert Rev. Clin. Pharmacol* **2008**, *1*, 547–558. [CrossRef]
62. Michaeloudes, C.; Sukkar, M.B.; Khorasani, N.M.; Bhavsar, P.K.; Chung, K.F. TGF-β regulates Nox4, MnSOD and catalase expression, and IL-6 release in airway smooth muscle cells. *Am. J. Physiol.-Lung Cell. Mol. Physiol.* **2011**, *300*, L295–L304 [CrossRef]
63. Repine, J.E.; Bast, A.A.L.T.; Lankhorst, I.D.A.; Oxidative Stress Study Group. Oxidative stress in chronic obstructive pulmonary disease. *Am. J. Respir. Crit. Care Med.* **1997**, *156*, 341–357. [CrossRef]
64. Lu, H.; Burns, D.; Garnier, P.; Wei, G.; Zhu, K.; Ying, W. P2X7 Receptors Mediate NADH Transport across the Plasma Membranes of Astrocytes. *Biochem. Biophys. Res. Commun.* **2007**, *362*, 946–950. [CrossRef]
65. Burnstock, G.; Knight, G.E. The Potential of P2X7 Receptors as a Therapeutic Target, Including Inflammation and Tumour Progression. *Purinergic Signal.* **2018**, *14*, 1–18. [CrossRef]
66. Lucattelli, M.; Cicko, S.; Müller, T.; Lommatzsch, M.; De Cunto, G.; Cardini, S.; Sundas, W.; Grimm, M.; Zeiser, R.; Dürk, T.; et al P2X7 Receptor Signaling in the Pathogenesis of Smoke-Induced Lung Inflammation and Emphysema. *Am. J. Respir. Cell Mol. Biol* **2011**, *44*, 423–429. [CrossRef]
67. Munk, S.H.N.; Merchut-Maya, J.M.; Adelantado Rubio, A.; Hall, A.; Pappas, G.; Milletti, G.; Lee, M.; Johnsen, L.G.; Guldberg, P. Bartek, J.; et al. NAD^+ Regulates Nucleotide Metabolism and Genomic DNA Replication. *Nat. Cell Biol.* **2023**, *25*, 1774–1786 [CrossRef]

68. Bruzzone, S.; Guida, L.; Zocchi, E.; Franco, L.; De Flora, A. Connexin 43 Hemi Channels Mediate Ca^{2+}-Regulated Transmembrane NAD^+ Fluxes in Intact Cells. *FASEB J.* **2001**, *15*, 10–12. [CrossRef]
69. Billington, R.A.; Travelli, C.; Ercolano, E.; Galli, U.; Roman, C.B.; Grolla, A.A.; Canonico, P.L.; Condorelli, F.; Genazzani, A.A. Characterization of NAD Uptake in Mammalian Cells. *J. Biol. Chem.* **2008**, *283*, 6367–6374. [CrossRef]

diseases

MDPI

Review

Target Role of Monocytes as Key Cells of Innate Immunity in Rheumatoid Arthritis

Diana I. Salnikova [1,*], Nikita G. Nikiforov [2,3,4], Anton Y. Postnov [3] and Alexander N. Orekhov [2,3,5]

[1] Laboratory of Oncoproteomics, Department of Experimental Tumor Biology, Institute of Carcinogenesis, Blokhin N.N. National Medical Research Center of Oncology, 24 Kashirskoe Highway, 115522 Moscow, Russia

[2] Laboratory of Angiopathology, The Institute of General Pathology and Pathophysiology, 8 Baltiyskaya Street, 125315 Moscow, Russia; nikiforov.mipt@googlemail.com (N.G.N.); ano.inat@mail.ru (A.N.O.)

[3] Laboratory of Cellular and Molecular Pathology of Cardiovascular System, Federal State Budgetary Scientific Institution "Petrovsky National Research Centre of Surgery", 3 Tsyurupa Street, 117418 Moscow, Russia; anton-5@mail.ru

[4] Center for Precision Genome Editing and Genetic Technologies for Biomedicine, Institute of Gene Biology, Russian Academy of Sciences, 34/5 Vavilova Street, 119334 Moscow, Russia

[5] Institute for Atherosclerosis Research, Osennyaya Street 4-1-207, 121609 Moscow, Russia

* Correspondence: dianasalnikova08@yandex.ru

Abstract: Rheumatoid arthritis (RA) is a chronic, systemic, and inflammatory autoimmune condition characterized by synovitis, pannus formation (with adjacent bone erosion), and joint destruction. In the perpetuation of RA, fibroblast-like synoviocytes (FLSs), macrophages, B cells, and CD4$^+$ T-cells—specifically Th1 and Th17 cells—play crucial roles. Additionally, dendritic cells, neutrophils, mast cells, and monocytes contribute to the disease progression. Monocytes, circulating cells primarily derived from the bone marrow, participate in RA pathogenesis. Notably, CCR2 interacts with CCL2, and CX3CR1 (expressed by monocytes) cooperates with CX3CL1 (produced by FLSs), facilitating the migration involved in RA. Canonical "classical" monocytes predominantly acquire the phenotype of an "intermediate" subset, which differentially expresses proinflammatory cytokines (IL-1β, IL-6, and TNF) and surface markers (CD14, CD16, HLA-DR, TLRs, and β1- and β2-integrins). However, classical monocytes have greater potential to differentiate into osteoclasts, which contribute to bone resorption in the inflammatory milieu; in RA, Th17 cells stimulate FLSs to produce RANKL, triggering osteoclastogenesis. This review aims to explore the monocyte heterogeneity, plasticity, antigenic expression, and their differentiation into macrophages and osteoclasts. Additionally, we investigate the monocyte migration into the synovium and the role of their cytokines in RA.

Keywords: monocyte subsets; macrophages; innate immunity; rheumatoid arthritis; chemokines; proinflammatory cytokines

1. Introduction

RA is a chronic, systemic, and autoimmune disease. The mechanisms of this condition are still being investigated. The illness is characterized by an inflammatory process in the synovial joints, which is called synovitis [1]. Moreover, RA is accompanied by the hyperplasia of the synovial tissue. The disease is complicated by the destruction of the cartilage structure and the formation of pannus [2]. Throughout the course of the pathology, bone erosion occurs and predominantly surrounds the peripheral synovial joints. The clinical symptoms of RA include pain, edema development, and tenderness of the synovial joints located symmetrically and peripherally [3]. A great deal of progress has been made in the treatment of RA with antagonists of proinflammatory cytokines, such as tumor necrosis factor (TNF), interleukin-6 (IL-6), and IL-1β. However, the disease remains refractory in some patients. Studies have demonstrated that prostaglandins, leukotrienes, reactive oxygen species, nitric oxide, lipoxins, and platelet-activating factors as small-molecule inflammatory mediators play an important role in RA development. Such compounds assist in inducing, maintaining, or reducing inflammation and could therefore be potential therapeutic targets [1].

Innate and adaptive autoimmune cells promote the continuation of RA pathogenesis. Among them are B cells and $CD4^+$ T cells, which include the T helper 1 (Th1), Th2, and Th17 cells. Moreover, monocytes/macrophages and resident macrophages participate in the disease development [4]. In addition, synovial cells and FLSs contribute to RA. Furthermore, dendritic cells (DCs), neutrophils, mast cells, and immunoregulatory cells, for example, regulatory T (Treg) cells, are involved in the complex interaction that leads to the preservation of chronic inflammation [5]. The above-mentioned cells stimulate the formation of the modulators of local inflammation, such as cytokines, chemokine ligands, and the appropriate receptors. These modulators take part in synovial inflammation and destruction [6].

Monocytes are a type of blood cell containing a horseshoe-shaped nucleus in their cytoplasm. They relate to the mononuclear phagocyte system and are much smaller than macrophages, which are in turn much smaller than multinucleated osteoclasts. Monocytes originate from bone marrow precursors [7]. Together with lymphocytes, monocytes were previously known as agranulocytes. Moreover, monocytes are defense cells of the second line after neutrophils in an innate immune system and are able to phagocytose foreign particles. They have the capability of differentiating into their own subsets and macrophages based on the necessity of the microenvironment. Additionally, monocytes produce cytokines and act as antigen-presenting cells (APCs) [8].

Monocytes differ from other autoimmune cells due to several reasons. First of all, they are capable of triggering, maintaining, and increasing the activity of inflammation in the synovial joints in RA. Moreover, chemokine receptors CCR2 (CD192) of $CD14^+$ monocytes and CX3CR1 (fractalkine receptor, GPR13) of $CD16^+$ monocytes interact with the corresponding ligands CCL2 (MCP-1) and CX3CL1 (fractalkine) released from FLSs, and this process contributes to the migration of monocytes from circulation and their recruitment into the RA synovium [9]. These chemoalkine receptors represent the differentiation markers of monocytes. A disintegrin and metalloproteinase domain-containing protein 10 and products of FLSs such as granulocyte–macrophage colony-stimulating factor (GM-CSF), TNF, and IL-1β promote monocyte migration. Next, monocytes are characterized by the increased expression of chemokine receptors and antigens on their cell surface [6]. Among them are CD14, CD16, toll-like receptors (TLRs), human leukocyte antigen DR (HLA-DR), and β1- and β2-integrins that are adhesion molecules. Moreover, they produce proinflammatory cytokines such as TNF, IL-1β, and IL-6. The differentiation of monocytes leads to the development of classical, intermediate, and non-classical monocyte subsets [10]. The intermediate monocytes are prevalent in RA, and they undergo differentiation into proinflammatory M1 macrophages. Proinflammatory macrophages are induced by TNF, GM-CSF, interferon (IFN)-γ, and lipopolysaccharide (LPS). M1 macrophages produce proinflammatory cytokines TNF, IL-1β, IL-6, and IL-12 and stimulate inflammation in the synovial joints [11]. Furthermore, classical monocytes expressing $CD14^{++}$ and $CD16^-$ have relatively greater potential to differentiate into osteoclasts and induce the erosion of the surrounding bones in the synovial joints in RA [12]. Osteoclastogenesis is the process by which osteoclasts are differentiated. Th17 cells trigger the formation of the receptor activator of the NF-κB (RANK) ligand (RANKL) by FLSs, which contributes to the differentiation of monocytes into osteoclasts [13]. Osteoclastogenesis is increased by cytokines such as TNF, IL-1β, and IL-6 [12,14].

The overview reveals the formation, classification, and specific markers of monocytes, their functioning as APCs and progenitors of macrophages and osteoclasts, the expression of chemokine receptors, and the production of cytokines in RA.

2. Monocytes in RA

2.1. Development of Monocytes

Monocytopoiesis, the process of monocyte production, originates from human stem cells, predominantly found in the bone marrow. Monocytes are part of the mononuclear phagocyte system and act as key innate immune cells in the organism. The process of monocytopoiesis occurs at a stage of embryonic development via definitive hematopoiesis. The ventral wall of the aorta is a site for the aorta gonad mesonephros emergence following three weeks of pregnancy in women and at the E-7 stage in mice. The aorta gonad mesonephros is the first location in the embryo where monocytes appear [15]. Hematopoietic stem cells differentiate into monoblasts under the influence of various cytokines, including GM-CSF and macrophage colony-stimulating factor (M-CSF). Hematopoietic stem cells undergo various stages of multipotent progenitor transformation into monocyte/macrophage and DC progenitors. These progenitors lose the ability to generate granulocytes and either give rise to "common monocyte progenitors" restricted to monocytes and their progeny or are directed to a common DC progenitor [15]. The subsequent stages involve further maturation and differentiation, giving rise to promonocytes and finally monocytes. These differentiated monocytes are released into the bloodstream, where they execute crucial functions such as phagocytosis, antigen presentation, and cytokine secretion, playing a pivotal role in immune surveillance and tissue homeostasis. Moreover, monocyte production happens in the liver, thymus, and spleen of the fetus. Since the late period of embryonic development, the formation of monocytes relocates to the bone marrow, which remains the main site for the monocyte production in adults and older people [16].

2.2. Human Monocyte Subsets and Their Role in RA

The expression of CD14 and CD16 markers on the cell surface of monocytes was used to identify and categorize the subsets of monocytes. According to the classification developed by Ziegler-Heitbrock et al., three types of monocyte subsets are presented in humans [7].

2.2.1. Classical Monocytes

Primarily, there are classical monocytes, which have high expression of the CD14 marker and, more importantly, do not express the CD16 marker. Furthermore, they produce the cytokines TNF, IL-1β, IL-6, and IL-10 in high concentrations. Several forms of inflammatory stimulus are capable of eliciting the cytokine expression from monocytes. For instance, this process occurs as a consequence of the LPS stimulation and activation of the immune complex [17]. This type of monocyte undergoes differentiation into intermediate monocytes, inflammatory macrophages, and osteoclasts in the regions of inflammation. Classical monocytes function as phagocytic scavenger cells and promote synovial inflammation and the osteoclastic erosion of bones. $CD16^-$, but not $CD16^+$, monocyte subsets represent circulating osteoclast progenitors that differentiate into osteoclasts [12]. Consequently, classical monocytes are able to be the circulating predecessors of osteoclasts in erosive RA.

2.2.2. Intermediate Monocytes

The second group refers to intermediate monocytes, which are characterized by the high expression of the CD14 marker and diminished expression of the CD16 marker. The number of these monocytes is highly upregulated in the peripheral blood and synovia in RA. They secrete TNF, IL-1β, and IL-6 in high quantities in the synovial joints in RA [18]. The differentiation of intermediate monocytes results in inflammatory monocyte subsets and proinflammatory M1 macrophages. They maintain the inflammation of the synovial joints and enhance the disease development. Additionally, intermediate monocytes lead to the direct activation of Th17 cells in the inflamed synovial joints and their expansion. The amount of these monocytes increases in the blood circulation over the course of the RA pathogenesis [19]. The enhanced level of classical and intermediate monocytes in an untreated RA patient is a prognostic factor for the decline or absence of susceptibility to methotrexate therapy [20].

2.2.3. Non-Classical Monocytes

In addition, there are non-classical monocytes that have diminished expression of the CD14 marker and high expression of the CD16 marker. Non-classical monocytes preferentially associated with the endothelial wall engage in "patrolling behavior" urgently in cases of tissue injury [21]. This process provides an early inflammatory response. Non-classical monocytes stimulate the adhesion of monocytes in the microvessels of joints. Resident anti-inflammatory M2 macrophages represent another product of monocyte differentiation and help to resolve inflammation. Among the monocyte subsets, the non-classical ones proliferate the least [10] and undergo senescence to a greater degree [22]. They are capable of acquiring a senescence-associated secreted phenotype (SASP) that transforms into a proinflammatory type and causes inflammation. Purchasing a phenotype occurs due to age-related chronic inflammation called inflammaging [23].

2.2.4. Disease-Modifying Antirheumatic Drugs

The prevalence of circulating monocytes subsets, particularly the CD16 expressing subsets, is associated with RA progression and assists in estimating treatment effectiveness, for example, in the case of disease-modifying antirheumatic drugs (DMARDs). Commonly prescribed DMARDs include methotrexate, sulfasalazine, and hydroxychloroquine. Methotrexate inhibits dihydrofolate reductase, an enzyme that converts dihydrofolic acid into tetrahydrofolic acid. This enzyme, in turn, is a donor of one-carbon groups in the synthesis of purine nucleotides and thymidylate required for DNA synthesis. As a result, methotrexate inhibits DNA synthesis and repair, cell mitosis, and, to a lesser extent, affects RNA and protein synthesis [24]. Sulfasalazine dissociates into 5-aminosalicylic acid in the connective tissue of the intestinal wall, and 5-aminosalicylic acid promotes the anti-inflammatory properties of sulfasalazine and sulfapyridine [25]. Sulfapyridine is a competitive antagonist of para-aminobenzoic acid. This drug stops the synthesis of folate in the cells of microorganisms and causes antibacterial activity. Hydroxychloroquine seals lysosomal membranes and prevents the exit of lysosomal enzymes. Moreover, this drug disrupts DNA replication, RNA synthesis, and hemoglobin utilization by erythrocytic forms of plasmodium. Hydroxychloroquine weakens the activity of proteolytic enzymes, which are protease and collagenase. Additionally, this drug decreases the activity of leukocytes and the chemotaxis of lymphocytes. DMARDs help to prevent joint deformity and functional impairment [26].

2.3. Murine Monocyte Subsets in RA

Murine monocytes are subdivided into Ly6C^{++} CD43^{+}, LY6C^{++} CD43^{++}, and Ly6C^{-} types. The first one is an analogue of human classical monocytes. Another type resembles the intermediate monocytes. Both of these monocyte types trigger synovial inflammation under sterile conditions. The third type is an equivalent of non-classical monocytes and manages the progression and termination of sterile synovial inflammation [27]. In the beginning, Ly6C^{-} monocytes develop into proinflammatory M1 macrophages, which induce and maintain the inflammation in the synovial joints. Further, M1 macrophages are exposed to polarization and acquire an alternative phenotype, M2, that suppresses synovial inflammation [28].

2.4. Monocyte Markers

Monocytes are characterized by numerous antigen expression types on their cell surface, with some alterations in dependence on the monocyte subset. These antigens manage RA development [8].

2.4.1. Markers of Double-Positive Monocytes/Macrophages

Double-positive monocytes/macrophages were revealed in human and rat peripheral blood. These cells express both CD4 and CD8. In addition, they possess activated phenotypes expressing M1 and M2 markers, producing proinflammatory cytokines and contributing to chronic inflammation. Double-positive monocytes/macrophages may be transferred to the inflammation area and be involved in the immune response of Th1 type [29]. These cells promote synovial hyperplasia and facilitate joint damage in RA (Figure 1).

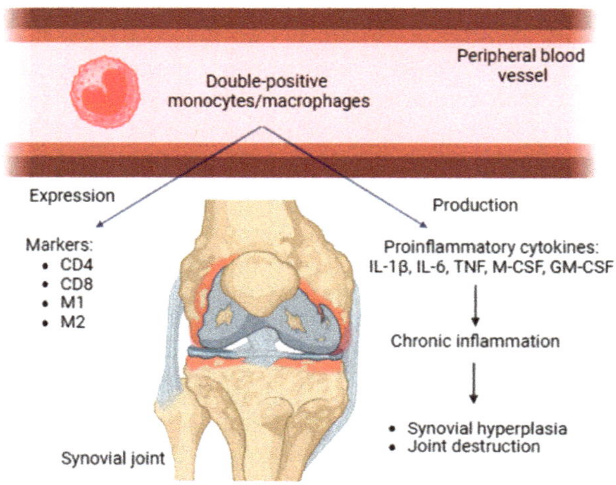

Figure 1. Double-positive monocytes/macrophages, expressed markers, proinflammatory (IL-1β, IL-6, TNF, M-CSF, and GM-CSF) cytokines, role in RA. CD, cluster of differentiation; IL, interleukin; TNF, tumor necrosis factor; GM-CSF, granulocyte–macrophage colony-stimulating factor.

2.4.2. Clusters of Differentiation

CD14 represents the LPS receptor, which is able to be linked to an LPS-binding protein. A CD14 interaction with an LPS–LPS binding protein complex initiates signaling pathways with the involvement of TLR-4. Further, TLR-4 triggers the formation and secretion of the proinflammatory chemokine IFN-γ inducible protein 10 and the cytokines TNF, IL-1β, and IL-6 [30]. CD16 designates the immunoglobulin (Ig) Fc-gamma receptor III (FcγRIII), which has a specific phagocytic activity. CD16$^+$ monocytes, mostly the intermediate ones, are more abundant than non-classical monocytes in RA [19]. IgG-containing immune complexes, for instance, containing anti-citrullinated protein antibody (ACPA), provoke a higher level of TNF in the case of FcγRIII/CD16$^+$ hyperexpression on CD14^{++} monocytes in RA. Magnetic microbeads for negative and positive selection with the use of anti-CD14 and anti-CD16 monoclonal antibodies allow separating the CD14 and CD16 markers [31]. CD56 is an adhesion molecule in neural cells. CD56$^+$ monocytes mainly belong to classical monocyte subsets and spread in RA. Under the influence of LPS stimulation, CD14^{bright} CD56$^+$ monocytes secrete greater amounts of TNF, IL-10, and IL-23. Anti-TNF therapy, for example, with the use of etanercept, diminishes the level of these cytokines [17]. Monocytes as well as myeloid series cells express the myeloid identification marker CD115 [32].

In addition to ACPAs, antibodies targeting various post-translational modifications such as carbamylation [33], acetylation, and malondialdehyde are found in RA. Approximately half of the ACPA clones in RA patients react with carbamylated antigens. Some antigens even show reactivity to acetylated peptides. The cross-reactivity may be due to similar electron density distributions at key recognized residues. Anti-malondialdehyde antibodies, although not cross-reactive with citrullinated antigens, can activate osteoclasts similar to ACPAs [34]. As a result, targeting antigens from different protein modifications trigger various pathways. Co-existing mechanisms and overlapping protein residues complicate the understanding of the key protein modifications for specific autoantibody effects. Various protein modifications can co-exist in the same tissues, cells, proteins, and even at the same peptide epitope. This co-existence explains the presence of autoantibodies targeting various post-translational modifications in RA and their similar functional effects. Colasanti T. et al. (2020) described the detection of antibodies targeting homocysteinylated alpha 1 antitrypsin in RA patients seropositive for the "classical" ACPA and RF. Alpha 1 antitrypsin is a protease inhibitor protein of the serpin superfamily and protects tissues from the effects of many enzymes secreted by inflammatory cells. Variation in the alpha 1 antitrypsin gene is associated with increased ACPA production, which leads to RA progression and joint destruction [35].

2.4.3. HLA-DR and Co-Stimulatory Molecules

The HLA-DR marker refers to the group of MHC II (CD68) molecules. HLA-DR activates $CD4^+$ cells via interaction with T cell receptors [36]. Intermediate monocytes produce a higher level of HLA-DR in comparison with other monocyte subsets in RA [37]. Furthermore, intermediate monocytes secrete a significant amount of TNF through Pam3Cys activation and binding to TLR2/TLR1. Classical monocytes increase the expression of HLA-DR over a period of low RA activity. Monocytes of the synovial joints are characterized by higher expression of HLA-DR than monocytes of the peripheral blood. Additionally, DCs demonstrate HLA-DR expression to a high degree and participate in antigen presentation to $CD4^+$ T cells. HLA-DR interacts with an antigen and passes the first signal to the T cell receptor on a $CD4^+$ T cell. Co-stimulatory molecules CD80 (B7-1) and CD86 (B7-2) are expressed on the monocyte surface and work as a second signal. To sum up, both signals stimulate $CD4^+$ T-cells and enable adaptive autoimmune responses that happen with the involvement of Th1 and Th17 cells in RA. The expression of HLA-DR and CD80 is enhanced on the intermediate monocyte surface in the RA synovial joints, and this process contributes to the activation of IL-17^+ and IFN-γ^+ $CD4^+$ T-cells under conditions of cocultivation [38]. Moreover, activated Th1 cells promote the expression of HLA-DR and CD80 on the surface of the monocytes in RA.

2.4.4. Toll-like Receptors

TLRs are expressed on the surface of innate immune cells, for instance, monocytes, macrophages, DCs, and neutrophils. TLRs identify inflammatory tissues, microbial products, and cellular debris that remains after cell necrosis. Lipoteichoic acid and peptidoglycan recognition activate TLR2. LPS identification provokes TLR4 functioning [39]. Moreover, signal transduction through TLR2 and TLR4 is stimulated by molecules of heat shock protein 60, hyaluronic acid, and fibronectin products that are synthesized endogenously. The TLR level intensifies in resident and infiltrating cells in the RA synovium. Furthermore, TNF secretion is enhanced by increasing the TLR2 expression in $CD16^+$ macrophages of blood and synovial origin in RA. The production of TLR2 grows with the assistance of classical and intermediate monocytes in the RA peripheral blood and synovial joints. All three monocyte subsets demonstrate a high TLR9 level on their surface independently of blood or synovial localization. TLR2 and TLR9 promote the early secretion of proinflammatory cytokines TNF and IL-1β [40]. Thereby, they induce inflammation that is maintained by their other products, such as the cytokine IL-6 and the chemokine macrophage inflammatory protein-1. Various levels of these proinflammatory factors are correlated with the involvement of TLR agonists. High expression of TLR3 and TLR4 is observed on fibroblasts in the RA synovial joints. In particular, continuous inflammation and joint damage cause this secretion [39].

Monocytes express the genes of type 1 interferons, especially in response to TLR signaling. Roelofs M.F. et al. (2009) described the co-expression of synovial TLR3/7 expression with IFN-α, IL-1β, and IL-18, but not with TNF, IL-12, or IL-17 [41]. The stimulation of TLR3/TLR7 on monocytes, monocyte-derived DCs, or synovial fibroblasts contributed to the secretion of type I IFN. However, no biologically active IL-1β or IL-18 could be revealed. Type I IFN-α increased the TLR3/7 mRNA expression, whereas IL-1β and IL-18 did not. In spite of the fact that the mRNA level of TLR4 remained unchanged, IFN-α enhanced the response to TLR4 agonists, a phenomenon that was clearly more marked in patients with RA. To conclude, type I IFNs are highly co-expressed with TLR3/TLR7 in RA synovium. They enhance TLR3/TLR7-mediated cytokine production and TLR4-mediated responses [41].

2.4.5. β1- and β2-Integrins

The migration of circulating monocytes proceeds after their adhesion into the vascular endothelium. β1- and β2-integrins are expressed in high concentrations on monocytes in RA and participate in the adhesion of monocytes to activated endothelial cells. The β1 subfamily of integrins includes very late antigen-4 (α4β1) and -5 (α5β1) that bind to fibronectin and vascular cell adhesion molecule-1 in the endothelium and provoke monocyte adhesion [42]. β2-integrins take part in the formation of $CD11_{a,b,c}$ (CD18) complexes in RA, which are mostly presented by $CD11_b$ molecules and associated with the ligands in the endothelial lining. Moreover, intercellular adhesion molecule-1 (CD54), -2 (CD102), and -3 (CD50) cause monocyte adhesion to endothelial cells. Inflammatory monocytes/macrophages migrate into the synovial joints in RA and result in local inflammation [43].

2.4.6. A Proliferation-Inducing Ligand

Two separate forms of a proliferation-inducing ligand (APRIL) are enhanced in the process of RA progression. The first form is a soluble one, which refers to the TNF superfamily and is secreted by myeloid cells, for instance, DCs, monocytes, macrophages, activated T cells, and B cells. Soluble APRIL operates as a proinflammatory cytokine and binds to receptors of two types. The first one is a transmembrane activator, calcium modulator and cyclophilin ligand interactor receptor (TACI), which is produced in B cells [44]. The second one is a B cell maturation antigen receptor (BCMA) that is secreted in plasma cells. The second form of APRIL is a receptor on the cell surface that is highly produced by the above-mentioned myeloid cells, including all the circulating monocyte subsets in RA. In the process of binding to TACI and BCMA, a surface form of APRIL functions as a ligand or receptor and provokes the formation and viability of B cells and plasma cells in RA. As a result, a B cell-mediated autoimmune response is provided [45].

2.4.7. Sialic Acid Binding Ig-like Lectin

Siglec-1 is a representative of the sialic acid binding Ig-like lectin family. These proteins undergo upregulation by the circulating monocytes and macrophages in RA, and their concentration rises with the development of RA and increasing level of C-reactive protein, erythrocyte sedimentation rate, and IgM-rheumatoid factor. Singlec-1 operates as an autoantigen, takes part in a cell-to-cell contact of autoimmunity, and induces inflammation in RA [46].

2.4.8. Transmembrane TNF

Transmembrane TNF is overexpressed on the monocyte surface in RA. Etanercept is a TNF inhibitor that binds to transmembrane TNF. Consequently, the anti-inflammatory cytokine IL-10 and soluble decoy receptors are produced. Thus, reverse signaling through transmembrane TNF occurs in monocytes and represents a prognostic factor for the pharmacological effect of anti-TNF agents in RA [47]. CD147 is an extracellular matrix metalloproteinase inducer, which promotes the production of matrix metalloproteinases (MMPs) by monocytes, for instance, MMP2, MMP3, and MMP9. MMPs provoke the dissolution of extracellular matrix, which leads to the destruction of synovium in RA. CD147 is hyperexpressed in $CD14^+$ monocytes in the RA peripheral blood and synovial joints. Infliximab is a TNF inhibitor that is supposed to block the CD147 secretion on the surface of CD14$^+$ monocytes in RA [48].

2.4.9. Other Monocyte Markers

α-Enolase is an anti-citrullinated autoantigen for anti-citrullinated protein autoantibodies and is also expressed on the surface of monocytes/macrophages in RA. The main function of α-enolase is to initiate the secretion of proinflammatory cytokines, for example, TNF, IFN-γ, prostaglandin E2, and IL-1α/β [49]. Proteinase-activated receptor-2 is a member of the G protein receptor family and is produced by monocytes and T lymphocytes. The expression of proteinase-activated receptor-2 is directly proportional to the RA activity. In addition, the C-reactive protein and erythrocyte sedimentation rate concentrations increase over the course of the disease. Proteinase-activated receptor-2 initiates the production of the proinflammatory cytokine IL-6 [50]. Allograft inflammatory factor-1 is produced in the cytoplasm of monocytes/macrophages, lymphocytes, and synovial fibroblasts. Its function is to initiate and preserve inflammation in the synovial joints in RA. Hyperexpressed allograft inflammatory factor-1 participates in the proliferation of inflammatory macrophages and activated T lymphocytes in the RA synovium [51]. Moreover, 50–60% of CD14$^+$ CD16^{++} non-classical monocytes have been shown to express the 6-sulfo LacNAc (SLAN) antigen, which is an O-linked glycosylated variant of P-selectin glycoprotein ligand-1 recognized by specific monoclonal antibodies, including macrophage-derived chemokine 8 and anti-D-dimers 1 and 2 [52,53]. In clinical studies, Hofer Th.P. et al. (2015) showed a fivefold depletion of SLAN-positive monocytes in patients with chronic inflammation [54]. SLAN is one of the monocyte markers stimulating the differentiation of non-classical monocytes into anti-inflammatory M2 macrophages, which, in turn, provide phagocytosis and resolution of inflammation.

Monocytes of the peripheral blood are progenitors of macrophages, and both of them mediate inflammation. Cardiovascular complications of RA are similar to synovitis and subclinical atherosclerosis, which have an inflammatory mechanism in the endothelium. Altered levels of the following receptor expression in circulating monocytes cause RA, accompanied by atherosclerotic complications, for instance, localized in a coronary artery. Specifically, low secretion of the scavenger receptor (CD36) is observed [55]. Moreover, a comorbidity is characterized by the high production of the calcium-sensing receptor and low-density lipoprotein-related receptor protein-1. The functional IL-25 receptor is secreted on the monocyte surface in RA and interacts with the cytokine IL-25, which is produced mostly by T cells. As a result, proinflammatory cytokine formation through the p38 mitogen-activated protein kinase (MAPK)-dependent Soc-3 pathway occurs. Additionally, this process signifies that IL-25 performs a negative control of monocyte-associated autoimmune disorders [56].

2.5. Cytokines

The cytokines participating in the RA pathways are subdivided into two types: proinflammatory and anti-inflammatory cytokines. The first type is responsible for the occurrence and development of synovial inflammation [57]. Conversely, the functioning of anti-inflammatory cytokines leads to a reduction in the inflammatory process. The cytokine environment of the RA synovium is formed by the cells of two groups. The first one includes resident synovial cells. The second group is represented by innate and adaptive autoimmunity cells. A higher secretion of cytokines is provided in the RA synovium to a greater extent by monocytes/macrophages and synovial fibroblasts than by T cells. The cytokines are involved in all the stages of RA development. Moreover, they unite the processes of immune regulation and inflammation that mediate the clinical symptoms and pathogenesis of RA [58].

2.5.1. Proinflammatory Cytokines

IL-2 and IFN-γ are the main proinflammatory cytokines of Th1 cells. IL-2 stimulates the maturation and viability of T cells. IFN-γ initiates the functioning of HLA-DR. Moreover, IFN-γ localized in the synovial joints in RA triggers the development of inflammatory M1 macrophages [59]. IL-17 is a pleiotropic cytokine secreted by Th17 cells. This cytokine maintains the synovial inflammation. In addition, IL-17 participates in the activation of monocytes and promotes their migration. Furthermore, the Th17 cytokine stimulates the formation of cytokines by monocytes. There is a synergistic effect between IL-17 and TNF participating in the distribution of RA processes. Moreover, TNF increases osteoclastogenesis, as well as between IL-17 and IL-1β. These advantageous interactions lead to the activation of fibroblasts in the synovial joints, resulting in the production of proinflammatory cytokines and MMPs. Additionally, the Th17 cytokine provokes the erosion in the RA synovial joints. IL-17, in addition to TGF-β, IL-1β, and IL-23, increases osteoclastogenesis in RA [60].

TNF is mostly secreted by activated synovial FLSs and inflammatory macrophages in RA. Moreover, this cytokine is secreted by intermediate monocytes, T cells, and B cells. TNF participates in the distribution of RA processes. Moreover, TNF increases osteoclastogenesis in synovial inflammation. Infliximab is an effective anti-TNF agent that demonstrates the central role of TNF in RA development [61]. The B cell activator factor is a representative of the TNF family. Along with a soluble form of APRIL secreted by peripheral blood mononuclear cells, the B cell activator factor is able to be linked to B cells, resulting in B cell proliferation. Next, plasma cells are developed from autoreactive B cells and lead to the formation of RF and ACPA. Consequently, a B cell-mediated response occurs in RA, particularly in the early stages. Atacicept is an antagonist of APRIL and the B cell activator factor and is undergoing clinical trials at the moment [62].

In addition, FLSs release other proinflammatory cytokines in the RA synovial joints, for example, GM-CSF, IL-1β, IL-6, and IL-18. M1 macrophages ordinarily produce high concentrations of TNF, IL-1β, IL-6, and IL-12. With the secretion of TNF, Il-1β, and IL-6, monocytes stimulate an inflammatory process in the RA synovium. Adhesion molecules β1- and β2-integrins are expressed on the monocyte surface under the effect of proinflammatory cytokines. Intermediate monocytes are prevalent among the monocyte subsets that form the proinflammatory cytokines Il-1β, IL-6, and TNF in RA. Moreover, classical monocytes secrete the above-mentioned cytokines in accordance with the TLR agonists functioning [63]. The cytokine IL-18 is released by mononuclear cells in RA and is able to synergize with Il-1β, IL-12, and IL-15. Next, these molecules trigger the IFN-γ formation by activated synovial T cells and mediate the realization of the Th1 response. Moreover, IL-18 is capable of acting as a straight proinflammatory cytokine in RA and causing the secretion of TNF and IL-1β under the control of macrophages [64].

NF-kB signaling plays an important role in RA pathogenesis. This statement is confirmed by the NF-kB participation in the production of macrophage inflammatory protein-1a and the chemokine IL-8 [65]. Additionally, IL-15 stimulates neutrophils and delays the apoptosis of FLSs and endothelial cells over the period of synovial inflammation. Synovial fibroblasts are the main cells producing IL-23 in RA. Moreover, monocytes secrete IL-23 and initiate Th17 cell distribution and IL-17 expression in the RA synovial tissue. TNF, IL-1β, and IL-32 trigger inflammation in the murine synovium that is supposed to indicate their proinflammatory activity. IL-33 is a cytoplasmic representative of the IL-1 family and is expressed in activated monocytes and fibroblasts in the RA synovium. IL-33 undergoes emission from injured or necrotic cells and participates in the inflammation process. For instance, this protein controls the formation of mast cells. Furthermore, it manages the secretion of Th2 cytokines, such as IL-4, IL-5, and IL-13. Next, IL-33 promotes Th2-regulated pathological conditions [66].

2.5.2. Anti-Inflammatory Cytokines

IL-1Ra is an IL-1 receptor antagonist formed by monocytes in RA. IL-1Ra and IL-10 are anti-inflammatory cytokines; therefore, their antagonistic action presupposes the decline and termination of inflammation. Nevertheless, IL-10 and TGF-β prevail among the products of Breg cells, Treg cells, and suppressor cells of myeloid origin. Il-4 and IL-10 are also secreted by Th2 cells. Moreover, Th2 cells enhance IL-1Ra expression. In addition, M2 macrophages secrete IL-10 and contribute to wound healing, tissue remodeling, and inflammation arrest. IL-10, as an anti-inflammatory cytokine, decreases inflammation. Therefore, a decrease in IL-10 production leads to the development of the inflammatory process and its transformation into a chronic form. IL-10 and M-CSF added to the cultivation medium promote monocyte survival, growth, and differentiation into macrophages [67]. Furthermore, monocytes express the cytokines IL-11, IL-19, IL-20, and IL-24. Additionally, the products of monocyte secretion are GM-CSF, G-CSF, and oncostatin M [68].

2.6. Chemokine Receptors

Chemokines binding to their receptors on the monocyte surface cause the return and migration of monocytes from the blood into the synovial tissue. CCR2 and CX3CR1 are chemokine receptors that are located on monocytes and trigger their chemotaxis. The first receptor is overexpressed on classical $CD14^{++}$ $CD16^{-}$ monocytes and binds to CCL2, which is a monocyte chemoattractant protein [69]. The second receptor undergoes high expression on predominantly intermediate $CD14^{++}$ $CD16^{+}$ monocytes and also non-classical $CD14^{+}$ $CD16^{++}$ monocytes in RA and interacts with CX3CL1. IL-1β cytokines and TNF induce the synovial fibroblasts to produce mainly CCL2, CX3CL1, and CCL20 in RA. CCL20, or macrophage inflammatory protein-3 alpha, is a different monocyte chemoattractant. Moreover, the c-Jun N-terminal kinase, extracellular signal-regulated kinase, and phosphatidylinositol 3′–kinase signaling pathways participate in the chemoattractant secretion by the Th17-associated cytokine IL-17. In addition, IL-17 has an indirect influence on monocyte migration [70].

Chemokine receptors undergo constitutive expression on peripheral blood and synovial monocytes/macrophages, mediate the monocyte chemotaxis, and maintain their level. The migration of peripheral blood monocytes to the synovial tissue during the inflammatory process promotes the increased concentration of chemokine receptors on their surface in RA [6]. Therefore, the regional inflammation and monocyte preservation in the synovium are defined by the overexpression of chemokine receptors on the RA monocytes. The increased expression of CCR1, CCR2, and CCR4 receptors is provided on peripheral blood monocytes, whereas synovial monocytes demonstrate high production of CCR3 and CCR5 in RA. Furthermore, the circulating monocytes secrete CCR9, which interacts with the CCL25 chemokine, or thymus-expressed chemokine. This binding results in monocytes' development into macrophages in RA. The CCR7 chemokine receptor is secreted by not only B lymphocytes, $CD4^{+}$ T lymphocytes, DCs, and FLSs but also circulating monocytes in RA. CCR7 binds to the CCL19 and CCL21 ligands that are characterized by hyperexpression in RA. The regulation of CCR7 and CCL19 is directly proportional to the RA progression. Moreover, the CCL19 concentration in plasma indicates the radiographic development of joint destruction. The DMARD therapy maintains the normal level of both components of the CCR7/CCL19 system [26].

3. Monocyte Functions in RA

The RA etiopathogenesis and its sensitivity to therapy are defined by genetic predisposition, environmental factors, infections, and the decline of autoimmune regulation. Frequent inflammation induces the development of autoimmune conditions. The pathogenesis of RA involves the activation and polarization of monocytes into proinflammatory M1 macrophages within the joint environment [71]. In the arthritic joint, monocytes are recruited by proinflammatory cytokines such as TNF, IL-1, and IL-6, which are produced by resident cells, including FLSs and macrophages. These cytokines promote the activation of monocytes through the binding of their receptors, leading to the upregulation of adhesion molecules and chemoattractant receptors on the monocyte surface. As a result, the monocytes adhere to the endothelium of blood vessels and migrate into the synovial tissue. Activated monocytes express increased levels of cell surface markers, such as CD80 and CD86, which facilitate interactions with T cells and promote antigen presentation [72]. M1-like macrophages are characterized by the production of proinflammatory cytokines and reactive oxygen species, which contribute to tissue damage and perpetuate inflammation in the joint. Furthermore, M1-like macrophages express high levels of surface markers, such as CD14 and CD16, which enhance their phagocytic and antigen-presenting capabilities.

3.1. Monocyte Interactions with Other Cells

Cells of innate and adaptive immunity work in cooperation to cause and maintain an inflammatory process in RA. The main cells taking part in this signaling are DCs, monocytes/macrophages, FLSs, $CD4^+$ T cells (Th1, Th2, and Th17 cells), B cells, mast cells, and neutrophils. When immunoregulatory cells are not capable of attenuating acute inflammation, a chronic form of the disease develops. DCs, macrophages, and FLSs are activated at the beginning of RA pathogenesis [73].

Circulating monocytes are precursors of macrophages. Additionally, monocytes are able to operate as APCs and activate T cells. Moreover, they are classified as monocyte-derived DCs due to their capacity to behave as classical DCs [7]. Monocyte-derived DCs perform hyperexpression of IL-6 and IL-23. Tolerogenic monocyte-derived DCs are another type of DC that are capable of triggering the formation of $Foxp3^+$ Treg cells in RA. Myeloid-derived suppressor cells (MDSCs), Breg cells, and Treg cells control and decrease the inflammatory process [74].

Among $CD4^+$ T cells, the role of the Th1 and Th2 cells in the RA progression was initially revealed. The cytokine IL-12 mediates the participation of monocytes/macrophages in the polarization of $CD4^+$ Th1 cells. Th2 cells and their cytokines mainly decrease Th1 activation. Intermediate monocytes prevail in the RA peripheral blood and synovium and are supposed to be the main monocyte subsets that modulate the Th17 cell functioning. Th17 cells were investigated as effectors in RA because of the ability of their pleiotropic cytokine IL-17 to synergize with TNF. IL-17A triggers the secretion of proinflammatory cytokines IL-1β, IL-6, and TNF in macrophages through the AP-1, NF-kB, and MAPK pathways [60]. IL-1β, IL-6, and IL-23 initiate the activation and control the polarization of Th17 cells. Activated T lymphocytes take part in cell-to-cell contact and trigger the secretion of TNF and IL-1β. Moreover, T lymphocytes release cytokine inhibitor secretory IL-1Ra in monocytes/macrophages [75].

Mast cells are a source of small-molecule inflammatory mediators. Neutrophils undergo chemotaxis into the RA synovial joints, mostly in the early period of inflammation, and release inflammatory mediators and enzymes. Over the period of joint effusion, the level of neutrophils predominates in the synovial fluid in comparison with the synovium [76].

A cytotoxic T-lymphocyte-associated antigen 4 (CTLA4) is a receptor for co-stimulatory molecules and is expressed on the surface of activated T cells [77]. CTLA4 binds with a high avidity to CD80 (B7-1) and CD86 (B7-2) on APCs. They are expressed on the APC surface and interact with T cell co-stimulatory receptor CD28 through signal 2 in order to activate the T cells. Moreover, CTLA4 promotes CD80 and CD86 transport to the CD28 receptor located on T cells for further activation of these co-stimulatory molecules [72]. CTLA4-Ig is a CTLA4 inhibitor and is registered as Abatacept. A blocking effect of Abatacept indicates a cell-to-cell contact mechanism of antigen presentation via T cell-monocyte/macrophage cooperation [77].

Moreover, a surface form of APRIL secreted by monocytes promotes cell communication with B cells and plasma cells that produce BCMA and TACI [44]. In addition, FLSs secrete soluble APRIL and, consequently, release BCMA. Furthermore, FLSs and synovial macrophages express CXCL16 and CCL20 chemokines, which interact with $CCR6^+$ memory T cells. This communication, along with IL-15 cytokines, mainly contributes to CD4$^+$ T cell migration and their involvement in the synovial tissue. Moreover, the enhanced transport of circulating monocytes into the RA synovial joints stimulates the participation of CXCR6$^+$ T cells in the RA progression. Additionally, the CCL20 expression by activated monocytes occurs in the synovium of mice. Stimulated monocytes secrete CCL20, which contacts the CCR6 chemokine receptors, a product of Th17 cells. This interaction increases the CCL20 involvement in the synovial tissue. To sum up, cooperation between monocytes/macrophages, DCs, B cells, Th1, and Th17 cells is related to a positive feedback loop and has an effect on the continuation of inflammation in the synovial joints [60].

FLSs are the resident cells presenting in the intimal lining of the synovium along with resident macrophages, which are synoviocytes of type A. FLSs are highly proliferated in the synovial tissue, thus stimulating the hyperplasia of the synovium and damage to the joints. FLSs express RANKL and participate in the differentiation of osteoclasts and bone erosion [78]. CCL2 and CX3CL1 are FLS chemokines and behave as chemoattractants for monocytes/macrophages. Moreover, the corresponding MMPs eliminate the extracellular matrix. IL-6, IL-18, TNF, and GM-CSF, as the FLS cytokines, promote the stimulation of innate and adaptive immune cells [61].

Treg cells primarily decrease inflammation and regulate adaptive immunity. The Treg cells are determined as CD4$^+$ CD25$^+$ CD127^{low} FOXP3$^+$ cells. There are two ways in which they cooperate with APCs and effector T cells. The first one is direct communication through cell-to-cell contact. The second way occurs with the help of anti-inflammatory cytokines, for instance, TGF-β, IL-4/IL-13, and IL-10. Furthermore, IL-10, as a potent anti-inflammatory cytokine, influences both the innate and adaptive immune cells [5]. CD8$^+$ FoxP3$^+$ Treg cells induced by anti-CD3 monoclonal antibodies decrease Th1 and Th17 cell activation through P38 phosphorylation inhibition and halt RA inflammation [74]. Monocytes promote the FoxP3 expression in CD8$^+$ FoxP3$^+$ Treg cells through direct cell contact. IL-10 decreases the Th17 cell amount and the IL-17 cytokine generation while simultaneously increasing the Foxp3$^+$ Treg cell development. Thus, IL-10 modifies the ratio of Th17 cells and Treg cells in the CD4$^+$ T cell population. Activated monocytes/macrophages are able to have both a positive and negative effect on the Treg cell phenotype and function, with the predominance of a negative one [74].

MDSCs are tumor-associated cells and take part in the formation of tumor-induced T regulatory cells and T cell anergy. There are two subsets of MDSCs. The first one is presented by monocytic MDSCs. Consequently, monocytes can be expanded and polarized towards MDSCs [13]. The second group includes granulocytic MDSCs. Both of these subsets suppress Th1 and Th17 cell proliferation. Moreover, they secrete IL-10 and contribute to the expansion of Treg cells in mice. To sum up, MDSCs possess immunoregulatory activity and repress RA synovial inflammation [4].

3.2. Monocyte Transport to the RA Synovial Tissue

Monocytes are the important innate effectors in the progression of RA. Circulating monocytes undergo chemotaxis and infiltration into the synovial tissue and stimulate synovial inflammation. Intermediate monocytes, and, to a high extent, the classical ones, are constantly involved in the local synovial inflammation development. This statement is confirmed by the increased presence of both of them in the RA synovium as well as the declining concentration of classical monocytes in the RA peripheral blood and a slightly enhanced number of intermediate monocytes there. M-CSF promotes the differentiation of classical monocytes into the intermediate subset, which indicates the heterogeneous character of the monocyte subsets and their possible polarization into their own other type [13]. The cooperation between CCL2/CCR2 and CX3CL1/CX3CR1 contributes to the migration of circulating monocytes and their functioning in the RA synovium. CCL2 is released by bone marrow mesenchymal stem cells and precursor cells. The CCR2/CCl2 complex on monocytes triggers their recruitment from the bone marrow into the bloodstream. The CX3CL1 production by FLSs is supported by disintegrin and metalloproteinase domain-containing protein 10 and disintegrin; therefore, they mediate the monocyte migration in RA [79].

3.3. Differentiation of Monocytes into Macrophages

In RA, monocytes are replaced by circulating monocytes, which constantly enter the synovium to support the local inflammation, although their part among the synovial macrophages is small. GM-CSF is released by activated synovial fibroblasts under the influence of IL-1β and TNF and provokes the survival of monocytes more than their polarization into macrophages [67]. The human stem cells from the fetal liver and erythro-myeloid predecessors supply the resident macrophages over the period of embryogenesis. However, circulating monocytes supply the recruited inflammatory macrophages when it is necessary, for example, in acute synovial inflammation. When the niche in the synovial tissue is free or unsaturated, macrophage development from circulating monocytes occurs. When there is no available niche, the macrophages are self-replenished by their own turnover. Intermediate monocyte subsets ($CD14^{++}$ $CD16^{+}$) are the prevailing monocytes in the RA synovial tissue, and they mainly differentiate into inflammatory M1 macrophages [30]. Synovial macrophages are located in the sub-lining and lining layers at the cartilage–pannus junction. The activated macrophages of the intimal lining release cytokines and provoke articular destruction. The rheumatoid factor autoantibodies and antigens form IgG-containing immune complexes, which stimulate the macrophages. Furthermore, innate immune cells, T cells, and fibroblasts secrete cytokines that have an impact on the stimulation of macrophages via cell-to-cell contact. The involved TLR-2 and TLR-4 activate macrophages and maintain their level in RA [39].

There are two major phenotypes of macrophages that are differentiated from monocytes in humans. The first is a proinflammatory type represented by classically activated M1 Mφ macrophages. They secrete high levels of IL-1 β, IL-6, IL-12, IL-23, TNF, and reactive oxygen species, which have the main impact on the continuation of the RA inflammation. The second type is anti-inflammatory and refers to alternatively activated Mφ M2 macrophages [80]. They, in turn, provide high concentrations of TGF-β, IL-1Ra, decoy IL-1RII, IL-10, and low IL-12 content. The Mφ M2 macrophage functions are anti-inflammatory activity, tissue remodeling, and wound healing. Both the proinflammatory and anti-inflammatory macrophage phenotypes take part in inflammation regulation. Their differentiation from monocytes with the use of the GM-CSF and M-CSF induction cytokines leads to Mø M1 and Mø2 M2 formation, correspondingly [68]. Moreover, activated Mφ M2 macrophages have three subsets according to their stimulating cytokines. There are three M2 forms. The first one is an alternative M2 form called M2a and triggered by IL-4 and IL-13. The second one is M2b, which is initiated by the impact of the IgG-containing immune complex and the TLR agonists or IL-1R. The third M2 form is M2c, which is induced by IL-10 and glucocorticoid hormones [60].

Th1 cells, Th2 cells, and Th17 cells, along with their associated cytokines, play a crucial role in the polarization, recruitment, activation, and differentiation of monocytes/macrophages [59]. The activation and differentiation of M1 macrophages are driven by the Th1 cytokine IFN-γ in the presence of LPS and TNF. On the other hand, M2 macrophages are driven by Th2 cytokines such as IL-4, IL-10, and IL-13. CXCL5, CXCL8, CXCL9, CXCL10, and CXCL13 are typical chemokines expressed by M1 macrophages. Notably, in vitro studies have demonstrated that M-CSF polarized M2 macrophages can produce proinflammatory cytokines in response to an IgG immune complex containing ACPA. This finding is also relevant in the context of RA since the synovium exhibits elevated levels of M-CSF [67]. Furthermore, activin A, found in RA synovial fluid, induces increased expression of MMP12 (a proinflammatory polarization marker) on monocytes/macrophages, polarizing them into proinflammatory M1 phenotypes. Given these findings, activin A levels may serve as a potential biomarker for various therapies.

The overexpression of the Silent Information Regulator-2 homolog, SIRT1, on monocytes has been shown to downregulate PU.1 phosphorylation, thereby inhibiting their differentiation into macrophages. SIRT1 overexpression can inhibit the production of proinflammatory cytokines by blocking the NF-kB pathway in RA patients. Consequently, SIRT1 has emerged as a significant therapeutic target of interest due to its role in regulating the inflammatory process in RA [81]. It is worth mentioning that monocytes/macrophages secrete the cytosolic phospholipase A2a enzyme, which plays a crucial role in generating prostaglandin E2 from cell membrane phospholipids [82]. Prostaglandin E2, in turn, contributes to the induction and maintenance of RA inflammation. In addition, under the influence of LPS, TNF, and IL-1β, osteoblastic stromal cells produce cytosolic phospholipase A2a, ultimately leading to the generation of prostaglandin E2. This process has been associated with the promotion of inflammatory bone resorption in RA.

3.4. Monocytes Are Osteoclast Predecessors

Periarticular osteopenia and bone erosion adjacent to the pannus formation of synovial joints are two of the most destructive events observed in RA with high disease activity. The main culprits responsible for this erosion are osteoclasts, the primary bone resorbing cells. Osteoclasts originate from circulating monocytes and resident macrophages, which continuously migrate into the inflamed synovium and differentiate into osteoclasts, particularly in active disease and bone erosion. Recent research has shown that monocytes expressing $CD14^+$ and lacking $CD16^-$ are the main precursors of osteoclast progenitors, as opposed to $CD16^+$ subsets [12]. These monocytes upregulate the RANK on their surface and interact with RANKL, which is predominantly expressed by FLSs, osteoblasts, and activated T cells. Th17 cells also play a significant role in promoting osteoclastogenesis as they stimulate the expression of RANKL, which preferably interacts with the $CD14^+$ monocytes expressing the surface marker CCR6, characteristic of Th17 cells [83]. Furthermore, the production of IL-17, along with TNF, IL-1β, and IL-6, can amplify osteoclastogenesis. Additionally, the mesenchymal stromal cells secreted by FLSs, when synergized with RANKL, also aid in promoting osteoclastogenesis [56].

The mature activated osteoclasts release hydrochloric acid near their ruffled border to dissolve the calcium from the bone matrix and also produce MMPs and cathepsin K, which break down the remaining bone matrix, resulting in bone erosion adjacent to the joints [48]. RA monocytes exhibit increased expression of the co-stimulatory osteoclast-associated receptor, which, upon interaction with the collagen type II and collagen type I ligands in the inflamed synovial articular cartilage, further promotes the formation of osteoclasts. However, the osteoblasts' soluble decoy receptor osteoprotegerin negatively affects osteoclastogenesis and disrupts the osteoprotegerin/RANK ratio, consequently favoring osteogenesis [12]. The activated T cells expressing the inducible costimulator, when interacting with the inducible costimulator ligand (CD275) expressed by monocyte-derived osteoclast-like cells, obstruct their differentiation into osteoclasts. This interaction suppresses the expression of tartrate-resistant acid phosphatase, the nuclear factor of activated T cells, and the osteoclast-associated receptors in monocyte-derived osteoclast-like cells during their maturation into osteoclasts. Thus, the CD275-inducible costimulator system directly interferes with osteoclastogenesis [84].

Clinical trials in RA focused on the monocytes that are of interest. The Chinese government approved sinomenine as an anti-inflammation drug for RA treatment. Liu W. et al. (2018) screened the various secretory cytokines in both LPS-induced and sinomenine-treated RAW264.7 cells, followed by an estimation of the sinomenine ability to modulate the cytokine secretion in a cell model, a collagen-induced arthritis mouse model, and RA patients [2]. The results demonstrated that sinomenine regulated the IL-6, GM-CSF, IL-12 p40, IL-1α, TNF, IL-1β, CXCL1, Eotaxin-2, IL-10, M-CSF, RANTES, and CCL2 secretion in vivo and in vitro and reduced the RA activity and the 28-joint disease activity score in a clinical setting. Moreover, sinomenine attenuated the $CD11b^+F4/80^+CD64^+$ resident macrophages in the synovial tissue, the $CD11b^+Ly6C^+CD43^+$ macrophages in the spleen, and draining the lymph nodes in collagen-induced arthritic mice. The percentage of $CD14^+CD16^+$ peripheral blood mononuclear cells was reduced by sinomenine in the

RA patients. In conclusion, sinomenine controls the secretion of multiple inflammatory cytokines and monocyte/macrophage subsets, thus decreasing RA development. Along with methotrexate, sinomenine could be an alternative as a cost-effective anti-inflammatory agent for treating RA [2].

4. Discussion

The innate and adaptive autoimmunity cells within the interconnected network drive the continuous progression of RA pathogenesis. Numerous studies conducted to date, as well as targeted therapies, have demonstrated that FLSs, macrophages, Th1 cells, and B cells play a pivotal role in initiating and advancing synovial inflammation [85]. Recently, Th17 cells have been implicated as the primary drivers of immune cell activation and cytokine production [60]. Furthermore, they are primarily responsible for inducing RANKL production by FLSs and osteoblasts, thereby promoting osteoclastogenesis [78]. Presently, the data suggest that monocyte activation occurs within the circulation of individuals with RA. These activated monocytes respond to chemotactic ligands such as CCL2 and CX3CL1, migrating from the circulation into the RA synovium and releasing proinflammatory cytokines [83]. Thus, their involvement in perpetuating synovial inflammation in RA cannot be disregarded. Additionally, they function as APCs, activating other autoimmune cells and stimulating the production of their respective cytokines. Evidently, they partake in a positive feedback loop with the other key cells involved in RA pathogenesis. The increased expression of various antigens on the monocyte membrane surface can be a potential target for therapy in RA. Evaluating the levels of total monocytes and their subsets in the peripheral blood of the RA patients, both before and after therapy, can provide rheumatologists with guidance in determining the preference for treatment with DMARDs or biologic agents [26]. Elevated levels of monocytes in the peripheral blood of RA patients may serve as an additional biomarker for high disease activity, as evidenced by the correlation with the disease activity score-28 scores and the serum levels of C-reactive protein and the erythrocyte sedimentation rate.

The display of a heterogeneous character by the monocytes enables the differentiation into subsets based on the microenvironment or inflammatory stages and, more importantly, the ability to transform into intermediate monocytes. This emphasizes the high plasticity of the monocytes in the pathogenesis of RA. Inflammatory M1 macrophages, which are crucial players in the development of RA, are primarily derived from circulating monocytes, specifically intermediate monocytes [2]. This raises the question of which chemical events, signals, or specific factors, apart from the arthritic joint environment, trigger the conversion of CD14 monocytes to $CD14^{++}$ $CD16^{+}$ intermediate inflammatory macrophages [86]. Focusing on these studies would not only benefit RA patients but also shed light on other diseases where $CD14^{++}$ $CD16^{+}$ macrophages play a significant role, such as atherosclerosis. Classical monocytes expressing $CD14^{++}$ and $CD16^{-}$ are responsible for the bone erosion observed in erosive RA [87]. Osteoclastogenesis, the formation of osteoclasts, is influenced by the presence of FLSs and Th17 cells. FLSs produce RANKL and M-CSF to promote osteoclastogenesis [67]. Additionally, IL-17, produced by Th17 cells, induces the production of RANKL by FLSs. Furthermore, IL-17, along with TNF, IL-1β, and IL-6, amplifies osteoclastogenesis [88]. However, it is equally important to consider the availability of classical monocytes in the RA synovium or microcirculation near RA synovial joints in erosive rheumatoid arthritis as they have been shown to be precursor cells capable of differentiating into osteoclasts.

5. Conclusions

Recent discussions have highlighted the significant advancements in our understanding of how innate immune cells and signaling play a crucial role in driving the pathogenesis of RA. This complexity of the disease underscores the importance of targeting the innate immune system and its components for potential therapeutic interventions that can reduce the incidence and enhance the quality of life for RA patients. To further explore this, additional research is needed to investigate how the heterogeneity and plasticity of monocytes, the antigenic expressions on their surface, the differentiation into macrophages and osteoclasts, the migration into the synovium, and the role of their cytokines in RA influence their function in RA development. Moreover, studying how macrophage polarization in inflamed joints changes during the course of RA can provide valuable insights into the intricate and pivotal role of these cells in the disease process.

Author Contributions: Conceptualization, D.I.S. and N.G.N.; methodology, A.N.O.; software, D.I.S.; validation, D.I.S., N.G.N. and A.N.O.; formal analysis, A.Y.P.; investigation, D.I.S.; resources, N.G.N.; data curation, D.I.S.; writing—original draft preparation, D.I.S.; writing—review and editing, N.G.N.; visualization, D.I.S.; supervision, N.G.N.; project administration, A.Y.P.; funding acquisition, A.Y.P. All authors have read and agreed to the published version of the manuscript.

Funding: This work was supported by Russian Science Foundation (Grant 22-15-00273).

Institutional Review Board Statement: Not applicable.

Informed Consent Statement: Not applicable.

Data Availability Statement: Data available from the authors.

Acknowledgments: The authors would like to thank Alina I. Salnikova, translator and interpreter at the European Medical Center (Moscow, Russia), for her kind assistance in English editing. Figure was created with Biorender.com, accessed on 1 January 2024.

Conflicts of Interest: The authors declare no conflicts of interest. The funders had no role in the design of the study; in the collection, analyses, or interpretation of data; in the writing of the manuscript; or in the decision to publish the results.

References

1. Cheng, Q.; Wu, H.; Du, Y. The roles of small-molecule inflammatory mediators in rheumatoid arthritis. *Scand. J. Immunol.* **2021**, *93*, e12982. [CrossRef] [PubMed]
2. Liu, W.; Zhang, Y.; Zhu, W.; Ma, C.; Ruan, J.; Long, H.; Wang, Y. Sinomenine Inhibits the Progression of Rheumatoid Arthritis by Regulating the Secretion of Inflammatory Cytokines and Monocyte/Macrophage Subsets. *Front. Immunol.* **2018**, *26*, 2228. [CrossRef] [PubMed]
3. Balchin, C.; Tan, A.L.; Golding, J.; Bissell, L.-A.; Wilson, O.J.; McKenna, J.; Stavropoulos-Kalinoglou, A. Acute effects of exercise on pain symptoms, clinical inflammatory markers and inflammatory cytokines in people with rheumatoid arthritis: A systematic literature review. *Ther. Adv. Musculoskelet. Dis.* **2022**, *14*, 1759720X221114104. [CrossRef] [PubMed]
4. Morell, M.; Varela, N.; Marañón, C. Myeloid Populations in Systemic Autoimmune Diseases. *Clin. Rev. Allergy Immunol.* **2017**, *53*, 198–218. [CrossRef] [PubMed]
5. Mishra, S.; Srinivasan, S.; Ma, C.; Zhang, N. CD8+ Regulatory T Cell—A Mystery to Be Revealed. *Front. Immunol.* **2021**, *12*, 708874. [CrossRef] [PubMed]
6. Choi, J.; Selmi, C.; Leung, P.S.C.; Kenny, T.P.; Roskams, T.; Gershwin, M.E. Chemokine and chemokine receptors in autoimmunity: The case of primary biliary cholangitis. *Expert Rev. Clin. Immunol.* **2016**, *12*, 661–672. [CrossRef] [PubMed]
7. Ziegler-Heitbrock, L.; Ancuta, P.; Crowe, S.; Dalod, M.; Grau, V.; Hart, D.N.; Leenen, P.J.M.; Liu, Y.-J.; MacPherson, G.; Randolph, G.J.; et al. Nomenclature of monocytes and dendritic cells in blood. *Blood* **2010**, *116*, e74–e80. [CrossRef] [PubMed]
8. Liu, E.G.; Yin, X.; Swaminathan, A.; Eisenbarth, S.C. Antigen-Presenting Cells in Food Tolerance and Allergy. *Front. Immunol.* **2021**, *11*, 616020. [CrossRef] [PubMed]
9. Li, L.; Huang, L.; Sung, S.-S.J.; Vergis, A.L.; Rosin, D.L.; Rose, C.E., Jr.; Lobo, P.I.; Okusa, M.D. The chemokine receptors CCR2 and CX3CR1 mediate monocyte/macrophage trafficking in kidney ischemia-reperfusion injury. *Kidney Int.* **2008**, *74*, 1526–1537. [CrossRef]
10. Wolf, A.A.; Yáñez, A.; Barman, P.K.; Goodridge, H.S. The Ontogeny of Monocyte Subsets. *Front. Immunol.* **2019**, *10*, 1642. [CrossRef]
11. Mushenkova, N.V.; Nikiforov, N.G.; Shakhpazyan, N.K.; Orekhova, V.A.; Sadykhov, N.K.; Orekhov, A.N. Phenotype Diversity of Macrophages in Osteoarthritis: Implications for Development of Macrophage Modulating Therapies. *Int. J. Mol. Sci.* **2022**, *23*, 8381. [CrossRef] [PubMed]
12. Komano, Y.; Nanki, T.; Hayashida, K.; Taniguchi, K.; Miyasaka, N. Identification of a human peripheral blood monocyte subset that differentiates into osteoclasts. *Arthritis Res. Ther.* **2006**, *8*, R152. [CrossRef] [PubMed]
13. Chen, S.; Guo, C.; Wang, R.; Feng, Z.; Liu, Z.; Wu, L.; Zhao, D.; Zheng, S.; Chen, F.; Zhang, D.; et al. Monocytic MDSCs skew Th17 cells toward a pro-osteoclastogenic phenotype and potentiate bone erosion in rheumatoid arthritis. *Rheumatology* **2021**, *60*, 2409–2420. [CrossRef] [PubMed]

14. Luukkonen, J.; Huhtakangas, J.; Palosaari, S.; Tuukkanen, J.; Vuolteenaho, O.; Lehenkari, P. Preliminary Report: Osteoarthritis and Rheumatoid Arthritis Synovial Fluid Increased Osteoclastogenesis In Vitro by Monocyte Differentiation Pathway Regulating Cytokines. *Mediators Inflamm.* **2022**, *2022*, 2606916. [CrossRef] [PubMed]
15. De Kleer, I.; Willems, F.; Lambrecht, B.; Goriely, S. Ontogeny of myeloid cells. *Front. Immunol.* **2014**, *5*, 423. [CrossRef] [PubMed]
16. Weaver, L.K.; Chu, N.; Behrens, E.M. TLR9-mediated inflammation drives a Ccr2-independent peripheral monocytosis through enhanced extramedullary monocytopoiesis. *Proc. Natl. Acad. Sci. USA* **2016**, *113*, 10944–10949. [CrossRef] [PubMed]
17. Krasselt, M.; Baerwald, C.; Wagner, U.; Rossol, M. CD56+ monocytes have a dysregulated cytokine response to lipopolysaccharide and accumulate in rheumatoid arthritis and immunosenescence. *Arthritis Res. Ther.* **2013**, *15*, R139. [CrossRef] [PubMed]
18. Sørensen, A.S.; Andersen, M.N.; Juul-Madsen, K.; Broksø, A.D.; Skejø, C.; Schmidt, H.; Vorup-Jensen, T.; Kragstrup, T.W. Tumor necrosis factor alpha neutralization attenuates immune checkpoint inhibitor-induced activation of intermediate monocytes in synovial fluid mononuclear cells from patients with inflammatory arthritis. *Arthritis Res. Ther.* **2022**, *24*, 43. [CrossRef] [PubMed]
19. Tsukamoto, M.; Seta, N.; Yoshimoto, K.; Suzuki, K.; Yamaoka, K.; Takeuchi, T. CD14brightCD16+ intermediate monocytes are induced by interleukin-10 and positively correlate with disease activity in rheumatoid arthritis. *Arthritis Res. Ther.* **2017**, *19*, 28. [CrossRef]
20. Chara, L.; Sánchez-Atrio, A.; Pérez, A.; Cuende, E.; Albarrán, F.; Turrión, A.; Chevarria, J.; del Barco, A.A.; Sánchez, M.A.; Monserrat, J.; et al. The number of circulating monocytes as biomarkers of the clinical response to methotrexate in untreated patients with rheumatoid arthritis. *J. Transl. Med.* **2015**, *13*, 2. [CrossRef]
21. Buscher, K.; Marcovecchio, P.; Hedrick, C.C.; Ley, K. Patrolling Mechanics of Non-Classical Monocytes in Vascular Inflammation. *Front. Cardiovasc. Med.* **2017**, *4*, 80. [CrossRef]
22. Ong, S.-M.; Hadadi, E.; Dang, T.-M.; Yeap, W.-H.; Tan, C.T.-Y.; Ng, T.-P.; Larbi, A.; Wong, S.-C. The pro-inflammatory phenotype of the human non-classical monocyte subset is attributed to senescence. *Cell Death Dis.* **2018**, *9*, 266. [CrossRef] [PubMed]
23. Rodríguez-Vargas, G.-S.; Santos-Moreno, P.; Rubio-Rubio, J.-A.; Bautista-Niño, P.-K.; Echeverri, D.; Gutiérrez-Castañeda, L.-D.; Sierra-Matamoros, F.; Navarrete, S.; Aparicio, A.; Saenz, L.; et al. Vascular Age, Metabolic Panel, Cardiovascular Risk and Inflammaging in Patients with Rheumatoid Arthritis Compared with Patients with Osteoarthritis. *Front. Cardiovasc. Med.* **2022**, *9*, 894577. [CrossRef] [PubMed]
24. Frouin, I.; Prosperi, E.; Denegri, M.; Negri, C.; Donzelli, M.; Rossi, L.; Riva, F.; Stefanini, M.; Scovassi, A.I. Different effects of methotrexate on DNA mismatch repair proficient and deficient cells. *Eur. J. Cancer* **2001**, *37*, 1173–1180. [CrossRef] [PubMed]
25. Greenstein, R.J.; Su, L.; Shahidi, A.; Brown, S.T. On the action of 5-amino-salicylic acid and sulfapyridine on M. avium including subspecies paratuberculosis. *PLoS ONE* **2007**, *2*, e516. [CrossRef] [PubMed]
26. Deng, G.; Chen, X.; Shao, L.; Wu, Q.; Wang, S. Effectiveness and safety of 99Tc-methylene diphosphonate as a disease-modifying anti-rheumatic drug (DMARD) in combination with conventional synthetic (cs) DMARDs in the treatment of rheumatoid arthritis: A systematic review and meta-analysis of 34 randomized controlled trials. *Heliyon* **2023**, *9*, e21691. [CrossRef] [PubMed]
27. Ammari, M.; Presumey, J.; Ponsolles, C.; Roussignol, G.; Roubert, C.; Escriou, V.; Toupet, K.; Mausset-Bonnefont, A.-L.; Cren, M.; Robin, M.; et al. Delivery of miR-146a to Ly6Chigh Monocytes Inhibits Pathogenic Bone Erosion in Inflammatory Arthritis. *Theranostics* **2018**, *8*, 5972–5985. [CrossRef] [PubMed]
28. Ledesma-Colunga, M.G.; Baschant, U.; Weidner, H.; Alves, T.C.; Mirtschink, P.; Hofbauer, L.C.; Rauner, M. Transferrin receptor 2 deficiency promotes macrophage polarization and inflammatory arthritis. *Redox Biol.* **2023**, *60*, 102616. [CrossRef] [PubMed]
29. Roberts, C.A.; Dickinson, A.K.; Taams, L.S. The Interplay Between Monocytes/Macrophages and CD4(+) T Cell Subsets in Rheumatoid Arthritis. *Front. Immunol.* **2015**, *6*, 571. [CrossRef]
30. Zamani, F.; Shahneh, F.Z.; Aghebati-Maleki, L.; Baradaran, B. Induction of CD14 Expression and Differentiation to Monocytes or Mature Macrophages in Promyelocytic Cell Lines: New Approach. *Adv. Pharm. Bull.* **2013**, *3*, 329–332. [CrossRef]
31. Rodrigues, C.P.; Ferreira, A.C.F.; Pinho, M.P.; de Moraes, C.J.; Bergami-Santos, P.C.; Barbuto, J.A.M. Tolerogenic IDO(+) Dendritic Cells Are Induced by PD-1-Expressing Mast Cells. *Front. Immunol.* **2016**, *7*, 9. [CrossRef] [PubMed]
32. Forget, A.; Gianni-Barrera, R.; Uccelli, A.; Sarem, M.; Kohler, E.; Fogli, B.; Muraro, M.G.; Bichet, S.; Aumann, K.; Banfi, A.; et al. Mechanically Defined Microenvironment Promotes Stabilization of Microvasculature, Which Correlates with the Enrichment of a Novel Piezo-1+ Population of Circulating CD11b+ /CD115+ Monocytes. *Adv. Mater.* **2019**, *31*, e1808050. [CrossRef] [PubMed]
33. Spinelli, F.R.; Pecani, A.; Conti, F.; Mancini, R.; Alessandri, C.; Valesini, G. Post-translational modifications in rheumatoid arthritis and atherosclerosis: Focus on citrullination and carbamylation. *J. Int. Med. Res.* **2016**, *44*, 81–84. [CrossRef] [PubMed]
34. Sakuraba, K.; Krishnamurthy, A.; Sun, J.; Zheng, X.; Xu, C.; Peng, B.; Engström, M.; Jakobsson, P.-J.; Wermeling, F.; Catrina, S.; et al. Autoantibodies targeting malondialdehyde-modifications in rheumatoid arthritis regulate osteoclasts via inducing glycolysis and lipid biosynthesis. *J. Autoimmun.* **2022**, *133*, 102903. [CrossRef] [PubMed]
35. Colasanti, T.; Sabatinelli, D.; Mancone, C.; Giorgi, A.; Pecani, A.; Spinelli, F.R.; Giamberardino, A.D.; Navarini, L.; Speziali, M.; Vomero, M.; et al. Homocysteinylated alpha 1 antitrypsin as an antigenic target of autoantibodies in seronegative rheumatoid arthritis patients. *J. Autoimmun.* **2020**, *113*, 102470. [CrossRef]
36. Costantino, C.M.; Ploegh, H.L.; Hafler, D.A. Cathepsin S regulates class II MHC processing in human CD4+ HLA-DR+ T cells. *J. Immunol.* **2009**, *183*, 945–952. [CrossRef]
37. Wahyurini, D.; Wibowo, H. Monocytic HLA-DR expression in type 2 diabetes mellitus: Impact on disease susceptibility. *World J. Adv. Res. Rev.* **2023**, *18*, 684–689. [CrossRef]

38. Iwamoto, N.; Kawakami, A. The monocyte-to-osteoclast transition in rheumatoid arthritis: Recent findings. *Front. Immunol.* **2022**, *13*, 998554. [CrossRef]
39. Hwang, S.; Sung, D.K.; Kim, Y.E.; Yang, M.; Ahn, S.Y.; Sung, S.I.; Chang, Y.S. Mesenchymal Stromal Cells Primed by Toll-like Receptors 3 and 4 Enhanced Anti-Inflammatory Effects against LPS-Induced Macrophages via Extracellular Vesicles. *Int. J. Mol. Sci.* **2023**, *24*, 16264. [CrossRef]
40. Wu, X.-Y.; Li, K.-T.; Yang, H.-X.; Yang, B.; Lu, X.; Zhao, L.-D.; Fei, Y.-Y.; Chen, H.; Wang, L.; Li, J.; et al. Complement C1q synergizes with PTX3 in promoting NLRP3 inflammasome over-activation and pyroptosis in rheumatoid arthritis. *J. Autoimmun.* **2020**, *106*, 102336. [CrossRef]
41. Roelofs, M.F.; Wenink, M.H.; Brentano, F.; Abdollahi-Roodsaz, S.; Oppers-Walgreen, B.; Barrera, P.; van Riel, P.L.C.M.; Joosten, L.A.B.; Kyburz, D.; van den Berg, W.B.; et al. Type I interferons might form the link between Toll-like receptor (TLR) 3/7 and TLR4-mediated synovial inflammation in rheumatoid arthritis (RA). *Ann. Rheum. Dis.* **2009**, *68*, 1486–1493. [CrossRef] [PubMed]
42. Park, J.-Y.; Park, H.-M.; Kim, S.; Jeon, K.-B.; Lim, C.-M.; Hong, J.T.; Yoon, D.-Y. Human IL-32θA94V mutant attenuates monocyte-endothelial adhesion by suppressing the expression of ICAM-1 and VCAM-1 via binding to cell surface receptor integrin αVβ3 and αVβ6 in TNF-α-stimulated HUVECs. *Front. Immunol.* **2023**, *14*, 1160301. [CrossRef] [PubMed]
43. Luo, Z.; The, E.; Zhang, P.; Zhai, Y.; Yao, Q.; Ao, L.; Zeng, Q.; Fullerton, D.A.; Meng, X. Monocytes augment inflammatory responses in human aortic valve interstitial cells via β2-integrin/ICAM-1-mediated signaling. *Inflamm. Res.* **2022**, *71*, 681–694. [CrossRef] [PubMed]
44. Mantchev, G.T.; Cortesão, C.S.; Rebrovich, M.; Cascalho, M.; Bram, R.J. TACI is required for efficient plasma cell differentiation in response to T-independent type 2 antigens. *J. Immunol.* **2007**, *179*, 2282–2288. [CrossRef] [PubMed]
45. Nagatani, K.; Itoh, K.; Nakajima, K.; Kuroki, H.; Katsuragawa, Y.; Mochizuki, M.; Aotsuka, S.; Mimori, A. Rheumatoid arthritis fibroblast-like synoviocytes express BCMA and are stimulated by APRIL. *Arthritis Rheum.* **2007**, *56*, 3554–3563. [CrossRef] [PubMed]
46. Xiong, Y.-S.; Cheng, Y.; Lin, Q.-S.; Wu, A.-L.; Yu, J.; Li, C.; Sun, Y.; Zhong, R.-Q.; Wu, L.-J. Increased expression of Siglec-1 on peripheral blood monocytes and its role in mononuclear cell reactivity to autoantigen in rheumatoid arthritis. *Rheumatology* **2014**, *53*, 250–259. [CrossRef]
47. Meusch, U.; Krasselt, M.; Rossol, M.; Baerwald, C.; Klingner, M.; Wagner, U. In vitro response pattern of monocytes after tmTNF reverse signaling predicts response to anti-TNF therapy in rheumatoid arthritis. *J. Transl. Med.* **2015**, *13*, 256. [CrossRef] [PubMed]
48. Huang, J.; Xie, B.; Li, Q.; Xie, X.; Zhu, S.; Wang, M.; Peng, W.; Gu, J. Infliximab reduces CD147, MMP-3, and MMP-9 expression in peripheral blood monocytes in patients with active rheumatoid arthritis. *Eur. J. Pharmacol.* **2013**, *698*, 429–434. [CrossRef]
49. Ebrahimi-Rad, M.; Khatami, S.; Akhbari, H.; Mahmoudzadeh-Niknam, H.; Valadbeigi, S.; Mahmoudi, M.; Jamshidi, A.; Riazi-Rad, F.; Saghiri, R. Evaluation of autoantibodies against vimentin and α-enolase in rheumatoid arthritis patients. *Reumatologia* **2020**, *58*, 350–356. [CrossRef]
50. Crilly, A.; Burns, E.; Nickdel, M.B.; Lockhart, J.C.; Perry, M.E.; Ferrell, P.W.; Baxter, D.; Dale, J.; Dunning, L.; Wilson, H.; et al. PAR(2) expression in peripheral blood monocytes of patients with rheumatoid arthritis. *Ann. Rheum. Dis.* **2012**, *71*, 1049–1054. [CrossRef]
51. Piotrowska, K.; Słuczanowska-Głabowska, S.; Kurzawski, M.; Dziedziejko, V.; Kopytko, P.; Paczkowska, E.; Rogińska, D.; Safranow, K.; Machaliński, B.; Pawlik, A. Over-Expression of Allograft Inflammatory Factor-1 (AIF-1) in Patients with Rheumatoid Arthritis. *Biomolecules* **2020**, *10*, 1064. [CrossRef] [PubMed]
52. Hofer, T.P.; van de Loosdrecht, A.A.; Stahl-Hennig, C.; Cassatella, M.A.; Ziegler-Heitbrock, L. 6-Sulfo LacNAc (Slan) as a Marker for Non-classical Monocytes. *Front. Immunol.* **2019**, *10*, 2052. [CrossRef] [PubMed]
53. Tamassia, N.; Bianchetto-Aguilera, F.; Gasperini, S.; Grimaldi, A.; Montaldo, C.; Calzetti, F.; Gardiman, E.; Signoretto, I.; Castellucci, M.; Barnaba, V.; et al. The slan antigen identifies the prototypical non-classical CD16+-monocytes in human blood. *Front. Immunol.* **2023**, *14*, 1287656. [CrossRef] [PubMed]
54. Hofer, T.P.; Zawada, A.M.; Frankenberger, M.; Skokann, K.; Satzl, A.A.; Gesierich, W.; Schuberth, M.; Levin, J.; Danek, A.; Rotter, B.; et al. slan-defined subsets of CD16-positive monocytes: Impact of granulomatous inflammation and M-CSF receptor mutation. *Blood* **2015**, *126*, 2601–2610. [CrossRef] [PubMed]
55. Gómez-Bañuelos, E.; Martín-Márquez, B.T.; Martínez-García, E.A.; Figueroa-Sanchez, M.; Nuñez-Atahualpa, L.; Rocha-Muñoz, A.D.; Sánchez-Hernández, P.E.; Navarro-Hernandez, R.E.; Madrigal-Ruiz, P.M.; Saldaña-Millan, A.A.; et al. Low levels of CD36 in peripheral blood monocytes in subclinical atherosclerosis in rheumatoid arthritis: A cross-sectional study in a Mexican population. *Biomed. Res. Int.* **2014**, *2014*, 736786. [CrossRef] [PubMed]
56. Min, H.K.; Won, J.-Y.; Kim, B.-M.; Lee, K.-A.; Lee, S.-J.; Lee, S.-H.; Kim, H.-R.; Kim, K.-W. Interleukin (IL)-25 suppresses IL-22-induced osteoclastogenesis in rheumatoid arthritis via STAT3 and p38 MAPK/IκBα pathway. *Arthritis Res. Ther.* **2020**, *22*, 222. [CrossRef] [PubMed]
57. Pan, S.; Wu, S.; Wei, Y.; Liu, J.; Zhou, C.; Chen, T.; Zhu, J.; Tan, W.; Huang, C.; Feng, S.; et al. Exploring the causal relationship between inflammatory cytokines and inflammatory arthritis: A Mendelian randomization study. *Cytokine* **2024**, *173*, 156446. [CrossRef] [PubMed]
58. Filali, S.; Noack, M.; Géloën, A.; Pirot, F.; Miossec, P. Effects of pro-inflammatory cytokines and cell interactions on cell area and cytoskeleton of rheumatoid arthritis synoviocytes and immune cells. *Eur. J. Cell Biol.* **2023**, *102*, 151303. [CrossRef] [PubMed]

59. Gloyer, L.; Golumba-Nagy, V.; Meyer, A.; Yan, S.; Schiller, J.; Breuninger, M.; Jochimsen, D.; Kofler, D.M. Adenosine receptor A2a blockade by caffeine increases IFN-gamma production in Th1 cells from patients with rheumatoid arthritis. *Scand. J. Rheumatol.* **2022**, *51*, 279–283. [CrossRef]
60. Park, J.-S.; Kim, N.-R.; Lim, M.-A.; Kim, S.-M.; Hwang, S.-H.; Jung, K.-A.; Choi, J.W.; Park, S.-H.; Cho, M.-L. Deficiency of IL-1 receptor antagonist suppresses IL-10-producing B cells in autoimmune arthritis in an IL-17/Th17-dependent manner. *Immunol. Lett.* **2018**, *199*, 44–52. [CrossRef]
61. Yan, J.; Yao, L.; Tan, Y.; Wang, Y. The protective effects of Phoenixin-20 in tumor necrosis factor α (TNF-α)-induced cell senescence of rheumatoid arthritis fibroblast-like synoviocytes (FLS). *Aging* **2023**, *15*, 14607–14616. [CrossRef] [PubMed]
62. Shabgah, A.G.; Shariati-Sarabi, Z.; Tavakkol-Afshari, J.; Ghasemi, A.; Ghoryani, M.; Mohammadi, M. A significant decrease of BAFF, APRIL, and BAFF receptors following mesenchymal stem cell transplantation in patients with refractory rheumatoid arthritis. *Gene* **2020**, *732*, 144336. [CrossRef]
63. Okamato, Y.; Ghosh, T.; Okamoto, T.; Schuyler, R.P.; Seifert, J.; Charry, L.L.; Visser, A.; Feser, M.; Fleischer, C.; Pedrick, C.; et al. Subjects at-risk for future development of rheumatoid arthritis demonstrate a PAD4-and TLR-dependent enhanced histone H3 citrullination and proinflammatory cytokine production in CD14hi monocytes. *J. Autoimmun.* **2021**, *117*, 102581. [CrossRef] [PubMed]
64. Stangl, H.; Krammetsvogl, A.; Lesiak, M.; Wolff, C.; Straub, R.H. MHC/class-II-positive cells inhibit corticosterone of adrenal gland cells in experimental arthritis: A role for IL-1β, IL-18, and the inflammasome. *Sci. Rep.* **2020**, *10*, 17071. [CrossRef] [PubMed]
65. Murphy, E.P.; Crean, D. Molecular Interactions between NR4A Orphan Nuclear Receptors and NF-κB Are Required for Appropriate Inflammatory Responses and Immune Cell Homeostasis. *Biomolecules* **2015**, *5*, 1302–1318. [CrossRef] [PubMed]
66. Yamamoto, T.; Endo, Y.; Onodera, A.; Hirahara, K.; Asou, H.K.; Nakajima, T.; Kanno, T.; Ouchi, Y.; Uematsu, S.; Nishimasu, H.; et al. DUSP10 constrains innate IL-33-mediated cytokine production in ST2hi memory-type pathogenic Th2 cells. *Nat. Commun.* **2018**, *9*, 4231. [CrossRef] [PubMed]
67. Chung, S.; Ranjan, R.; Lee, Y.G.; Park, G.Y.; Karpurapu, M.; Deng, J.; Xiao, L.; Kim, J.Y.; Unterman, T.G.; Christman, J.W. Distinct role of FoxO1 in M-CSF- and GM-CSF-differentiated macrophages contributes LPS-mediated IL-10: Implication in hyperglycemia. *J. Leukoc. Biol.* **2015**, *97*, 327–339. [CrossRef] [PubMed]
68. Elbjeirami, W.M.; Donnachie, E.M.; Burns, A.R.; Smith, C.W. Endothelium-derived GM-CSF influences expression of oncostatin M. *Am. J. Physiol. Cell Physiol.* **2011**, *301*, C947–C953. [CrossRef]
69. Haringman, J.J.; Gerlag, D.M.; Smeets, T.J.M.; Baeten, D.; van den Bosch, F.; Bresnihan, B.; Breedveld, F.C.; Dinant, H.J.; Legay, F.; Gram, H.; et al. A randomized controlled trial with an anti-CCL2 (anti-monocyte chemotactic protein 1) monoclonal antibody in patients with RA. *Arthritis Rheum.* **2006**, *54*, 2387–2392. [CrossRef]
70. Tsai, C.-H.; Liu, S.-C.; Wang, Y.-H.; Su, C.-M.; Huang, C.-C.; Hsu, C.-J.; Tang, C.-H. Osteopontin inhibition of miR-129-3p enhances IL-17 expression and monocyte migration in rheumatoid arthritis. *Biochim. Biophys. Acta Gen. Subj.* **2017**, *1861*, 15–22. [CrossRef]
71. Wu, Y.-J.; Zhang, S.-S.; Yin, Q.; Lei, M.; Wang, Q.-H.; Chen, W.-G.; Luo, T.-T.; Zhou, P.; Ji, C.-L. α-Mangostin Inhibited M1 Polarization of Macrophages/Monocytes in Antigen-Induced Arthritis Mice by Up-Regulating Silent Information Regulator 1 and Peroxisome Proliferators-Activated Receptor γ Simultaneously. *Drug Des. Devel Ther.* **2023**, *17*, 563–577. [CrossRef] [PubMed]
72. Vasilevko, V.; Ghochikyan, A.; Holterman, M.J.; Agadjanyan, M.G. CD80 (B7-1) and CD86 (B7-2) are functionally equivalent in the initiation and maintenance of CD4+ T-cell proliferation after activation with suboptimal doses of PHA. *DNA Cell Biol.* **2002**, *21*, 137–149. [CrossRef] [PubMed]
73. Moghaddami, M.; Cleland, L.G.; Radisic, G.; Mayrhofer, G. Recruitment of dendritic cells and macrophages during T cell-mediated synovial inflammation. *Arthritis Res. Ther.* **2007**, *9*, R120. [CrossRef] [PubMed]
74. König, M.; Rharbaoui, F.; Aigner, S.; Dälken, B.; Schüttrumpf, J. Tregalizumab—A Monoclonal Antibody to Target Regulatory T Cells. *Front. Immunol.* **2016**, *7*, 11. [CrossRef] [PubMed]
75. Bossi, G. Mutant p53 and sIL-1Ra. *Aging* **2015**, *7*, 742–743. [CrossRef] [PubMed]
76. Wang, M.; Zhao, H.; Zhao, H.; Huo, C.; Yuan, Y.; Zhu, Y. Moxibustion-mediated alleviation of synovitis in rats with rheumatoid arthritis through the regulation of NLRP3 inflammasome by modulating neutrophil extracellular traps. *Heliyon* **2023**, *10*, e23633. [CrossRef] [PubMed]
77. Jiang, F.-Y.; Zhang, Y.-Z.; Tai, Y.-H.; Chou, C.-Y.; Hsieh, Y.-C.; Chang, Y.-C.; Huang, H.-C.; Li, Z.-Q.; Hsieh, Y.-C.; Chen, I.-J.; et al. A lesion-selective albumin-CTLA4Ig as a safe and effective treatment for collagen-induced arthritis. *Inflamm. Regen.* **2023**, *43*, 13. [CrossRef] [PubMed]
78. Tian, Y.; Ming, J. Melatonin inhibits osteoclastogenesis via RANKL/OPG suppression mediated by Rev-Erbα in osteoblasts. *J. Cell Mol. Med.* **2022**, *26*, 4032–4047. [CrossRef] [PubMed]
79. Isozaki, T.; Nishimi, S.; Nishimi, A.; Saito, M.; Miwa, Y.; Toyoshima, Y.; Inagaki, K.; Kasama, T. A disintegrin and metalloproteinase (ADAM)-10 as a predictive factor for tocilizumab effectiveness in rheumatoid arthritis. *Mod. Rheumatol.* **2017**, *27*, 782–786. [CrossRef]
80. Li, S.; Wang, Y.; Wu, M.; Younis, M.H.; Olson, A.P.; Barnhart, T.E.; Engle, J.W.; Zhu, X.; Cai, W. Spleen-Targeted Glabridin-Loaded Nanoparticles Regulate Polarization of Monocyte/Macrophage (Mo/Mφ) for the Treatment of Cerebral Ischemia-Reperfusion Injury. *Adv. Mater.* **2022**, *34*, e2204976. [CrossRef]

31. Wang, D.-D.; He, C.-Y.; Wu, Y.-J.; Xu, L.; Shi, C.; Olatunji, O.J.; Zuo, J.; Ji, C.-L. AMPK/SIRT1 Deficiency Drives Adjuvant-Induced Arthritis in Rats by Promoting Glycolysis-Mediated Monocytes Inflammatory Polarization. *J. Inflamm. Res.* **2022**, *15*, 4663–4675. [CrossRef] [PubMed]
32. Pang, X.; Yin, P.; Han, J.; Wang, Z.; Zheng, F.; Chen, X. cPLA2a correlates with metastasis and poor prognosis of osteosarcoma by facilitating epithelial-mesenchymal transition. *Pathol. Res. Pract.* **2019**, *215*, 152398. [CrossRef] [PubMed]
33. Lee, A.Y.S.; Eri, R.; Lyons, A.B.; Grimm, M.C.; Korner, H. CC chemokine ligand 20 and its cognate receptor CCR6 in mucosal T cell immunology and inflammatory bowel disease: Odd couple or axis of evil? *Front. Immunol.* **2013**, *4*, 194. [CrossRef] [PubMed]
34. Riella, L.V.; Dada, S.; Chabtini, L.; Smith, B.; Huang, L.; Dakle, P.; Mfarrej, B.; D'Addio, F.; Adams, L.-T.; Kochupurakkal, N.; et al. B7h (ICOS-L) maintains tolerance at the fetomaternal interface. *Am. J. Pathol.* **2013**, *182*, 2204–2213. [CrossRef] [PubMed]
35. Blagov, A.V.; Grechko, A.V.; Nikiforov, N.G.; Zhuravlev, A.D.; Sadykhov, N.K.; Orekhov, A.N. Effects of Metabolic Disorders in Immune Cells and Synoviocytes on the Development of Rheumatoid Arthritis. *Metabolites* **2022**, *12*, 634. [CrossRef] [PubMed]
36. Amoruso, A.; Sola, D.; Rossi, L.; Obeng, J.A.; Fresu, L.G.; Sainaghi, P.P.; Pirisi, M.; Brunelleschi, S. Relation among anti-rheumatic drug therapy, CD14(+)CD16(+) blood monocytes and disease activity markers (DAS28 and US7 scores) in rheumatoid arthritis: A pilot study. *Pharmacol. Res.* **2016**, *107*, 308–314. [CrossRef] [PubMed]
37. Batko, B.; Schramm-Luc, A.; Skiba, D.S.; Mikolajczyk, T.P.; Siedlinski, M. TNF-α Inhibitors Decrease Classical CD14hiCD16- Monocyte Subsets in Highly Active, Conventional Treatment Refractory Rheumatoid Arthritis and Ankylosing Spondylitis. *Int. J. Mol. Sci.* **2019**, *20*, 291. [CrossRef]
38. Du, Z.; Cong, W.; Tang, K.; Zheng, Q.; Song, Z.; Chen, Y.; Yang, S.; Zhang, C.; Ye, T. Electroacupuncture stimulating Zusanli (ST36), Sanyinjiao (SP6) in mice with collagen-induced arthritis leads to adenosine A2A receptor-mediated alteration of p38α mitogen-activated protein kinase signaling and inhibition of osteoclastogenesis. *J. Tradit. Chin. Med.* **2023**, *43*, 1103–1109. [CrossRef]

cells

MDPI

Review

Cellular Senescence, Mitochondrial Dysfunction, and Their Link to Cardiovascular Disease

Maria Camacho-Encina [1,*], Laura K. Booth [2], Rachael E. Redgrave [1], Omowumi Folaranmi [1], Ioakim Spyridopoulos [2] and Gavin D. Richardson [1]

1 Vascular Medicine and Biology Theme, Bioscience Institute, Newcastle University, Newcastle upon Tyne NE1 3BZ, UK; rachael.redgrave@newcastle.ac.uk (R.E.R.); o.folaranmi2@newcastle.ac.uk (O.F.); gavin.richardson@ncl.ac.uk (G.D.R.)

2 Vascular Medicine and Biology Theme, Translational and Clinical Research Institute, Newcastle University, Newcastle upon Tyne NE1 3BZ, UK; l.booth2@newcastle.ac.uk (L.K.B.); ioakim.spyridopoulos@ncl.ac.uk (I.S.)

* Correspondence: maria.camacho-encina@newcastle.ac.uk; Tel.: +44-(0)191-241-8615

Abstract: Cardiovascular diseases (CVDs), a group of disorders affecting the heart or blood vessels, are the primary cause of death worldwide, with an immense impact on patient quality of life and disability. According to the World Health Organization, CVD takes an estimated 17.9 million lives each year, where more than four out of five CVD deaths are due to heart attacks and strokes. In the decades to come, an increased prevalence of age-related CVD, such as atherosclerosis, coronary artery stenosis, myocardial infarction (MI), valvular heart disease, and heart failure (HF) will contribute to an even greater health and economic burden as the global average life expectancy increases and consequently the world's population continues to age. Considering this, it is important to focus our research efforts on understanding the fundamental mechanisms underlying CVD. In this review, we focus on cellular senescence and mitochondrial dysfunction, which have long been established to contribute to CVD. We also assess the recent advances in targeting mitochondrial dysfunction including energy starvation and oxidative stress, mitochondria dynamics imbalance, cell apoptosis, mitophagy, and senescence with a focus on therapies that influence both and therefore perhaps represent strategies with the most clinical potential, range, and utility.

Keywords: senescence; mitochondrial dysfunction; cardiac cardiomyocyte; cardiac ischemia reperfusion

1. Cellular Senescence

Cellular senescence was originally defined as the irreversible exit from the cell cycle [1]. However, over recent years the definition of senescence has evolved and now includes many other characteristics such, as mitochondrial dysfunction, resistance to apoptosis, and the activation of a hypersecretory phenotype termed the senescence-associated secretory phenotype (SASP) [2]. Arguably, these characteristics more accurately define senescence given the substantive evidence that non-proliferative, post-mitotic cells, such as cardiomyocytes, can become senescent [3–6]. Similarly, while originally described as a consequence of telomere attrition following extensive proliferation [7,8], it is now accepted that numerous types of stresses which result in DNA damage within the genome or within the telomeres can activate pathways controlling senescence [9] (Figure 1). However, in both proliferative and post-mitotic cell populations, senescence induction is associated with the activation of either, or both, p21 and p16, cyclin-dependent kinase inhibitors that are components of the tumour suppressor pathways governed by the transcription factor p53 and the retinoblastoma protein (RB), respectively [10]. The traditional view that cellular senescence evolved as a tumour-suppressive mechanism has recently been challenged, as evidence suggests that senescent cells contribute to several important physiological processes throughout life, including tissue development, wound healing, and tissue repair [11]. In addition to these beneficial roles, cellular senescence has also been shown to be crucial in tissue pathophysiology, representing a key driver of ageing and age-related diseases [12–14]. Therefore, cellular senescence can be viewed as an example of antagonistic pleiotropy, which is a cellular program which is beneficial in one setting but deleterious in another [15].

Within the cardiovascular system, models of induced and attenuated senescence have implicated senescence in the pathophysiology of myocardial remodelling (age-related, chemotherapy-induced [16], and post-injury) [3,4,17–19], hypertension, atherosclerosis [20], and the development of aortic aneurysms [21], and have been extensively reviewed [22–27].

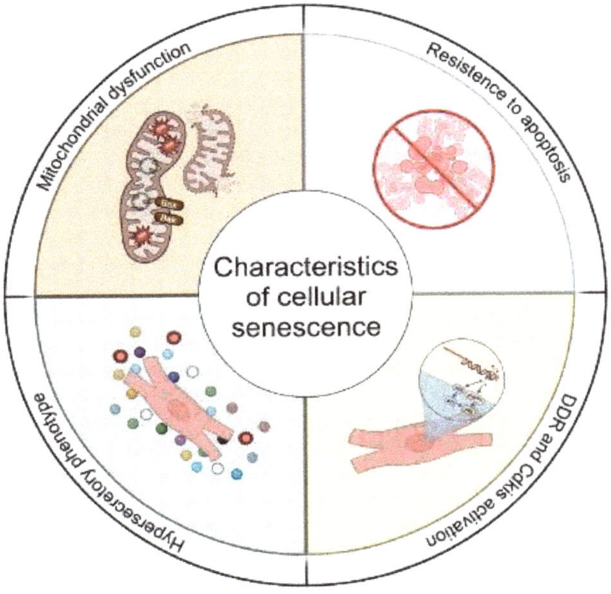

Figure 1. Common characteristics that define mitotic and post-mitotic senescent cells. DNA Damage Response (DDR) and Cyclin Dependant Kinase Inhibitors (Cdkis).

2. Mitochondrial Abnormalities in Cardiovascular Diseases

Mitochondria are double-membraned organelles with their own circular genome, mitochondrial DNA (mtDNA), which is replicated independently of the host genome [28]. Mitochondria are involved in diverse yet interconnected functions, including the production of adenosine triphosphate (ATP), and the regulation of nutritional metabolism, calcium homeostasis, and programmed cell death [29–31]. They are found in the cytoplasm of nearly all eukaryotic cells as highly dynamic networks, undergoing coordinated cycles of biogenesis, fusion, fission, and degradation (mitophagy) to sustain their homeostasis and to adapt energy production based on the cell's needs [32]. Proper mitochondrial function and dynamics are particularly necessary in tissues and cells with high energy demands such as the heart, and particularly in cardiomyocytes, which continuously require ATP to sustain cardiac activity. In adult cardiomyocytes, mitochondria occupy nearly one-third of the total intracellular volume [33] and provide approximately 95% of the ATP consumed by the heart [34]. It is, therefore, unsurprising that functional abnormalities in cardiac mitochondria have emerged as a key factor in cardiovascular disease (CVD) leading to decreased ATP production and energy supply, increased reactive oxygen species (ROS) production, cell apoptosis, and mitochondrial dynamic imbalance [35].

2.1. Energy Starvation and Oxidative Stress

Decreased energy supply is considered to be a leading consequence of mitochondrial dysfunction. The heart's voracious requirement for energy, in the form of ATP, mainly relies on oxidative phosphorylation (OXPHOS) or β-oxidation of fatty acids and the tricarboxylic acid (TCA) cycle in the mitochondria. During pathological myocardial remodelling, there is a reduction in the levels of carnitine in the heart [36], an essential cofactor for mediating the entry of fatty acids into the mitochondria at the site of β-oxidation [37]. Due to this reduction in fatty acids' availability within the mitochondria, cardiac metabolism is reprogrammed towards increased reliance on glucose as the energy resource with a significant increase in glycolysis, to maintain ATP production. However, ATP generated from glycolysis contributes less than 5% of the total ATP consumed [36], which is not enough to compensate for the reduction in fatty acid oxidation, and therefore, cardiac ATP is progressively depleted. The role of energy deprivation in the induction and pathogenesis of heart failure (HF) is well supported by clinical evidence, in which therapeutic measures to reduce energy consumption have been demonstrated to improve survival while treatment increasing energy demand is detrimental [38]. In the mitochondria, the synthesis of ATP takes place in the electron transport chain (ETC) [39]. Reduced nicotinamide adenine dinucleotide (NADH) and reduced flavin adenine dinucleotide ($FADH_2$) generated from the Krebs cycle, and from β-oxidation, transfer protons and electrons through the ETC, creating an electrochemical gradient that is then used to activate ATP synthase and produces ATP. Alterations in mtDNA genes such as NADH-dehydrogenase genes (*MT-ND1*, *MT-ND5* and *MT-ND6*), cytochrome b (*MT-CYB*), cytochrome c oxidase I and II (*MT-CO1* and *MT-CO2*), and ATP synthase 6 (*MT-ATP6*), have been described in dilated cardiomyopathies [40]. Reduced activities of complexes I and IV, as well as of the NADH phosphate (NADPH)-transhydrogenase and the Krebs cycle enzymes have been also observed in patients with HF [41,42]. Interestingly, some studies suggest that mtDNA mutations induce cardiovascular senescence and CVD, as demonstrated by the observation that $Polg^{m/m}$ mice, which are prone to the accumulation of mitochondrial DNA mutations, have increased expression of senescent markers $p16^{ink4a}$ and display early onset cardiomyopathy [43,44]. It remains unclear what mechanism mediates this induction, but an increase in mitochondrial ROS (mtROS) has been proposed as a causal factor.

Mitochondrial ATP production is accompanied by the generation of ROS (Figure 2), a generic term for an array of short-lived and unstable free radicals that contain oxygen with vastly different properties and biological functions that range from signalling (when strictly regulated) to causing cell damage [45]. Physiologically, ROS-mediated signalling pathways are associated with cell survival and proliferation, combatting infectious agents, and have mitogenic effects on cells [46,47]. However, excessive ROS production drives oxidative stress, a deleterious process that potentially causes irreversible damage to various molecules and structures within the cell [48], leading to further mitochondrial dysfunction, oxidative stress, and cell death [30,49]. Increased ROS appears to be capable of inducing senescence through several mechanisms. Telomeres are particularly sensitive to ROS-induced damage, possibly due to their guanine-rich regions, which increase their susceptibility to oxidation [50,51], and increased ROS can accelerate telomere attrition contributing to telomere dysfunction, premature senescence, and accelerated ageing [52]. ROS also generate DNA lesions in the form of single-stranded DNA and/or double-stranded breaks (DSBs) within the genomic or telomeric DNA. Eventually, as a result of telomere shortening or DNA damage, activation of the DNA damage response (DDR) occurs [53]. The DDR is an evolutionarily conserved signal transduction pathway required for genome integrity preservation. It coordinates cellular efforts to repair DNA damage, which, if unsuccessful, directs cell fate towards apoptosis or senescence thereby impeding the propagation of corrupted genetic information [54]. The DDR is characterised by the recruitment and activation of two large protein sensor kinases at the site of the lesion: ataxia telangiectasia and Rad3-related (ATR) protein when single-stranded DNA is exposed, and ataxia-telangiectasia mutated (ATM) protein at DSBs. The recruitment of ATR or ATM to the lesion causes the local formation of DNA damage foci containing the phosphorylated form of the histone H2AX (γH2AX) and ultimately inducing cell-cycle arrest through the activation of checkpoint proteins, including p53 [55]. Furthermore, once senescent, cells exhibit a decreased mitochondrial membrane potential, increased proton leak, and enhanced production of mtROS [56]. As such, the elevated ROS observed in senescent cells may drive mtDNA damage creating a positive feedback loop leading to further increases in ROS and DNA damage highlighting the cyclical interactions between mitochondrial dysfunction, oxidative stress, and senescence, and illustrating how the initiation of any of these processes could lead to a downward spiral in tissue function.

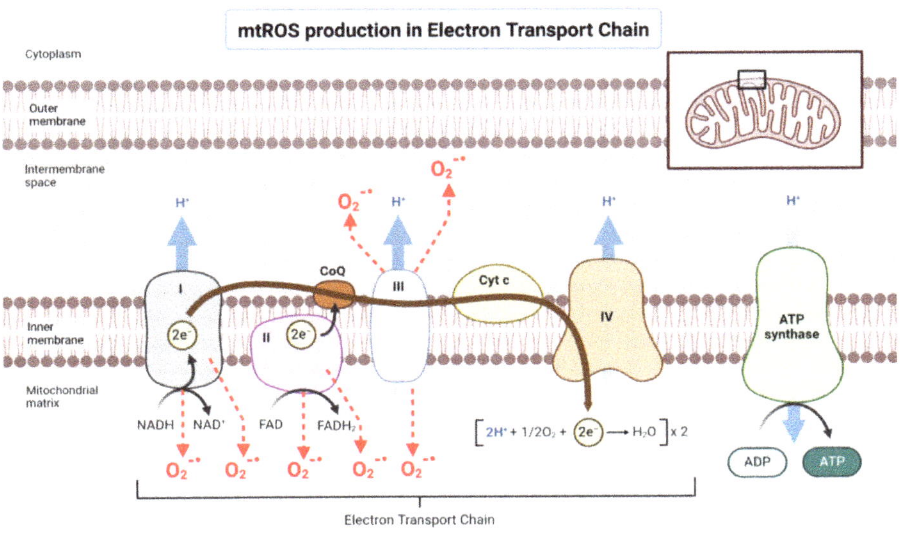

Figure 2. Illustrates mitochondrial reactive oxygen species (mtROS) production within the electron transport chain (ETC). Electrons, initially provided by NADH in complex I and FADH2 in complex II, traverse through ubiquinone to reach complex III. Subsequently, they move to complex IV via cytochrome c, where they combine with molecular oxygen to generate water. Proton-pumping activities by complex I, complex III, and complex IV into the intermembrane space establish a proton gradient crucial for ATP synthesis. During oxidative phosphorylation, electron leakage occurs, leading to the interaction with molecular oxygen and the formation of superoxide ($O_2^{-\cdot}$). Complex I and complex III serve as the primary sites for ROS production within the mitochondria, while complex II also contributes. Complex III directs superoxide production both towards the matrix and the intermembrane space, whereas complex I and complex II exclusively produce ROS towards the matrix. Key components and molecules involved include coenzyme Q (CoQ), cytochrome c (Cyt c), electrons (e−), protons (H+), adenosine diphosphate (ADP), adenosine triphosphate (ATP), reduced (NADH) and oxidized (NAD+) nicotinamide adenine dinucleotide, flavin adenine dinucleotide (FAD), oxygen (O_2).

Perhaps unsurprisingly, given the high-volume density of mitochondria required to fulfil the heart's energy demand, the heart has both high mtROS production and elevated mtROS, which have been shown to contribute to the pathophysiology of a variety of CVDs, including atherosclerosis, cardiac ischemia/reperfusion (IR) injury, HF, cardiac hypertrophy, and degenerative aortic valve disease [30,34,49,57]. ROS has also been shown to be a powerful inducer of senescence in multiple tissues and cell types, including the heart. Monoamine oxidase A (MAO-A) is a protein linked with driving oxidative stress; it is located at the outer mitochondrial membrane, involved in catalysing the oxidative deamination of monoamines, and produces hydrogen peroxide as one of its by-products [58].

Interestingly, cardiomyocyte-specific overexpression of MAO-A results in elevated ROS, increased senescence and mice display a dilated cardiomyopathy and myocardial dysfunction [59]. All of these can be rescued by treatment with antioxidants [4]. Similarly, the accelerated ageing mouse model *nfkb1*$^{-/-}$ showed increased ROS, telomere dysfunction, and cardiomyocyte hypertrophy [60]. Similar observations have been reported in more clinically relevant models: aged mice treated with the mitochondrial-targeted peptide SS-31 elamipretide had reduced myocardial ROS and improved cardiac function, which was associated with reduced senescence [61]. Furthermore, aged, senescent cardiomyocytes demonstrated an overall decline in the expression of most mitochondrial genes—particularly those genes involved in the ETC—and mitochondrial ultrastructural defects detected by transmission electron microscopy [61]. Myocardial infarction (MI) results in alterations to mitochondrial dynamics, culminating in increased ROS production and increased oxidative stress, particularly when followed by the clinical gold-standard treatment of reperfusion [62]. Several studies have shown that, even in this acute setting of increased oxidative stress, senescence is induced in multiple cell populations, including cardiomyocytes, and that these cells are active participants in post-MI myocardial remodelling since their elimination attenuates inflammation remodelling and improves functional outcomes [17,19].

Being so closely associated with cardiomyocyte dysfunction, mitochondrial damage is of major interest when exploring the mechanisms underpinning the cardiotoxicity of many otherwise beneficial therapeutics. This is relevant to both preclinical drug development, where cardiac liabilities remain a leading cause of drug attrition [63,64], but also to therapies approved for clinical use today which risk future withdrawal from the market due to cardiac adverse drug reactions (ADRs) [65]. Both traditional and new-generation oncology treatments are plagued by off-target cardiotoxic effects [66]. With cardiovascular disease being a leading noncancer cause of death in an ever-growing population of cancer survivors, understanding the mechanisms behind these cardiotoxicities is increasingly important [67]. As a case in point, anthracycline chemotherapies are notoriously chronically cardiotoxic and have been shown to deleteriously affect mitochondrial function in many ways.

Doxorubicin (DOX), an anthracycline commonly used in clinics, was historically shown to redox cycle via interactions with mitochondrial complex I, generating excessive ROS as a result [68,69]. Studies have subsequently demonstrated that DOX has a high affinity for cardiolipin, a lipid housed in the inner mitochondrial membrane which is essential for effective energy metabolism and proper mitochondrial function [70]. Notably, DOX becomes concentrated in the mitochondria of isolated neonatal rat cardiomyocytes, supporting the notion that this organelle is particularly vulnerable to off-target anthracycline toxicity [71]. Zhang and colleagues showed that mitochondrial function and oxidative phosphorylation pathways were disturbed in cardiomyocytes isolated from DOX-dosed mice, and that this was dependent on the topoisomerase IIβ (TopIIβ) enzyme which is thought to be crucial in the cardiotoxicity of this drug [72]. It has since been shown that DOX intercalates into mtDNA, which aids its accumulation in cardiomyocyte mitochondria in the same model [73]. Furthermore, Ichikawa and colleagues showed that DOX causes iron accumulation in cardiomyocyte mitochondria, leading to downstream toxicity. DOX treatment is associated with the depletion and mutation of mtDNA, as identified in the hearts of cancer patients [74]. The interplay between DOX-induced mitochondrial damage and cardiomyocyte senescence within this cardiotoxicity is less well-understood, but it has been shown that the two phenomena go hand-in-hand using in vitro and in vivo studies, as evidenced by Mitry et. al., amongst others [75–77]. As a long-established therapy, the impact of DOX upon cardiomyocyte mitochondria has been well reviewed [78], but newer oncology therapies are far less well-understood. For example, though tyrosine kinase inhibitors (TKIs) provide more targeted anticancer actions, the TKI sorafenib has historically been shown to impair cardiomyocyte mitochondrial function at clinically relevant doses in vitro, and more recent reports highlight that sunitinib may also induce cardiomyocyte mitochondrial damage via ROS accumulation [79,80]. Several other oncology therapies display off-target cardiovascular effects and mitochondrial toxicities [81] and it is clear the changing landscape of cancer survivorship necessitates thorough investigations into the long-term cardiac effects of both established and emerging antineoplastic therapies, and mitochondrial toxicity remains an attractive avenue of research.

2.2. Mitochondria Dynamics Imbalance

In physiological conditions, mitochondria constantly undergo co-ordinated cycles of fusion and fission, also referred to as mitochondrial dynamics [82]. Mitochondrial fusion is characterised by the union of two mitochondria resulting in one elongated mitochondrion, which allows for the dynamic repair of reversibly damaged mitochondria. Conversely, mitochondrial fission is characterised by the fragmentation of one irreversibly damaged and potentially harmful mitochondrion into small and spherical mitochondria that can be isolated and removed by mitophagy [83,84]. The coordination of these events is essential for the maintenance of mitochondrial quantity and quality, and therefore, the balance between them plays a vital role in the normal function of the cardiovascular system. Indeed, accumulating evidence has confirmed the influence of mitochondrial dynamics on the pathogenesis of CVD [82].

Mitochondrial fusion is first mediated by the transmembrane guanine triphosphatase (GTPase) proteins, mitofusin 1 (MFN1) and MFN2 in the outer mitochondrial membrane, and then by the optic atrophy protein 1 (OPA1) in the inner membrane [85]. Decreased levels of MFN1 and MFN2 have been found in animal models of atherosclerosis [86], and a decreased expression of OPA1 has been observed in post-MI hearts, which correlated with the downregulation of mtDNA and antioxidant genes [87]. Suggesting a causal role of fusion in CVD, ablation of the murine *Mfn1* and *Mfn2* genes in adult hearts induced mitochondrial fragmentation and dysfunction, and rapidly progressive and lethal dilated cardiomyopathy [88,89]. Different cardiac pathologies have also been associated with the formation of giant mitochondria or megamitochondria, as reviewed in [70], which evolve by fusion of the membranes of numerous large individual organelles due to the overexpression of protein fusion [90]. The opposing process, mitochondrial fission, is controlled by Mitochondrial fission protein 1 (Fis1) and Dynamin-related protein 1 (Drp1). It has been reported that Drp1 activation during cardiac IR results in left ventricular dysfunction and that Drp1 inhibition reduces cell death, preserves mitochondrial morphology, and inhibits the mitochondrial permeability transition pore [91,92]. While the relationship between mitochondrial fusion and myocardial senescence has yet to be investigated, elongated mitochondria have been observed in several senescent cell types, including fibroblasts, and are relevant to CVD, iPSC-derived and primary rat cardiomyocytes in vitro [93,94], and the depletion of *Fis1* mRNA levels leads to mitochondrial elongation, induces senescence, and increases ROS production [93,95].

Fusion and fission events control mitochondria biogenesis [96], a process that increases the number of mitochondria, improves the replication and repair of mtDNA, and induces the synthesis of mitochondrial enzymes and proteins [30]. The co-transcriptional regulator factor peroxisome-proliferator-activated receptor γ co-activator-1α (PGC-1α) induces mitochondrial biogenesis by activating the mitochondrial transcription factor A (TFAM), which drives the transcription and replication of mtDNA [97]. Reduced gene expression of PGC-1α has been associated with failing human hearts [98] and there is evidence that sirtuin-1 (SIRT1), a protein involved in metabolic regulation, delays the molecular characteristics of myocardial ageing by mediating the deacetylation of PGC-1α and the activation of mitochondrial biogenesis [99]. The *PGC-1*$\alpha^{+/-}$/*ApoE*$^{-/-}$ mouse model has shown that *PGC-1*α deficiency promotes vascular senescence, which is associated with increased oxidative stress, mitochondrial abnormalities, and reduced telomerase activity [100]. Mitochondrial biogenesis is also accompanied by variations in mitochondrial morphology [101]. Generally, various aspects of cardiovascular biology, including cardiac development, the response to cardiac IR injury and HF, are related to morphological and structural changes in mitochondria [87,91,102]. Dramatic changes in mitochondrial morphology have also been found in senescent cells, where mitochondria exist in a state of hyper-fusion as a response to reduced expression of mediators of the fission process and an overall reduction in the frequency of the fission and fusion events [103].

2.3. Cell Apoptosis and Mitophagy

Mitochondria are pivotal in controlling apoptosis, including the release of caspase activators and the participation of B-cell lymphoma-2 (BCL-2) family proteins [104,105]. Cardiomyocyte apoptosis plays a critical role in the pathogenesis and progression of all types of heart disease, particularly in ischemic heart disease and HF of various aetiologies [106]. For example, cardiac IR injury is related to the apoptotic death of cardiac muscle cells by activating the pro-apoptotic BCL-2 regulators BAX and BAK to change the integrity of the mitochondrial membrane and the cytosolic release of pro-apoptotic factors, which triggers caspase-dependent cell death [107]. In hypertension, the hormone angiotensin II, which plays an important role in volume and blood pressure control, has been linked to cardiomyocyte apoptosis in rats, and treatment with losartan has been associated with a reduction in cardiomyocyte apoptosis in both spontaneous hypertensive rats and hypertensive patients [108]. The subfamily of pro-apoptotic BCL-2 homology (BH) BH3-only proteins, BCL2/adenovirus E1B 19 kDa protein-interacting protein 3 (BNIP3) and its homologue BNIP3-like (BNIP3L or Nix), also induce apoptosis [109] and the forced expression of these genes is sufficient to induce cardiomyopathy in murine models [35,110,111]. Mitochondria are also important in other forms of cell death including necrosis. The mitochondrial permeability transition pore (MPTP), localized on the inner membrane of mitochondria, is the main player in oxidative stress-dependent cell death and increased mPTP is associated with ageing and age-associated disease [112]. In the context of the heart, mPTP activation is fundamental in causing myocardial damage following ischaemia-reperfusion (I/R) both as a result of myocardial infarction and transplantation. At the onset of ischaemia, oxidative phosphorylation is arrested due to a lack of oxygen which leads to the depolarisation of the mitochondrial membrane and loss of ATP. As the cellular metabolism rapidly shifts to anaerobic glycolysis, lactic acid is generated and the associated accumulation of hydrogen ions reduces intracellular pH levels, inhibiting myofibril contraction and closure of the mPTP. Upon reperfusion, the respiratory chain is rapidly exposed to oxygen, leading to oxidative stress, and Ca^{2+} accumulates due to rapid mitochondrial membrane potential restoration and pH is neutralized, which all contribute to the opening of the mPTP. The opening of the mPTP allows the free passage of molecules, including protons, through the inner mitochondrial membrane, uncoupling oxidative phosphorylation and disrupting ATP production. Impaired energy metabolism further results in a continuous cycle of increasing Ca^{2+} and mPTP causing osmotic swelling and damage and mitochondrial disruption and cellular necrosis [113]. Furthermore, this mitochondrial membrane disruption may also lead to a release of proapoptotic proteins, including cytochrome c, thereby also inducing apoptosis [112].

To prevent cardiomyocytes containing damaged mitochondria from undergoing apoptosis, mitophagy, a cargo-specific form of autophagy selectively targets the degradation of dysfunctional and damaged, and hence potentially cytotoxic, mitochondria within a cell [30]. There are two mechanisms described for mitophagy: adaptor-mediated and receptor-mediated. The former pathway functions via Phosphatase and Tensin Homolog (PTEN)-induced putative kinase 1 (PINK1) and Parkin-mediated mitophagy [114]. PINK1 is a serine/threonine kinase that continuously monitors mitochondrial health and provides a rapid response when mitochondrial function collapses [115]. When mitochondria lose membrane potential or amass unfolded protein, PINK1 accumulates on the outer membrane and both recruits and directly phosphorylates E3 ubiquitin ligase [115,116] or phosphorylates E3 ubiquitin via the intermediate phosphorylation of MFN2 [116]. The accumulation of ubiquitin in key mitochondria-associated proteins on the outer mitochondrial membrane, amplifies a signalling cascade involved in the recruitment of autophagosomes to target the damaged mitochondria. The mitochondria-containing autophagosome is trafficked to, and fused with, a lysosome and degraded [117]. In healthy young hearts, there is an underlying level of baseline mitophagy which is essential for maintaining cellular homeostasis in an energy-efficient heart, and for responding and adapting to stress [118]. However, decreased mitophagy is associated with CVD, as an accumulation of "old" defective mitochondria may reduce the heart's potential to adapt to stress. Indeed, multiple animal studies have linked the deletion of mitophagy-related genes at the whole-body level or cardiomyocytes with the spontaneous development of cardiovascular disorders [119]. For example, mice bearing a cardiomyocyte-specific deletion of *Mnf2* prematurely succumbed to progressive cardiomyopathy, which could be partially reversed by restoring mitophagy in cardiomyocytes via the expression of the antioxidant enzyme catalase [120]. The whole-body $Pink1^{-/-}$ mice experienced left ventricular dysfunction and pathological cardiac hypertrophy by 2 months of age [121]. Mitophagy is also essential for reducing cardiac injury following MI. Under baseline conditions, *Parkin*-deficient mice hearts were shown to have smaller and disorganised mitochondria as revealed by ultrastructural analysis, but mitochondrial and cardiac function were unaffected [122]. However, after MI, these mice had reduced survival and developed larger infarcts when compared to control mice, which was associated with the rapid accumulation of dysfunctional mitochondria in the infarct border zone [122]. In patients with late-stage heart disease, a low number of autophagosomes in cardiomyocytes is associated with a poor prognosis [123]. Damaging events (e.g., acute cardiac IR injury) lead to the reduction in the autophagy flux, and as a consequence, damaged dysfunctional mitochondria accumulate in cardiomyocytes, leading to severe oxidative stress and apoptosis [124]. The destabilisation of atherosclerotic plaques has also been associated with deficient mitophagy [125,126]. Furthermore, a reduced expression of autophagic markers p62 and microtubule-associated protein light chain (LC3)-II has been detected within atherosclerotic plaques from human samples and mouse models [127,128]. In mouse models, the activation of mitophagy through antioxidant therapeutic strategies has been explored to stabilise atherosclerotic plaques [129].

Aside from the conventional forms of mitophagy, there are additional specialized pathways including a process which exhibits a notable level of specificity and involves mitochondrial-derived vesicles, as well as the selective removal of mitochondrial fragments containing specific cargo rather than the entire organelle. This mechanism relies on the coordination of mitochondrial dynamics, mitophagy, and the vacuolar protein sorting (VPS) or retromer complex. In this process, alterations to mitochondrial membrane potential and the oxidation state of mitochondrial sub-compartments induce membrane curvature. This, in turn, leads to the recruitment of PINK1 and Parkin. The retromer complex, comprised of the VPS26, VPS29, and VPS35 proteins, plays a crucial role by providing the force needed to generate a vesicle. Importantly, these vesicles are subsequently delivered to lysosomes or peroxisomes, and this delivery process operates independently of the autophagy proteins Autophagy related 5 or Microtubule-associated protein 1A/1B-light chain 3 [130]. It remains to be seen if changes in the dynamics of this non-canonical form of mitophagy are associated with CVD or senescence.

Interestingly, despite and perhaps because of mitochondrial dysfunction, senescent cells express pro-survival pathways, enhancing survival and increasing resistance to apoptosis. Senescent cells are more resistant to apoptosis in response to stimuli, including serum withdrawal, ultraviolet damage, oxidative stress, and treatment with cytotoxic drugs [131]. While there is a heterogeneity between cell types and senescence stimuli, enhanced activation of several pathways including BCL-2 family members, p53/p21Cip, ephrins (EFNB1 or 3), the phosphatidylinositol-4,5-bisphosphate 3-kinase delta catalytic subunit (PI3KCD), plasminogen-activated inhibitor-1 and 2 (PAI1 and 2), and hypoxia-inducible factor-1α (HIF1α) can be involved [132–134] and are referred to as senescent cell anti-apoptotic pathways (SCAPs). As discussed below, the activation of these pathways may contribute to the proinflammatory nature of senescent cells.

3. Mitochondria Dysfunction, Senescence, and Inflammation in CVD

The role of inflammation in promoting CVD is increasingly recognised. Recent discoveries have demonstrated that mitochondria are key elements that stimulate innate immune signalling cascades which trigger inflammation and promote pathology in an expanding list of diseases, including cardiac pathologies [135]. Many investigations have revealed that, when mitochondrial integrity is compromised, mtROS and mtDNA act as damage-associated molecular patterns (DAMPs), endogenous molecules that are isolated within intracellular compartments and discharged to the extracellular space in response to damaged or dying cells [136], promoting pathological inflammatory responses by binding with pattern-recognition receptors (PRRs). For example, a study on mice found that mtDNA released by dying ischemic cells during MI activates the Interferon regulatory factor 3 (IRF3)-dependent innate immune response, which has a harmful effect on ventricular remodelling after MI [137]. The Stimulator of interferon genes (STING)-IRF3 pathway might also facilitate chronic inflammation and dysfunction in endothelial cells via sensing mtDNA [138], which are key events in the development of atherosclerosis and are associated with an elevated risk of many cardiovascular events [139]. Furthermore, cytoplasmic mtDNA which escapes from autophagy-mediated degradation cell-autonomously has been linked with the activation of the immune system via Toll-like receptor 9 (TLR9), which has been associated with elevated arterial pressure and vascular dysfunction in spontaneously hypertensive rats [140], and with exacerbated HF in mice [141]. Accumulating evidence has also shown that mtROS and mtDNA contribute to molecular inflammation events during the pathogenesis of CVDs, activating the Nod-like receptor (NLR) family, pyrin domain containing 3 (NLRP3) inflammasome [142,143], although how this unfolds remains unknown. For example, excessive mtROS and dysfunctional mitochondria are considered critical drivers responsible for NLRP3 activation during the progression of atherosclerosis, and the level of the inflammasome has been found to be highly associated with the severity of disease [144]. Upon activation, NLRP3 inflammasome activates caspase-1, which cleaves and matures the pro-inflammatory cytokines interleukin (IL)-1β and IL-18, which contribute to cardiac fibrosis and HF [145]. Elevated IL-1β levels have been also correlated with age-related CVD [143]. Furthermore, the suppression of NLRP3 extends the lifespan of obese adult mice by reducing liver steatosis and cardiac damage [146]. In turn, PRRs might also modulate mitochondrial dysfunction and apoptosis, protecting against mortality as occurs with the receptor NLR family member X1 (NLRX1) during IR injury [147].

A significant characteristic of senescent cells is the acquisition of a hypersecretory phenotype or SASP, a collection of many biologically active factors, such as inflammatory cytokines, chemokines, matrix remodelling proteases, extracellular vesicles, and growth factors [148]. This heterogeneous group of secreted proteins self-reinforce and spread senescence in an autocrine and paracrine manner, respectively, or affect the local tissue environment of senescent cells, and possibly, the entire organism [9]. Although some SASP factors are common to all senescent cells, its composition varies depending on the cell type and the nature of the stimulus [149]. In senescent cardiomyocytes, increased expression of SASP factors such as cellular communication network protein family member 1 (CCN1), interleukins (IL1α, IL1β, and IL6), tumour necrosis factor-alpha (TNFα), monocyte chemoattractant protein-1 (MCP1), endothelin 3 (Edn3), tumour growth factor-beta (TGFβ), and growth and differentiation factor 15 (GDF15) have been clinically linked with age-related myocardial ischemia and infarction [4,17,150]. mtROS are a component of the SASP [151], and functional mitochondria are critical for SASP production. As would be expected, senescent cells with depleted mitochondria have reduced ROS generation and also lose their proinflammatory phenotype yet remain in cell cycle arrest [77]. SASP production appears to involve mitochondria through several interconnected mechanisms. mtROS can induce c-Jun N-terminal kinase (JNK) signalling and the release of cytoplasmic chromatin fragments, triggering the innate immunity cytosolic DNA-sensing cyclic GMP-AMP synthase (cGAS)-STING pathway [152]. This, in turn, activates nuclear factor-κB (NFκB) signalling, switching on the transcription of proinflammatory genes and the

SASP [152]. Recent studies suggest that expression of pro-survival pathways in senescent cells leads to sublethal apoptosis and minority mitochondrial outer membrane permeabilization (miMOMP). This miMOMP allows the release of mtDNA into the cytosol which activates the cGAS–STING pathway, resulting in the increased expression of inflammatory mediators and SASP [153]. The sublethal release of cytochrome c and caspase activation, associated with miMOMP may also contribute to further DNA damage, increased genetic instability, and perhaps deeper senescence [154]. Similarly, oxidative stress-dependent, but sub-lethal activation of mPTP may allow the release of solutes and ions, including superoxide, hydrogen peroxide, and calcium, resulting in damage to both mitochondrial and cellular proteins, lipids, and DNA, and thus accelerating cell aging [155].

4. Mitochondrial and Senescent Cells Targeted Therapies for CVD

4.1. Therapeutically Targeting Mitochondrial Dysfunction

In recent years, an increasing number of cardiac mitochondrial targets have shown their cardioprotective effects in experimental and clinical studies. Mitochondria are not only the site of OXPHOS; their dysfunction is also commonly associated with ATP deficiency and excessive ROS generation. Therefore, restoring their ATP-producing capacity and counteracting the damaging effects of ROS to reduce oxidative stress and chronic inflammation have been suggested as primary therapeutic targets to improve mitochondrial dysfunction [31].

AMP-activated protein kinase (AMPK) is an exclusive kinase of eukaryotes that plays a major role in regulating energy balance by monitoring changes in the level of intracellular ATP and coupling these changes to phosphorylation of downstream substrates, leading to an increase in ATP synthesis and/or a restriction of ATP depletion [156]. Thus, targeting the AMPK pathway has attracted widespread interest [30]. A well-known AMPK agonist is the first-line drug for treating Type 2 diabetes mellitus (T2DM), metformin [157]. Mechanistically, it has been widely accepted that metformin exerts beneficial effects through the inhibition of the respiratory chain at the level of Complex 1, leading to an increased AMP/ATP ratio and activation of the signalling kinase AMPK [158], which in turn, induces muscles to take up glucose from the blood. However, this mechanism requires higher doses of metformin than those used in the clinical routine [159]. Recently, it has been reported that clinically relevant doses of metformin activate AMPK through the lysosomal pathway, without perturbing AMP/ATP levels [159]. The authors demonstrated that metformin targeted lysosomal presenilin enhancer protein 2 (PEN2), which then inhibited the vacuolar H^+-ATPase (v-ATPase) on the lysosome by binding to its AT6AP1 subunit. The formation of the PEN2-AT6AP1 axis initiates the lysosomal glucose-sensing pathway for AMPK activation [160]. Metformin also improves mitochondrial function and quality, as AMPK activation phosphorylates a range of target proteins involved in the regulation of mitochondrial biogenesis (PCG-1α), mitochondrial dynamics (Drp1, MFF), and mitophagy (PINK1-Parkin pathway) [161–164]. Interestingly, metformin has been described as senomorphic, being able to modulate SASP secretion from senescent cells and improve senescent cell function [165,166]. Metformin is inhibitory to SASP expression due to its inhibition of IκB kinase and IKKα/β phosphorylation, thereby preventing the NF-κB nuclear translocation [167]. Furthermore, metformin can attenuate senescence in human diploid fibroblasts and mesenchymal stem cells [168], and in healthy mice, metformin has been observed to extend health span and lifespan [169].

Indicating that metformin may have similar effects clinically, a recent meta-analysis has identified that patients with diabetes taking metformin have a significantly increased survival rate and a reduced incidence of age-related diseases, including CVD [170]. Several clinical studies have shown the beneficial effects of metformin in diabetes-related atherosclerosis, IR injury, and arrhythmia (as discussed by Bu et al.) [171]. For example, in the Reversing with MetfOrmin Vascular Adverse Lesions (REMOVAL) trial, a double-blind placebo-controlled randomized controlled trial to evaluate the cardiovascular effects of metformin in adults with T1DM, atherosclerosis progression was significantly reduced in metformin-treated patients [172]. In another randomized, placebo-controlled trial involving 390 patients with T2DM treated with insulin, metformin treatment improved endothelial function [173]. In non-diabetes patients, clinical studies are more controversial when evaluating the benefits of metformin in CVD. In a small clinical study consisting of 33 women who did not have diabetes, metformin reduced myocardial ischemia and improved endothelium-dependent microvascular responses in patients with angina, compared to the placebo [174]. However, in a subsequent clinical study consisting of 173 patients without diabetes with coronary heart disease treated with statins, Preiss et al. [175] found that metformin had no effect on disease progression and little or no effect on several surrogate markers of CVD. Although it remains unclear if the senomorphic activity of metformin contributes to any of these cardioprotective effects, in patients with carotid artery atherosclerosis, metformin ameliorates the proinflammatory state, which includes a reduction in serval SASP related proteins including IL-6 and TNF-α [176]. Metformin also influences other hallmarks of biological ageing. For example, nutrient-signalling pathways both through AMPK and SIRT1 activation, as well as downregulating insulin/insulin-like growth factor 1 (IGF-1) signalling and mechanistic targeting of rapamycin complex 1 (mTORC1). Metformin also attenuates oxidative damage and genome instability by enhancing DNA damage response and repair mechanisms, improving proteostasis by enhancing autophagy and inhibiting protein synthesis, and ameliorating mitochondrial dysfunction via mitochondrial complex I inhibition and PGC-1α upregulation. Furthermore, metformin treatment reduces telomere shortening by activating telomeric repeat-containing RNA [177]. Metformin is now being evaluated for its age-targeting effects in the TAME (Targeting Ageing with Metformin) clinical trial [178].

Because of the role of ROS in CVD, a reduction in oxidative stress through the supplementation with antioxidants such as Coenzyme Q10 (CoQ10), vitamin E, vitamin C, and β-carotene has been clinically studied in humans for the treatment of CVD, including HF, atherosclerosis, and acute MI [179–182]. However, with the sole exception of CoQ10, no clinically significant benefits were reported. CoQ10 is a lipid-soluble and biologically active quinone whose principal role is to participate in the ETC, where it functions as an electron carrier [183]. In a study including 420 patients with moderate to severe HF, Svend et al. [179] reported that long-term treatment with CoQ10, in addition to standard therapy, was safe, and associated with an improvement in symptoms and a reduction in mortality from cardiovascular events. Zeb et al. [180] reported beneficial effects on inflammatory markers and reduced progression of coronary atherosclerosis in patients treated with a capsule containing aged garlic extract and CoQ10 daily for 1 year. In a meta-analysis of 14 studies with 2149 enrolled subjects Lei et al. [184] found that patients with HF who used coQ10 had lower mortality.

One possible explanation for the ineffectiveness of common antioxidants to show beneficial effects is their inability to enter the mitochondria, the primary source of ROS [185]. There are several approaches to targeting molecules towards the mitochondria and one of the most versatile is to develop synthetically modified antioxidants with lipophilic cationic compounds, such as triphenylphosphonium (TPP+) [186]. TPP+ is a membrane-permeant cation that is accumulated within the mitochondria up to several-hundredfold-fold because of the negative potential (-140 to −180 mV) generated across the inner mitochondrial membrane by the proton pumping action of the ETC [187]. Mitoquinone (MitoQ) is CoQ10 conjugated to TPP^+ and has been shown to display impressive benefits in the treatment of CVD. It has been reported that 100 μM MitoQ in drinking water rescues the cardiac function of pressure-overloaded HF in a mouse model by decreasing hydrogen peroxide formation, improving mitochondrial respiration and mitochondrial permeability transition pore opening [188]. In mice and rat studies, MitoQ protected against IR injury by blocking oxidative damage within the mitochondria [189,190]. Treatment with MitoQ also prevented the development of hypertension, improved endothelial function, and limited cardiac hypertrophy in eight-week-old male spontaneously hypertensive rats [191]. Furthermore, MitoQ controls the expression levels of cardiac hypertrophy-associated transcript (*Chast*) and myosin heavy chain-associated transcript (*Mhrt*), two long non-coding RNAs involved in cardiac remodelling. It also attenuates adverse cardiac remodelling, and prevents HF in mice by inhibiting the interplay between TGF-β1 and mitochondrial-associated redox signalling [192]. In humans, a randomized, placebo-controlled, double-blind, crossover study of 20 healthy adults (60–79 years) with endothelial dysfunction demonstrated that oral supplementation with 20 mg/day of MitoQ was well tolerated and significantly improved endothelial function and reduced arterial stiffness and plasma-oxidized low-density lipoprotein (LDL), a marker of oxidative stress, through a reduction in mtROS [193]. Currently, in the USA, there are two ongoing clinical trials focused on the effects of MitoQ on cardiac function: the MitoQ Supplementation and Cardiovascular Function in Healthy Men and Women study (NCT03960073), and the Chronic Kidney Disease and Heart Failure With Preserved Ejection Fraction: The Role of Mitochondrial Dysfunction study (NCT03586414). Given that ROS is both an inducer and a consequence of senescence, it is perhaps unsurprising that, in a wide range of diseases and models, anti-oxidants (including those that are mitochondrial targeted) are demonstrated to attenuate senescence and SASP [194].

4.2. Senolytics, Senomorphics and Future Approaches

Despite active DNA damage responses, increased mitochondrial dysfunction, increased mitochondrial membrane permeability, and increased ROS production, senescent cells remain resistant to apoptosis. Based on these findings, Zhu and colleagues hypothesized that pharmacologically inhibiting the pro-survival networks could eliminate senescent cells [132]. This gave rise to the advent of compounds collectively termed senolytics, which target various components of anti-apoptotic pathways, including BCL-2 family members, to promote senescent cell apoptosis.

In the context of heart health, studies have largely investigated the senolytic effects of the combination therapy dasatinib and quercetin (D&Q), and navitoclax (ABT-263). Dasatinib is a second-generation tyrosine kinase inhibitor, shown to inhibit ephrins, disrupting the pro-survival network that includes BCL-XL, PI3K, p21Cip, PAI1, and PAI2 [132,195,196]. Quercetin, a natural flavanol, inhibits multiple pro-survival proteins, including PAIs and PI3K, ultimately reducing BCL-W expression [197,198]. Navitoclax, a BH3 mimetic, induces senescent cell apoptosis by inhibiting anti-apoptotic proteins BCL-2, BCL-XL, and BCL-W [199,200].

Use of these senolytics in several animal models of CVD, such as age-related myocardial dysfunction, MI, anthracycline-induced cardiotoxicity and atherosclerosis, has provided proof-of-principle data that promoting mitochondrial mediated apoptosis in senescent cells reduces inflammation and attenuates disease pathophysiology [17,19,132,201–204]. On the other hand, as increased apoptosis has been implicated in age-related myocardial dysfunction, and after MI the primary objective of reperfusion therapy is to save as much myocardium as possible, concerns have been raised regarding the long-term outcomes of increased cell death [3]. However, recent studies have demonstrated that senescent cardiomyocytes are indeed detrimental to the outcome, and that the inhibition/modulation of the senescent phenotype may be beneficial in the senescent cardiomyocyte context: inhibition of *p16* in murine cardiomyocytes improved outcome following MI with reperfusion [3].

In the future, the modulation/inhibition of the senescent phenotype may be a more feasible route to successful intervention in this disease context, rather than the promotion of senescent cardiomyocyte apoptosis. As such, a senomorphic approach, modulating the senescent phenotype and attenuating the SASP, may consequently have more translational potential than senotherapies. Alternatively, specific inhibition of miMOMP-induced inflammation [153], may have therapeutic utility. For instance, the inhibition of the mitochondrial membrane BAX and BAK nanopores with small-molecule BAX inhibitor BAI1 was shown to decrease systemic inflammation and improve health span in aged mice [153]. Underpinning all these findings, the evaluation of a drug's senolytic and/or senomorphic capabilities must be approached with rigour and caution, as emphasised in Niedernhofer and Robbins' 2018 correspondence [204].

5. Conclusions

In the complex realm of cardiovascular diseases, mitochondrial dysfunction, and oxidative stress (in isolation or within the context of senescence induction and senescent cell function) play a key role in pathophysiology (Figure 3). A better understanding of these interconnected phenomena will enable the development of novel therapies for CVD. Ongoing research and clinical trials signal a new frontier in cardiovascular medicine, promising innovative treatments that could transform patient outcomes. These developments mark a significant stride towards enhancing both the quality and duration of life for those affected by cardiovascular diseases.

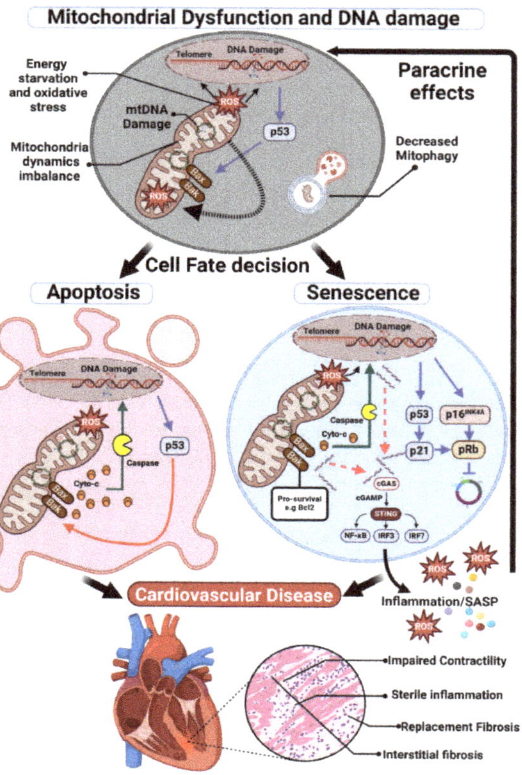

Figure 3. Mitochondrial dysfunction contributes to cardiovascular disease through apoptosis and senescence. Mitochondrial dysfunction and increased ROS production promote DNA damage, both chromosomal and mitochondrial. DNA damage leads to p53 activation and a cell-fate decision between apoptosis and senescence. In apoptotic cells p53 induces mitochondrial outer membrane permeabilization via formation of the apoptotic pore which allows cytochrome c release, activation of the caspase cascade, and cell death. While not yet completely understood, but perhaps as a result as less severe stress, DNA damage and p53 can lead to expression of the p21 (a negative regulator of apoptosis and the cell cycle), activation of the p16 pathway, or activation of both p21 and p16 pathways resulting in cellular senescence. Upregulation of pro-survival pathways in senescent cells suppresses apoptotic pore formation leading to miMOMP, sublethal apoptosis and the release of mtDNA into the cytoplasm. mtDNA fragments are sensed by the cGAS-STING pathway, upregulating expression of inflammatory mediators. Sublethal activation of the caspase cascade may also promote additional DNA damage. A combination of apoptosis and senescence will drive pathological myocardial remodelling.

Author Contributions: M.C.-E., I.S. and G.D.R. conceptualized and supervised the draft, and M.C.-E., L.K.B., G.D.R. and O.F. looked for, read, and made a first selection of the most relevant articles, and M.C.-E., L.K.B. and G.D.R. wrote the draft, and L.K.B. and R.E.R. reviewed and edited the draft. All authors have read and agreed to the published version of the manuscript.

Funding: This work has been funded by the British Heart Foundation (PG/23/11571, PG/21/10761 and PG/22/10788), Heart Research UK (PHD23-100007) and the MRC.

Acknowledgments: Figures made in Biorender.

Conflicts of Interest: The authors declare no conflicts of interest.

eferences

1. Hayflick, L.; Moorhead, P.S. The serial cultivation of human diploid cell strains. *Exp. Cell Res.* **1961**, *25*, 585–621. [CrossRef] [PubMed]
2. Coppe, J.P.; Desprez, P.Y.; Krtolica, A.; Campisi, J. The senescence-associated secretory phenotype: The dark side of tumor suppression. *Annu. Rev. Pathol.* **2010**, *5*, 99–118. [CrossRef] [PubMed]
3. Redgrave, R.; Dookun, E.; Booth, L.; Folaranm, O.; Tual-Chalot, S.; Gill, J.; Owens, A.; Spyridopoulos, I.; Passos, J.; Richardson, G. Senescent cardiomyocytes contribute to cardiac dysfunction following myocardial infarction. *NPJ Aging* **2023**, *9*, 15. [CrossRef]
4. Anderson, R.; Lagnado, A.; Maggiorani, D.; Walaszczyk, A.; Dookun, E.; Chapman, J.; Birch, J.; Salmonowicz, H.; Ogrodnik, M.; Jurk, D.; et al. Length-independent telomere damage drives post-mitotic cardiomyocyte senescence. *EMBO J.* **2019**, *38*, e100492. [CrossRef] [PubMed]
5. Jurk, D.; Wang, C.; Miwa, S.; Maddick, M.; Korolchuk, V.; Tsolou, A.; Gonos, E.S.; Thrasivoulou, C.; Saffrey, M.J.; Cameron, K.; et al. Postmitotic neurons develop a p21-dependent senescence-like phenotype driven by a DNA damage response. *Aging Cell* **2012**, *11*, 996–1004. [CrossRef]
6. Richardson, G.D. Simultaneous Assessment of Cardiomyocyte DNA Synthesis and Ploidy: A Method to Assist Quantification of Cardiomyocyte Regeneration and Turnover. *J. Vis. Exp.* 2016. [CrossRef]
7. de Lange, T.; Shiue, L.; Myers, R.M.; Cox, D.R.; Naylor, S.L.; Killery, A.M.; Varmus, H.E. Structure and variability of human chromosome ends. *Mol. Cell. Biol.* **1990**, *10*, 518–527. [CrossRef]
8. Szostak, J.W.; Blackburn, E.H. Cloning yeast telomeres on linear plasmid vectors. *Cell* **1982**, *29*, 245–255. [CrossRef]
9. Di Micco, R.; Krizhanovsky, V.; Baker, D.; d'Adda di Fagagna, F. Cellular senescence in ageing: From mechanisms to therapeutic opportunities. *Nat. Rev. Mol. Cell Biol.* **2021**, *22*, 75–95. [CrossRef]
10. van Deursen, J.M. The role of senescent cells in ageing. *Nature* **2014**, *509*, 439–446. [CrossRef]
11. Anderson, R.; Richardson, G.D.; Passos, J.F. Mechanisms driving the ageing heart. *Exp. Gerontol.* **2018**, *109*, 5–15. [CrossRef] [PubMed]
12. López-Otín, C.; Blasco, M.A.; Partridge, L.; Serrano, M.; Kroemer, G. Hallmarks of aging: An expanding universe. *Cell* **2023**, *186*, 243–278. [CrossRef] [PubMed]
13. Muñoz-Espín, D.; Serrano, M. Cellular senescence: From physiology to pathology. *Nat. Rev. Mol. Cell Biol.* **2014**, *15*, 482–496. [CrossRef] [PubMed]
14. Childs, B.G.; Durik, M.; Baker, D.J.; van Deursen, J.M. Cellular senescence in aging and age-related disease: From mechanisms to therapy. *Nat. Med.* **2015**, *21*, 1424–1435. [CrossRef]
15. Gorgoulis, V.; Adams, P.D.; Alimonti, A.; Bennett, D.C.; Bischof, O.; Bishop, C.; Campisi, J.; Collado, M.; Evangelou, K.; Ferbeyre, G.; et al. Cellular Senescence: Defining a Path Forward. *Cell* **2019**, *179*, 813–827. [CrossRef] [PubMed]
16. Demaria, M.; O'Leary, M.N.; Chang, J.; Shao, L.; Liu, S.; Alimirah, F.; Koenig, K.; Le, C.; Mitin, N.; Deal, A.M.; et al. Cellular Senescence Promotes Adverse Effects of Chemotherapy and Cancer Relapse. *Cancer Discov.* **2017**, *7*, 165–176. [CrossRef] [PubMed]
17. Dookun, E.; Walaszczyk, A.; Redgrave, R.; Palmowski, P.; Tual-Chalot, S.; Suwana, A.; Chapman, J.; Jirkovsky, E.; Donastorg Sosa, L.; Gill, E.; et al. Clearance of senescent cells during cardiac ischemia-reperfusion injury improves recovery. *Aging Cell* **2020**, *19*, e13249. [CrossRef] [PubMed]
18. Walaszczyk, A.; Dookun, E.; Redgrave, R.; Tual-Chalot, S.; Victorelli, S.; Spyridopoulos, I.; Owens, A.; Arthur, H.M.; Passos, J.F.; Richardson, G.D. Pharmacological clearance of senescent cells improves survival and recovery in aged mice following acute myocardial infarction. *Aging Cell* **2019**, *18*, e12945. [CrossRef]
19. Salerno, N.; Marino, F.; Scalise, M.; Salerno, L.; Molinaro, C.; Filardo, A.; Chiefalo, A.; Panuccio, G.; De Angelis, A.; Urbanek, K.; et al. Pharmacological clearance of senescent cells improves cardiac remodeling and function after myocardial infarction in female aged mice. *Mech. Ageing Dev.* **2022**, *208*, 111740. [CrossRef]
20. Roos, C.M.; Zhang, B.; Palmer, A.K.; Ogrodnik, M.B.; Pirtskhalava, T.; Thalji, N.M.; Hagler, M.; Jurk, D.; Smith, L.A.; Casaclang-Verzosa, G.; et al. Chronic senolytic treatment alleviates established vasomotor dysfunction in aged or atherosclerotic mice. *Aging Cell* **2016**, *15*, 973–977. [CrossRef]
21. Balint, B.; Yin, H.; Nong, Z.; Arpino, J.M.; O'Neil, C.; Rogers, S.R.; Randhawa, V.K.; Fox, S.A.; Chevalier, J.; Lee, J.J.; et al. Seno-destructive smooth muscle cells in the ascending aorta of patients with bicuspid aortic valve disease. *EBioMedicine* **2019**, *43*, 54–66. [CrossRef] [PubMed]

22. Witham, M.D.; Granic, A.; Miwa, S.; Passos, J.F.; Richardson, G.D.; Sayer, A.A. New Horizons in cellular senescence for cliniciar *Age Ageing* **2023**, *52*, afad127. [CrossRef]
23. Booth, L.K.; Redgrave, R.E.; Tual-Chalot, S.; Spyridopoulos, I.; Phillips, H.M.; Richardson, G.D. Heart Disease and Ageing: Th Roles of Senescence, Mitochondria, and Telomerase in Cardiovascular Disease. *Subcell. Biochem.* **2023**, *103*, 45–78. [CrossRe [PubMed]
24. Booth, L.K.; Redgrave, R.E.; Folaranmi, O.; Gill, J.H.; Richardson, G.D. Anthracycline-induced cardiotoxicity and senescenc *Front. Aging* **2022**, *3*, 1058435. [CrossRef]
25. Dookun, E.; Passos, J.F.; Arthur, H.M.; Richardson, G.D. Therapeutic Potential of Senolytics in Cardiovascular Disease. *Cardiovas Drugs Ther.* **2022**, *36*, 187–196. [CrossRef] [PubMed]
26. Owens, W.A.; Walaszczyk, A.; Spyridopoulos, I.; Dookun, E.; Richardson, G.D. Senescence and senolytics in cardiovascul disease: Promise and potential pitfalls. *Mech. Ageing Dev.* **2021**, *198*, 111540. [CrossRef]
27. Hoffmann, J.; Richardson, G.; Haendeler, J.; Altschmied, J.; Andrés, V.; Spyridopoulos, I. Telomerase as a Therapeutic Target i Cardiovascular Disease. *Arterioscler. Thromb. Vasc. Biol.* **2021**, *41*, 1047–1061. [CrossRef]
28. Cooper, G.M. *The Cell: A Molecular Approach*, 2nd ed.; Sinauer Associates: Sunderland, MA, USA, 2000.
29. Ramaccini, D.; Montoya-Uribe, V.; Aan, F.J.; Modesti, L.; Potes, Y.; Wieckowski, M.R.; Krga, I.; Glibetić, M.; Pinton, P.; Giorgi, C et al. Mitochondrial Function and Dysfunction in Dilated Cardiomyopathy. *Front. Cell Dev. Biol.* **2020**, *8*, 624216. [CrossRef]
30. Yang, J.; Guo, Q.; Feng, X.; Liu, Y.; Zhou, Y. Mitochondrial Dysfunction in Cardiovascular Diseases: Potential Targets for Treatmen *Front. Cell Dev. Biol.* **2022**, *10*, 841523. [CrossRef]
31. Stamerra, C.A.; Di Giosia, P.; Giorgini, P.; Ferri, C.; Sukhorukov, V.N.; Sahebkar, A. Mitochondrial Dysfunction and Cardiovascul Disease: Pathophysiology and Emerging Therapies. *Oxid. Med. Cell. Longev.* **2022**, *2022*, 9530007. [CrossRef]
32. Tilokani, L.; Nagashima, S.; Paupe, V.; Prudent, J. Mitochondrial dynamics: Overview of molecular mechanisms. *Essays Biochem* **2018**, *62*, 341–360. [CrossRef] [PubMed]
33. Jennings, R.B.; Ganote, C.E. Mitochondrial structure and function in acute myocardial ischemic injury. *Circ. Res.* **1976**, *38*, I80–I9 [PubMed]
34. Murphy, E.; Ardehali, H.; Balaban, R.S.; DiLisa, F.; Dorn, G.W., 2nd; Kitsis, R.N.; Otsu, K.; Ping, P.; Rizzuto, R.; Sack, M.N.; et a Mitochondrial Function, Biology, and Role in Disease: A Scientific Statement From the American Heart Association. *Circ. Re* **2016**, *118*, 1960–1991. [CrossRef] [PubMed]
35. Chistiakov, D.A.; Shkurat, T.P.; Melnichenko, A.A.; Grechko, A.V.; Orekhov, A.N. The role of mitochondrial dysfunction i cardiovascular disease: A brief review. *Ann. Med.* **2018**, *50*, 121–127. [CrossRef] [PubMed]
36. Allard, M.F.; Schönekess, B.O.; Henning, S.L.; English, D.R.; Lopaschuk, G.D. Contribution of oxidative metabolism and glycolysi to ATP production in hypertrophied hearts. *Am. J. Physiol.* **1994**, *267*, H742–H750. [CrossRef] [PubMed]
37. Wang, Z.Y.; Liu, Y.Y.; Liu, G.H.; Lu, H.B.; Mao, C.Y. l-Carnitine and heart disease. *Life Sci.* **2018**, *194*, 88–97. [CrossRef] [PubMed
38. Zhou, B.; Tian, R. Mitochondrial dysfunction in pathophysiology of heart failure. *J. Clin. Investig.* **2018**, *128*, 3716–3726. [CrossRef
39. Kühlbrandt, W. Structure and function of mitochondrial membrane protein complexes. *BMC Biol.* **2015**, *13*, 89. [CrossRef]
40. Casademont, J.; Miró, O. Electron transport chain defects in heart failure. *Heart Fail. Rev.* **2002**, *7*, 131–139. [CrossRef]
41. Arbustini, E.; Diegoli, M.; Fasani, R.; Grasso, M.; Morbini, P.; Banchieri, N.; Bellini, O.; Dal Bello, B.; Pilotto, A.; Magrini, G.; et al Mitochondrial DNA mutations and mitochondrial abnormalities in dilated cardiomyopathy. *Am. J. Pathol.* **1998**, *153*, 1501–1510 [CrossRef] [PubMed]
42. Sheeran, F.L.; Pepe, S. Mitochondrial Bioenergetics and Dysfunction in Failing Heart. *Adv. Exp. Med. Biol.* **2017**, *982*, 65–80 [CrossRef]
43. Dai, D.F.; Chen, T.; Wanagat, J.; Laflamme, M.; Marcinek, D.J.; Emond, M.J.; Ngo, C.P.; Prolla, T.A.; Rabinovitch, P.S. Age dependent cardiomyopathy in mitochondrial mutator mice is attenuated by overexpression of catalase targeted to mitochondria *Aging Cell* **2010**, *9*, 536–544. [CrossRef]
44. Kang, S.; Louboutin, J.P.; Datta, P.; Landel, C.P.; Martinez, D.; Zervos, A.S.; Strayer, D.S.; Fernandes-Alnemri, T.; Alnemri, E.S Loss of HtrA2/Omi activity in non-neuronal tissues of adult mice causes premature aging. *Cell Death Differ.* **2013**, *20*, 259–269 [CrossRef]
45. Li, R.; Jia, Z.; Trush, M.A. Defining ROS in Biology and Medicine. *React. Oxyg. Species* **2016**, *1*, 9–21. [CrossRef]
46. McCubrey, J.A.; Lahair, M.M.; Franklin, R.A. Reactive oxygen species-induced activation of the MAP kinase signaling pathways *Antioxid. Redox Signal* **2006**, *8*, 1775–1789. [CrossRef]
47. Valko, M.; Leibfritz, D.; Moncol, J.; Cronin, M.T.; Mazur, M.; Telser, J. Free radicals and antioxidants in normal physiological functions and human disease. *Int. J. Biochem. Cell Biol.* **2007**, *39*, 44–84. [CrossRef]
48. Cui, H.; Kong, Y.; Zhang, H. Oxidative stress, mitochondrial dysfunction, and aging. *J. Signal Transduct.* **2012**, *2012*, 646354 [CrossRef]
49. Peoples, J.N.; Saraf, A.; Ghazal, N.; Pham, T.T.; Kwong, J.Q. Mitochondrial dysfunction and oxidative stress in heart disease. *Exp. Mol. Med.* **2019**, *51*, 1–13. [CrossRef]
50. Grollman, A.P.; Moriya, M. Mutagenesis by 8-oxoguanine: An enemy within. *Trends Genet.* **1993**, *9*, 246–249. [CrossRef]
51. David, S.S.; O'Shea, V.L.; Kundu, S. Base-excision repair of oxidative DNA damage. *Nature* **2007**, *447*, 941–950. [CrossRef]

52. Passos, J.F.; Saretzki, G.; Ahmed, S.; Nelson, G.; Richter, T.; Peters, H.; Wappler, I.; Birket, M.J.; Harold, G.; Schaeuble, K.; et al. Mitochondrial Dysfunction Accounts for the Stochastic Heterogeneity in Telomere-Dependent Senescence. *PLoS Biol.* **2007**, *5*, e110. [CrossRef] [PubMed]
53. Hewitt, G.; Jurk, D.; Marques, F.D.M.; Correia-Melo, C.; Hardy, T.; Gackowska, A.; Anderson, R.; Taschuk, M.; Mann, J.; Passos, J.F. Telomeres are favoured targets of a persistent DNA damage response in ageing and stress-induced senescence. *Nat. Commun.* **2012**, *3*, 708. [CrossRef] [PubMed]
54. Malaquin, N.; Carrier-Leclerc, A.; Dessureault, M.; Rodier, F. DDR-mediated crosstalk between DNA-damaged cells and their microenvironment. *Front. Genet.* **2015**, *6*, 94. [CrossRef] [PubMed]
55. d'Adda di Fagagna, F. Living on a break: Cellular senescence as a DNA-damage response. *Nat. Rev. Cancer* **2008**, *8*, 512–522. [CrossRef] [PubMed]
56. Martini, H.; Passos, J.F. Cellular senescence: All roads lead to mitochondria. *FEBS J.* **2023**, *290*, 1186–1202. [CrossRef] [PubMed]
57. Hertz, D.G. Trauma and nostalgia: New aspects on the coping of aging Holocaust survivors. *Isr. J. Psychiatry Relat. Sci.* **1990**, *27*, 189–198. [PubMed]
58. Youdim, M.B.; Bakhle, Y.S. Monoamine oxidase: Isoforms and inhibitors in Parkinson's disease and depressive illness. *Br. J. Pharmacol.* **2006**, *147* (Suppl. 1), S287–S296. [CrossRef]
59. Villeneuve, C.; Guilbeau-Frugier, C.; Sicard, P.; Lairez, O.; Ordener, C.; Duparc, T.; De Paulis, D.; Couderc, B.; Spreux-Varoquaux, O.; Tortosa, F.; et al. p53-PGC-1α pathway mediates oxidative mitochondrial damage and cardiomyocyte necrosis induced by monoamine oxidase-A upregulation: Role in chronic left ventricular dysfunction in mice. *Antioxid. Redox Signal* **2013**, *18*, 5–18. [CrossRef]
60. Correia-Melo, C.; Birch, J.; Fielder, E.; Rahmatika, D.; Taylor, J.; Chapman, J.; Lagnado, A.; Carroll, B.M.; Miwa, S.; Richardson, G.; et al. Rapamycin improves healthspan but not inflammaging in nfκb1$^{-/-}$ mice. *Aging Cell* **2019**, *18*, e12882. [CrossRef]
61. Chiao, Y.A.; Zhang, H.; Sweetwyne, M.; Whitson, J.; Ting, Y.S.; Basisty, N.; Pino, L.K.; Quarles, E.; Nguyen, N.H.; Campbell, M.D.; et al. Late-life restoration of mitochondrial function reverses cardiac dysfunction in old mice. *Elife* **2020**, *9*, e55513. [CrossRef]
62. Windecker, S. Chapter 30—Acute Coronary Syndromes. In *Clinical Critical Care Medicine*; Albert, R.K., Slutsky, A.S., Ranieri, V.M., Takala, J., Torres, A., Eds.; Mosby: Philadelphia, PA, USA, 2006; pp. 301–318.
63. Gintant, G.; Sager, P.T.; Stockbridge, N. Evolution of strategies to improve preclinical cardiac safety testing. *Nat. Rev. Drug Discov.* **2016**, *15*, 457–471. [CrossRef]
64. Laverty, H.; Benson, C.; Cartwright, E.; Cross, M.; Garland, C.; Hammond, T.; Holloway, C.; McMahon, N.; Milligan, J.; Park, B.; et al. How can we improve our understanding of cardiovascular safety liabilities to develop safer medicines? *Br. J. Pharmacol.* **2011**, *163*, 675–693. [CrossRef]
65. Onakpoya, I.J.; Heneghan, C.J.; Aronson, J.K. Post-marketing withdrawal of analgesic medications because of adverse drug reactions: A systematic review. *Expert. Opin. Drug Saf.* **2018**, *17*, 63–72. [CrossRef]
66. Ewer, M.S.; Ewer, S.M. Cardiotoxicity of anticancer treatments. *Nat. Rev. Cardiol.* **2015**, *12*, 547–558. [CrossRef]
67. Chow, E.J.; Leger, K.J.; Bhatt, N.S.; Mulrooney, D.A.; Ross, C.J.; Aggarwal, S.; Bansal, N.; Ehrhardt, M.J.; Armenian, S.H.; Scott, J.M.; et al. Paediatric cardio-oncology: Epidemiology, screening, prevention, and treatment. *Cardiovasc. Res.* **2019**, *115*, 922–934. [CrossRef]
68. Davies, K.J.; Doroshow, J.H. Redox cycling of anthracyclines by cardiac mitochondria. I. Anthracycline radical formation by NADH dehydrogenase. *J. Biol. Chem.* **1986**, *261*, 3060–3067. [CrossRef]
69. Doroshow, J.H.; Davies, K.J. Redox cycling of anthracyclines by cardiac mitochondria. II. Formation of superoxide anion, hydrogen peroxide, and hydroxyl radical. *J. Biol. Chem.* **1986**, *261*, 3068–3074. [CrossRef]
70. Parker, M.A.; King, V.; Howard, K.P. Nuclear magnetic resonance study of doxorubicin binding to cardiolipin containing magnetically oriented phospholipid bilayers. *Biochim. Biophys. Acta (BBA) Biomembr.* **2001**, *1514*, 206–216. [CrossRef]
71. Ichikawa, Y.; Ghanefar, M.; Bayeva, M.; Wu, R.; Khechaduri, A.; Naga Prasad, S.V.; Mutharasan, R.K.; Naik, T.J.; Ardehali, H. Cardiotoxicity of doxorubicin is mediated through mitochondrial iron accumulation. *J. Clin. Investig.* **2014**, *124*, 617–630. [CrossRef]
72. Zhang, S.; Liu, X.; Bawa-Khalfe, T.; Lu, L.S.; Lyu, Y.L.; Liu, L.F.; Yeh, E.T. Identification of the molecular basis of doxorubicin-induced cardiotoxicity. *Nat. Med.* **2012**, *18*, 1639–1642. [CrossRef]
73. Abe, K.; Ikeda, M.; Ide, T.; Tadokoro, T.; Miyamoto, H.D.; Furusawa, S.; Tsutsui, Y.; Miyake, R.; Ishimaru, K.; Watanabe, M.; et al. Doxorubicin causes ferroptosis and cardiotoxicity by intercalating into mitochondrial DNA and disrupting Alas1-dependent heme synthesis. *Sci. Signal* **2022**, *15*, eabn8017. [CrossRef]
74. Lebrecht, D.; Kokkori, A.; Ketelsen, U.P.; Setzer, B.; Walker, U.A. Tissue-specific mtDNA lesions and radical-associated mitochondrial dysfunction in human hearts exposed to doxorubicin. *J. Pathol.* **2005**, *207*, 436–444. [CrossRef]
75. Mitry, M.A.; Laurent, D.; Keith, B.L.; Sira, E.; Eisenberg, C.A.; Eisenberg, L.M.; Joshi, S.; Gupte, S.; Edwards, J.G. Accelerated cardiomyocyte senescence contributes to late-onset doxorubicin-induced cardiotoxicity. *Am. J. Physiol. Cell Physiol.* **2020**, *318*, C380–C391. [CrossRef]
76. Chapman, J.; Fielder, E.; Passos, J.F. Mitochondrial dysfunction and cell senescence: Deciphering a complex relationship. *FEBS Lett.* **2019**, *593*, 1566–1579. [CrossRef]
77. Correia-Melo, C.; Marques, F.D.; Anderson, R.; Hewitt, G.; Hewitt, R.; Cole, J.; Carroll, B.M.; Miwa, S.; Birch, J.; Merz, A.; et al. Mitochondria are required for pro-ageing features of the senescent phenotype. *EMBO J.* **2016**, *35*, 724–742. [CrossRef]

78. Wallace, K.B.; Sardão, V.A.; Oliveira, P.J. Mitochondrial Determinants of Doxorubicin-Induced Cardiomyopathy. *Circ. Res.* **202** *126*, 926–941. [CrossRef]
79. Will, Y.; Dykens, J.A.; Nadanaciva, S.; Hirakawa, B.; Jamieson, J.; Marroquin, L.D.; Hynes, J.; Patyna, S.; Jessen, B.A. Effect of th multitargeted tyrosine kinase inhibitors imatinib, dasatinib, sunitinib, and sorafenib on mitochondrial function in isolated ra heart mitochondria and H9c2 cells. *Toxicol. Sci.* **2008**, *106*, 153–161. [CrossRef]
80. Bouitbir, J.; Alshaikhali, A.; Panajatovic, M.V.; Abegg, V.F.; Paech, F.; Krähenbühl, S. Mitochondrial oxidative stress plays critical role in the cardiotoxicity of sunitinib: Running title: Sunitinib and oxidative stress in hearts. *Toxicology* **2019**, *426*, 15228 [CrossRef] [PubMed]
81. Rocca, C.; De Francesco, E.M.; Pasqua, T.; Granieri, M.C.; De Bartolo, A.; Gallo Cantafio, M.E.; Muoio, M.G.; Gentile, M.; Ner A.; Angelone, T.; et al. Mitochondrial Determinants of Anti-Cancer Drug-Induced Cardiotoxicity. *Biomedicines* **2022**, *10*, 52 [CrossRef]
82. Forte, M.; Schirone, L.; Ameri, P.; Basso, C.; Catalucci, D.; Modica, J.; Chimenti, C.; Crotti, L.; Frati, G.; Rubattu, S.; et al. The rol of mitochondrial dynamics in cardiovascular diseases. *Br. J. Pharmacol.* **2021**, *178*, 2060–2076. [CrossRef] [PubMed]
83. Fu, W.; Liu, Y.; Yin, H. Mitochondrial Dynamics: Biogenesis, Fission, Fusion, and Mitophagy in the Regulation of Stem Cel Behaviors. *Stem Cells Int.* **2019**, *2019*, 9757201. [CrossRef]
84. Fenton, A.R.; Jongens, T.A.; Holzbaur, E.L.F. Mitochondrial dynamics: Shaping and remodeling an organelle network. *Curr. Opin Cell Biol.* **2021**, *68*, 28–36. [CrossRef]
85. Luan, Y.; Ren, K.D.; Luan, Y.; Chen, X.; Yang, Y. Mitochondrial Dynamics: Pathogenesis and Therapeutic Targets of Vascula Diseases. *Front. Cardiovasc. Med.* **2021**, *8*, 770574. [CrossRef]
86. de Brito, O.M.; Scorrano, L. Mitofusin 2: A mitochondria-shaping protein with signaling roles beyond fusion. *Antioxid. Redox Signal* **2008**, *10*, 621–633. [CrossRef]
87. Chen, L.; Gong, Q.; Stice, J.P.; Knowlton, A.A. Mitochondrial OPA1, apoptosis, and heart failure. *Cardiovasc. Res.* **2009**, *84*, 91–99 [CrossRef]
88. Chen, Y.; Liu, Y.; Dorn, G.W., 2nd. Mitochondrial fusion is essential for organelle function and cardiac homeostasis. *Circ. Res* **2011**, *109*, 1327–1331. [CrossRef]
89. Papanicolaou, K.N.; Kikuchi, R.; Ngoh, G.A.; Coughlan, K.A.; Dominguez, I.; Stanley, W.C.; Walsh, K. Mitofusins 1 and 2 are essential for postnatal metabolic remodeling in heart. *Circ. Res.* **2012**, *111*, 1012–1026. [CrossRef]
90. Santel, A.; Fuller, M.T. Control of mitochondrial morphology by a human mitofusin. *J. Cell Sci.* **2001**, *114*, 867–874. [CrossRef]
91. Ong, S.B.; Subrayan, S.; Lim, S.Y.; Yellon, D.M.; Davidson, S.M.; Hausenloy, D.J. Inhibiting mitochondrial fission protects the heart against ischemia/reperfusion injury. *Circulation* **2010**, *121*, 2012–2022. [CrossRef]
92. Sharp, W.W.; Fang, Y.H.; Han, M.; Zhang, H.J.; Hong, Z.; Banathy, A.; Morrow, E.; Ryan, J.J.; Archer, S.L. Dynamin-related protein 1 (Drp1)-mediated diastolic dysfunction in myocardial ischemia-reperfusion injury: Therapeutic benefits of Drp1 inhibition to reduce mitochondrial fission. *FASEB J.* **2014**, *28*, 316–326. [CrossRef]
93. Morris, S.; Molina-Riquelme, I.; Barrientos, G.; Bravo, F.; Aedo, G.; Gómez, W.; Lagos, D.; Verdejo, H.; Peischard, S.; Seebohm, G.; et al. Inner mitochondrial membrane structure and fusion dynamics are altered in senescent human iPSC-derived and primary rat cardiomyocytes. *Biochim. Biophys. Acta (BBA) Bioenerg.* **2023**, *1864*, 148949. [CrossRef]
94. Lee, H.C.; Yin, P.H.; Chi, C.W.; Wei, Y.H. Increase in mitochondrial mass in human fibroblasts under oxidative stress and during replicative cell senescence. *J. Biomed. Sci.* **2002**, *9*, 517–526. [CrossRef]
95. Lee, S.; Jeong, S.Y.; Lim, W.C.; Kim, S.; Park, Y.Y.; Sun, X.; Youle, R.J.; Cho, H. Mitochondrial fission and fusion mediators, hFis1 and OPA1, modulate cellular senescence. *J. Biol. Chem.* **2007**, *282*, 22977–22983. [CrossRef]
96. Yu, R.; Lendahl, U.; Nistér, M.; Zhao, J. Regulation of Mammalian Mitochondrial Dynamics: Opportunities and Challenges. *Front. Endocrinol.* **2020**, *11*, 374. [CrossRef]
97. Virbasius, J.V.; Scarpulla, R.C. Activation of the human mitochondrial transcription factor A gene by nuclear respiratory factors: A potential regulatory link between nuclear and mitochondrial gene expression in organelle biogenesis. *Proc. Natl. Acad. Sci. USA* **1994**, *91*, 1309–1313. [CrossRef]
98. Sihag, S.; Cresci, S.; Li, A.Y.; Sucharov, C.C.; Lehman, J.J. PGC-1alpha and ERRalpha target gene downregulation is a signature of the failing human heart. *J. Mol. Cell. Cardiol.* **2009**, *46*, 201–212. [CrossRef]
99. Wang, J.; Li, S.; Wang, J.; Wu, F.; Chen, Y.; Zhang, H.; Guo, Y.; Lin, Y.; Li, L.; Yu, X.; et al. Spermidine alleviates cardiac aging by improving mitochondrial biogenesis and function. *Aging* **2020**, *12*, 650–671. [CrossRef]
100. Xiong, S.; Salazar, G.; Patrushev, N.; Ma, M.; Forouzandeh, F.; Hilenski, L.; Alexander, R.W. Peroxisome proliferator-activated receptor γ coactivator-1α is a central negative regulator of vascular senescence. *Arterioscler. Thromb. Vasc. Biol.* **2013**, *33*, 988–998. [CrossRef]
101. Ong, S.B.; Hausenloy, D.J. Mitochondrial morphology and cardiovascular disease. *Cardiovasc. Res.* **2010**, *88*, 16–29. [CrossRef]
102. Brady, N.R.; Hamacher-Brady, A.; Gottlieb, R.A. Proapoptotic BCL-2 family members and mitochondrial dysfunction during ischemia/reperfusion injury, a study employing cardiac HL-1 cells and GFP biosensors. *Biochim. Biophys. Acta* **2006**, *1757*, 667–678. [CrossRef]
103. Mai, S.; Klinkenberg, M.; Auburger, G.; Bereiter-Hahn, J.; Jendrach, M. Decreased expression of Drp1 and Fis1 mediates mitochondrial elongation in senescent cells and enhances resistance to oxidative stress through PINK1. *J. Cell Sci.* **2010**, *123*, 917–926. [CrossRef]

4. Green, D.R.; Reed, J.C. Mitochondria and apoptosis. *Science* **1998**, *281*, 1309–1312. [CrossRef]
5. Newmeyer, D.D.; Farschon, D.M.; Reed, J.C. Cell-free apoptosis in Xenopus egg extracts: Inhibition by Bcl-2 and requirement for an organelle fraction enriched in mitochondria. *Cell* **1994**, *79*, 353–364. [CrossRef]
6. Takemura, G.; Kanoh, M.; Minatoguchi, S.; Fujiwara, H. Cardiomyocyte apoptosis in the failing heart--a critical review from definition and classification of cell death. *Int. J. Cardiol.* **2013**, *167*, 2373–2386. [CrossRef]
7. Wu, M.Y.; Yiang, G.T.; Liao, W.T.; Tsai, A.P.; Cheng, Y.L.; Cheng, P.W.; Li, C.Y.; Li, C.J. Current Mechanistic Concepts in Ischemia and Reperfusion Injury. *Cell. Physiol. Biochem.* **2018**, *46*, 1650–1667. [CrossRef]
8. González, A.; Fortuño, M.A.; Querejeta, R.; Ravassa, S.; López, B.; López, N.; Díez, J. Cardiomyocyte apoptosis in hypertensive cardiomyopathy. *Cardiovasc. Res.* **2003**, *59*, 549–562. [CrossRef]
9. Zhang, J.; Ney, P.A. Role of BNIP3 and NIX in cell death, autophagy, and mitophagy. *Cell Death Differ.* **2009**, *16*, 939–946. [CrossRef]
10. Dorn, G.W., 2nd. Mitochondrial pruning by Nix and BNip3: An essential function for cardiac-expressed death factors. *J. Cardiovasc. Transl. Res.* **2010**, *3*, 374–383. [CrossRef]
11. Diwan, A.; Wansapura, J.; Syed, F.M.; Matkovich, S.J.; Lorenz, J.N.; Dorn, G.W., 2nd. Nix-mediated apoptosis links myocardial fibrosis, cardiac remodeling, and hypertrophy decompensation. *Circulation* **2008**, *117*, 396–404. [CrossRef]
12. Rottenberg, H.; Hoek, J.B. The Mitochondrial Permeability Transition: Nexus of Aging, Disease and Longevity. *Cells* **2021**, *10*, 79. [CrossRef]
13. Morciano, G.; Bonora, M.; Campo, G.; Aquila, G.; Rizzo, P.; Giorgi, C.; Wieckowski, M.R.; Pinton, P. Mechanistic Role of mPTP in Ischemia-Reperfusion Injury. *Adv. Exp. Med. Biol.* **2017**, *982*, 169–189. [CrossRef]
14. Greene, A.W.; Grenier, K.; Aguileta, M.A.; Muise, S.; Farazifard, R.; Haque, M.E.; McBride, H.M.; Park, D.S.; Fon, E.A. Mitochondrial processing peptidase regulates PINK1 processing, import and Parkin recruitment. *EMBO Rep.* **2012**, *13*, 378–385. [CrossRef]
15. Nguyen, T.N.; Padman, B.S.; Lazarou, M. Deciphering the Molecular Signals of PINK1/Parkin Mitophagy. *Trends Cell Biol.* **2016**, *26*, 733–744. [CrossRef]
16. Kane, L.A.; Lazarou, M.; Fogel, A.I.; Li, Y.; Yamano, K.; Sarraf, S.A.; Banerjee, S.; Youle, R.J. PINK1 phosphorylates ubiquitin to activate Parkin E3 ubiquitin ligase activity. *J. Cell Biol.* **2014**, *205*, 143–153. [CrossRef]
17. Lazarou, M.; Sliter, D.A.; Kane, L.A.; Sarraf, S.A.; Wang, C.; Burman, J.L.; Sideris, D.P.; Fogel, A.I.; Youle, R.J. The ubiquitin kinase PINK1 recruits autophagy receptors to induce mitophagy. *Nature* **2015**, *524*, 309–314. [CrossRef]
18. Song, M.; Gong, G.; Burelle, Y.; Gustafsson, Å.B.; Kitsis, R.N.; Matkovich, S.J.; Dorn, G.W., 2nd. Interdependence of Parkin-Mediated Mitophagy and Mitochondrial Fission in Adult Mouse Hearts. *Circ. Res.* **2015**, *117*, 346–351. [CrossRef]
19. Bravo-San Pedro, J.M.; Kroemer, G.; Galluzzi, L. Autophagy and Mitophagy in Cardiovascular Disease. *Circ. Res.* **2017**, *120*, 1812–1824. [CrossRef]
20. Song, M.; Chen, Y.; Gong, G.; Murphy, E.; Rabinovitch, P.S.; Dorn, G.W., 2nd. Super-suppression of mitochondrial reactive oxygen species signaling impairs compensatory autophagy in primary mitophagic cardiomyopathy. *Circ. Res.* **2014**, *115*, 348–353. [CrossRef]
21. Billia, F.; Hauck, L.; Konecny, F.; Rao, V.; Shen, J.; Mak, T.W. PTEN-inducible kinase 1 (PINK1)/Park6 is indispensable for normal heart function. *Proc. Natl. Acad. Sci. USA* **2011**, *108*, 9572–9577. [CrossRef]
22. Kubli, D.A.; Zhang, X.; Lee, Y.; Hanna, R.A.; Quinsay, M.N.; Nguyen, C.K.; Jimenez, R.; Petrosyan, S.; Murphy, A.N.; Gustafsson, A.B. Parkin protein deficiency exacerbates cardiac injury and reduces survival following myocardial infarction. *J. Biol. Chem.* **2013**, *288*, 915–926. [CrossRef]
23. Saito, T.; Asai, K.; Sato, S.; Hayashi, M.; Adachi, A.; Sasaki, Y.; Takano, H.; Mizuno, K.; Shimizu, W. Autophagic vacuoles in cardiomyocytes of dilated cardiomyopathy with initially decompensated heart failure predict improved prognosis. *Autophagy* **2016**, *12*, 579–587. [CrossRef]
124. Campos, J.C.; Bozi, L.H.; Bechara, L.R.; Lima, V.M.; Ferreira, J.C. Mitochondrial Quality Control in Cardiac Diseases. *Front. Physiol.* **2016**, *7*, 479. [CrossRef]
125. Madamanchi, N.R.; Runge, M.S. Mitochondrial dysfunction in atherosclerosis. *Circ. Res.* **2007**, *100*, 460–473. [CrossRef]
126. Grootaert, M.O.J.; Roth, L.; Schrijvers, D.M.; De Meyer, G.R.Y.; Martinet, W. Defective Autophagy in Atherosclerosis: To Die or to Senesce? *Oxid. Med. Cell. Longev.* **2018**, *2018*, 7687083. [CrossRef]
127. Sergin, I.; Bhattacharya, S.; Emanuel, R.; Esen, E.; Stokes, C.J.; Evans, T.D.; Arif, B.; Curci, J.A.; Razani, B. Inclusion bodies enriched for p62 and polyubiquitinated proteins in macrophages protect against atherosclerosis. *Sci. Signal* **2016**, *9*, ra2. [CrossRef]
128. Swaminathan, B.; Goikuria, H.; Vega, R.; Rodríguez-Antigüedad, A.; López Medina, A.; Freijo Mdel, M.; Vandenbroeck, K.; Alloza, I. Autophagic marker MAP1LC3B expression levels are associated with carotid atherosclerosis symptomatology. *PLoS ONE* **2014**, *9*, e115176. [CrossRef]
129. Ma, S.; Chen, J.; Feng, J.; Zhang, R.; Fan, M.; Han, D.; Li, X.; Li, C.; Ren, J.; Wang, Y.; et al. Melatonin Ameliorates the Progression of Atherosclerosis via Mitophagy Activation and NLRP3 Inflammasome Inhibition. *Oxid. Med. Cell. Longev.* **2018**, *2018*, 9286458. [CrossRef]
130. Sen, A.; Kallabis, S.; Gaedke, F.; Jüngst, C.; Boix, J.; Nüchel, J.; Maliphol, K.; Hofmann, J.; Schauss, A.C.; Krüger, M.; et al. Mitochondrial membrane proteins and VPS35 orchestrate selective removal of mtDNA. *Nat. Commun.* **2022**, *13*, 6704. [CrossRef]
131. Soto-Gamez, A.; Quax, W.J.; Demaria, M. Regulation of Survival Networks in Senescent Cells: From Mechanisms to Interventions. *J. Mol. Biol.* **2019**, *431*, 2629–2643. [CrossRef]

132. Zhu, Y.; Tchkonia, T.; Pirtskhalava, T.; Gower, A.C.; Ding, H.; Giorgadze, N.; Palmer, A.K.; Ikeno, Y.; Hubbard, G.B.; Lenburg, M. et al. The Achilles' heel of senescent cells: From transcriptome to senolytic drugs. *Aging Cell* **2015**, *14*, 644–658. [CrossRef]
133. Kirkland, J.L.; Tchkonia, T. Cellular Senescence: A Translational Perspective. *EBioMedicine* **2017**, *21*, 21–28. [CrossRef]
134. Short, S.; Fielder, E.; Miwa, S.; von Zglinicki, T. Senolytics and senostatics as adjuvant tumour therapy. *EBioMedicine* **2019**, *4* 683–692. [CrossRef] [PubMed]
135. Nakayama, H.; Otsu, K. Mitochondrial DNA as an inflammatory mediator in cardiovascular diseases. *Biochem. J.* **2018**, *47* 839–852. [CrossRef]
136. Chen, G.Y.; Nuñez, G. Sterile inflammation: Sensing and reacting to damage. *Nat. Rev. Immunol.* **2010**, *10*, 826–837. [CrossRef]
137. King, K.R.; Aguirre, A.D.; Ye, Y.X.; Sun, Y.; Roh, J.D.; Ng, R.P., Jr.; Kohler, R.H.; Arlauckas, S.P.; Iwamoto, Y.; Savol, A.; et al. IRF and type I interferons fuel a fatal response to myocardial infarction. *Nat. Med.* **2017**, *23*, 1481–1487. [CrossRef] [PubMed]
138. Mao, Y.; Luo, W.; Zhang, L.; Wu, W.; Yuan, L.; Xu, H.; Song, J.; Fujiwara, K.; Abe, J.I.; LeMaire, S.A.; et al. STING-IRF3 Trigger Endothelial Inflammation in Response to Free Fatty Acid-Induced Mitochondrial Damage in Diet-Induced Obesity. *Arterioscle Thromb. Vasc. Biol.* **2017**, *37*, 920–929. [CrossRef]
139. Heitzer, T.; Schlinzig, T.; Krohn, K.; Meinertz, T.; Münzel, T. Endothelial Dysfunction, Oxidative Stress, and Risk of Cardiovascula Events in Patients With Coronary Artery Disease. *Circulation* **2001**, *104*, 2673–2678. [CrossRef]
140. McCarthy, C.G.; Wenceslau, C.F.; Goulopoulou, S.; Ogbi, S.; Baban, B.; Sullivan, J.C.; Matsumoto, T.; Webb, R.C. Circulatin mitochondrial DNA and Toll-like receptor 9 are associated with vascular dysfunction in spontaneously hypertensive rat *Cardiovasc. Res.* **2015**, *107*, 119–130. [CrossRef]
141. Oka, T.; Hikoso, S.; Yamaguchi, O.; Taneike, M.; Takeda, T.; Tamai, T.; Oyabu, J.; Murakawa, T.; Nakayama, H.; Nishida, K.; et a Mitochondrial DNA that escapes from autophagy causes inflammation and heart failure. *Nature* **2012**, *485*, 251–255. [CrossRef] [PubMed]
142. Wang, Y.; Liu, X.; Shi, H.; Yu, Y.; Yu, Y.; Li, M.; Chen, R. NLRP3 inflammasome, an immune-inflammatory target in pathogenesi and treatment of cardiovascular diseases. *Clin. Transl. Med.* **2020**, *10*, 91–106. [CrossRef]
143. Keshavarz-Bahaghighat, H.; Darwesh, A.M.; Sosnowski, D.K.; Seubert, J.M. Mitochondrial Dysfunction and Inflammaging in Heart Failure: Novel Roles of CYP-Derived Epoxylipids. *Cells* **2020**, *9*, 1565. [CrossRef]
144. Liberale, L.; Montecucco, F.; Tardif, J.C.; Libby, P.; Camici, G.G. Inflamm-ageing: The role of inflammation in age-dependen cardiovascular disease. *Eur. Heart J.* **2020**, *41*, 2974–2982. [CrossRef] [PubMed]
145. Li, X.; Geng, J.; Zhao, J.; Ni, Q.; Zhao, C.; Zheng, Y.; Chen, X.; Wang, L. Trimethylamine N-Oxide Exacerbates Cardiac Fibrosis via Activating the NLRP3 Inflammasome. *Front. Physiol.* **2019**, *10*, 866. [CrossRef] [PubMed]
146. Cañadas-Lozano, D.; Marín-Aguilar, F.; Castejón-Vega, B.; Ryffel, B.; Navarro-Pando, J.M.; Ruiz-Cabello, J.; Alcocer-Gómez E.; Bullón, P.; Cordero, M.D. Blockade of the NLRP3 inflammasome improves metabolic health and lifespan in obese mice *Geroscience* **2020**, *42*, 715–725. [CrossRef] [PubMed]
147. Stokman, G.; Kors, L.; Bakker, P.J.; Rampanelli, E.; Claessen, N.; Teske, G.J.D.; Butter, L.; van Andel, H.; van den Bergh Weerman M.A.; Larsen, P.W.B.; et al. NLRX1 dampens oxidative stress and apoptosis in tissue injury via control of mitochondrial activity *J. Exp. Med.* **2017**, *214*, 2405–2420. [CrossRef] [PubMed]
148. Hernandez-Segura, A.; Nehme, J.; Demaria, M. Hallmarks of Cellular Senescence. *Trends Cell Biol.* **2018**, *28*, 436–453. [CrossRef]
149. Sikora, E.; Bielak-Zmijewska, A.; Mosieniak, G. A common signature of cellular senescence; does it exist? *Ageing Res. Rev.* **2021** *71*, 101458. [CrossRef]
150. Tang, X.; Li, P.H.; Chen, H.Z. Cardiomyocyte Senescence and Cellular Communications Within Myocardial Microenvironments *Front. Endocrinol.* **2020**, *11*, 280. [CrossRef]
151. Nelson, G.; Kucheryavenko, O.; Wordsworth, J.; von Zglinicki, T. The senescent bystander effect is caused by ROS-activated NF-κB signalling. *Mech. Ageing Dev.* **2018**, *170*, 30–36. [CrossRef]
152. Vizioli, M.G.; Liu, T.; Miller, K.N.; Robertson, N.A.; Gilroy, K.; Lagnado, A.B.; Perez-Garcia, A.; Kiourtis, C.; Dasgupta, N.; Lei, X. et al. Mitochondria-to-nucleus retrograde signaling drives formation of cytoplasmic chromatin and inflammation in senescence *Genes. Dev.* **2020**, *34*, 428–445. [CrossRef]
153. Victorelli, S.; Salmonowicz, H.; Chapman, J.; Martini, H.; Vizioli, M.G.; Riley, J.S.; Cloix, C.; Hall-Younger, E.; Machado Espindola-Netto, J.; Jurk, D.; et al. Apoptotic stress causes mtDNA release during senescence and drives the SASP. *Nature* **2023**, *622*, 627–636 [CrossRef] [PubMed]
154. Birch, J.; Passos, J.F. Targeting the SASP to combat ageing: Mitochondria as possible intracellular allies? *Bioessays* **2017**, *39*, 1600235. [CrossRef] [PubMed]
155. Rottenberg, H.; Hoek, J.B. The path from mitochondrial ROS to aging runs through the mitochondrial permeability transition pore. *Aging Cell* **2017**, *16*, 943–955. [CrossRef] [PubMed]
156. Carling, D. AMPK signalling in health and disease. *Curr. Opin. Cell Biol.* **2017**, *45*, 31–37. [CrossRef] [PubMed]
157. LaMoia, T.E.; Shulman, G.I. Cellular and Molecular Mechanisms of Metformin Action. *Endocr. Rev.* **2021**, *42*, 77–96. [CrossRef]
158. Agius, L.; Ford, B.E.; Chachra, S.S. The Metformin Mechanism on Gluconeogenesis and AMPK Activation: The Metabolite Perspective. *Int. J. Mol. Sci.* **2020**, *21*, 3240. [CrossRef]
159. Ma, T.; Tian, X.; Zhang, B.; Li, M.; Wang, Y.; Yang, C.; Wu, J.; Wei, X.; Qu, Q.; Yu, Y.; et al. Low-dose metformin targets the lysosomal AMPK pathway through PEN2. *Nature* **2022**, *603*, 159–165. [CrossRef]

160. Zhang, C.S.; Li, M.; Ma, T.; Zong, Y.; Cui, J.; Feng, J.W.; Wu, Y.Q.; Lin, S.Y.; Lin, S.C. Metformin Activates AMPK through the Lysosomal Pathway. *Cell Metab.* **2016**, *24*, 521–522. [CrossRef]
161. Wang, Q.; Zhang, M.; Torres, G.; Wu, S.; Ouyang, C.; Xie, Z.; Zou, M.H. Metformin Suppresses Diabetes-Accelerated Atherosclerosis via the Inhibition of Drp1-Mediated Mitochondrial Fission. *Diabetes* **2017**, *66*, 193–205. [CrossRef]
162. Scarpulla, R.C. Metabolic control of mitochondrial biogenesis through the PGC-1 family regulatory network. *Biochim. Biophys. Acta* **2011**, *1813*, 1269–1278. [CrossRef]
163. Ducommun, S.; Deak, M.; Sumpton, D.; Ford, R.J.; Núñez Galindo, A.; Kussmann, M.; Viollet, B.; Steinberg, G.R.; Foretz, M.; Dayon, L.; et al. Motif affinity and mass spectrometry proteomic approach for the discovery of cellular AMPK targets: Identification of mitochondrial fission factor as a new AMPK substrate. *Cell. Signal* **2015**, *27*, 978–988. [CrossRef] [PubMed]
164. Wang, B.; Nie, J.; Wu, L.; Hu, Y.; Wen, Z.; Dong, L.; Zou, M.H.; Chen, C.; Wang, D.W. AMPKα2 Protects Against the Development of Heart Failure by Enhancing Mitophagy via PINK1 Phosphorylation. *Circ. Res.* **2018**, *122*, 712–729. [CrossRef]
165. Laberge, R.M.; Sun, Y.; Orjalo, A.V.; Patil, C.K.; Freund, A.; Zhou, L.; Curran, S.C.; Davalos, A.R.; Wilson-Edell, K.A.; Liu, S.; et al. MTOR regulates the pro-tumorigenic senescence-associated secretory phenotype by promoting IL1A translation. *Nat. Cell Biol.* **2015**, *17*, 1049–1061. [CrossRef]
166. Abdelgawad, I.Y.; Agostinucci, K.; Sadaf, B.; Grant, M.K.O.; Zordoky, B.N. Metformin mitigates SASP secretion and LPS-triggered hyper-inflammation in Doxorubicin-induced senescent endothelial cells. *Front. Aging* **2023**, *4*, 1170434. [CrossRef]
167. Moiseeva, O.; Deschênes-Simard, X.; St-Germain, E.; Igelmann, S.; Huot, G.; Cadar, A.E.; Bourdeau, V.; Pollak, M.N.; Ferbeyre, G. Metformin inhibits the senescence-associated secretory phenotype by interfering with IKK/NF-κB activation. *Aging Cell* **2013**, *12*, 489–498. [CrossRef] [PubMed]
168. Fang, J.; Yang, J.; Wu, X.; Zhang, G.; Li, T.; Wang, X.; Zhang, H.; Wang, C.C.; Liu, G.H.; Wang, L. Metformin alleviates human cellular aging by upregulating the endoplasmic reticulum glutathione peroxidase 7. *Aging Cell* **2018**, *17*, e12765. [CrossRef]
169. Martin-Montalvo, A.; Mercken, E.M.; Mitchell, S.J.; Palacios, H.H.; Mote, P.L.; Scheibye-Knudsen, M.; Gomes, A.P.; Ward, T.M.; Minor, R.K.; Blouin, M.J.; et al. Metformin improves healthspan and lifespan in mice. *Nat. Commun.* **2013**, *4*, 2192. [CrossRef]
170. Campbell, J.M.; Bellman, S.M.; Stephenson, M.D.; Lisy, K. Metformin reduces all-cause mortality and diseases of ageing independent of its effect on diabetes control: A systematic review and meta-analysis. *Ageing Res. Rev.* **2017**, *40*, 31–44. [CrossRef] [PubMed]
171. Bu, Y.; Peng, M.; Tang, X.; Xu, X.; Wu, Y.; Chen, A.F.; Yang, X. Protective effects of metformin in various cardiovascular diseases: Clinical evidence and AMPK-dependent mechanisms. *J. Cell. Mol. Med.* **2022**, *26*, 4886–4903. [CrossRef]
172. Petrie, J.R.; Chaturvedi, N.; Ford, I.; Brouwers, M.; Greenlaw, N.; Tillin, T.; Hramiak, I.; Hughes, A.D.; Jenkins, A.J.; Klein, B.E.K.; et al. Cardiovascular and metabolic effects of metformin in patients with type 1 diabetes (REMOVAL): A double-blind, randomised, placebo-controlled trial. *Lancet Diabetes Endocrinol.* **2017**, *5*, 597–609. [CrossRef]
173. De Jager, J.; Kooy, A.; Lehert, P.; Bets, D.; Wulffelé, M.G.; Teerlink, T.; Scheffer, P.G.; Schalkwijk, C.G.; Donker, A.J.; Stehouwer, C.D. Effects of short-term treatment with metformin on markers of endothelial function and inflammatory activity in type 2 diabetes mellitus: A randomized, placebo-controlled trial. *J. Intern. Med.* **2005**, *257*, 100–109. [CrossRef]
174. Jadhav, S.; Ferrell, W.; Greer, I.A.; Petrie, J.R.; Cobbe, S.M.; Sattar, N. Effects of metformin on microvascular function and exercise tolerance in women with angina and normal coronary arteries: A randomized, double-blind, placebo-controlled study. *J. Am. Coll. Cardiol.* **2006**, *48*, 956–963. [CrossRef]
175. Preiss, D.; Lloyd, S.M.; Ford, I.; McMurray, J.J.; Holman, R.R.; Welsh, P.; Fisher, M.; Packard, C.J.; Sattar, N. Metformin for non-diabetic patients with coronary heart disease (the CAMERA study): A randomised controlled trial. *Lancet Diabetes Endocrinol.* **2014**, *2*, 116–124. [CrossRef]
176. Xu, W.; Deng, Y.Y.; Yang, L.; Zhao, S.; Liu, J.; Zhao, Z.; Wang, L.; Maharjan, P.; Gao, S.; Tian, Y.; et al. Metformin ameliorates the proinflammatory state in patients with carotid artery atherosclerosis through sirtuin 1 induction. *Transl. Res.* **2015**, *166*, 451–458. [CrossRef]
177. Zhang, L.; Pitcher, L.E.; Prahalad, V.; Niedernhofer, L.J.; Robbins, P.D. Targeting cellular senescence with senotherapeutics: Senolytics and senomorphics. *FEBS J.* **2023**, *290*, 1362–1383. [CrossRef]
178. Barzilai, N.; Crandall, J.P.; Kritchevsky, S.B.; Espeland, M.A. Metformin as a Tool to Target Aging. *Cell Metab.* **2016**, *23*, 1060–1065. [CrossRef]
179. Mortensen, S.A.; Rosenfeldt, F.; Kumar, A.; Dolliner, P.; Filipiak, K.J.; Pella, D.; Alehagen, U.; Steurer, G.; Littarru, G.P. The effect of coenzyme Q10 on morbidity and mortality in chronic heart failure: Results from Q-SYMBIO: A randomized double-blind trial. *JACC Heart Fail.* **2014**, *2*, 641–649. [CrossRef]
180. Zeb, I.; Ahmadi, N.; Nasir, K.; Kadakia, J.; Larijani, V.N.; Flores, F.; Li, D.; Budoff, M.J. Aged garlic extract and coenzyme Q10 have favorable effect on inflammatory markers and coronary atherosclerosis progression: A randomized clinical trial. *J. Cardiovasc. Dis. Res.* **2012**, *3*, 185–190. [CrossRef]
181. MRC/BHF Heart Protection Study of antioxidant vitamin supplementation in 20,536 high-risk individuals: A randomised placebo-controlled trial. *Lancet* **2002**, *360*, 23–33. [CrossRef]
182. Sesso, H.D.; Buring, J.E.; Christen, W.G.; Kurth, T.; Belanger, C.; MacFadyen, J.; Bubes, V.; Manson, J.E.; Glynn, R.J.; Gaziano, J.M. Vitamins E and C in the prevention of cardiovascular disease in men: The Physicians' Health Study II randomized controlled trial. *JAMA* **2008**, *300*, 2123–2133. [CrossRef] [PubMed]

183. Gutierrez-Mariscal, F.M.; de la Cruz-Ares, S.; Torres-Peña, J.D.; Alcalá-Diaz, J.F.; Yubero-Serrano, E.M.; López-Miranda, Coenzyme Q(10) and Cardiovascular Diseases. *Antioxidants* **2021**, *10*, 906. [CrossRef] [PubMed]
184. Lei, L.; Liu, Y. Efficacy of coenzyme Q10 in patients with cardiac failure: A meta-analysis of clinical trials. *BMC Cardiovasc. Disor.* **2017**, *17*, 196. [CrossRef] [PubMed]
185. Sheu, S.S.; Nauduri, D.; Anders, M.W. Targeting antioxidants to mitochondria: A new therapeutic direction. *Biochim. Biophy Acta* **2006**, *1762*, 256–265. [CrossRef]
186. Reily, C.; Mitchell, T.; Chacko, B.K.; Benavides, G.; Murphy, M.P.; Darley-Usmar, V. Mitochondrially targeted compounds an their impact on cellular bioenergetics. *Redox Biol.* **2013**, *1*, 86–93. [CrossRef]
187. Kulkarni, C.A.; Fink, B.D.; Gibbs, B.E.; Chheda, P.R.; Wu, M.; Sivitz, W.I.; Kerns, R.J. A Novel Triphenylphosphonium Carrier t Target Mitochondria without Uncoupling Oxidative Phosphorylation. *J. Med. Chem.* **2021**, *64*, 662–676. [CrossRef]
188. Ribeiro Junior, R.F.; Dabkowski, E.R.; Shekar, K.C.; KA, O.C.; Hecker, P.A.; Murphy, M.P. MitoQ improves mitochondria dysfunction in heart failure induced by pressure overload. *Free Radic. Biol. Med.* **2018**, *117*, 18–29. [CrossRef]
189. Adlam, V.J.; Harrison, J.C.; Porteous, C.M.; James, A.M.; Smith, R.A.; Murphy, M.P.; Sammut, I.A. Targeting an antioxidant to mitochondria decreases cardiac ischemia-reperfusion injury. *FASEB J.* **2005**, *19*, 1088–1095. [CrossRef]
190. Dare, A.J.; Logan, A.; Prime, T.A.; Rogatti, S.; Goddard, M.; Bolton, E.M.; Bradley, J.A.; Pettigrew, G.J.; Murphy, M.P.; Saeb-Parsy K. The mitochondria-targeted anti-oxidant MitoQ decreases ischemia-reperfusion injury in a murine syngeneic heart transplan model. *J. Heart Lung Transplant.* **2015**, *34*, 1471–1480. [CrossRef]
191. Graham, D.; Huynh, N.N.; Hamilton, C.A.; Beattie, E.; Smith, R.A.; Cochemé, H.M.; Murphy, M.P.; Dominiczak, A.F. Mitochondria targeted antioxidant MitoQ10 improves endothelial function and attenuates cardiac hypertrophy. *Hypertension* **2009**, *54*, 322–328 [CrossRef]
192. Goh, K.Y.; He, L.; Song, J.; Jinno, M.; Rogers, A.J.; Sethu, P.; Halade, G.V.; Rajasekaran, N.S.; Liu, X.; Prabhu, S.D.; et al Mitoquinone ameliorates pressure overload-induced cardiac fibrosis and left ventricular dysfunction in mice. *Redox Biol.* **2019**, *21* 101100. [CrossRef]
193. Rossman, M.J.; Santos-Parker, J.R.; Steward, C.A.C.; Bispham, N.Z.; Cuevas, L.M.; Rosenberg, H.L.; Woodward, K.A.; Chonchol M.; Gioscia-Ryan, R.A.; Murphy, M.P.; et al. Chronic Supplementation With a Mitochondrial Antioxidant (MitoQ) Improves Vascular Function in Healthy Older Adults. *Hypertension* **2018**, *71*, 1056–1063. [CrossRef]
194. Varesi, A.; Chirumbolo, S.; Campagnoli, L.I.M.; Pierella, E.; Piccini, G.B.; Carrara, A.; Ricevuti, G.; Scassellati, C.; Bonvicini C.; Pascale, A. The Role of Antioxidants in the Interplay between Oxidative Stress and Senescence. *Antioxidants* **2022**, *11*, 1224 [CrossRef]
195. Breccia, M.; Alimena, G. Activity and safety of dasatinib as second-line treatment or in newly diagnosed chronic phase chronic myeloid leukemia patients. *BioDrugs* **2011**, *25*, 147–157. [CrossRef]
196. Chan, C.M.; Jing, X.; Pike, L.A.; Zhou, Q.; Lim, D.J.; Sams, S.B.; Lund, G.S.; Sharma, V.; Haugen, B.R.; Schweppe, R.E. Targeted inhibition of Src kinase with dasatinib blocks thyroid cancer growth and metastasis. *Clin. Cancer Res.* **2012**, *18*, 3580–3591. [CrossRef]
197. Bruning, A. Inhibition of mTOR signaling by quercetin in cancer treatment and prevention. *Anti-Cancer Agents Med. Chem.* **2013**, *13*, 1025–1031. [CrossRef]
198. Olave, N.C.; Grenett, M.H.; Cadeiras, M.; Grenett, H.E.; Higgins, P.J. Upstream stimulatory factor-2 mediates quercetin-induced suppression of PAI-1 gene expression in human endothelial cells. *J. Cell. Biochem.* **2010**, *111*, 720–726. [CrossRef]
199. Chang, J.; Wang, Y.; Shao, L.; Laberge, R.M.; Demaria, M.; Campisi, J.; Janakiraman, K.; Sharpless, N.E.; Ding, S.; Feng, W.; et al. Clearance of senescent cells by ABT263 rejuvenates aged hematopoietic stem cells in mice. *Nat. Med.* **2016**, *22*, 78–83. [CrossRef] [PubMed]
200. Zhu, Y.; Tchkonia, T.; Fuhrmann-Stroissnigg, H.; Dai, H.M.; Ling, Y.Y.; Stout, M.B.; Pirtskhalava, T.; Giorgadze, N.; Johnson, K.O.; Giles, C.B.; et al. Identification of a novel senolytic agent, navitoclax, targeting the Bcl-2 family of anti-apoptotic factors. *Aging Cell* **2016**, *15*, 428–435. [CrossRef] [PubMed]
201. Lérida-Viso, A.; Estepa-Fernández, A.; Morellá-Aucejo, Á.; Lozano-Torres, B.; Alfonso, M.; Blandez, J.F.; Bisbal, V.; Sepúlveda, P.; García-Fernández, A.; Orzáez, M.; et al. Pharmacological senolysis reduces doxorubicin-induced cardiotoxicity and improves cardiac function in mice. *Pharmacol. Res.* **2022**, *183*, 106356. [CrossRef] [PubMed]
202. Garrido, A.M.; Kaistha, A.; Uryga, A.K.; Oc, S.; Foote, K.; Shah, A.; Finigan, A.; Figg, N.; Dobnikar, L.; Jørgensen, H.; et al. Efficacy and limitations of senolysis in atherosclerosis. *Cardiovasc. Res.* **2022**, *118*, 1713–1727. [CrossRef] [PubMed]
203. Lewis-McDougall, F.C.; Ruchaya, P.J.; Domenjo-Vila, E.; Shin Teoh, T.; Prata, L.; Cottle, B.J.; Clark, J.E.; Punjabi, P.P.; Awad, W.; Torella, D.; et al. Aged-senescent cells contribute to impaired heart regeneration. *Aging Cell* **2019**, *18*, e12931. [CrossRef]
204. Niedernhofer, L.J.; Robbins, P.D. Senotherapeutics for healthy ageing. *Nat. Rev. Drug Discov.* **2018**, *17*, 377. [CrossRef] [PubMed]

diseases

MDPI

Article

Impact of Non-Surgical Periodontal Treatment on the Concentration and Level of MRP-8/14 (Calprotectin) as an Inflammatory Biomarker in Women with Periodontitis and Rheumatoid Arthritis: A Quasi-Experimental Study

Elena Aurora Popoca-Hernández [1,2], Rita Elizabeth Martínez-Martínez [2,*], Roberto Fidencio González-Amaro [3,4], Perla del Carmen Niño-Moreno [4], José Luis Ayala-Herrera [5], Alberto Vinicio Jerezano-Domínguez [6], Leon Francisco Espinosa-Cristóbal [7], María de Lourdes Márquez-Corona [8], Irene Aurora Espinosa-de Santillana [6] and Carlo Eduardo Medina-Solís [8]

1 Doctoral Program in Basic Biomedical Sciences, Faculty of Medicine, Autonomous University of San Luis Potosi, San Luis Potosi 78210, Mexico; elena.popoca@correo.buap.mx
2 Master Program in Advanced Dentistry, Faculty of Dentistry, Autonomous University of San Luis Potosi, San Luis Potosi 78290, Mexico
3 Department of Immunology, Faculty of Medicine, Autonomous University of San Luis Potosi, San Luis Potosi 78210, Mexico; rgonzale@uaslp.mx
4 Center of Research in Health Sciences and Biomedicine, Faculty of Medicine, Autonomous University of San Luis Potosi, San Luis Potosi 78210, Mexico; ncarmenp@uaslp.mx
5 School of Dentistry, Universidad De La Salle Bajío, Leon 37150, Mexico; jayala@delasalle.edu.mx
6 School of Stomatology, Meritorious Autonomous University of Puebla, Puebla 72410, Mexico; alberto.jerezano@correo.buap.mx (A.V.J.-D.); irene.espinosa@correo.buap.mx (I.A.E.-d.S.)
7 Master Program in Dental Sciences, Stomatology Department, Institute of Biomedical Sciences, Autonomous University of Juarez City, Ciudad Juárez 32310, Mexico; leon.espinosa@uacj.mx
8 Academic Area of Dentistry, Health Sciences Institute, Autonomous University of Hidalgo State, Pachuca 42160, Mexico; lmarquez@uaeh.edu.mx (M.d.L.M.-C.); cemedinas@uaeh.edu.mx (C.E.M.-S.)
* Correspondence: rita.martinez@uaslp.mx

Abstract: The aim of this study was to evaluate the impact of non-surgical periodontal treatment (NS-PT) on periodontal parameters and inflammatory biomarkers in the concentration and level of calprotectin (CLP) in women with periodontitis and rheumatoid arthritis (RA). In this quasi-experimental study, we evaluated 30 women (mean age: 52.0 ± 5.8 years) with periodontitis and RA who had been diagnosed and treated for RA for more than 3 years and whose activity markers remained at similar values without significant reduction over three consecutive months. Patients underwent NS-PT, which included plaque control, scaling, and root planing. Serum and saliva samples, periodontal indices, RA activity markers, Disease Activity Score-28 (DAS28), the erythrocyte sedimentation rate (ESR), and the C-reactive protein (CRP) and CLP contents were measured at the beginning of the study and 6 and 12 weeks after NS-PT. Parametric and nonparametric tests were used in the analysis. The mean age was 52.0 ± 5.8 years. Compared to the baseline results, all periodontal indices were significantly reduced 6 and 12 weeks after NS-PT ($p < 0.001$). DAS28 was also significantly reduced after 12 weeks ($p < 0.0001$). Similarly, the serum CLP concentration decreased 6 and 12 weeks after NS-PT ($p < 0.0001$). Of the patients, 100% presented lower levels of CRP and ESR ($p < 0.0001$). Overall, NS-PT reduced inflammation and disease activity, highlighting the importance of oral health in the control and treatment of systemic diseases such as RA and confirming that NS-PT effectively reduces periodontitis activity and plays a key role in modulating RA activity. Therefore, NS-PT should be considered as an adjunct treatment for RA.

Keywords: oral health; periodontitis; periodontal treatment; inflammatory biomarkers; rheumatoid arthritis

1. Introduction

According to the Global Burden of Disease Study 2017, periodontal disease, a chronic inflammatory disease, is considered the 11th most prevalent condition [1]. It affects tooth-supporting tissues and has effects ranging from gingivitis to the most aggressive forms of periodontitis (PE) that result in tooth loss [2,3]. Following caries, PE is considered the second-most-frequent oral disease. On a global scale, the prevalence of severe periodontal disease has experienced a progressive increase, despite ongoing attempts to prevent and manage the advancement of this condition, and gingivitis and periodontitis now have a global prevalence ranging from 20% to 50% [4]. Periodontal disease affects the tissues that both surround and support the teeth. The disease is characterized by bleeding or swollen gums (gingivitis), pain, and sometimes bad breath. In its more severe form, the gum can come away from the tooth and supporting bone, causing teeth to become loose and sometimes fall out. The main risk factors for periodontal disease are poor oral hygiene and tobacco use. The origin of periodontitis is multifactorial and involves multiple component causes, genetics, epigenetic influences, and modifiable factors such as environmental factors, habits, and medications that establish and propagate periodontitis lesions [5,6]. The appearance of dysbiosis of the subgingival microbiome triggers an inflammatory response. This results in the expression of several mediators that can lead to alveolar bone loss and tooth mobility. In this situation, oral hygiene is essential; however, this is not achieved adequately in the majority of patients, because many of them do not prioritize oral care and hygiene [7,8].

The first step in the chronological sequence of periodontal procedures is termed non-surgical periodontal treatment (NS-PT), the cornerstone of periodontal therapy. It includes plaque removal and control, scaling and root planing, and occasionally, the use of chemical agents [9,10]. The goal of NS-PT is to control periodontal infection by removing bacteria and calculus from periodontally involved root surfaces. However, when periodontal tissues require remodeling, surgical periodontal treatment is also indicated. Periodontitis does not only affect dentition; it also represents a threat to general health. Indeed, periodontitis has been associated with different systemic conditions, including adverse pregnancy outcomes [11,12], metabolic syndrome [13], diabetes mellitus [14], osteoporosis [14], cardiovascular disease [15–17], Alzheimer's disease [18], and chronic obstructive pulmonary disease [19]. As a disease in which inflammation is triggered, it has also been associated with the presence of oral, colorectal, or breast cancers [20].

In addition, periodontal bacteria and related inflammatory mediators have been demonstrated to modulate systemic inflammatory and autoimmune responses in various diseases, including RA, a chronic inflammatory disease of autoimmune origin [11–23], and studies have demonstrated a correlation between periodontitis and RA [21–23]. RA, a systemic disease, is characterized by the accumulation of an inflammatory infiltrate in the synovial membrane, which leads to the destruction of the joint's architecture, typically affecting the small joints of the hands and feet, among others, causing losses in function and a decreased quality of life or even death [24,25].The diagnosis of RA and its level of activity are determined using a combination of clinical and laboratory tests, most commonly the Disease Activity Score-28 (DAS28) index, the erythrocyte sedimentation rate (ESR), and the serum level of C-reactive protein (CRP), to establish the baseline values in order to assess the evolution of the disease [26].

Several reports have provided evidence of an association between RA and periodontitis [21–23]. Currently, the possible etiopathogenic relationship between RA and PE is being investigated. This is not only limited to the sharing of inflammatory mechanisms but also the importance of periodontal infections due to the role they play in the citrullination of peptides (post-production modification of arginine residues into citrulline) and the associated development of antibodies against citrullinated proteins that are specific to RA and are related to the pathogenesis and severity of the disease. The prevalence of periodontitis is high, and the presence of bacterial DNA from periodontal bacteria has been identified in the synovial fluid, as well as in the serum of patients with RA [27]. The gram-negative bacterium *Porphyromonas gingivalis* is a significant factor in the development of PE and is the only bacterium that expresses the enzyme peptidyl arginine deiminase (PAD), which is responsible for the citrullination process. It has been suggested that infection with this microorganism could accelerate the onset and progression of RA by facilitating the presentation of autoantigens and the expression of autoantibodies against citrullinated peptides (ACPA) that are specific and almost exclusive to RA [26–30].

Some biomarkers common to both diseases have also been detected. However, there is a paucity of information about the effects of periodontal treatment on the evolution and activity level of RA [21,22,27,31]. Common biomarkers of periodontitis and RA activity include calprotectin (CLP), also known as a myeloid-related protein (MRP-8/14) or leukocyte protein L1, which is a heterodimer formed by two calcium-binding proteins S100A8 and S100A9 [27,32]. CLP is predominantly expressed in myeloid cells, such as neutrophils, monocytes, and macrophages [33]. Recently, CLP has been demonstrated to play a role in modulating host adaptive immunity and has been associated with various inflammatory diseases such as RA, systemic lupus erythematosus, Sjögren's syndrome, pulmonary fibroma, colorectal cancer, and periodontitis [34]. CLP is a highly regulated protein in RA and has been identified in tissues and synovial fluid at sites of active joint destruction produced by macrophages, synovial fibroblasts, and chondrocytes. These cells are involved in the amplification of the inflammatory process, cartilage destruction, and bone resorption [35,36]. In periodontitis, CLP has been identified in crevicular fluid in areas with gingival inflammation. It binds to specific receptors involved in different transduction signals, such as advanced glycation end-products (RAGE) and toll-like 4 receptors (TLR4). These receptors detect pathogen-associated and/or damage-associated molecular patterns (DAMPs) and immediately trigger an inflammatory cascade [37,38]. Their concentrations are correlated with periodontal parameters such as the pocket depth (PD), bleeding on probing (BOP), and gingival index (GI). Notably, human S100A8 is a potent and specific autocrine chemotactic factor in periodontal ligament cells. Accordingly, it may be an attractive therapeutic candidate for the treatment of periodontal disease [39].

Given the association of CLP with RA and periodontitis, the aim of this study was to evaluate the impact of non-surgical periodontal treatment (NS-PT) on periodontal parameters and inflammatory biomarkers in the concentration and level of CLP in women with periodontitis and rheumatoid arthritis (RA).

2. Materials and Methods

2.1. Study Design

This quasi-experimental study included 30 female consecutive patients with PE and RA who provided their informed consent. Quasi-experimental study designs are often described as non-randomized, before-and-after, or pre- and post-intervention studies (pretest-posttest). They comprise a broad range of clinical-epidemiological studies in which, for ethical or logistical reasons, it is not possible to carry out randomization or, because the patients need the treatment, a pure experimental study cannot be carried out. They are those studies in which the control and experimental groups comprise the same subjects. Similar to randomized trials, the aim of quasi-experiments aim is to demonstrate causality between an intervention and an outcome. Although the randomized controlled trial is generally considered to have the highest level of credibility with respect to assessing causality, researchers often choose not to randomize the intervention for one or more reasons: (1) ethical considerations, (2) difficulty in randomizing subjects, (3) difficulty in randomizing by locations, and (4) small available sample size [40]. The patients were recruited from the clinics of the Faculty of Dentistry and the Department of Rheumatology of University Hospital of the Meritorious Autonomous University of Puebla, Mexico, in the period from January 2018 to February 2020. Samples were processed as part of the Master's Laboratory Degree in Dental Sciences from the Autonomous University of San Luis Potosí, San Luis Potosí, SLP, Mexico.

The inclusion criteria were the following: adult women with a minimum of 20 teeth who had been treated with the disease-modifying antirheumatic drug (DMARD) methotrexate for a minimum of 3 years; had at least a 5-year history of RA with similar RA indicator values, without a significant decrease in the last 3 months and rheumatoid factor seropositive and anti-cyclic citrullinated peptide (anti-CCP) antibodies; and had no other diagnosed systemic disease, including Sjögren's syndrome. Pregnant or lactating women and patients who had undergone prior periodontal treatment were excluded from the study.

2.2. Rheumatoid Arthritis Diagnosis and DAS28

The diagnosis of RA was made by an expert rheumatologist, who applied the criteria of the American College of Rheumatology and the European League Against Rheumatism established in 2010 [41]. The DAS28 index was employed to identify the level of disease activity and was performed as previously described in the literature [42]. The RA activity level was considered low, moderate, and high when the DAS28 score was 2.6–3.2, 3.2–5.1, and >5.1, respectively [41].

2.3. Periodontal Diagnosis

The diagnosis of periodontitis was made by a single examiner based on criteria previously standardized by an expert periodontist. Patients were diagnosed with generalized chronic periodontitis according to the 1999 Classification of Periodontal Diseases [42]. Patients corresponded to stage II and grade A based on the application of the periodontitis staging and grading system [43].

Other periodontal measurements such as PD and clinical attachment loss (CAL) were performed at six sites per tooth using the standard North Carolina manual periodontal probe (HuFriedy, Chicago, IL, USA) graduated in mm. CAL was calculated by adding the probing depth to the gingival margin level at the recession sites and subtracting the gingival margin level from the probing depth where the margin covered enamel; at the normal level, CAL was coincident with the PD [43]. Periodontal indices, including the oral hygiene index (OHI) [44], GI [45], BOP [46], plaque index (PI) [47], periodontal inflamed surface area (PISA), and periodontal epithelial surface area (PESA) [48], were obtained.

2.4. NS-PT

All patients underwent NS-PT. At the first appointment, patients received a verbal explanation about the treatment. A baseline evaluation of the periodontal indices was performed, and blood and saliva samples were collected. Subsequently, patients received oral hygiene instructions and education about the modified Bass technique. Supragingival deposits (plaque and calculus) were then removed using an ultrasonic scaler (Various 350, NSK, Shimohinata, Kanuma, Japan). Patients were instructed to maintain adequate oral hygiene in order to reduce the OHI, PI, BOP, and GI by at least 25% and to be able to continue with the treatment in order to ensure the success of NS-PT during the 12-week study period [49]. At the second appointment, if this reduction had been achieved, patients were treated with full-mouth scaling and root planing (SRP). Patients attended follow-up appointments every 2 weeks. In weeks 6 and 12 post-treatment, samples were recollected, and the indices were re-evaluated. The treatment was carried out on all participants. If, after a week, they did not exhibit reductions of 25%, instructions were given again, and NS-PT was performed until this was achieved. This served as confirmation that the patient already knew the correct techniques to maintain good oral hygiene.

In addition to measurements at the baseline, 6 weeks, and 12 weeks after NS-PT, records were obtained on the day of SRP. "Baseline" refers to the first time the patient arrived and had her periodontal indices checked before the oral hygiene techniques were explained to her and "Day of NS-PT" is the day on which there was already a 25% reduction and the patient underwent NS-PT.

2.5. Serum and Saliva Samples

To measure serum concentrations of CLP and CRP, peripheral blood samples were collected from the cubital vein in citrated vacuum tubes. The ESR was determined routinely. Samples were centrifuged at 1500 g for 10 min to obtain the serum [49]. Stimulated saliva samples were collected to measure the CLP concentration. Samples were obtained at the baseline and 6 and 12 weeks after NS-PT. The samples were stored at −40 °C until the performance of enzyme-linked immunosorbent assays (ELISAs) [50].

2.6. Enzyme-Linked Immunosorbent Assay

The serum and saliva levels of CLP and CRP were measured using commercial ELISA kits (S100A8/9 Human Elisa Kit 96 test, Invitrogen ThermoFisher, Madison, WI, USA, and CRP Human Instant ELISA Kit 128 test, Invitrogen ThermoFisher, Madison, WI, USA, respectively) according to the manufacturer's instructions using 50 μL serum or saliva samples. Absorbance was measured and analyzed with a microplate spectrophotometer (Thermo Scientific Multiskan FC Microplate Photometer, Vantaa, Finland).

2.7. Statistical Analysis

The examiner was calibrated by an expert in the diagnosis of periodontitis through an intraclass correlation coefficient analysis (k = 0.80). Qualitative data are expressed as frequencies and proportions. Quantitative data are presented as means, standard deviations, and ranges. The Shapiro–Wilk test was performed to determine the normality of the distribution of the variables. Friedman, ANOVA, and Wilcoxon tests were performed to compare the differences between examination periods. The significance level was set to $p < 0.05$. For the data analysis, the statistical program Prism-GraphPad was used.

2.8. Ethical Issues

This study was approved by the Research Ethics Committee of the Faculty of Dentistry of the Autonomous University of San Luis Potosi, Mexico (CEI-FE-044-018), and the Research Committee of the Faculty of Dentistry of the Meritorious Autonomous University of Puebla, Mexico (2019110). The study was performed in accordance with the Declaration of Helsinki and the CONSORT guidelines.

3. Results

3.1. Patients

The interobserver consistency for the results of the 30 patients was >0.80.

3.2. Periodontal Findings

The criterion of reductions of at least 25% in the values of the OHI, PI, GI, and BOP was attained ($p < 0.0001$). Significant reductions were observed in all indices 6 and 12 weeks after NS-PT compared to the baseline ($p < 0.001$) (Table 1). No significant differences were noted between 6 and 12 weeks after treatment ($p > 0.05$). A reduction of >50% was observed for PD (4.0, 1.8, and 1.8 mm; $p < 0.0001$). CAL also exhibited a significant reduction among samples ($p < 0.0001$).

The PESA values represent the surface area of the periodontal epithelium, including healthy and inflamed tissues. This index demonstrated a reduction of approximately 70% from the baseline to 6–12 weeks after NS-PT (556.4, 174.1, and 161.1 mm^2; $p < 0.0001$). The PISA values, which correspond only to the inflamed surface area, exhibited a decrease of >95% from the baseline measurements (352 mm^2) to 6–12 weeks after NS-PT (16.5 mm^2) ($p < 0.0001$).

Table 1. Periodontal evaluation before and after non-surgical periodontal treatment (NS-PT).

	Baseline Mean ± SD (Range)	6 Weeks after NS-PT Mean ± SD (Range)	12 Weeks after NS-PT Mean ± SD (Range)	*p* Value
PD (mm)	4.0 ± 0.11 (3.7–4.2)	1.8 ± 0.12 (1.7–2.1)	1.8 ± 0.1 (1.6–1.9)	<0.0001 *
CAL (mm)	2.6 ± 0.14 (2.4–3.1)	2.0 ± 0.23 (1.8–2.8)	1.7 ± 0.08 (1.6–1.8)	<0.0001 *
PESA (mm^2)	556.4 ± 28.8 (487.6–597.0)	174.1± 14.8 (156.6–208.8)	161.1 ± 9.1 (150.5–183.5)	<0.0001 **
PISA (mm^2)	351.1 ± 29.7 (292.5–398.3)	16.5 ± 6.7 (6.3–28.9)	16.5 ± 6.7 (5.5–29.9)	<0.0001 **

SD: standard deviation, PD: pocket depth, CAL: clinical attachment loss, PESA: periodontal epithelial surface area, PISA: periodontal inflamed surface area. * Friedman test, ** ANOVA repeated measurements. n = 30. The PD, CAL, PESA, and PISA results were measured at the baseline and 6 and 12 weeks after NS-PT. Data are presented as the mean ± standard deviation. PD and CAL were compared using the Friedman test ($p < 0.0001$). PESA and PISA were analyzed using repeated-measures ANOVA ($p < 0.0001$).

The OHI and dental PI values were reduced from 1.2 ± 0.15 and 2.1 ± 0.09 to 0.3 ± 0.04 and 0.5 ± 0.03, respectively, on the day of the SRP ($p < 0.0001$). These values were maintained at similar levels 6 and 12 weeks after NS-PT ($p > 0.05$) (Table 2).

Table 2. Periodontal indexes at different time points.

	Baseline Mean ± SD (Range)	At Scaling and Root Planing Mean ± SD (Range)	6 Weeks after NS-PT Mean ± SD (Range)	12 Weeks after NS-PT Mean ± SD (Range)	*p* Value *
OHI	1.2 ± 0.15 (1.0–1.6)	0.3 ± 0.04 (0.2–0.4)	0.3 ± 0.04 (0.2–0.4)	0.2 ± 0.04 (0.2–0.3)	<0.0001
PI	2.1 ± 0.09 (1.8–2.2)	0.5 ± 0.03 (0.4–0.5)	0.5 ± 0.03 (0.4–0.5)	0.4 ± 0.05 (0.3–0.5)	<0.0001
GI	2.8 ± 0.17 (2.5–3.0)	1.2 ± 0.1 (1.0–1.5) **	0.8 ± 0.35 (0.2–1.3)	0.6 ± 0.27 (0.0–1.0)	<0.0001
BOP	3.8 ± 0.19 (3.5–4.0)	0.8 ± 0.09 (0.7–1.0) **	0.5 ± 0.20 (0.2–0.8)	0.4 ± 0.22 (0.0–0.8)	<0.0001

SD: standard deviation, OHI: oral hygiene index, PI: plaque index, GI: gingival index, BOP: bleeding on probing. * Friedman test, ** $p < 0.0001$ Wilcoxon test. n = 30. The results of the periodontal indices, OHI, GI, and BOP were measured and compared at four different timepoints (baseline, day of NS-PT, and 6 weeks and 12 weeks after NS-PT). Data are presented as the mean ± standard deviation. The analysis was performed using the Friedman test ($p < 0.0001$). Wilcoxon testing was used to analyze the GI and BOP on the day of the NS-PT and 6 weeks post-treatment.

GI and BOP decreased from 2.8 ± 0.17 and 3.8 ± 0.19 to 1.2 ± 0.1 and 0.8 ± 0.09 on the day of the SRP, respectively ($p < 0.0001$). These two indices were significantly lower 6 and 12 weeks post-NS-PT ($p < 0.0001$). The GI values obtained 6 and 12 weeks after NS-PT were 0.8 ± 0.35 and 0.6 ± 0.27, respectively. The BOP values were 0.5 ± 0.20 and 0.4 ± 0.22 6 and 12 weeks after NS-PT, respectively ($p > 0.05$) (Table 2).

3.3. RA Activity Level

The mean ESR values at the baseline and 12 weeks after NS-PT were significantly different (70.5 mm vs. 42.3 mm; $p < 0.0001$), reaching almost-normal values over this period. The DAS28 scores exhibited a significant decrease from 5.4 ± 0.47 at the baseline to 3.2 ± 0.28 12 weeks post-treatment ($p < 0.0001$), representing a decline of >40%. The level of RA activity at the baseline was high in 61.5% and moderate in 38.5% of patients. None of the patients exhibited low levels of RA activity. This situation improved 12 weeks after NS-PT with 57.7% of patients exhibiting reduced RA activity and reaching a moderate level, and 42.3% reaching a low level ($p < 0.0001$). No patient demonstrated a high level of activity post-treatment. Of the patients, 100% exhibited a reduction in the RA activity level, and only one patient demonstrated a reduction from high to low (Table 3, Figure 1).

Table 3. Disease Activity Score-28 (DAS28) and erythrocyte sedimentation rate (ESR).

	Before Treatment Mean ± SD (Range)	12 Weeks after NS-PT Mean ± SD (Range)	p Value
ESR (mm per hour)	70.5 ± 8.01 (60–82)	42.3 ± 4.81 (36–49.2)	<0.0001 *
DAS28	5.4 ± 0.47 (4.8–6.0)	3.2 ± 0.28 (2.8–3.6)	<0.0001 *
	Frequency (%)	**Frequency (%)**	
RA activity level			
Low (DAS28: 2.6–3.2)	0 (0)	11 (42.3)	
Moderate (DAS28: 3.2–5.1)	10 (38.5)	15 (57.7)	< 0.0001 **
High (DAS28: 5.1–8.4)	16 (61.5)	0 (0)	

NS-PT: non-surgical periodontal treatment, SD: standard deviation, RA: rheumatoid arthritis. * Wilcoxon test, ** Fisher's exact test. AR activity level, comparison of DAS28 and ESR measured at baseline and 12 weeks after NS-PT. Data were analyzed using a Wilcoxon test ($p < 0.0001$). RA activity was divided into low, moderate, and high activity levels based on DAS28 scores. Comparisons were performed using Fisher's exact test ($p < 0.0001$).

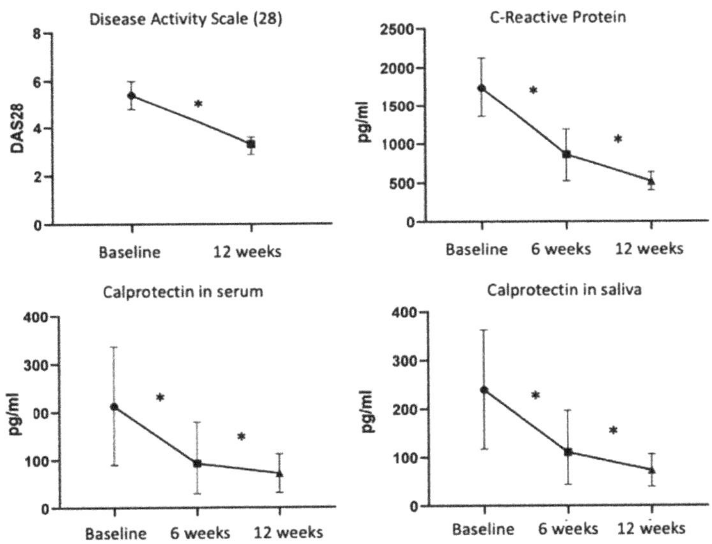

Figure 1. Comparison of AR activity and DAS-28 before treatment and 12 weeks after NS-PT using a Wilcoxon test (* $p < 0.0001$). C-reactive protein (CRP) levels were measured in pg/mL. Values at baseline and 6 and 12 weeks after NS-PT were compared using a repeated-measures ANOVA (* $p < 0.0001$). A comparison of calprotectin in serum and saliva (in pg/mL) at baseline and 6 and 12 weeks after NS-PT was conducted using the Friedman test (* $p < 0.0001$).

3.4. CLP and CRP

The serum concentration of CRP demonstrated a significant decrease 6 weeks after NS-PT relative to the value at the baseline (861.9 ± 200.1 pg/mL vs. 1739 ± 383.1 pg/mL; $p < 0.0001$). This reduction persisted up to 12 weeks post-intervention, reaching a value of 521.7 ± 114.9 pg/mL ($p < 0.0001$) (Table 4).

Serum CLP was significantly different between the baseline and 6-week post-treatment time points (234.4 ± 113.4 pg/mL vs. 105.6 ± 49.6 pg/mL; $p < 0.0001$) and exhibited a continuous reduction up to 12 weeks after treatment (70.6 pg/mL; $p < 0.0001$). These results are similar to those observed in saliva (baseline: 234.4 pg/mL, 6 weeks: 105.6 ± 49.6 pg/mL, and 12 weeks: 70.6 ± 113.4 pg/mL; $p < 0.0001$). The results obtained for serum were similar to those observed for saliva for the three different samples obtained ($p < 0.0001$).

Table 4. Inflammatory biomarkers before and after NS-PT.

	Baseline Mean ± SD (Range)	6 Weeks after NS-PT Mean ± SD (Range)	12 Weeks after NS-PT Mean ± SD (Range)	*p* Value
C-reactive protein	1739 ± 383.1 (1106–2298)	861.9 ± 200.1 †† (522.8–663.4)	521.7 ± 114.9 (331.7–689.5)	<0.0001 *
Serum calprotectin	205.0 ± 114.0 (90.5–391.1)	87.5 ± 48.6 †† (29.3–178.9)	66.8 ± 38.1 (18.5–141.2)	<0.0001 **
Saliva calprotectin	234.4 ± 113.4 (107.3–411.9)	105.6 ± 49.6 †† (43.0–197.0)	70.6 ± 32.4 (20.6–120.5)	<0.0001 **
Calprotectin serum vs. saliva	0.3564 †	0.1881 †	0.7059 †	

SD: standard deviation, results expressed in pg/mL. * Repeated-measures ANOVA, ** Friedman test, † Mann–Whitney U test, †† Wilcoxon test. n = 30. A comparison of inflammatory CRP was performed using a repeated-measures ANOVA ($p < 0.0001$). Serum and saliva CLP levels at baseline and at 6 weeks and 12 weeks were compared using the Friedman test ($p < 0.0001$). A comparison of calprotectin results in serum and saliva was performed using the Mann–Whitney test. All baseline and 6-week results were compared using the Wilcoxon test.

4. Discussion

This study investigated the effects of NS-PT as a treatment for RA. In accordance with our hypothesis, decreases in RA activity (DAS28), serum and saliva concentrations of CLP, ESR, serum CRP levels, and periodontal indices of patients with RA were measured 6–12 weeks post-treatment. A large number of patients were examined in the present study, but only 30 met the inclusion criteria and were included in the final analysis. In addition, some other patients also received NS-PT because they had PE and it was important to perform the treatment; however, they could not be included in the study. In this quasi-experimental study, a control group was not included in accordance with ethical recommendations, and each patient was used as their own control. To proceed with NS-PT, a 25% reduction in periodontal indices was required, as carried out by Walter, since this ensured that the patients were taking care of their oral hygiene. Patients who did not reduce their indices by 25% were taught the techniques again and were evaluated again; i.e., they all received the treatment until they reached a 25% reduction. Only females were evaluated in the study, since, in the biology of autoimmune disorders, it is generally accepted that females constitute a large majority of patients. Autoimmune disorders are characterized by a condition in which the host's immune system attacks itself by mistake. The mechanism of autoimmune diseases is not clear; however, they present a clear sex bias with a greater prevalence (2 to 1) among females. We assume that the results could also be beneficial for males [50].

Periodontitis is an inflammatory disease with a high global prevalence [7]. Periodontal bacteria and related inflammatory mediators have been demonstrated to modulate systemic inflammatory and autoimmune responses in various diseases, including RA [11–22]. Several reports have demonstrated an association between periodontitis and RA activity levels [14,20–27]. NS-PT is performed to eliminate the presence of periodontal bacteria and other local factors such as calculus, which trigger an inflammatory reaction. This procedure involves the control of dental plaque, oral hygiene instructions, and SRP [10].

In the current study, significant decreases were observed in periodontal indices (Tables 1 and 2), highlighting the effectiveness of NS-PT for reducing gingival inflammation. This is in accordance with previous reports demonstrating similar reductions in PD at 3 and 6 months to almost-normal levels [51,52]. Gonzalez et al. conducted a study in which 99 female patients (47.8 ± 15.5 years) were treated with synthetic disease-modifying antirheumatic drugs, and evaluations were performed 3-, 6-, and 12-months post-treatment. A total of 85% of the patients had evaluations 3 months, 58% 6 months, and 53% one year post-treatment. During a 3-month follow-up period, significant decreases were observed in DAS28 scores and the clinical activity of the disease compared to the values at the baseline visit ($p < 0.05$). We used this study as a guide to estimate the results 12 weeks after the treatment [53].

The PESA and PISA indices provide quantitative measures of the inflamed periodontal tissue (mm^2). In the current study, a reduction of approximately 70% in the PESA and a decrease of >95% in the PISA were observed from the baseline to 6–12 weeks after NS-PT. A significant reduction in the PISA index clearly demonstrates a reduction in the inflammatory component that impacts the levels of systemic biomarkers and response to pharmacological treatment of RA [54].

Measurement of the DAS28 index demonstrated a clinical decrease in the RA activity level after NS-PT. This index is considered the gold standard in the clinical evaluation of RA activity. We observed a significant reduction 12 weeks after NS-PT, in agreement with previous studies that reported a significant decrease in DAS28 3 months after NS-PT that remained constant at 6 months compared to an untreated control group [25,53,55]. Before treatment, most of the patients had a high level of RA activity and none of them demonstrated a low level. However, this changed drastically 12 weeks after treatment. During this period, all patients exhibited a decrease in the DAS28 index by one level, and one patient also exhibited a decrease by two levels (from high to low). Notably, none of the patients continued to exhibit high clinical levels of RA activity. This coincides with the report of Cosgarea et al. [52], in which NS-PT was performed on 18 patients with moderate-to-high RA activity (DAS28 $\geq$ 3.2). After 6 months, RA activity was reduced from moderate to remission (DAS28 < 2.6).

ESR is a laboratory test that reflects inflammatory processes and is used to identify increases in the plasma concentrations of two types of proteins, globulins and fibrinogen, which promote the more rapid sedimentation of erythrocytes during inflammation [56]. This assessment is necessary to determine the DAS28 index. In the present study, we observed a significant reduction at 3 months after NS-PT, in agreement with the results of Zhao et al. [57], who observed decreases in RA indicators (ESR, CRP, and DAS28 index) 3 months after NS-PT.

CRP is a protein produced by the liver that is secreted into the bloodstream within a few hours of the onset of an inflammatory process. Measurement of CRP is a useful tool to monitor the activity of chronic inflammatory diseases such as RA and periodontitis. In our study, NS-PT resulted in a decrease in this biomarker, similar to other studies presented in the literature [53–55].

The CLP biomarker is considered a key acute-phase protein that is produced by activated polymorphonuclear leukocytes (PMNs) in vascular tissue and inflammatory lesions. It is relatively stable and easy to measure [33]. CLP is found primarily in human plasma, urine, cerebrospinal fluid, feces, synovial fluid, gingival crevicular fluid, and saliva. It plays major roles in diverse biological functions, such as cell proliferation and differentiation, immunoregulation, oncogenesis, and apoptosis [58]. CLP levels increase significantly in individuals with various infectious and inflammatory diseases, such as pneumonia, septicemia, urinary tract infections, inflammatory bowel diseases (mainly Crohn's disease and ulcerative colitis), and RA [59]. Elevated CLP levels have been observed in the synovial fluid and plasma of patients with RA compared to healthy individuals. Notably, this outcome is closely associated with the level of disease activity [7]. CLP has recently been considered a key endogenous danger signal or DAMP and is an excellent biomarker for inflammatory processes that trigger intracellular signaling cascades in adjacent cells, thereby inducing inflammatory processes and the release of essential mediators [34]. In the current study, CLP concentrations in both the serum and saliva decreased significantly post-treatment. A search of the literature failed to reveal a similar study that measured the impact of NS-PT on CLP levels in the serum and saliva of patients with RA. Zhou et al. [60] investigated the levels of inflammatory biomarkers including CLP in saliva in individuals with experimental plaque-induced gingivitis. Their results demonstrated that CLP levels in saliva gradually increased and reached a peak on day 21, indicating that CLP levels in saliva may reflect the degree of gingival inflammation.

Other reports have demonstrated significant differences in the salivary CLP concentration between periodontally healthy individuals and those with periodontal disease [61]. A study of 969 patients with RA by Jarlborg et al. demonstrated an association between CLP levels and increased RA activity and severity measured using the swollen joint count, DAS, evaluation of health questionnaire joint radiographs, and the ultrasound power Doppler score (USPD) for RA [62].

In terms of limitations, this study was quasi-experimental, only one study was evaluated before, during, and twice after the treatment, and there was no control group. Additionally, the sample size was small. This was because patients had to have a weekly follow-up for 3 months; unfortunately, during this process, the COVID-19 pandemic began and it was no longer possible to continue with the follow-up of the other patients who had begun treatment. It is also likely that the Hawthorne effect occurred; this is a type of human behavioral reactivity in which individuals modify an aspect of their behavior in response to their awareness of being observed. This provides us with guidelines by which to continue the study and expand the sample to verify the results and observe the impact of this treatment in a larger population and for a longer time.

5. Conclusions

This study demonstrates that NS-PT is associated with a decrease in RA activity levels based on a significant decrease in the main clinical criterion of RA activity (DAS28 index) and several parameters such as CRP and ESR. NS-PT was also associated with reductions in serum and saliva concentrations of CLP, a key biomarker of RA activity. Collectively, these findings suggest that periodontal health is essential for the adequate control of RA activity. Rheumatologists may consider NS-PT as a tool to provide more effective rheumatologic treatment. Crucially, our study underscores the need to educate patients and professionals about the importance of oral health for their general well-being.

Author Contributions: Conceptualization, E.A.P.-H., R.F.G.-A., P.d.C.N.-M., A.V.J.-D., J.L.A.-H., L.F.E.-C., R.E.M.-M., M.d.L.M.-C., I.A.E.-d.S. and C.E.M.-S.; data curation, E.A.P.-H. and R.E.M.-M.; formal analysis, E.A.P.-H., R.F.G.-A., P.d.C.N.-M., A.V.J.-D., J.L.A.-H., L.F.E.-C., R.E.M.-M., M.d.L.M.-C., I.A.E.-d.S. and C.E.M.-S.; funding acquisition, R.E.M.-M.; investigation, E.A.P.-H. and R.E.M.-M.; methodology, E.A.P.-H., R.F.G.-A., P.d.C.N.-M., A.V.J.-D., J.L.A.-H., L.F.E.-C., R.E.M.-M., M.d.L.M.-C., I.A.E.-d.S. and C.E.M.-S.; project administration, E.A.P.-H.; resources, E.A.P.-H.; supervision, R.E.M.-M.; validation, E.A.P.-H. and R.E.M.-M.; writing—original draft, E.A.P.-H., R.F.G.-A., P.d.C.N.-M., A.V.J.-D., J.L.A.-H., L.F.E.-C., R.E.M.-M., M.d.L.M.-C., I.A.E.-d.S. and C.E.M.-S.; writing—review and editing, E.A.P.-H., R.F.G.-A., P.d.C.N.-M., A.V.J.-D., J.L.A.-H., L.F.E.-C., R.E.M.-M., M.d.L.M.-C., I.A.E.-d.S. and C.E.M.-S. All authors have read and agreed to the published version of the manuscript.

Funding: This investigation was supported by CONACYT CB-2014-01 (grant No. 242939) and CONACYT INFR-2014-01 (grant No. 226467).

Institutional Review Board Statement: All procedures involving human participants were in accordance with the ethical standards of the research committees of the two institutions where the study was conducted, i.e., UASLP (CEI-FE-044-018) and BUAP (2019110), and with the Declaration of Helsinki.

Informed Consent Statement: Informed consent was obtained from all subjects involved in the study.

Data Availability Statement: The datasets generated and/or analyzed during the current study are available from the corresponding author upon reasonable request.

Conflicts of Interest: The authors declare that they have no conflict of interest.

References

1. Murray, C.J.L. The Global Burden of Disease Study at 30 years. *Nat. Med.* **2022**, *28*, 2019–2026. [CrossRef] [PubMed]
2. Jiang, W.; Wang, Y.; Cao, Z.; Chen, Y.; Si, C.; Sun, X.; Huang, S. The role of mitochondrial dysfunction in periodontitis: From mechanisms to therapeutic strategy. *J. Periodontal Res.* **2023**, *58*, 853–863. [CrossRef] [PubMed]

GBD 2016 Disease and Injury Incidence and Prevalence Collaborators. Global, regional, and national incidence, prevalence, and years lived with disability for 328 diseases and injuries for 195 countries, 1990–2016: A systematic analysis for the global burden of disease study 2016. *Lancet* **2017**, *390*, 1211–1259. [CrossRef] [PubMed]

Nazir, M.; Al-Ansari, A.; Al-Khalifa, K.; Alhareky, M.; Gaffar, B.; Almas, K. Global prevalence of periodontal disease and lack of its surveillance. *Sci. World J.* **2020**, *2020*, 2146160. [CrossRef] [PubMed]

Laberge, S.; Akoum, D.; Wlodarczyk, P.; Massé, J.-D.; Fournier, D.; Semlali, A. The potential role of epigenetic modifications on different facets in the periodontal pathogenesis. *Genes* **2023**, *14*, 1202. [CrossRef] [PubMed]

Hung, M.; Kelly, R.; Mohajeri, A.; Reese, L.; Badawi, S.; Frost, C.; Sevathas, T.; Lipsky, M.S. Factors associated with periodontitis in younger individuals: A scoping review. *J. Clin. Med.* **2023**, *12*, 6442. [CrossRef] [PubMed]

Choi, I.A.; Kim, J.H.; Kim, Y.M.; Lee, J.Y.; Kim, K.H.; Lee, E.Y.; Lee, E.B.; Lee, Y.M.; Song, Y.W. Periodontitis is associated with rheumatoid arthritis: A study with longstanding rheumatoid arthritis patients in Korea. *Korean J. Intern. Med.* **2016**, *31*, 977–986. [CrossRef]

Herrera-Cruz, C.J.; Medina-Solís, C.E.; Pontigo-Loyola, A.P.; Navarrete-Hernández, J.J.; González-López, B.S.; Acuña-González, G.R.; Márquez-Corona, M.L. La disbiosis en la aparición y progresión de la periodontitis: Una revisión de la literatura. *Gac. Med. Caracas* **2023**, *131*, 381–386. [CrossRef]

Buwembo, W.; Munabi, I.G.; Kaddumukasa, M.; Kiryowa, H.; Mbabali, M.; Nankya, E.; Johnson, W.E.; Okello, E.; Sewankambo, N.K. Non-surgical oral hygiene interventions on disease activity of rheumatoid arthritis patients with periodontitis: A randomized controlled trial. *J. Dent. Res. Dent. Clin. Dent. Prospect.* **2020**, *14*, 26–36. [CrossRef]

10. Ehizele, A.; Akhionbare, O. Effect of non-surgical periodontal therapy on the concentration of volatile sulfur compound in mouth air of a group of Nigerian young adults. *Ann. Med. Health Sci. Res.* **2013**, *3*, 433–437. [CrossRef]
11. AlSharief, M.; Alabdurubalnabi, E. Periodontal pathogens and adverse pregnancy outcomes: A narrative review. *Life* **2023**, *13*, 1559. [CrossRef] [PubMed]
12. Téllez-Girón Valdez, A.; Veras-Hernández, M.A.; Espinosa-de Santillana, I.A.; Kubodera-Ito, T.; Sosa-Velasco, T.A.; Canseco-Prado, G.; Acuña-González, G.A.; Mendoza-Rodríguez, M.; Lucas-Rincón, S.E.; Medina-Solís, C.E. Efecto de indicadores de salud bucal maternos sobre partos prematuros con bajo peso al nacer: Un estudio de casos y controles. *Gac. Med. Caracas* **2023**, *131*, 268–277.
13. Aizenbud, I.; Wilensky, A.; Almoznino, G. Periodontal disease and its association with metabolic syndrome-A comprehensive review. *Int. J. Mol. Sci.* **2023**, *24*, 13011. [CrossRef] [PubMed]
14. Larvin, H.; Kang, J.; Aggarwal, V.R.; Pavitt, S.; Wu, J. Periodontitis and risk of immune-mediated systemic conditions: A systematic review and meta-analysis. *Community Dent. Oral. Epidemiol.* **2023**, *51*, 705–717. [CrossRef] [PubMed]
15. Ponce-Díaz, M.E.; Rodríguez-Hernández, A.P.; González-López, B.S.; Robles-Bermeo, N.L.; Medina-Solís, C.E.; Sámano-Valencia, C.; Márquez-Corona, M.L. Factores de virulencia de porphyromonas gingivalis en la evolución de enfermedades cardiovasculares. *Acta Bioclínica* **2023**, *13*, 21–55. [CrossRef]
16. Iwashita, M. Association between periodontal disease and arteriosclerosis-related diseases. *J. Atheroscler. Thromb.* **2023**, *30*, 1517–1524. [CrossRef] [PubMed]
17. Bassani, B.; Cucchiara, M.; Butera, A.; Kayali, O.; Chiesa, A.; Palano, M.T.; Olmeo, F.; Gallazzi, M.; Dellavia, C.P.B.; Mortara, L.; et al. Neutrophils' contribution to periodontitis and periodontitis-associated cardiovascular diseases. *Int. J. Mol. Sci.* **2023**, *24*, 15370. [CrossRef]
18. Salhi, L.; Al Taep, Y.; Salmon, E.; Van Hede, D.; Lambert, F. How periodontitis or periodontal bacteria can influence alzheimer's disease features? A systematic review of pre-clinical studies. *J. Alzheimers Dis.* 2023; *in press*. [CrossRef]
19. Tamiya, H.; Mitani, A.; Abe, M.; Nagase, T. Putative bidirectionality of chronic obstructive pulmonary disease and periodontal disease: A review of the literature. *J. Clin. Med.* **2023**, *12*, 5935. [CrossRef]
20. Murphy, S. Is there an association between periodontitis and breast cancer? *Evid. Based Dent.* **2023**, *24*, 75–76. [CrossRef]
21. Kobayashi, T.; Bartold, P.M. Periodontitis and periodontopathic bacteria as risk factors for rheumatoid arthritis: A review of the last 10 years. *Jpn. Dent. Sci. Rev.* **2023**, *59*, 263–272. [CrossRef] [PubMed]
22. Batool, A.; Vaithilingam, R.D.; Mohamad Hassan, N.H.; Safii, S.H.; Saub, R. Evaluating the potential of matrix metalloproteinase as a diagnostic biomarker in rheumatoid arthritis and periodontitis: A systematic review and meta-analysis. *Medicine* **2023**, *102*, e35340. [CrossRef] [PubMed]
23. Hascoët, E.; Blanchard, F.; Blin-Wakkach, C.; Guicheux, J.; Lesclous, P.; Cloitre, A. New insights into inflammatory osteoclast precursors as therapeutic targets for rheumatoid arthritis and periodontitis. *Bone Res.* **2023**, *11*, 26. [CrossRef] [PubMed]
24. Gravallese, E.M.; Firestein, G.S. Rheumatoid arthritis—Common origins, divergent mechanisms. *N. Engl. J. Med.* **2023**, *388*, 529–542. [CrossRef] [PubMed]
25. Atarbashi-Moghadam, F.; Rashidi Maybodi, F.; Dehghan, A.; Haerian Ardakani, A. Effect of non-surgical periodontal treatment on clinical signs of rheumatoid arthritis. *J. Adv. Periodontol. Implant. Dent.* **2018**, *10*, 13–17. [CrossRef]
26. Roman-Torres, C.V.; Neto, J.S.; Souza, M.A.; Schwartz-Filho, H.O.; Brandt, W.C.; Diniz, R.E. An Evaluation of non-surgical periodontal therapy in patients with rheumatoid arthritis. *Open Dent. J.* **2015**, *9*, 150–153. [CrossRef] [PubMed]
27. Martinez-Martinez, R.E.; Abud-Mendoza, C.; Patiño-Marin, N.; Rizo-Rodríguez, J.C.; Little, J.W.; Loyola-Rodríguez, J.P. Detection of periodontal bacterial DNA in serum and synovial fluid in refractory rheumatoid arthritis patients. *J. Clin. Periodontol.* **2009**, *36*, 1004–1010. [CrossRef]

28. Detert, J.; Pischon, N.; Burmester, G.; Buttgereit, F. The association between rheumatoid arthritis and periodontal disease. *Arthritis Res. Ther.* **2010**, *12*, 218. [CrossRef]
29. Bartold, P.M.; Marshall, R.I.; Haynes, D.R. Periodontitis and rheumatoid arthritis: A review. *J. Periodontol.* **2005**, *76* (Suppl. S1 2066–2074. [CrossRef]
30. Smolik, I.; Robinson, D.; El-Gabalawy, H.S. Periodontitis and rheumatoid arthritis: Epidemiologic, clinical, and immunologic associations. *Compend. Contin. Educ. Dent.* **2009**, *30*, 188–190.
31. de Smit, M.J.; Brouwer, E.; Vissink, A.; van Winkelhoff, A.J. Rheumatoid arthritis and periodontitis; a possible link via citrullination *Anaerobe* **2011**, *17*, 196–200. [CrossRef] [PubMed]
32. Caproli, A.; Pina, S.D.; Vezzoli, M.; Cavazzana, I.; Airò, P.; Brugnoni, D.; Franceschini, F.; Garrafa, E.; Piantoni, S. Calprotectin a biomarker in rheumatoid arthritis: The potential predictive value of response to treatment. *Bioanalysis* **2023**, *15*, 1111–111 [CrossRef] [PubMed]
33. Zheng, Y.; Hou, J.; Peng, L.; Zhang, X.; Jia, L.; Wang, X.; Wei, S.; Meng, H. The pro-apoptotic and pro-inflammatory effects of calprotectin on human periodontal ligament cells. *PLoS ONE* **2014**, *9*, e110421. [CrossRef] [PubMed]
34. Ahn, S.H.; Shin, K.H.; Oh, J.T.; Park, S.C.; Rha, M.S.; Kim, S.I.; Cho, H.J.; Yoon, J.H.; Kim, C.H. Calprotectin in chronic rhinosinusitis eosinophil extracellular traps. *Int. Forum Allergy Rhinol.* **2023**, *13*, 1926–1936. [CrossRef] [PubMed]
35. Wang, S.; Song, R.; Wang, Z.; Jing, Z.; Wang, S.; Ma, J. S100A8/A9 in Inflammation. *Front. Immunol.* **2018**, *9*, 1298. [CrossRef]
36. Manfredi, M.; Van Hoovels, L.; Benucci, M.; De Luca, R.; Coccia, C.; Bernardini, P.; Russo, E.; Amedei, A.; Guiducci, S.; Grossi, V. et al. Circulating calprotectin (cCLP) in autoimmune diseases. *Autoimmun. Rev.* **2023**, *22*, 103295. [CrossRef]
37. von Wulffen, M.; Luehrmann, V.; Robeck, S.; Russo, A.; Fischer-Riepe, L.; van den Bosch, M.; van Lent, P.; Loser, K.; Gabrilovich D.I.; Hermann, S.; et al. S100A8/A9-alarmin promotes local myeloid-derived suppressor cell activation restricting severe autoimmune arthritis. *Cell Rep.* **2023**, *42*, 113006. [CrossRef]
38. Shabani, F.; Farasat, A.; Mahdavi, M.; Gheibi, N. Calprotectin (S100A8/S100A9): A key protein between inflammation and cancer *Inflamm. Res.* **2018**, *67*, 801–812. [CrossRef]
39. George, A.K.; Malaiappan, S.; Joseph, B.; Anil, S. Calprotectin, S100A8, and S100A9: Potential biomarkers of periodontal inflammation: A scoping review. *World J. Dent.* **2023**, *14*, 559–567. [CrossRef]
40. Harris, A.D.; McGregor, J.C.; Perencevich, E.N.; Furuno, J.P.; Zhu, J.; Peterson, D.E.; Finkelstein, J. The use and interpretation of quasi-experimental studies in medical informatics. *J. Am. Med. Inform. Assoc.* **2006**, *3*, 16–23. [CrossRef]
41. Aletaha, D.; Neogi, T.; Silman, A.J.; Funovits, J.; Felson, D.T.; Bingham, C.O., 3rd; Birnbaum, N.S.; Burmester, G.R.; Bykerk, V.P. Cohen, M.D.; et al. 2010 Rheumatoid arthritis classification criteria: An american college of rheumatology/european league against rheumatism collaborative initiative. *Arthritis Rheum.* **2010**, *62*, 2569–2581. [CrossRef] [PubMed]
42. Prevoo, M.L.; van't Hof, M.A.; Kuper, H.H.; van Leeuwen, M.A.; van de Putte, L.B.; van Riel, P.L. Modified disease activity scores that include twenty-eight-joint counts. Development and validation in a prospective longitudinal study of patients with rheumatoid arthritis. *Arthritis Rheum.* **1995**, *38*, 44–48. [CrossRef] [PubMed]
43. Armitage, G.C. Development of a classification system for periodontal diseases and conditions. *Ann. Periodontol.* **1999**, *4*, 1–6 [CrossRef] [PubMed]
44. Tonetti, M.S.; Greenwell, H.; Kornman, K.S. Staging and grading of periodontitis: Framework and proposal of a new classification and case definition. *J. Periodontol.* **2018**, *89* (Suppl. S1), S159–S172. [CrossRef] [PubMed]
45. Löe, H. The gingival index, the plaque index and the retention index systems. *J. Periodontol.* **1967**, *38*, 610–616. [CrossRef] [PubMed]
46. Newbrun, E. Indices to measure gingival bleeding. *J. Periodontol.* **1996**, *67*, 555–561. [CrossRef]
47. O'Leary, T.J.; Drake, R.B.; Naylor, J.E. The plaque control record. *J. Periodontol.* **1972**, *43*, 38. [CrossRef]
48. Nesse, W.; Abbas, F.; van der Ploeg, I.; Spijkervet, F.K.; Dijkstra, P.U.; Vissink, A. Periodontal inflamed surface area: Quantifying inflammatory burden. *J. Clin. Periodontol.* **2008**, *35*, 668–673. [CrossRef]
49. Walter, C.; Buset, S.; Thillainathan, L.; Weiger, R.; Zitzmann, N.U. Evaluation of periodontal therapy in undergraduate courses of the University of Basle. A retrospective study. *Schweiz. Monatsschr Zahnmed.* **2013**, *123*, 861–877.
50. Angum, F.; Khan, T.; Kaler, J.; Siddiqui, L.; Hussain, A. The prevalence of autoimmune disorders in women: A narrative review. *Cureus* **2020**, *12*, e8094. [CrossRef]
51. Cuida, M.; Halse, A.K.; Johannessen, A.C.; Tynning, T.; Jonsson, R. Indicators of salivary gland inflammation in primary Sjogren's syndrome. *Eur. J. Oral. Sci.* **1997**, *105*, 228–233. [CrossRef] [PubMed]
52. Cosgarea, R.; Tristiu, R.; Dumitru, R.B.; Arweiler, N.B.; Rednic, S.; Sirbu, C.I.; Lascu, L.; Sculean, A.; Eick, S. Effects of non-surgical periodontal therapy on periodontal laboratory and clinical data as well as on disease activity in patients with rheumatoid arthritis *Clin. Oral. Investig.* **2019**, *23*, 141–151. [CrossRef] [PubMed]
53. González, M.L.; Ruedab, J.; González, H.; Cantor, E.; Martínez, A. Artritis reumatoide temprana: Resultados clínicos y funcionales de una cohorte en un centro de alta complejidad, Cali-Colombia. *Rev. Colomb Reumatol.* **2016**, *23*, 148–154. [CrossRef]
54. Yamashita, M.; Kobayashi, T.; Ito, S.; Kaneko, C.; Murasawa, A.; Ishikawa, H.; Tabeta, K. The periodontal inflamed surface area is associated with the clinical response to biological disease-modifying antirheumatic drugs in rheumatoid arthritis: A retrospective study. *Mod. Rheumatol.* **2020**, *30*, 990–996. [CrossRef] [PubMed]
55. Erciyas, K.; Sezer, U.; Ustün, K.; Pehlivan, Y.; Kisacik, B.; Senyurt, S.Z.; Tarakçioğlu, M.; Onat, A.M. Effects of periodontal therapy on disease activity and systemic inflammation in rheumatoid arthritis patients. *Oral. Dis.* **2013**, *19*, 394–400. [CrossRef]

56. Tishkowski, K.; Gupta, V. Erythrocyte sedimentation rate. 2023. In *StatPearls*; StatPearls Publishing: St. Petersburg, FL, USA, 2023.
57. Zhao, X.; Liu, Z.; Shu, D.; Xiong, Y.; He, M.; Xu, S.; Si, S.; Guo, B. Association of periodontitis with rheumatoid arthritis and the effect of non-surgical periodontal treatment on disease activity in patients with rheumatoid arthritis. *Med. Sci. Monit.* **2018**, *24*, 5802–5810. [CrossRef]
58. Pathirana, W.G.W.; Chubb, S.P.; Gillett, M.J.; Vasikaran, S.D. Faecal calprotectin. *Clin. Biochem. Rev.* **2018**, *39*, 77–90.
59. Stríz, I.; Trebichavský, I. Calprotectin—A pleiotropic molecule in acute and chronic inflammation. *Physiol. Res.* **2004**, *53*, 245–253. [CrossRef]
60. Zhou, M.; Meng, H.X.; Zhao, Y.B.; Chen, Z.B. Changes of four proinflammatory proteins in whole saliva during experimental gingivitis. *Chin. J. Dent. Res.* **2012**, *15*, 121–127.
61. Haririan, H.; Andrukhov, O.; Pablik, E.; Neuhofer, M.; Moritz, A.; Rausch-Fan, X. Comparative analysis of calcium-binding myeloid-related protein-8/14 in saliva and serum of patients with periodontitis and healthy individuals. *J. Periodontol.* **2016**, *87*, 184–192. [CrossRef]
62. Jarlborg, M.; Courvoisier, D.S.; Lamacchia, C.; Martinez Prat, L.; Mahler, M.; Bentow, C.; Finckh, A.; Gabay, C.; Nissen, M.J. Physicians of the swiss clinical quality management (SCQM) registry. Serum calprotectin: A promising biomarker in rheumatoid arthritis and axial spondyloarthritis. *Arthritis Res. Ther.* **2020**, *22*, 105. [CrossRef] [PubMed]

MDPI AG
Grosspeteranlage 5
4052 Basel
Switzerland
Tel.: +41 61 683 77 34

MDPI Books Editorial Office
E-mail: books@mdpi.com
www.mdpi.com/books

www.ingramcontent.com/pod-product-compliance
Lightning Source LLC
Chambersburg PA
CBHW061827210926
51850CB00006B/831
9783725861835